Berry & Kohn's Introduction to Operating Room Technique

Berry & Kohn's Introduction to Operating Room Technique

Fifth Edition

Lucy Jo Atkinson, B.S.N., R.N., M.S.

Director of Educational Services, Ethicon, Inc.
Formerly Assistant Director of Nursing
for Operating Rooms and Recovery Room,
Cedars of Lebanon Hospital, Los Angeles

Mary Louise Kohn, A.B., R.N., M.N.

Formerly Instructor in Operating Room Technique
Frances Payne Bolton School of Nursing
Case Western Reserve University, Cleveland

McGraw-Hill Book Company

New York St. Louis San Francisco Auckland Bogotá Düsseldorf
Johannesburg London Madrid Mexico Montreal New Delhi Panama
Paris São Paulo Singapore Sydney Tokyo Toronto

To Edna Cornelia Berry,
whose dedication to teaching was surpassed only by her devotion to the care of surgical patients in the operating room.

Library of Congress Cataloging in Publication Data

Berry, Edna Cornelia.
Berry and Kohn's Introduction to operating room technique.

Bibliography: p.
Includes index.
1. Operating room nursing. I. Kohn, Mary Louise, joint author. II. Atkinson, Lucy Jo. III. Title: Introduction to operating room technique. [DNLM: 1. Operating room nursing. WY162 B534i]
RD32.3.B4 1978 617'.91 78-4956
ISBN 0-07-002540-1

BERRY & KOHN'S INTRODUCTION
TO OPERATING ROOM TECHNIQUE

1 2 3 4 5 6 7 8 9 0 WCWC 7 8 3 2 1 0 9 8

This book was set in English Times by Allen Wayne Technical Corp. The editor was Orville W. Haberman, Jr., and the production supervisor was Jeanne Selzam. Webcrafters, Inc., was printer and binder.

NOTICE

Medicine is an ever-changing science. As new research and clinical experience broaden our knowledge, changes in treatment and drug therapy are required. The editors and the publisher of this work have made every effort to ensure that the drug dosage schedules herein are accurate and in accord with the standards accepted at the time of publication. Readers are advised, however, to check the product information sheet included in the package of each drug they plan to administer to be certain that changes have not been made in the recommended dose or in the contraindications for administration. This recommendation is of particular importance in regard to new or infrequently used drugs.

Contents

Preface to the Fifth Edition

This edition marks the retirement of Edna C. Berry, one of the original authors and a teacher of the present authors, who regard her with affection and respect. The senior author welcomes Lucy Jo Atkinson, R.N., M.S., a well-known contributor to nursing literature, as associate author.

The text is addressed to all learners of operating room technology, primarily student and new graduate nurses and technicians, all of whom should remain learners and humanitarians throughout their careers. Although the material has been updated, the fundamental purposes remain unchanged: to develop perfection in carrying out aseptic and sterile techniques, and to appreciate nursing care of the patient in the operating room. Primary emphasis is directed to total patient care and to the necessity for integrity of the health care team.

While it is a major revision, the fifth edition generally retains the format of and considerable material from previous editions. The content is broader in volume and scope, and the number of illustrations has been increased. Important facts are repeated throughout the text to emphasize basic principles. New chapters include material on the patient, work simplification, microsurgery, oncology, transplantation, and potential complications in surgical patients. To present an overview, all surgical specialties are included in chapters appropriately titled. Although it is assumed that the learner has a foundation in the basic sciences, some anatomy, physiology, and bacteriology are added to improve understanding.

The comprehensive bibliography is intended as an entree to current literature for the learner and as an aid to the instructor. Checking a regular set of leading journals as well as the periodicals and special publications of associations, institutions, and industrial companies is one of the most efficient methods for both basic learner and specialist practitioner to keep abreast of developments.

The authors hope this internationally used text will continue to be of value to learners everywhere.

Grateful acknowledgement is extended to June Lorig, B.S.N., R.N., for her major contribution in the writing of Chapter 17 and a section of Chapter 21; Judith Grieg, R.N., M.S.N., for contributing a segment of Chapter 17; to Marcia R. Kohn, A.B., B.S.N., R.N., for authoring Chapter 29; to Geraldine Mink, A.B., B.S. in Library Science, for verifying and helping with the preparation of the bibliography; and to Anita Rogoff, M.A., for continuing as illustrator.

The authors give sincere appreciation to the following persons who graciously reviewed specific material: Brenda Sovero, A.B., B.S.N., R.N., for reading portions from the viewpoint of the new graduate nurse in the OR, Robert Crumrine, M.D., Ralph G. DePalma, M.D., Richard P. Glove, M.D., John R. Hannan, M.D., Howard D. Kohn, M.D., Robert S. Rhodes, M.D., John P. Storaasli, M.D., James Sturm, M.D., and W. Budd Wentz, M.D., all associated with University Hospitals of Cleveland and/or the faculty of the School of Medicine, Case Western Reserve University, Cleveland.

Other reviewers to whom we are indebted are Mary Senna, R.N., Westfield Orthopaedic Group, Westfield, New Jersey, Dwight C. Hanna, M.D., Western Pennsylvania Hospital, Pittsburgh, Daniel M. Lavigna, M.D., formerly of Ohio State University Medical School faculty, and Ellen V. Mausser, M.D., St. Luke's Hospital, Cleveland.

The authors are particularly grateful to Grace Plumbo and Corley Owen for diligence in typing most of the manuscript, assisted by Joan Avolio, Corinne Frensdorf, and Doris Blackmon.

Lucy Jo Atkinson
Mary Louise Kohn

Preface to the First Edition

The material in this text is the outgrowth of the coauthors' experience in the operating room—one as instructor of students, the other as head nurse with some responsibility for instructing and guiding students. It is an adaptation of the instructor's teaching outline for which there have been many requests.

The aim of the book is to facilitate the nurse's study of aseptic technique and care of the patient in the operating room. Although this text is intended primarily for the student, the authors hope it may prove useful to the graduate nurse as well.

Since it is assumed that the student has studied pathological conditions necessitating surgical treatment, these conditions are not discussed. When applicable, and as a matter of emphasis, there is a reiteration of principles of sterile technique and safety factors for the patient. It is hoped this will aid in fixing the principles as patterns of thought and work.

While operative routines vary in different hospitals, underlying principles are the same. Consequently, basic principles are stressed and the authors have endeavored to keep the material as general as possible. Principles must be adapted to suit the situations found in individual hospitals. Specific linen, equipment, and procedures are mentioned merely to serve as a framework upon which to demonstrate principles or as samples for points of departure. However, the specific examples mentioned are workable procedures that have evolved. They are kept as uncomplicated as possible for student teaching and for use in the practical situation.

Instruments for operations are not listed and few are mentioned, because each hospital has its instrument lists, standardized for each case, to which students can refer.

Emphasis is placed upon meeting the psychological as well as the physical needs of the surgical patient. An endeavor is made where possible to correlate briefly the preoperative and postoperative care with the operative procedure, to give the student a complete concept of patient care.

The frequent use of the imperative mood is for the purpose of brevity, organization, and emphasis. Questions and assignments in each chapter are to aid the student in reviewing the material, in recalling pertinent facts, and in applying the principles to her specific situation.

Obviously, if the student starts scrubbing for cases with an older nurse after her first day or two in the operating room and if her operating-room theory is given concurrently with the practice, much of the material in this book will have been covered by individual instruction before class discussion.

The authors have attempted to maintain simplicity and brevity, and to present a concise outline for preliminary study. They suggest that the student supplement this material by reference reading.

The authors wish to express their grateful appreciation and thanks to those persons who by their interest and cooperation supported them:

To Miss Edythe Angell, Supervisor of the Operating Rooms at University Hospitals of Cleveland, for helpful suggestions during the preparation of the manuscript and for reading, critically, the entire manuscript. We are gratefully indebted to her because we have learned from her much of what appears in this text.

To Miss Janet McMahon, Educational Director, School of Anesthesia, University Hospitals of Cleveland, for valuable assistance in preparing Chapter 21. Also, to Dr. Edward Depp, Anesthesiologist, Euclid-Glenville Hospital, Cleveland, who offered suggestions on this chapter and reviewed it.

To Dr. C. C. Roe Jackson, of the faculty of Western Reserve University School of Medicine, for constructive criticism in reviewing Chapter 17. To Dr. Howard D. Kohn, also of the faculty, who has been most helpful in reading the manuscript and offering suggestions.

To Mrs. Geraldine Mink, Librarian, for her assistance; to Mrs. Leona Peck for her patience in typing the manuscript and for her helpful suggestions; to Miss Ruth Elmenthaler and Miss Margaret Sanderson of the operating-room staff for their assistance in making the photographs; and to Mrs. Anita Rogoff for drawing the illustrations.

Edna Cornelia Berry
Mary Louise Kohn

Chapter 1

Introduction for the Learner

MODERN SURGERY

Health is a personal and economic asset. Needs are altered in proportion to one's ability to function normally. *Optimal health* has been defined as the best an individual can feel and function in the particular circumstances or with a disease process. *Disease* is a failure of the adaptive mechanisms to adequately counteract stimuli or stresses, resulting in disturbance in function or structure of any part, organ, or system of the body. Illness is often a composite of many reactions or diseases.

Jean-Martin Charcot, the eminent nineteenth-century French neurologist, once stated, "Disease is from old and nothing about it has changed. It is we who change as we learn to recognize what was formerly imperceptible."

Since time immemorial human beings have searched for the causes of illnesses and ways to relieve suffering. To participate as a health care worker increases one's awareness of some basic facts:

1 No one is immune to suffering, but to alleviate it is worth the effort and cost, for life is priceless.

2 One should not try to face suffering alone; let others help.

3 Vulnerability is an important component of life. Anne Morrow Lindberg's insight is most applicable. "Suffering is certainly individual . . . to suffer is to be alone. . . To suffering must be added mourning, understanding, patience, love, openness, and the willingness to remain vulnerable."*

Fifty years ago only a small percentage of hospitalized patients were admitted for operations. Today, surgical intervention, one step in the total process of restoring or maintaining health, brings a population of all ages to the hospital with conditions that can be treated surgically. The number of operations performed and of anesthetics administered increases annually. This is due to the population explosion, the increased incidence of congenital abnormalities, the ever-increasing number of aged persons, and the rapid progress in all facets of medicine. Many former contraindications to surgery have changed and, because of better supportive and drug therapies, many persons are now considered candidates for surgery.

The word *surgery* designates the branch of medicine that encompasses preoperative care, intraoperative judgment and management, and postoperative care of patients. Surgery as a discipline is total care of illness with an extra

*AM Lindberg, *Hour of Gold, Hour of Lead: Diaries and Letters of Anne Morrow Lindberg 1929–1932,* New York: Harcourt Brace Jovanovich, 1973, p. 212.

modality of treatment, the *operation,* for correction of deformities and defects, repair of injuries, diagnosis and cure of disease processes, relief of suffering, and prolongation of life. At the time of operation, pathologic conditions are documented and treated. Surgical intervention encompasses more than technical performance of an operative procedure. In fact, the operation may constitute a minor part of the total therapy for surgical patients.

Surgical science has progressed far beyond what was envisioned years ago. Modern surgery is safer and surer than ever before. Reliable diagnostic techniques and equipment enable physicians to more precisely measure the effects of illness and injury and to more accurately make diagnoses and predict surgical outcomes. Surgeons and equipment manufacturers consult together constantly to develop and perfect instrumentation. Improvement in the knowledge and management of the surgical patient's nutritional and physiological condition, plus the many complex, precise skills of the surgeon are also beneficial to the effectiveness and safety of surgical care. Specialization in all areas of medicine, and increasingly in nursing too, brings to patient care a vast augmentation of available consultative services for helping to determine what is wrong, what needs to be done, and how best to do it. Some of the greatest gains have been in methods of preparing patients for operation, and of caring for them postoperatively in the rehabilitation period. These new methods of patient care are based on the premise that each patient is a unique individual requiring individualized care. Exceptionally rapid advances have been made in the development of safe anesthesia, which is so vital to a favorable surgical outcome.

Patients come to the operating room for a variety of reasons, including:

1 To preserve life, e.g., relief of intestinal obstruction or decompression of a skull fracture

2 To maintain dynamic bodily equilibrium, e.g., removal of a diseased kidney

3 To undergo diagnostic procedures, e.g., breast biopsy, bronchoscopy

4 To prevent infection and to promote healing, e.g., burn debridement

5 To obtain comfort and to ensure the ability to earn a living, e.g., elective herniorrhaphy

Ambulatory Surgery

Most, but not all, operations are performed in hospitals. Many are performed in surgeons' offices or in independent, non-hospital based, freestanding surgical facilities if they are not complex enough to require hospitalization of the patients. Not all patients operated on in a hospital-contained operating room unit are admitted to the hospital. Surgeons view activity as beneficial rather than hazardous for surgical patients. Consequently, operation on an outpatient or ambulatory basis is feasible and safe for carefully selected patients. *Ambulatory surgery* refers to a method of delivering surgical care whereby patients enter the facility, are operated on either with or without anesthesia, and are cared for postoperatively in anticipation of being discharged to return home the same day. If patients develop complications, they are admitted as inpatients.

Patients eligible for ambulatory surgery are carefully selected. Criteria considered by the surgeon include:

1 Age. Children and young or middle-age adults who do not have complex health problems may be candidates for ambulatory surgery.

2 General health status. Patients are evaluated physically and emotionally to determine the possibility of complications occurring during or after operations.

3 Willingness of the patient and agreement of the surgeon that a minimal risk is involved.

Most hospitals utilize ambulatory surgery for a limited number of comparatively simple procedures. Others allow the surgeon to perform relatively extensive operations, ones for which patients are customarily admitted as inpatients in most hospitals. Ambulatory surgery has proved to be practical for many operations. The advantages of ambulatory surgery include:

1 Staff and resources may concentrate on patients with more serious problems. Ambulatory surgery withdraws relatively minor procedures from the inpatient operating room (OR) schedule.

2 It is less costly because it eliminates the need to occupy expensive bed space and many customary expenses that go with hospitalization.

3 It reserves inpatient bed space for those who need it in geographical areas where a critical shortage of hospital beds exists.

4 It is particularly beneficial for children as it eliminates the psychological trauma of an overnight hospital stay.

5 Patients appreciate returning quickly to familiar surroundings that are less stressful than a hospital environment.

Daily Schedule

The types of operations performed in a hospital or other facility vary according to the expertise of the surgeons on the staff, the community in which the facility is located, and the equipment available. The daily schedule of operations is as variable as the type of facility and the types of operations performed. Regardless of the circumstances that bring patients to the operating room, care in the operating room becomes an integral part of nursing service, filling a need that cannot be met by the individual patient or his or her family. In the operating room you must accept the challenge of this critical phase of nursing care upon which the patient's ultimate recovery is so dependent. Nursing care of patients undergoing surgical intervention as the therapeutic modality of choice is carried out at two levels: professional and technical.

PROFESSIONAL NURSING

Characteristics of a Profession

The characteristics of a profession are that:

1 It defines its own rules.
2 It sets its own standards and conducts its own affairs.
3 It identifies and develops its own body of knowledge unique to its role.
4 It engages in periodic self-evaluation and peer review to control and alter its practices and behaviors.

The members of a profession must act responsibly in accord with their commitment to public trust and service. However, professional conduct is not synonymous with ritualism, detachment, or denial of feeling. Simply stated the word *profession* implies a combination and coordination of knowledge, skills, and ideals that are communicated through a highly specialized educational discipline. In this way education sets the standards for practice.

Professional Nursing

Professional and legal standards extend the nurse's responsibility and accountability beyond procedural steps. Their purpose is to fulfill the profession's obligation to provide and improve practice. Standards have been established by professional organizations, federal and state governments, and the Joint Commission on the Accreditation of Hospitals (JCAH). Definitions and standards give guidance to nursing service and nursing education. The standards of education and training have been progressively elevated and are continually assessed, maintained, and improved.

Data have shown that care tends to move to the lowest level of preparation of personnel. Therefore, the better prepared the staff, the higher the quality of care given. Professional education should be built upon a solid base of general education. The RN, educated to assess the total patient, is an indispensable member of the OR professional team. A person with quality education approaches challenges creatively and with confidence that solutions can be found. As changes occur with surprising rapidity, and nursing develops as a profession in its own right, its responsibilities to the patient, to itself, and to its correlated professions increase as well. The source of professional authority is an understanding of the role functions of the professional.

Professional nursing is dedicated to the promotion of optimal health for all human beings in their various environments. In addition to performing many other roles including teaching health-seeking behaviors, promoting preventive medicine, taking part in patient rehabilitation, and participating in nursing research, the professional nurse in the acute care setting performs functions that are primarily curative and restorative in nature. The professional nurse practitioner's role, as defined by the American Nurses' Association (ANA), includes planning, providing, directing, collaborating in, and evaluating direct patient care.

As a helping profession, nursing's ideal characteristics include the ability and commitment to respond with compassion to, and to care for, dependent people in need, whether they are curable or not. If we deny humanity to others, we dehumanize ourselves as well. The professional nurse is deeply committed to life and health. In practice she helps each patient to attain his or her highest possible level of general health.

Operating Room Nursing

New developments are constantly taking place in the field of surgery. As diagnostic and supportive services have become increasingly complex, so have surgical procedures. Intricate procedures have now become part of daily surgical routine. It is therefore essential that nurses have extensive specialized knowledge and training, and the ability to apply them humanistically. They must have the critical judgment and skills needed to be equal to their responsibilities. Concurrently, the role of the OR nurse is expanding as nurses relinquish non-nursing activities in order to accept newer nursing responsibilities. The OR presents an opportunity for the nurse to practice professional nursing at its finest to the full benefit of the patient. Nursing care of surgical patients extends behind and beyond the doors of the operating room.

Professional nursing in the operating room has been defined as "the identification of the physiological, psychological and sociological needs of the patient, and the implementation of an individualized program of nursing care that coordinates the nursing actions, based on a knowledge of the natural and behavioral sciences, in order to restore, or maintain, the health and welfare of the patient before, during, and after surgical intervention."*

The professional operating room nurse practitioner, a duly licensed registered nurse (RN), is legally responsible for the nature and quality of the nursing care patients receive during surgical intervention, i.e., the operation itself. The scope of operating room nursing practice encompasses those nursing activities that assist the individual surgical patient. These activities are directed toward providing continuity of care through preoperative assessment and preparation, intraoperative intervention, and postoperative evaluation. The program for nursing care prescribes:

1 What nursing actions are to be performed
2 How the nursing actions are to be done
3 When the nursing actions are to be performed
4 Where the nursing actions are to be performed
5 Who is to perform the nursing actions†

Nursing actions, the functions of professional nursing, provide the foundation of the nursing process used in assessing, planning, implementing, and evaluating patient care. These actions are:

1 Application and execution of the physician's legal orders
2 Observation of the patient's symptoms and reactions
3 Supervision of the patient
4 Supervision of others who contribute to the care of the patient
5 Reporting and recording
6 Application and execution of nursing procedures and techniques
7 Promotion of the patient's physical and emotional health by directing and teaching

The first action is dependent upon the physician, and the other six are independently taken by the nurse. The activities of registered professional nurses are supplemented and complemented by the services of allied technical health personnel who function as assistants to nurses.

The concepts of total patient care and continuity of nursing care encompass the *perioperative role* of the OR nurse. This role has both technical and professional components in carrying out the nursing process preoperatively, intraoperatively, and postoperatively. The preoperative phase of a surgical patient's care extends to the time the patient is moved onto the operating table. The intraoperative phase begins at this time and ends when the patient is admitted to the recovery room. Postoperative care continues through the immediate recovery period to complete rehabilitation. The scope of the nursing activities that the OR nurse assumes in the perioperative role is contingent upon his or her personal knowledge, skills, and experience, and upon the expectations delineated in the job description of the nurse's position.

OR nursing is an intellectually and physically demanding yet rewarding acute care specialty of clinical nursing practice. The OR is a dynamic, ever-changing critical care setting where the care given is a decisive factor in postoperative outcome. Since no 2 days are alike, OR nursing is always challenging, never tedious.

A wise physician once said that the physician's role is to cure sometimes, to relieve often, to comfort always. The same can be said for the OR nurse who embodies all the word *nurse* has traditionally meant to a patient—provider of safety and comfort, supporter and confidante—no less so because the practice environment within the OR suite is geographically separated from most of the hospital complex to reduce traffic, noise, and sources of bacterial contamination. The professional OR nurse holds a unique position. Patients' safety and welfare are entrusted to the nurse from the moment of their arrival in the operating room until their departure and until the transfer of responsibility for their care has been made to

*AORN Statement Committee: Definition and objective for clinical practice of professional operating room nursing, AORN J 10(5):48, Nov. 1969.

†Association of Operating Room Nurses and American Nurses' Association Division on Medical-Surgical Nursing Practice: *Standards of Nursing Practice: Operating Room,* American Nurses' Association, Kansas City, Missouri, 1975. Reprinted with permission of ANA.

another professional health care team member. The primary emphasis of the nurse's responsibility is that of total nursing care. He or she is accountable to patients and responsible for the scope of nursing practice whether it is accomplished personally or by qualified assisting personnel. The patient relies on the nurse:

1 To provide competent, skilled, trustworthy care during the operation
2 To mitigate anxiety and pain
3 To meet aggregate needs for which the nurse is qualified through extensive, in-depth education and training

The nurse fulfills a vital function in the continuity of care of the surgical patient as he or she pursues goals to enable persons to experience ever more healthy, productive lives.

TECHNICAL NURSING

The activities of registered professional nurses are supplemented and complemented by the services of allied technical health care personnel who function as assistants to nurses. *Technical nursing practice* has been defined as the carrying out of delegated techniques with a high degree of skill through the use of principles learned through didactic and clinical training. Technical nursing practice is unlimited in depth but limited in scope. The *operating room technician* (ORT) works with the surgeon, anesthesiologist or anesthetist, and professional registered nurse as a member of the direct patient care team during surgical intervention. This team is referred to as the *OR team.* The OR technician assists by preparing and handling supplies and equipment to maintain an aseptic environment through a system of specific techniques and practices designed to exclude all pathogenic microorganisms from the operative wound.

Operating room technicians who successfully pass an examination attesting to their theoretical knowledge are certified by the Association of Surgical Technologists, formerly the Association of Operating Room Technicians, Inc.

OBJECTIVES FOR LEARNING

The operation itself is the focal point of all that happens to the surgical patient. Management of this critical act requires a team whose members understand the principles of the problems at hand, the methods being used, and the gravity of the situation. All team members must have theoretical knowledge of the principles of technique in order to provide an environment free from microorganisms, referred to as *aseptic* or *sterile technique,* and they must be able to apply these principles in this clinical setting. These principles are applicable, in various measures, to nursing in general. The need for knowledge of aseptic and sterile technique is greatly intensified and emphasized in the operating room as it is nowhere else. Through it surgeons are able to use their skill effectively to the highest degree.

This is a text of the basic principles of the technology carried out during surgical intervention. These principles must be thoroughly learned by the nurses and technicians who work in the operating room. They are the essence of the basic training of OR technicians. Education for first-level entry into professional practice prepares nurses to be knowledgeable generalists and leaders capable of working with and through others in all clinical settings. After graduation from a generalist program, the nurse needs further preparation in the clinical area of specialization. This may take the form of formal preparation in a postbasic operating room nursing course. Or it may be provided through well-planned and well-taught on-the-job inservice training, plus self-study, the purpose of which is to meet the nurse's needs for theoretical and technical knowledge and clinical experience. The RN in the OR must have full knowledge and experience in all the roles that are tangentially connected and interdependent with the care of the surgical patient. Therefore, the concepts to be learned and the objectives to be met for all beginning learners who want to specialize in operating room technology must include the following:

1 To increase and clarify knowledge of anatomy and physiology in normal structure and function, and in patterns altered by disease processes. This knowledge will be demonstrated by ability to correctly position patients on the operating table and to select appropriate instrumentation, equipment, and supplies.
2 To demonstrate an understanding of the more common operations by anticipating the needs of members of the OR team and by organizing work efficiently in the best interests of patient safety and welfare.
3 To understand the action and use of anesthetic agents, fluids, and electrolytes and patient responses to them by having appropriate supplies available in the event of adverse reactions.

4 To understand and apply the principles of sterilization, disinfection, and aseptic and sterile technique in the preparation and use of all supplies and equipment under all conditions and circumstances imperative to patient safety.

5 To recognize the trauma inflicted, and consequent legal implications involved, on each patient undergoing surgical intervention and to carry out the care required to ensure safety for the patient.

6 To identify the potential environmental dangers to the patient through an understanding of the function and care of surgical instruments, supplies, and equipment, so as to prevent hazards to patient safety and subsequent incidents of negligence.

7 To develop manual dexterity and the ability to manage personal anxiety by learning basic techniques so well that correct activity response is quickly carried out in life-threatening emergency or stressful situations as well as in normal circumstances.

8 To identify factors that create stress and the coping mechanisms exhibited by members of the OR team in their cooperative effort as a basis for evaluating and modifying your own behavior in order to enhance your personal participation in the team effort on behalf of the patient.

9 To function as a team member by showing consideration for and cooperation with others within the OR and by communicating with the interdependent departments of the hospital that work together for the well-being of the surgical patient.

10 To develop flexibility, adaptability, and self-reliance as a team member by acquiring a working knowledge of all aspects of the operating room environment and the functions of all personnel.

11 To exert a conscientious effort to carry out all duties accurately and with integrity, in compliance with hospital policies and recognized standards of practice, and thus to develop pride in performance consistent with personal, professional, and vocational ethical and moral values.

12 To help control patient and hospital costs through the correct, safe, and economical use of supplies and equipment and personal efficiency in time and motion.

A basic understanding of operating room technique and intraoperative procedures is essential for the total care of the surgical patient. To plan and manage the preoperative, intraoperative, or postoperative nursing care regimen of the surgical patient in order to meet individualized needs, the professional nurse must have a knowledge of the operative site and procedure, the effects of operative trauma and anesthesia on the body, and the problems of recovery and rehabilitation. The operating room can be used as a clinical laboratory for learning generalist nursing behaviors by focusing on what happens to the patient during surgical intervention. Participation in and observation of operating room nursing process can help the nurse:

1 To investigate the nursing care process through assessment and implementation of nursing actions in the OR that correlate the operative procedure with other aspects of patient care.

2 To promote an understanding of the patient's total surgical experience by demonstrating the ability to assess physiological, psychological, and sociological patient needs through preparation of a nursing care plan.

3 To reinforce basic knowledge of anatomy and physiology and to gain knowledge of the total patient experience as a basis for management of preoperative patient anxiety related to body image and postoperative pain related to site of incision and intraoperative procedure.

4 To assist patients with the management of anxiety by assessing their needs for psychological support preoperatively and by anticipating their psychological and physiological needs in the postoperative recovery period through an understanding of the total surgical experience.

5 To recognize the effects of preoperative medication, anesthesia, positioning on the operating table, site of incision, and operative procedure as the basis for planning the patient's postoperative recovery and rehabilitation.

6 To develop an appreciation of the meaning of the surgical experience for patients and their families as a basis for correlating the intraoperative phase with establishment of priorities for teaching and planning all aspects of surgical patient care to promote continuity of care.

7 To become a more effective communicator with patients through pre- and postoperative teaching based on knowledge of the intraoperative procedure as it relates to each individual patient and his or her family.

8 To identify the members of the OR team and the legal responsibility of each member for the care of the conscious or the unconscious patient as a basis for establishing and maintaining inter- and intradepartmental functions that ensure continuity of surgical patient care.

9 To participate in making collaborative decisions that demonstrate his or her willingness to cooperate with members of the OR team on behalf of the patient.

10 To decrease the potential eventuality of an environmentally acquired infection by understanding the principles of aseptic and sterile technique and by demonstrating the ability to adhere to them. The principles learned in the OR apply in other clinical settings to procedures requiring isolation or a sterile field to prevent hospital or self-acquired infection.

CORRELATION OF THEORY AND PRACTICE

Knowledge and technology advance so rapidly that physicians, nurses, and other health care personnel must remain learners throughout their professional or vocational careers or face obsolescence in 5 to 10 years. The types of learners in any setting are as varied as their backgrounds, personalities, experiences, and abilities to learn. For this reason, the methods of teaching must be equally varied.

Some learning of OR technique can take place in the classroom setting or the self-study laboratory. Lecture/demonstration may be given to learners who then practice the procedure, which, in turn, is followed by the instructor's evaluation of their work. Books, journals, films, slides, and videotapes may supplement the lecture approach. Many audiovisual materials are self-contained units that provide adequate basic knowledge through self-study. A bibliography in a text such as this is only a start. Each reference leads on through many paths to add to and broaden the learner's theoretical knowledge. The amount of literature is almost without limit. Each instructor plans classes or self-study units according to available materials and learner needs.

Reading the literature and using audiovisual teaching aids are only part of providing adequate preparation for clinical practice. Nursing skills are gained by active participation. Theory becomes meaningful and of value only when it is put to practical use. In the operating room, some learning will be accomplished through observation, but skills will be learned through actual experience in which you will apply the theory learned in the classroom or self-study laboratory.

The operating room is an exciting department. Here you will see living anatomy, its alteration by congenital deformities, disease, or injury, and its restoration or reconstruction. You will see the important part operative procedures play in the care of life-threatening emergencies and you will learn to act in these situations for the patient's welfare.

Your practice in the operating room will give you opportunity to apply your knowledge of the basic sciences. Much theory is translated into practice, and can be observed, such as the effect of a tourniquet in creating a dry operative site, the effect of warm tapes in restoring circulation to a strangulated bowel, the gangrene that results from prolonged strangulation, the dark appearance of blood not properly oxygenated, the expansion of the lungs, the movement of the diaphragm, etc.

Operating room nursing is an invaluable experience in preparing one to be a more understanding, observing, efficient nurse. In close teamwork with surgeons and anesthesiologists, the nurse participates in vital resuscitative measures, and learns to evaluate their effectiveness and to care for anesthetized, unconscious, and/or critically ill patients. In addition, the learner discovers that such emergencies as cardiac arrest are more easily prevented than treated. He or she gains valuable experience applicable to any nursing situation by learning:

1 To fully realize what surgical intervention in all its aspects means to a patient. When one is familiar with operative procedures, the *whys* of postoperative pain, complications, and care are clearly apparent.

2 To realize the importance of optimal physical and emotional preoperative preparation for all patients and the need for constant patient observation intraoperatively. One deficiency can have a snowballing effect. For example, if an adequate blood volume is not maintained, cardiac output is reduced, the blood pressure then falls, and renal function is impaired; retained body wastes then further disturb delicate acid-base, potassium-sodium balances. The heat-regulating mechanism is also upset. Fluid and electrolyte maintenance is important to prevent dehydration and acid-base imbalance in blood and tissues.

3 To differentiate between innocuous occurrences and situations that, if unrecognized and allowed to progress, will lead to disaster. For example, a slowing pulse may indicate progression toward bradycardia and an impending cardiac arrest.

4 To cope with any eventuality in a calm, efficient manner; to think clearly and act quickly in crisis situations.

5 To attend to every pertinent detail, to keenly observe, and to anticipate the needs of the patient and of colleagues.

6 To know the need for and to comprehensively practice aseptic and sterile techniques.

Above all, operating room experience teaches that *no operation is minor*! The only predictable element in the operating room is the potential for the unpredictable occurrence. Operations may be classified as major or minor by hospitals for practical use but in reality no such distinction exists. An operation has a deep personal meaning for each patient and the possibility of death cannot be ruled out completely. Every operative procedure carries an element of inherent risk. A supposedly relatively safe procedure can rapidly become a catastrophic one, even a fatal one, if the patient is allergic to medication or anesthetic drug, develops uncontrollable bleeding, irreversible shock, overwhelming postoperative infection, or experiences a cardiac arrest on the operating table. While every precaution is taken to foresee and prevent adverse reactions, such reactions do occur on occasion. No matter how simple a procedure, an experienced OR team member has indelibly inscribed in memory such occurrences and gives undivided attention to the patient at *all* times.

During your experience, you may participate in or observe the preparation of operating room supplies and learn their use. You will gain an appreciation of the precision with which surgical instruments and equipment are made for particular functions. You will learn the proper care of these expensive instruments and equipment and the economical use of all materials. Also, in helping to carry out a daily schedule of operations, you will become aware of the interdependence of the various departments of the hospital, and how they work together for the well-being of the patient. One of the most valuable learning experiences in the OR is the opportunity to see and become a part of real teamwork in action. This will be discussed in Chapter 2.

THE CLINICAL INSTRUCTOR

Experience in the OR clinical setting must be planned and supervised. A designated resource person, either a faculty member or nursing staff member employed by the hospital, is available to guide and assist you in competently applying newly acquired knowledge. *The term "instructor" will be used throughout this text to refer to the resource person responsible for planning, implementing, and evaluating learners' experiences, both in the classroom or self-study laboratory and in the clinical setting.* The instructor who is a faculty member employed by a teaching institution may not be a member of the hospital staff. Hospitals offering the clinical setting for educational and training programs have their own policies and procedures that must be adapted and adhered to by both the instructor and the learner. During clinical experience, the instructor supervises learner activities.

The instructor must objectively assess your skills and knowledge. When your deficiencies are identified, you must be provided with learning experience to enable you to reach your highest potential. You must be involved in the teaching/learning process too. Effective education develops from the needs of the learner. It is essential for the instructor to discover what the learner wants to know as well as what will be required for the learner to know.

The instructor must determine in what areas the learner is knowledgeable and in what areas additional training is needed. A written knowledge and skills inventory checklist can assist in identifying learning needs. This involves rating the actual skills and knowledge of the learner against a standardized listing of the skills and knowledge required for optimum performance. Learners usually understand and respond well to training plans and instruction sessions developed through this framework. It provides a means for the learner to identify his or her own learning needs as well as to request new learning experiences.

The instructor must use a variety of approaches with learners to achieve the desired results, such as formulation of clear-cut explicit behavioral objectives; use of skill in questioning and encouraging learners to make discoveries and correlations; employment of written guidelines and assignment for feedback to assure that learning has taken place. Learner conferences should be held on a regular basis to discuss procedures as well as problems.

The instructor must work closely with the *OR nursing supervisor* (ORS). Classroom hours and clinical experience assignments are worked out together. The supervisor offers suggestions and criticism for the benefit of the learner. The instructor offers suggestions to the supervisor for the experiences of the learner. The ORS is aware of the planned program for the learner. An effort is made to confer and to coordinate any changes in the program. This fosters a friendly and cooperative relationship. The ORS is advised of each learner's progress.

The instructor must also acquaint the entire operating room staff with the proposed learning experiences. Everyone should be familiar with the level of the learners, the learning goals, and the roles that staff members will be expected to assume with respect to teaching. All staff members should assist in teaching the learners.

THE LEARNER

The beginning learner in the OR may be either a student nurse or technician enrolled in a formalized educational program or a registered nurse, recently graduated or reentering the profession, learning first-level beginning OR nursing skills.

Each hospital has its learner level of work more or less defined. In most hospitals, beginning learners are not used to fill staff positions. Learners actually help prepare for, assist during, and clean up following operations. Novices will not be expected to assume responsibilities for which they are not fully prepared. Only through continued study and experience can individuals qualify as team members during the most complex operations.

The learner is usually taught the scrub nurse functions early in the OR experience. These functions are discussed in detail throughout this text. At first, an experienced instructor or staff member scrubs with the new person, gradually permitting the learner to take over more of the work in the sterile field until the learner is able to function without help. The types of operations to which the novice may be assigned vary from hospital to hospital, depending upon many factors peculiar to each. However, rarely does the beginning learner scrub on operations of the heart, lung, or brain.

Since one of the objectives of learning is to gain a thorough knowledge of sterile technique, repetition of the scrub nurse functions serves a valuable purpose by impressing it indelibly in the mind of the learner. It is better to learn the fundamentals in a thorough manner and to retain them than to try to cover the many complicated operations by observing and retaining little. Knowing how to do a procedure is not enough. You will feel greater satisfaction when you gain skill in performing it. To make the experience as profitable as possible, the learner should circulate during operations as well as scrub. This necessitates constant supervision and help from the instructor or another experienced RN. All OR procedures must be practiced. Contribution to the accomplishment of the work of the entire team becomes real and is a necessary, important part of the learning process.

The learner is not the only one who benefits from this learning process. The OR team gains from each learner contact. The surgeons actively participate in the learning experience by acquainting the learner with patients' situations, by explaining why operations are being performed, and by answering questions.

By learning as many procedures as the course of study permits, you can benefit in the following ways:

1 As you learn various assignments, you will be able to teach others who have not yet had those particular assignments. In helping others, you will be stimulated to increased effort and will feel more a part of the department.

2 After completion of formal study, you must know how to do the work in order to teach others.

3 If you perform the job yourself, you will learn the proper care of expensive instruments and appreciate the need for economy in the use of all supplies.

4 You will be better able to evaluate and compare other methods for the purpose of improvement, if you know the methods in use.

5 You will be better qualified to supervise others and to evaluate their performance if you know the time and labor involved in their work.

BEHAVIOR OF O.R. NURSING PERSONNEL

Nurses are expected to be both human and humane, as well as competent in their work, and the standard for the behavior of all OR nursing personnel is no less high. The ability to successfully discharge duties contributes to efficient teamwork and, even more importantly, to patient confidence and sense of security. *Behavior makes a lasting impression that the patient will always associate with his or her experience in the operating room.* It reveals a justified self-confidence (or lack of it), interest (or indifference), or proficiency and authority (or ineptitude). In addition to possessing special technical expertise, nursing personnel in the OR must have many personal attributes that inspire confidence, trust, and honesty in patients and team members. OR nursing personnel must be:

1 *Empathic.* A feeling person can put one's own self in another's place. Nurses as allies of patients convey compassion and a sense of personal worth. They understand and are sensitive to feelings, values, points of views, and actions, yet they do not let emotions indiscriminately obscure or override professional judgment and rationale, or interfere with care. Caring can be painful and caring nurses are vulnerable. However, nurses must never so insulate or steel themselves against anxiety, suffering, or even death that they lose their ability to interact with patients or colleagues.

Human beings react through their senses. Research has documented the positive effects of *touch* on seriously ill persons as a helpful nonverbal communication in establishing nurse-patient rapport within a short time. Touch says that someone is there and cares. Gentle touch can bridge a language barrier through the establishment of human contact. Warmly holding a patient's hand or laying a hand on an arm during induction of anesthesia or a painful procedure can do much to alleviate that patient's anxiety and elicit his or her trust. A smile has been called the universal language. Above one's mask one's eyes can convey a smile, hope, or amusement. Likewise, they can reveal fear, anger, or hostility. Physiognomy, the ancient Chinese art of discovering qualities of the mind and temperament from the expression of facial features, still has relevance today. In *Macbeth,* Shakespeare says that "your face is like a book where man can read strange matters." Facial expressions, eye contacts, and body movements all have a positive or negative effect on the patient. Warmth and solicitude can be conveyed by a pleasant manner and the expression of the eyes.

The sedated patient is not totally unaware of the OR milieu. Softly spoken, reassuring words are another valuable way to express concern. Never be reticent to communicate your empathy to a patient.

2 *Conscientious.* These persons will not compromise or sacrifice their principles and they adhere to the principle of self-accountability to ensure quality in practice.

3 *Efficient and well organized.* Such people develop coherent, organized work habits. They know, and know that they know. Patients are properly prepared and the OR ready for operations on schedule with the required equipment in working order. They anticipate the needs of patients and team members, and save time and energy. They are prepared for the unexpected. Their efficiency provides reassurance and comfort to patients and surgeons alike.

4 *Flexible and adaptable.* Team members react quickly to changing circumstances in a calm manner and rearrange routine accordingly with one or more acceptable alternative methods. Discriminating judgment prepares adaptable people to cope with all situations with professional decorum.

5 *Sensitive and perceptive.* Nursing personnel are responsive at all times to areas of need and to problems that need to be solved. Perception is based on previous learning. Perceptive persons exhibit genuine interest and kindness. It has been said that the secret of patient care lies in caring for patients or about them, in looking after them and letting them know that they mean something to you. OR nurses are sensitive to the special kind of caring that their patients need.

6 *Understanding, reassuring, and supportive.* In a kind and emotionally controlled way, team members allow others to express their feelings. This conveys to patients the team's ability to relieve physical and emotional discomfort.

7 *Skilled listeners, keen observers, and able communicators.* Such people watch, look, listen, and act. Listening to what another person says can be an effective measure in preventing errors. Unless conclusions are based on observation and full knowledge they should only be considered tentative and subject to revision. Aware personnel will not underestimate the importance of communications in their relationships with patients and colleagues.

"People often talk of the nurse who has been ten years with the sick as being an experienced nurse. But it is observation only which makes experience. The woman who does not observe might be 50 or 60 years with the sick and never be wiser."*

8 *Considerate.* These individuals respect other people's concepts and do not automatically reject those different from their own. Consideration extends to all interpersonal relationships.

9 *Informative and sincere.* Nursing personnel should answer questions and share pertinent information for the mutual benefit of patients, families, and colleagues. All health team members must have the same information to deal honestly and factually with patients and their families. Shared information and forewarning can avoid problems. Nurses should explain procedures before touching patients and give the rationale for them. Patients must never be permitted to feel lost, confined, or abandoned. Control and trust are enhanced by knowledge. Patients have greater confidence when an open, facilitating approach is used. Nurses should reinforce the physicians' explanations.

10 *Aware of individuality.* All personnel convey to patients and colleagues an interest in them as unique persons and act accordingly.

11 *Manually and intellectually dextrous.* These people have quick hands, sharp minds, and keen eyes. Manual dexterity, inherent in most OR team members, is perfected with experience.

12 *Objective.* Such individuals assemble factual data before making a judgment. They view situations from all sides before taking action. Objectivity requires experience and self-discipline. This attribute does not exclude concern but is combined with empathy. Nurses should remain sen-

*F Nightingale, *Notes on Nursing: What It Is and What It Is Not,* London: Harrison, 1860, p. 63.

sitive to problems while acknowledging their own feelings. However, fear must never be obvious to patients whom it would affect adversely.

13 *Impartial, nonjudgmental, open-minded.* These individuals set value judgments aside when making decisions and do not permit their own values and attitudes to distort observations. Judgments can be detrimental to interpersonal relationships. Accept others as they are without attaching conditions to acceptance.

14 *Versatile.* These persons have a comprehensive knowledge of an extensive amount of instrumentation and equipment. They are familiar with numerous diverse operative procedures and care for many diverse patients.

15 *Analytical.* These persons are competent in analyzing and correlating significant data. *They know the "why" as well as the "how" of surgical intervention.* Patients depend on their judgment.

16 *Creative.* These individuals are innovative, using a fluency of ideas to devise effective methods of approach to meeting individual needs and helping patients and colleagues utilize available resources.

17 *Humanistic.* OR team members act in a humane way toward others, which is a quality not easy to computerize. They consider the patient as a person as opposed to someone hooked up to technology.

18 *Sense of humor.* These are the people who can maintain a balance for their own mental health through their perception of the ironies in life situations.

19 *Enduring.* Personnel with endurance maximize their physical and emotional capacities and stamina. OR personnel interact with a large number of people in a critical setting in constant contact with stress, often for prolonged periods of time. Continual demands are made on them for keen observation, rapid judgment, and fast action. All personnel must be disaster-prepared and work rapidly, often under pressure, without sacrificing competency.

20 *Intellectually eager and curious.* Florence Nightingale emphasized that nursing is a progressive art in which to stand still is to have gone back. Nurses have a legal responsibility to keep current in their knowledge, to be present-oriented and informed. Documented proof of continuing education and demonstrated competence in performing nursing functions are of value in litigation. Educational development is a dynamic, ongoing process. Continuing education is a shared responsibility of the hospital, the nursing service, and the individual nurse. The instructional environment should be individually designed. Learning is not just subject-centered, but more problem-centered. Participating in research improves nursing practice and patient care.

NECESSITY FOR STANDARDIZED PROCEDURES AND TECHNIQUES

Standardized procedures and techniques are essential. While there are different ways of arriving at the same ends, it is necessary that one method in each hospital be established and practiced. This prevents chaos for learners and other new personnel. When you are expected to follow accepted procedures, you may sometimes feel that you are being regimented, but that is not the case. Standardized procedures are a great aid in the development of skill and efficiency because:

1 They have as their chief aim the safety and welfare of the patient.

2 It is easier for the instructor or nursing staff member to teach the learners if there is a clearly defined method of work.

3 Learning is easier if everyone does the procedures in the same way.

4 When procedures are kept up-to-date, they set a high standard of work performance.

5 Deviations show a need for evaluation of the procedures and the staff. Do the procedures need revision? Or have staff members become careless?

6 They provide an efficient check during the preparation for any operation. They supplement the memory of the OR staff.

7 One person can take over for another at any time during the operation, if necessary, and know exactly where to find instruments and supplies.

8 Routine procedures establish patterns of habit that increase speed in thought and action. These habits act as motives for doing work in a certain way, which means a high level of proficiency when keyed to high standards of performance.

All personnel involved in the care of patients during the critical surgical intervention phase of their hospital stay must be thoroughly familiar not only with setups, policies, and procedures, but also with equipment and surgeons' routines. OR nursing personnel must be able to cope with all situations in order to provide patients with the utmost in skill, knowledge, and abilities. The enhancement of each individual's potential will provide the best guarantee of high quality patient care.

Inasmuch as details vary from hospital to hospital, discussion of specific equipment has

SURGEON:	PROCEDURE:
GLOVE SIZE: ____________	POSITION OF PATIENT: ____________
SKIN PREP:	DRAPES:
SUTURES AND NEEDLES	**INSTRUMENTS AND EQUIPMENT**
TIES:	BASIC:
PERITONEUM:	
FASCIA:	SPECIAL:
SUB-CU:	
SKIN:	
RETENTION:	
OTHER:	
DRESSINGS:	

Figure 1-1 Surgeon Preference Card. (*Reproduced by permission of Ethicon, Inc.*)

been avoided in this text. However, certain items and techniques for handling are basic. Comparable if not identical equipment is in use in all hospitals. Efficiency is increased by knowledge of equipment and its use. Many items are a part of the operation only. Others are returned to units with patients, and their use carries over to the nursing care and safety of patients there. You must have a broad scope of general knowledge concerning OR procedures and equipment and you must be able to bring it into immediate use as the need arises.

The following is a list of *reference sources* and *learning aids* that all personnel will find useful in mastering and carrying out accepted procedures and techniques:

Hospital Policy Manual. This book contains written basic and general administrative and patient care policies that apply to all hospital personnel. A copy is retained on each nursing unit and in all departments of the hospital.

Operating Room Policy Manual. This book, usually a hardcover ringed binder, contains the policies pertaining solely to the administration and operation of the OR department. A copy is available for reference either in the supervisor's office or at the control desk or both.

Operating Room Procedure Manual. Procedure manuals are assembled for the OR department, as for other hospital departments, to ensure the optimum safety of patients. The primary purpose of the OR procedure manual is to detail how procedures should be specifically performed within the OR suite. It includes those procedures involving direct patient care and supportive procedures.

Instrument Book. The instruments for each operation may be listed in a separate book, which is kept in the instrument room. Photographs or catalog illustrations help learners to identify the vast number of instruments used.

Surgeon Preference Cards. A preference card is maintained for each operation that each surgeon performs. A set of cards is kept in a central file under the surgeon's name. The file is kept where it is readily available, usually in the instrument room. Each day the cards are pulled for operations scheduled and are taken into the appropriate OR. The nurses and technicians consult them, along with the procedure book, as they prepare for each operation. The surgeon's specific preference and any variance from the procedures in the procedure book are noted on the card. It is inexcusable for nurses and technicians to fail to prepare the equipment and supplies that a surgeon routinely uses.

These cards are revised as necessary as procedures and personal preferences for new technology change. These cards permit surgeons to maintain their individuality. Figure 1-1 is a sample surgeon's preference card.

Directories. Alphabetical listings of the location of supplies and equipment are maintained for the instrument room, general workroom, sterile supply room, and general operating room suite storage areas. Regardless of where the storage areas are located, personnel must know the location of supplies and equipment. Directories save valuable time in trying to locate items.

Checklist for learners. The instructor provides a checklist of work assignments for the learners. Learners check off their assignment as they observe or complete it. New assignments are made each day from this list, according to the experience needs of each learner. Learners should avail themselves of every opportunity to learn by observation and practice to enhance their competency.

Checklist of operations. The instructor also provides a record sheet for operations on which learners have scrubbed or circulated. It contains a list of operations for each surgical service. Learners check off their daily experience. This enables the supervisor, when making out assignments, to see at a glance the experience needed by each learner. This record is for the purpose of assignment only.

Library and literature file. Books and current periodicals are available for learner reference in the department library. These may be found in the supervisor's office, the nursing staff lounge area, or in the classroom or conference room if there is such a facility within the OR suite. In addition to books and periodicals, educational literature is available from surgical supply and instrument manufacturers. The literature that accompanies new equipment is of inestimable value to all the staff as well as to learners. This literature is filed and kept available as part of the inservice educational program.

NOTE. 1. Medical Literature Analysis and Retrieval System On-Line (MEDLINE) is a computer-based reference system available at more than 700 libraries in medical schools, institutions, government agencies in the United States and Canada. Over 3000 biomedical journals, including 200 nursing journals, are referenced.
2. Audiovisual aids have become increasingly important in teaching and continuing education. The National Library of Medicine has established Audiovisuals On-Line (AVLINE), a data base of references to audiovisual aids in the health sciences. AVLINE is available through the same on-line network as MEDLINE.

Self-help aids. Habit patterns are formed early in one's learning. Carry in your pocket a memorandum book and pencil. After the completion of an operation, as a reminder, write down in a notebook any questions concerning the patient, or the operation and duties regarding it, and discuss them with the instructor before going off duty. Whenever in doubt, ask for clarification and direction. Always complete an assignment thoroughly and neatly. Ask for help or consult the procedure book when in doubt. Report any assignment as finished or unfinished and ask to have it checked. Seek new experiences. This demonstrates your interest. Remember your purpose: to learn about the nursing care of patients during surgical intervention, the critical phase of surgical patient care, so that you can be a functional member of the operating room team.

Chapter 2

The Health Care Team

TEAM CONCEPT

This text is directed to the health care personnel who care for the surgical patient primarily during the most critical phase of intervention — the operative procedure. When the patient is reconciled to and has given consent for surgical intervention, the patient is dependent on the health care team. A *team* is a group of two or more persons who recognize common goals and coordinate their efforts to achieve them. Broadly defined, the *health care team* includes all personnel relating to the patient, those in direct patient contact as well as those who are not but whose services are essential and contribute to patient care.

The team's approach to patient care must be harmonious and involve impeccable personal ethics. A hospital unit takes on a personality from the individuals in it. This personality gives the unit a reputation for good or otherwise. Unethical discussions or conduct, carelessness, or forgetfulness make an impression on a patient or visitor, who takes it as an index of the total picture and may carry his or her impression to others outside of the hospital. Pride in one's work and in the unit as a whole leads to dissatisfaction with anything short of the very best. A high morale is facilitated by adequate staff orientation, staff participation in departmental decision making and problem solving, receipt of deserved praise, opportunity for continuing education, and motivation to reach and practice at one's highest potential. For patient safety the OR staff, like any other staff, requires instructions, assistance, supervision, motivation, and evaluation.

The team's common goal is the efficient and effective delivery of care to the individual patient for the relief of suffering, the restoration of bodily structure and function, and a favorable postoperative outcome contributing to the patient's optimal health and return to society.

TOTAL DEPENDENCE OF THE PATIENT ON THE O.R. TEAM

At no other time during the hospital experience will the patient be so well attended as during the operation. The patient is surrounded by a surgeon and one or two assistants, a scrub nurse or technician, an anesthesiologist or anesthetist, and a circulating nurse. These individuals, each with specific functions to perform, comprise the operating team. *Reference will be made throughout this text to this direct patient care team as the OR team.* This team literally has the patient's life in its hand. The OR team is like a symphony orchestra; each person is an integral entity in unison and harmony with his or her colleagues for the total accomplishment of a successful outcome.

Persons who function in stressful situations, such as those who work in acute and critical care units, are among the most qualified of professionals and allied technical personnel. They are motivated to maintain high standards. There is no place for mediocrity in the OR! For the welfare and safety of the patient, all persons need to work rapidly, and efficiently as a functioning single unit of *one,* often under tension in a critical setting. They must be thoroughly familiar with procedures, setups, equipment, and policies and must be able to cope with the unpredictable. They must have high morale, mutual understanding, trust, cooperation, and consideration. Anyone who cannot function wholeheartedly as a qualified team member, practicing at his or her optimum level at all times, has no place in the OR! This team works to promote the best interests of the patient every single minute.

O.R. Team

The OR team is subdivided according to the functions of its members:

1 The *scrubbed sterile* team
  a Operating surgeon
  b Assistants to the surgeon
  c Scrub nurse or technician

These team members scrub (wash) their hands and arms, don sterile gown and gloves (see Chap. 7), and enter the sterile field. The *sterile field* is the area of the operating room that immediately surrounds and is especially prepared for the patient. To establish the sterile field, all items needed for the operation are *sterilized,* which are the processes by which all microorganisms are killed (see Chap. 5). Thereafter, the scrubbed, sterile team members function within this limited area and handle only sterile items (see Chaps. 4 and 8).

2 The *unscrubbed unsterile* team
  a Anesthesiologist or anesthetist
  b Circulating nurse
  c Others: In complicated, critical operations such as those in which the chest is opened for procedures on the heart or lungs, the OR team is enlarged to include biomedical engineers or technicians who may be needed to set up and operate the heart-lung machine, monitoring devices, and other instruments that safeguard patient welfare during the operation.

These team members do not enter the sterile field. They function outside and around it. They must assume responsibility for maintaining sterile technique during the operation, but they handle supplies and equipment not considered sterile. Using the principles of aseptic technique, they keep the sterile team supplied, give direct patient care, and handle other requirements that may come up during the opeation.

STERILE TEAM MEMBERS

Operating Surgeon

The surgeon must have the knowledge, skill, and judgment required to successfully perform the intended operation and any deviation in procedure necessitated by unforeseen difficulties. The American College of Surgeons has stated principles of patient care that dictate ethical surgical practice. Protection of the patient and quality care are preeminent in these principles. The surgeon's responsibilities include preoperative diagnosis and care, selection and performance of the operation, and postoperative management of care. The care of many surgical patients is so complex that considerably more than technical skill is required of a surgeon. Advance prediction of simple and uncomplicated operations is uncertain. A surgeon must be prepared for the unexpected with a knowledge of the fundamentals of several basic sciences and the ability to apply them to the diagnosis and management of the patient before, during, and after surgical intervention.

The surgeon assumes full responsibility for all medical acts of judgment and for the management of the surgical patient. The surgeon is a licensed physician (MD), osteopath (DO), or oral surgeon (DDS) especially trained and qualified by knowledge and experience to perform operative procedures.

Most surgeons, by virtue of their postgraduate surgical education, engage in practice within a specific surgical specialty. Qualification for surgical practice, although not a rigid requirement, is certification by an American surgical specialty board approved by the American Board of Medical Specialists or fellowship in the American College of Surgeons. Ten American Specialty Boards grant certification for surgical practice or include surgery. Highly trained and qualified surgeons limit themselves to their specialty except perhaps in emergency situations.

Operations may also be performed by physicians who do not meet these criteria. These physicians include: a physican who received the MD degree prior to 1968 and who has had surgical privileges for over 5 years in a hospital approved by the Joint Commission on Accreditation of Hospitals where most of his or her surgical practice is conducted; a physician who renders surgical care in an emergency or in an area of limited population where a surgical specialist is not available; or a physician who by reason of education, training, and experience is eligible but who has not yet obtained certification or fellowship.

The surgeon must become a member of the medical staff and be granted surgical privileges by each hospital in which he or she wishes to practice. Standards for admission to staff membership, and retention of that membership, are clearly delineated in the bylaws formulated by the medical staff and approved by the governing body of the hospital. The credentials committee has the primary responsibility for investigating thoroughly not only the training of an applicant but also the surgeon's integrity and surgical judgment. In making its recommendations, the committee sets any limitations it sees fit on the surgeon's privileges. The fact that the hospital has assigned privileges does not mean that the surgeon has a free hand. Each hospital sets specific rules, which must be strictly adhered to by each member of the medical staff.

Patients are entitled to the protection and assurance of knowing that surgical privileges are limited to those for which the surgeon has been educated and in which his or her competence has been demonstrated. The patient's choice of and confidence in a surgeon, as well as adherence to directions and advice, are potent factors in the outcome of surgical intervention. A discerning patient will check the qualifications of a surgeon preoperatively.

Assistants to the Surgeon

Under the operating surgeon's direction, one or two assistants hold retractors in the wound to expose the operative site, place clamps on blood vessels, and assist in suturing during the operation. Ideally, another competent surgeon should back up the operating surgeon during every operation in the event of an unanticipated accident to the latter. Such sudden incapacities are, however, rare. For many simple procedures it is clearly not feasible to have a second surgeon, or even another physician as assistant, on the operating team. It would be superfluous to insist upon a physician as assistant at all operations. The degree of hazard of an operation is not so much in the nature of the procedure itself as in the condition of the patient. The operating surgeon must evaluate all individual patient factors to determine the needs for adequate assistance during the operation. The surgeon must be prepared to defend his or her decision before the medical staff and the governing body of the hospital.

In most medical staff bylaws, a section reads, "A qualified physician shall assist during all major operations." The surgical staff of some hospitals maintains a listing of operations by classification as major or minor. If policy stipulates that a physician must assist on all major operations, the surgeon should not be allowed to operate unless a qualified MD assistant is present. Differentiation of major versus minor begs the question. In any operation with unusual hazard to life, a qualified physician must be present and scrubbed as first assistant. Determination of what constitutes unusual hazard rests with the conscience of the operating surgeon and is part of his or her responsibility to the patient.

First Assistant to the Surgeon The first assistant should be capable of assuming the responsibility of the operating surgeon in case of an emergency. A qualified assistant is an individual acknowledged by the credentials committee of the medical staff as having sufficient knowledge, skill, and experience to properly and adequately assist and act for the benefit of the patient.

When the magnitude of the situation warrants, the surgeon may employ another surgeon to first assist. This may be an associate with whom surgical practice is shared and to whom part of the care of the patient may be delegated.

A referring staff physician who is not a surgeon by education and training, but who has a contractural relationship with the patient, may assist the surgeon if granted this privilege by the medical staff. These physicians are usually engaged in general or family practice and have had some training in basic operative principles and techniques. Specially trained nonmedical personnel such as oral surgeons and podiatrists perform or assist with operative procedures in a hospital only under the authority of the medical staff and the surgeon responsible for the surgical service.

In hospitals with approved postdoctoral surgical education and training programs, the surgical resident in the third or more postdoctoral year usually acts as first assistant. The resident is given sufficient responsibility under supervision at the operating table to acquire skill and judgment. This experience is progressively graded so that on completion of training the resident is able to assume individual responsibility for operations.

The 10 boards governing the surgical specialties all require at least 3 years of approved formal residency training, and most set the minimum at 4 or 5 years. Any physician who aspires to become recognized as a surgeon must meet these requirements, under close supervision, while assuming increasing responsibility in the care of surgical patients.

It is proper for the responsible surgeon to delegate the performance of part of an operation to a resident assistant, provided the surgeon is an active participant throughout the essential part of the operation. If a resident is to operate on and take care of the patient under the general supervision of an attending surgeon who will not participate actively, the patient should be so informed and give consent prior to the operation.

The medical staff may approve privileges for a nonphysician allied health practitioner, physician's assistant, or surgeon's assistant. A *nonphysician surgeon's assistant* is qualified by academic and clinical training to perform designated procedures in the operating room and in other areas of surgical patient care. Authorization by the medical staff is based upon the individual's training, experience, and demonstrated competency. Eligibility for appointment as an allied health nonphysician assistant for specified services is determined by the following criteria:

1 Exercising judgment within areas of competence, with the physician member of the medical staff having the ultimate responsibility for patient care

2 Participating directly in the management of patients under the supervision or direction of a member of the medical staff

3 Recording reports and progress notes on patients' records and writing orders to the extent established by the medical staff

4 Performing services in conformity with the applicable provisions of the medical staff bylaws

A member of an allied health profession is individually assigned to an appropriate clinical department as a staff affiliate to carry out activities subject to departmental policies and procedures. The surgeon's assistant must perform duties under the direct supervision of the surgeon. The assistant may help take care of patients in any setting for which the surgeon assumes responsibility and may perform tasks delegated by the surgeon. The ultimate role of the surgeon's assistant cannot be rigidly defined because of variations in practice requirements due to geographic, economic, and sociological factors. The high degree of responsibility an assistant may assume requires that at the conclusion of formal education he or she will possess the knowledge, skills, and abilities necessary to provide those services appropriate to the surgical setting, which may include those of first assistant at the operating table.

The surgeon's assistant may become highly trained and specialized in the areas in which the immediate supervisor has interest, or may remain in an area of surgery requiring a wide variety of procedures such as those performed by a general surgeon in a community hospital. The frequency of performance of certain duties will in part determine the degree of special expertise such an individual acquires in the care of patients. A surgeon's assistant usually is employed by the surgeon, not the hospital, but must receive approval from the medical staff, which delineates the assistant's practice privileges within the hospital under the direct supervision of the surgeon who is on the premises.

The surgeon's assistant is not the same as the operating room technician nor is the role of the surgeon's assistant an extension of the role of the registered nurse in the OR. A nurse may not be compelled to perform an action outside the scope of capacity or the legal limits of nursing practice. He or she is free to refuse to act as first assistant, out of concern both for the well-being of the patient and for one's own professional responsibility. Before any nurse or technician acts as a first assistant at the operating table, he or she should check to be sure a written hospital policy permits this action. *If RNs and/or OR technicians are expected to act as first assistants, this should be part of their written job descriptions and inservice training.*

Second Assistant to the Surgeon Qualified nurses and technicians may be utilized as second or third assistants during operations requiring a physician first assistant or as first assistant during operations in which the surgeon deems this assistance is adequate and for which they have been trained.

Prior to entering postdoctoral programs in the surgical specialties, physicians complete at least 1 year of general surgical training immediately following graduation from medical school. Medical students also receive some exposure to the operating room during surgical clinical experience. These first postdoctoral year general surgical residents and medical students usually function as second assistants at the operating table.

Scrub Nurse

Scrub nurse is a term used to designate the nursing member of the sterile team who actually may or may not be a nurse. The role of scrub nurse may be filled by a registered nurse, a practical nurse, or an operating room technician. The scrub nurse may also be called the *sterile nurse, instrument nurse,* or *suture nurse. The term "scrub nurse" will be used throughout this text to designate this role and to elaborate the specific functions of the individual performing in this capacity.*

The scrub nurse is responsible for maintaining the integrity, safety, and efficiency of the sterile field throughout the operation. Knowledge of and experience with aseptic technique qualify the scrub nurse to prepare and arrange instruments and supplies, and to assist the surgeon and assistants throughout the operation by providing the sterile instruments and supplies required. This demands that the scrub nurse anticipate, plan for, and respond to the needs of the surgeons and other members of the team by *constantly watching the sterile field.* Manual skill and dexterity, along with physical stamina, are important. A stable temperament and ability to work under pressure are also important assets of the scrub nurse, as well as a keen sense of responsibility and concern for accuracy in performing all duties in a manner consistent with good patient care and operative technique.

During extremely complicated or hazardous operations or in teaching situations, two scrub nurses may join the team. One may pass instruments and supplies to the surgeon while the other prepares supplies. An experienced nurse often joins the team to teach, guide, and assist the learner to function in the scrub nurse role. When unexpected, unusual, or emergency situations arise, specific instructions and guidance are received from the surgeon or registered nurse. The OR technician provides services under the supervision and responsibility of a registered nurse at all times.

UNSCRUBBED TEAM MEMBERS

Anesthesiologist or Anesthetist

An *anesthesiologist* is an MD, certified by the American Board of Anesthesiology, who specializes in the art and science of administering anesthetics to produce the various states of anesthesia. An *anesthetist* is a person, not necessarily a physician, who administers anesthetics. When a drug or gas is administered by an anesthetist, this individual works under the direct supervision of the surgeon or of an anesthesiologist. It has been said that no anesthetic agent is safer than its worst administrator, and the value of well-trained anesthetists is inestimable. Excellent training programs are offered to both nurses and physicians. *Throughout this text the term "anesthesiologist" will be used to refer to the person responsible for inducing anesthesia, maintaining anesthesia at the required levels, and managing untoward reactions to anesthesia throughout the operation.*

Anesthesia and surgery are not two separate specialties; they are the two parts of one. These parts must not go their independent ways but must go together and remain together. Adequate communication between the surgeon and the anesthesiologist is the greatest safeguard the patient has. The anesthesiologist is an indispensable member of the OR team (see Chap. 9).

Modern anesthesia is vastly superior to anesthesia of previous years. A continuing increase in the number of anesthetic agents available and refinements of adminstration techniques have broadened its scope. The anesthesiologist's armamentarium is increasing all the time. Improvement in understanding of the pharmacologic actions of anesthetic drugs has led to safer anesthesia. The choice and application of an appropriate agent and a suitable technique of administration, monitoring of vital signs, and maintenance of fluid balance and replacement are all an essential part of the anesthesiologist's responsibility. He or she is also responsible for minimizing the hazards of fire and explosion in areas in which flammable anesthetic agents are used. Appropriate precautions must be taken to ensure the safe administration of anesthetic agents. All team members, as a unit, are working for the safety and recovery of the patient. Functioning as guardian of the patient, the anesthesiologist must also observe the principles of aseptic technique.

With the broadening of the field of anesthesiology, anesthesiologists are not confined to the operating room although this is their primary arena. Their role includes that of overseer of the recovery room to provide resuscitative care until the patient has regained control of vital functions. Anesthesiologists may also participate in the hospital's program of cardiopulmonary resuscitation, act as consultants or managers of problems of acute and chronic respiratory insufficiency, and act as consultants on a variety of other diagnostic and therapeutic measures related to patient care. Their advice may be sought in the total care of unconscious patients, those with acute circulatory disorders, and those with respiratory ventilation problems requiring inhalation therapy.

Circulating Nurse

The *circulating nurse* plays a role that is vital to the smooth flow of events before, during, and after the operation. Patients undergoing surgical intervention experience physical and psychosocial trauma. They enter an alien environment removed from the personal contact of family and friends. Physical and psychological needs reach ultimate proportions. Because most patients are unconscious, they are powerless and unable to make decisions concerning their welfare. At this critical time, patients need the professional judgment of others who must function on their behalf. These advocates must be within close physical and social proximity. The surgeon is in charge at the operating table, but he or she relies upon the circulating nurse to take care of the activities of the room outside the sterile field and to manage the nursing care required for each patient. To some extent, the circulating nurse controls both the physical and emotional atmosphere in the room. The role of the OR nurse as the patient's advocate, protector, guardian angel, and provider cannot be stressed enough. Therefore, the circulating nurse must always be a registered nurse.

The role of the circulating nurse is vital to the provision of that care that includes but is not limited to:

1 Application of the nursing process in directing and coordinating all nursing activities related to the care and support of the patient within the OR to meet individualized patient needs. Nursing judgment and decision-making skill are requisites to assessing, planning, implementing, and evaluating nursing care before, during, and after surgical intervention. This is the professional role of the circulating nurse.

2 Creation and maintenance of a safe and comfortable environment for the patient through implementing the principles of asepsis (see Chap. 4). The circulating nurse must see the OR as a whole and be so "technique conscious" that any break or near-break on the part of anyone in the room is evident to her instantly. Although sterile technique is the responsibility of everyone in the room, the circulating nurse must be on the alert to catch any breaks that others may not have seen. Because she stands farther away from the sterile field than others, she is better able to see any break.

3 Provision of assistance to any member of the OR team in any manner in which the circulating nurse is qualified. This requires current knowledge of the legal implications of surgical intervention. The circulating nurse must know the organization of the work and the relative importance of factors involved in accomplishing it. The effective circulating nurse will know the fine points of performance as a scrub nurse to be able to anticipate the needs of the scrubbed team. She must be alert to these needs and see that the team is supplied with every item necessary to perform the operation efficiently. The circulating nurse must know all supplies, instruments, and equipment, be able to get them quickly, and guard against inadvertent hazards in their use and care. She must direct the scrub nurse and stay close to assist with unfamiliar equipment.

4 Identification of any potential environmental dangers or stressful situations involving the patient and/or other team members. This requires constant flexibility to meet the unexpected and to act in an efficient, rational manner in emergency situations.

5 Maintenance of the communication link between events and team members at the sterile field and persons not in the OR but concerned with the outcome of the operation. The latter includes the patient's family and other personnel in the OR suite and in other departments of the hospital. The ability to recognize and effectively communicate situations involving the patient and/or other team members is a vital link in the continuity of patient care.

6 Direction of the activity of the scrub nurse. The circulating nurse usually is the more experienced nursing team member. In an OR suite in which there are many learners, RNs frequently assume responsibility for the individual learner assigned with them. Kindly help builds up the learner's confidence. In this capacity the circulating nurse acts as supervisor, advisor, and teacher.

DIRECT PATIENT CARE TEAM IS PART OF TOTAL DEPARTMENT

The OR team, as described, immediately surrounds the patient throughout the operation. This direct patient care team functions within the physical confines of a specific room, *the operating room* (OR). This room is one part of the physical facilities that comprise the total *operating room suite.* Similarly, this team makes up only one part of the human activity directed toward the care of the surgical patient. Many other people function in an indirect relationship with the patient, contributing vital supporting services toward the common goal of ensuring a safe, comfortable, and effective environment for the safety and welfare of the patient within the OR suite. All of the nursing personnel assigned to work in the operating room suite are collectively referred to as *the operating room nursing staff of the OR department.* The relationship and duties of those staff members within the OR department will vary from hospital to hospital depending on the size and extent of the physical facilities and the number of personnel employed. No one's job is small! Each staff member fits into the general scheme of the department, and each has important functions to perform. A high state of morale exists when each person performs his or her duties and feels responsible for assuming a part of the total workload of the OR department.

Job Descriptions

Each OR staff member must understand his or her own functions and responsibilities. A *job description* provides a written summary of the job to be done, lists the duties and requirements of the job as it must be performed in order to fulfill the department's requirements, and states to whom the employee is accountable.

The staffing plan must delineate those functions for which nursing service is responsible, and indicate all positions to carry out these functions. Job descriptions delineate the functions, responsibilities, and desired qualifications of each classification of professional, allied technical, and ancillary personnel. They serve as a guide for individual employees as well as for the supervisor; give order to individual work assignments and orderly, intelligent direction to the activities of the department; and prevent duplication of effort or neglect of duties.

Job descriptions must be written by each hospital for its own OR department staff to plan and coordinate work, and to establish methods of accomplishing it. An employee is not required to assume responsibility not specified in the job description. Work satisfaction is promoted by giving members of the staff basic duties and fixed responsibilities. Because the job description spells out each job requirement, it provides the supervisor with a means of checking that the employee understands the assignments and carries them out.

Performance Standards

Performance standards complement job descriptions. They are precise criteria for evaluating what an employee must do under present working conditions to perform a specific duty in a manner that is completely satisfactory. They are the measurements by which the employee's performance is judged in terms of quality, quantity, and manner. Standards of acceptable practice in the OR department are based on sound principles of the natural and behavioral sciences.

A standard developed by a profession or regulatory body is an authoritative statement of the range of acceptable variation from a norm or criterion by which quality can be judged. Standards of nursing practice are a means of determining the quality of nursing care that a patient receives regardless of whether such care is provided solely by professional nurses or by nurses in conjunction with allied technical and/or ancillary assistants. For the individual practitioner, standards provide a yardstick for the day-to-day evaluation of patient care. Since the professional nurse is primarily accountable to the patient, the standards focus on the nursing process and reflect a systematic approach to nursing practice. Standards for the practice of nursing are intended to provide safe individualized patient care, detect inadequacy of care, prevent legal implications resulting from alleged nursing malpractice or negligence, and improve the integrated nursing care program offered each patient.

Nursing Administrative Personnel

The *operating room supervisor* is responsible for the administration and supervision of nursing service in the OR department. The title is not used universally in all hospitals; neither is it always representative of the position's major functions. In large hospitals, the title *director of operating rooms* or *assistant director of nursing service* may be given to this position because of the extent and complexity of its administrative responsibilities. Actual supervision of personnel is then delegated to an assistant or assistants who may be titled *supervisor.* In smaller hospitals, where the volume of administrative and supervisory work is limited, the operating room supervisor often approaches the level of head nurse and may bear this title. In other situations, one nursing supervisor may be responsible for the administration and supervision of more than one clinical service such as OR department, central service department, recovery room, and/or emergency department.

The title should indicate the scope of the responsibilities of the nurse who is accountable for coordination of all nursing care given and all related supporting services of the OR department and its staff. *"Operating room supervisor" (ORS) will be used throughout this text to designate this position.*

Operating Room Supervisor

An operating room supervisor must have thorough knowledge of general nursing theory and practice and specialized knowledge of operating room technique and management. The ORS must be an RN in order to supervise and direct all nursing care given to patients, both directly and indirectly by nursing service personnel within the OR department, according to nursing principles and standards. The main function of the ORS is that of leadership—of promoting cooperative effort. To be a leader requires an additional set of skills and knowledge. These concern functions of management that include planning, organizing, staffing, directing, and controlling, plus the connecting processes of decision making, coordinating, and communicating.

The ORS is responsible for the allocation and completion of work, but does not do it all or make all of the decisions. Capable personnel are employed and given increasing responsibility as they develop competence in their work under the guidance of the ORS. He or she develops the will and desire among all staff members to cooperate with one another. The ORS creates an organization that can function well in his or her absence.

Personnel must know the direction of the entire organizational effort. This knowledge is a prerequisite for their successful functioning. The ORS interprets the hospital and departmental philosophy, objectives, policies, and procedures, as defined below, to the OR staff.

Philosophy Statement of beliefs regarding patient care and the nature of perioperative nursing care that clarifies the overall responsibilities to be fulfilled.

Objectives Statements of specific goals to be accomplished during the course of action and definitions of criteria for acceptable performance.

Policies Specific authoritative statements of governing principles or actions, within the context of the philosophy and objectives, that assist in decision making by providing guidelines for action to be taken or, in some situations, for what is not to be done.

Basic Policies Statements of the principles of administration and its approach to functioning.

General Policies Guidelines of the principles dealing with everyday situations that affect all personnel within the hospital.

Departmental Policies Guidelines structured to meet the needs of a specific work unit, i.e., OR policies.

Procedures Statements of actions to be taken in the implementation of policies.

The ORS must implement and enforce these hospital and departmental policies and procedures. He or she also analyzes and evaluates continuously all nursing services rendered and, through participation in research, seeks to improve the quality of patient care given. The ORS retains accountability for all nursing care given, all related activities in the OR department, and all aspects of environmental control in the OR suite. Areas of this accountability include:

1 Assistance to surgeons in operations through provision of adequately prepared OR team members

2 Delegation of responsibilities and duties to professional, allied technical, and ancillary personnel

3 Responsibility for performance evaluation of all department personnel

4 Provision of educational opportunities to increase knowledge of all personnel

5 Coordination of administrative duties to ensure proper functioning of the staff

6 Provision and control of materials, supplies, and equipment

7 Coordination of activities within the OR suite with other departments of the hospital

Assistant Operating Room Supervisor

The *assistant operating room supervisor* (AORS) aids in the administration and supervision of nursing service in the OR department and is directly responsible to the OR supervisor. This person acts as the administrative head in the absence of the supervisor. The position usually does not exist in small hospitals.

Head Nurse

The *head nurse* functions in a middle management position as liaison between staff members and administrative personnel. In some hospitals, the title of head nurse is given to the person whose position is comparable to an AORS. In other hospitals, usually smaller ones, the ORS functions more or less in the capacity of head nurse.

In large hospitals with many surgical specialty services, a head nurse may be responsible for the administration and direct supervision of nursing service in a designated room or rooms within the OR suite assigned to a particular specialty service, such as ophthalmology, neurosurgery, cardiovascular surgery, urology, etc. With this structure, there will be several head nurses in the department. These head nurses should have the technical proficiency required for the specialty service for which they are responsible and should have sufficient management ability to plan for and administer effectively the nursing service activities.

The duties of the head nurse will include, but are not limited to:

1 Planning for and supervising the nursing activities within the entire OR suite or specific room(s) to which assigned
2 Coordinating nursing activities with those of the surgeons and anesthesiologists to provide for the care of patients
3 Surveying and maintaining adequate supplies and equipment and providing for their economical use
4 Observing the performance of all staff members pertaining to nursing activities
5 Interpreting to personnel all aseptic techniques, procedures, and policies adopted by the department and hospital administration
6 Informing the ORS of needs and problems arising in the department

Functions vary in different hospitals, but the head nurse always has the responsibility for learners. She assists in implementing orientation and teaching programs for new personnel and staff members during operations and related services. The position of head nurse, with its direct and continuous responsibility for both patients and staff, is an important one.

Master Clinician

The traditional administrative pattern of the lines of authority within the OR nursing department has been outlined to describe the overall functions that establish the working relationship of the staff. Within any organization a formal structure of authority and responsibility exists. However, the evolution of nursing as a profession has changed the focus of functions for many nurses within the hospital organization. With experience and advanced study, a nurse can become recognized as a *master clinician* capable of organizing and providing complex care, and of using initiative and independent judgment. Specific job titles vary considerably from one locale and one hospital to another. The master clinician may hold the title of *team leader, senior clinical nurse, nurse clinician,* or *clinical nurse specialist.* Although the *term "master clinician" will be used to describe any or all of these roles,* differentiation is made within the profession on the basis of formal academic educational preparation.

In general, minimal preparation for this role is a baccalaureate degree in nursing. The *clinical nurse specialist,* however, has been defined as a graduate of a master's program in nursing, with a major in a clinical specialty, who enhances the quality of nursing care directly with patients and indirectly through guidance and planning of care with other nursing personnel. It is expected that the clinical nurse specialist serves as a role model by being involved in teaching patients and personnel, and by demonstrating the highest level of interpersonal skills and promoting collegial relationships. These skills can be utilized as effectively in the OR as in any nursing unit.

The master clinician is capable of exercising a high degree of discriminative judgment in planning, executing, and evaluating nursing care based upon the assessed needs of patients having one or more common clinical manifestations. A master clinician may develop the nursing care plan for a group of orthopaedic patients, for example.

The master clinician develops and implements a nursing care plan for each patient in her group. This plan is coordinated with the surgeon, other professional personnel, and allied technical personnel who assist in the performance of functions related to the nursing care plan. Clinical nursing is not necessarily performed by the master clinician. She decides what needs to be done and determines which nursing functions can be done by others and which she must do herself. The important point is that the decision is based upon personal interaction with each patient and a knowledge of the clinical condition. The master clinician exercises a degree of autonomy and independent nursing action within the clinical setting.

Since a master clinician is one who has had extensive academic preparation in theoretical knowledge and clinical experience in a particular clinical nursing setting and who is an expert in nursing situations in that setting, then qualified OR supervisors may function as master clinicians. In this role, they assist in planning a program of total nursing care for each surgical patient, coordinating nursing and supportive services, participating in the orientation, development, and evaluation of nursing personnel assigned to direct patient care functions in the OR, and conducting research studies to evaluate nursing interventions. Supervisors who also assess individual patient needs through personal patient interviews and who plan for individualized nursing care in the OR truly function as master clinicians. They have the title of *OR nurse clinician* or *OR clinical specialist* in some hospitals. These supervisors make decisions relative to the direct and indirect nursing care of the patient in the OR setting, utilizing specialized judgments and skills. Decision making is the heart of professional management and professional leadership.

The OR master clinician, whatever the organizational title may be, may not be the nurse charged with the overall management and leadership functions in the OR department. OR nurses may be assigned to work solely or primarily with the surgeons in a specific surgical specialty. This concept of nursing specialization coincides with the specialization of surgeons. With practice and formal or informal study, nurses develop expertise in planning and implementing nursing care for patients with similar surgical problems. Skills and knowledge become highly specialized, and the surgeons in that particular specialty rely on such nurses to supervise the nursing care of their patients and to direct less-experienced nursing personnel on the OR team. Master clinicians may fulfill the circulating nurse duties in one OR or serve as consultant-coordinators for several rooms in which patients are being operated on by surgeons within a given surgical specialty. The job title for the nurse and the assignment structure will vary with the size of the hospital and the manner in which it is organized. With either type of assignment, these nurses are master clinicians of very narrow scope unless they visit patients preoperatively to assess their individual needs, plan nursing care on the basis of need assessment, and evaluate the quality of nursing care postoperatively through direct patient interaction. Then they are master clinicians in the broader context.

Inservice Educational Coordinator

Inservice training is a planned educational experience provided in the job setting and closely identified with service designed to help each staff member perform more effectively and knowledgeably as a person and as an employee. The *inservice educational coordinator,* a hospital employee and member of the administrative staff, is responsible for planning, scheduling, and coordinating orientation, staff development, and other educational programs within the OR department. These programs are held on a continuing basis.

STAFF NURSING PERSONNEL

General Duty Registered Nurse

Under the immediate supervision of the head nurse and/or OR supervisor, *general duty professional staff nurses* provide direct care to patients utilizing the nursing process and discriminative judgment in making independent nursing decisions. They work in a collaborative relationship with surgeons and anesthesiologists to determine the needs of patients during the operation and assume responsibility for planning nursing care. Preoperatively they help alleviate patient anxiety and identify nursing care problems (see Chap. 3).

Staff nurses perform either scrub nurse or circulating nurse functions. In general, the more experienced nurse functions as the circulating nurse to supervise the management of all nursing activities in the room assigned. If staffing does not permit an RN staff nurse in both positions, the RN must circulate.

As part of their professional practice in the OR, staff nurses assess the effectiveness of nursing actions taken, identify and carry out systematic investigations of clinical problems, and engage in periodic review of their own contributions to nursing care and those of their professional peers. To assure a safe environment for patients, they assist other nursing staff members through teaching and supervising to carry out aseptic techniques and procedures as adopted by the department and based on sound scientific principles. They also assist in the control and maintenance of drugs, supplies, equipment, and records. Staff nurses assist all members of the OR team and work cooperatively with members of the nursing staff and other departments to promote continuity of patient care.

By actively participating in the operation, scrubbing, or circulating, teaching, and directing, the OR staff nurse maintains nursing skills, extends area of competence, and keeps abreast of current developments in patient care and treatment. OR nursing is a specialty of clinical nursing practice.

The professional nurse serves as a role model for others to emulate. Since she influences others by her own nursing practice, behavior, and appearance, her conduct must be exemplary. Her demeanor should express dignity, self-confidence, and *genuine concern for each individual.*

Licensed Practical/Vocational Nurses

Licensed practical/vocational nurses (LPN/LVNs) who are qualified by training, experience, and demonstrated ability may be utilized to give nursing care that does not require the skill and judgment of a registered nurse. With specialized training in OR technology, these nurses may be permitted to serve as scrub nurses under the direct supervision of a professional registered nurse. LPN/LVNs are not permitted to function independently as circulating nurses in the OR. They may second assist in implementing the nursing care plan by working with a qualified professional nurse. *Throughout this text the functions of the LPN/LVN on the OR staff will be considered the same as those of operating room technicians.*

OR Technician/Surgical Technologist

Operating room technicians (ORTs) are responsible for their own acts, but must function under the supervision of a registered nurse at all times. OR technicians assist with the nursing care of patients in the OR by performing routine and delegated duties according to the standards of practice and the policies of the hospital and department. They are restricted from administering medications, completing patient records, or carrying out direct physician orders regarding treatment of patients. ORTs are permitted to serve as scrub nurses, but they are not permitted to function as circulating nurses in the OR.* They may be permitted to second assist the surgeon at the operating table or second assist the RN circulating nurse.

Routine duties of OR technicians also include stocking, replenishing, preparing and/or selecting supplies and equipment for storage or for immediate use during operations. OR technicians also assist with housekeeping duties to maintain cleanliness in the OR suite in order to ensure a safe patient environment.

Ancillary Personnel

Ancillary personnel are lay workers trained through an inservice educational program.

Clerical Personnel One or more ancillary workers may perform clerical duties associated with activities within the OR suite. These duties may include assisting with preparation of the schedule of operations, ordering supplies, and maintaining records and reports.

*HEW Code of Federal Regulations, Title 20, Chapter III, Part 405, Social Security Act.

A control desk is usually located at the entrance to the OR suite where a clerk-receptionist can see and check all visitors and personnel. Unauthorized persons can be intercepted.

Clerical personnel serve as vital communication links between the OR department and other departments. They receive and send messages by telephone, intercommunication system, and mail.

The hospital telephone exchange operators frequently relay messages for surgeons while they are operating. The clerk in the OR suite must be aware of the arrival and departure of the surgeons in order to be certain that they receive their messages without being disturbed during operations.

Most hospitals have an intercommunication system between the OR and other areas in the OR suite. Clerical personnel coordinate messages through this system. They can arrange for transportation of patients to and from the OR, obtain supplies or additional personnel for the OR team if needed, etc.

Many hospitals have a pneumatic-tube system that provides a quick means for the delivery of written communications and small, nonbreakable supplies to all parts of the hospital. The clerk operates this system.

Clerical personnel relieve nurses of much paper work by doing the departmental record keeping.

Nursing Assistants Ancillary personnel are employed to perform certain indirect nursing care activities. A *nursing assistant* may be male or female. Most OR departments have both. Their duties include, but are not limited to:

1 Assisting with transporting, moving, and positioning of patients
2 Performing errands to other departments as needed
3 Cleaning, processing, and storing instruments and supplies
4 Maintaining assigned work area in a clean and orderly condition

A male assistant, sometimes titled an *orderly,* may be asked to do the heavier work in the department, such as lifting patients and moving or setting up large pieces of equipment.

INTERDEPARTMENTAL RELATIONSHIPS

The operating room is one of many departments within the total hospital organization, just as the operation is one segment of total surgical patient care. To provide continuity in total patient care, the staffs of many departments must cooperate. Their efforts are coordinated through the administration of the formal organizational structure of the hospital.

Every hospital has a *governing body* that appoints a chief executive officer, usually titled the *hospital administrator,* to provide appropriate physical resources and personnel to meet the needs of patients. Administrative lines of authority, responsibility, and accountability are defined to establish the working relationships between departments and personnel.

The *director of nursing service* reports to the hospital administrator. The OR supervisor will report to the director of nursing if the OR department is structured as a unit within nursing service. In some hospitals, the OR is considered an independent department separate from nursing service. This OR supervisor then reports directly to the hospital administrator or an assistant administrator. Through either channel of administration, many activities in the OR department must be coordinated with other nursing units and hospital departments.

Nursing Units

Patients come to the OR directly from the emergency department, inpatient nursing units, or outpatient ambulatory care department. It is vital that channels of communication be kept open between OR personnel and nursing personnel in these other nursing units in order to coordinate preoperative preparation and transportation of patients. Many hospitals use a checklist to assure adequate preparation of surgical patients. An RN or LPN/LVN signs or initials for each item accomplished. By the time the patient leaves for the OR suite, all the preparations have been completed.

Recovery Room

The inestimable value of a good recovery room to provide maximal safety for patients immediately following their operation is undisputed. Recovery rooms evolved to meet a need for trained personnel to constantly observe patients within facilities equipped for specialized care until recovery from anesthesia is stabilized sufficiently for safe transfer to their rooms elsewhere in the hospital. Because this is the purpose, the *recovery room* (RR) is referred to as the *postanesthesia room* (PAR) in some hospitals.

The recovery room is usually physically adjacent to the OR suite. Included in the RR may be partitioned isolation areas for patients with known infectious organisms or patients who are highly susceptible to infection, such as burn patients. These patients need the same postoperative care as others do. They should be sent to the RR unless they can receive the same care in an isolation room on the nursing unit. Hospital policy should determine this. If the RR does not have a partitioned isolation area, patients may be placed at the end of the room, separated from others by screens or curtains. Extra care must be used in handling bedding and equipment. Hand washing is essential after each patient contact to prevent cross contamination.

In large hospitals, the recovery room may be open for 24 hours. In other hospitals, especially if most of the operations are performed in the morning hours, the RR may be open only during the day. The extent of utilization of the operating rooms will determine the routine hours of available recovery room care. Special arrangements for constant observation must be made for patients during hours in which the recovery room is closed. These arrangements are established by hospital policy.

The recovery room is under the supervision of an anesthesiologist in coordination with a nursing supervisor. This supervisor may be the OR supervisor who has a head nurse assigned to the recovery room to directly supervise the activities in this specialized area.

The recovery room is staffed by specially trained registered nurses and other nursing personnel. The patients are under their constant observation. Respiratory and circulatory depressions are at once detected and corrected. Monitoring and emergency resuscitation equipment is always at hand. An intercommunication system or emergency call system connects the recovery room personnel with the OR suite so that additional personnel are readily available in situations that are life-threatening to patients.

Patients remain in the recovery room until they have reacted from anesthesia and their vital signs have become stabilized following the operation. Clinical evaluation of patients by listening, watching, and feeling is augmented by electronic devices to monitor respiratory and cardiac functions. Monitors are used in the recovery room to aid personnel in keeping a careful check on patients during the critical postoperative period.

When patients have regained consciousness and

it is deemed safe to transfer them, they are returned to their rooms. There family and friends may visit them. The period of time spent in the recovery room postpones these visits until patients are better able to see visitors. Family members are notified when the patient is admitted to the recovery room so that they will know the operation is over. This helps to relieve their anxiety during the hours of waiting.

Intensive Care Units

As surgery has become more specialized and operations of great magnitude have been developed and perfected, specialized facilities where concentrated treatment can bring the patient to a satisfactory recovery have become a necessity. This care is provided in an *intensive care unit* (ICU) open 24 hours a day, 7 days a week. It is staffed by highly trained and specialized registered nurses. Critically ill patients who need constant care for several days are admitted directly from the operating room, recovery room, emergency department, or other nursing unit. Each bedside is equipped with therapeutic and monitoring equipment.

Depending on the size of the hospital and its specialty services, more than one specially designed and equipped intensive care unit may be provided. One ICU may admit only cardiovascular surgical patients, another burn patients, another only pediatric patients, another transplant patients. In addition to surgical intensive care units, most hospitals also have a *coronary care unit* (CCU) and/or a unit for nonsurgical (medical) patients. The increased efficiency these units afford serves the best interests of both the hospital and the patient. They create the most effective utilization of personnel and equipment, and lower morbidity and mortality rates.

Movements of patients to and from the surgical intensive care units must be closely coordinated with the operating room schedule, the OR team, and the recovery room personnel. If the surgeon anticipates that a patient will need intensive care postoperatively, a bed in the ICU must be reserved before the patient is scheduled for operation. Sometimes the patient must wait in the OR or recovery room for another patient to be transferred out of the ICU when the former's condition warrants intensive care that was unanticipated.

Many surgeons prefer to transfer their patients directly from the operating room to the intensive care unit, thus bypassing the recovery room. This facilitates immediate initiation of treatment that will be prolonged in the postoperative period and eliminates the stress that additional movement causes patients.

Medical Records

Clinical records must be complete. They include the admitting diagnosis, the patient's chief complaint, complete history and physical examination, the records of laboratory examinations, and the physicians' and nurses' care plans. Records must state therapy employed including operations, progress notes, consultation remarks, condition on discharge or observations in case of death, and a summary of the hospitalization experience also must be complete. These records are signed by all physicians and nurses attending the patient.

Notes about the operation must be explicit, dictated promptly after the operation, and incorporated into the record of each surgical patient. For the surgeons' convenience, many hospitals have dictating machines or a phone hookup with the medical records department installed within the OR suite, usually located in the dressing room or lounge. Details of the pre- and postoperative diagnosis and the operation itself may have medical and legal significance. It is the responsibility of the medical records department to accurately transcribe the surgeon's dictation and maintain the patient's chart after his or her discharge from the hospital.

The anesthesia record completed during the operation by the anesthesiologist also becomes part of the patient's record. Nursing care must also be documented on the patient's chart. Therefore, the circulating nurse should write pertinent remarks pertaining to nursing care rendered in the OR and the patient's response to care on the nurses' note sheet or the progress notes. Documentation is a responsibility of all professional team members implementing direct patient care.

Radiology and Nuclear Medicine Departments

Frequently, personnel from the radiology (x-ray) and nuclear medicine (radiation therapy) departments assist with diagnostic or therapeutic procedures in the OR. For some procedures it may be necessary for OR nursing personnel to go to the x-ray department to assist the surgeon during a procedure requiring sterile technique. Whenever a diagnostic procedure or operation is scheduled that will require use of x-ray or a radioactive implant, all departments must be notified at least the day before. This is not only common courtesy, but facilitates the scheduling of personnel and the workload in all departments.

Pharmacy

Many drugs are routinely stocked in the OR suite for the anesthesiologists' use and some for use by the surgeons during operations. These are obtained by requisition from the pharmacy. When received, narcotics are always kept under lock and each dosage is recorded as dispensed.

The pharmacy is not an isolated department but an integral part of the hospital. Pharmacists are resource persons who convey drug information to physicians and nurses. They cooperate with physicians in obtaining new, unusual, or special drugs for patients and in providing information about actions and interactions. They also recommend new or improved products or forms of packaging drugs. Pharmacists should be responsible for the preparation of all admixtures and for the quality control of associated drug product services throughout the hospital.

Blood Bank

If the surgeon anticipates in advance of the operation that blood loss replacement may be necessary, a sample of the patient's blood is sent to the blood bank for type and cross match. In emergency situations this sample may be sent from the emergency department or the OR. The units of blood products ordered by the surgeon are prepared and labeled with the patient's name and blood data.

Blood products for transfusion are kept in a special refrigerator at a constant temperature between 2 and 6°C, which is verified by a recording thermometer. Blood banks usually dispense whole blood, plasma, or packed cells only as they are needed.

Pathology Department

The *pathologist,* an MD who specializes in the cause and effect of disease, may be on call at a few minutes' notice to examine tissue while the patient is under anesthesia. This enables the surgeon to proceed immediately with a definitive operation, if malignant tumor cells are found, without subjecting the patient to a second operation at a later time. A small laboratory may be located within the OR suite with equipment for microscopic tissue examination. This laboratory may be used for other tests and/or for taking photographs of tissue specimens removed from patients.

All tissue removed during operations ultimately is sent to the pathology department for routine examination. These tissues may be stored in a refrigerator in the laboratory or some other location within the OR suite until they are taken to the pathology department at the end of or at intervals during each day's schedule of operations.

Bacteriology Laboratory

Biological testing of the OR environment and sterile supplies is done periodically according to hospital routine and always when a problem of contamination is suspected. The *bacteriologist,* who specializes in the study of microorganisms, may come into the OR suite to collect samples for testing or samples may be collected and sent to the laboratory by OR personnel. The results provide a method for evaluating the effectiveness of procedures and the degree of adherence to environmental standards.

OR Unit Manager

To relieve the OR supervisor of nonnursing duties, some hospitals employ an *OR unit manager.* This manager may report to the ORS or directly to the hospital administrator. Lines of authority and responsibility between the unit manager and the ORS must be clearly defined regardless of the organizational structure. The OR unit manager directs the management of the nonnursing and nondirect patient care functions in the OR suite, while the OR nursing supervisor and other administrative nursing personnel direct and supervise patient care and the professional and allied technical nursing personnel.

In addition to directing and supervising all nursing care given to patients within the OR, administrative duties must include maintaining a clean, orderly, safe environment within the OR suite for patients and personnel. The maintenance of a clean and safe environment entails more than removing visible dust and dirt. A safe environment is one that is free of contamination, free of electrical and explosive hazards, and free of negligence. Formulation of procedures is necessary. Personnel must be trained. But inspection and followup are equally important. The OR unit manager coordinates these efforts with the supporting service departments: housekeeping, maintenance, central service, laundry, central storeroom, and purchasing. If the hospital does not employ an OR unit manager, the ORS must assume responsibility for these duties.

Housekeeping Department

Housekeeping functions are recognized as important preventive measures to eliminate microorganisms from the hospital environment. Each hospital establishes a routine for its particular needs. Usually housekeeping department personnel and nursing personnel share the housekeeping duties in the OR suite. The amount of cleaning done by the OR personnel varies from one hospital to another. In many, the members of the housekeeping department clean all furniture, flat surfaces, lights, and floors once a day at the end of the operating schedule. In others, they also clean the furniture and floors before the schedule starts and between each operation throughout the day. Whatever plan they follow, housekeeping personnel must have a storage area within the OR suite in which to keep their equipment and supplies. Equipment used for cleaning in the OR is not taken outside the suite.

The *executive housekeeper,* who is the head of the housekeeping department, and the OR supervisor or unit manager plan the division of work. Personnel in each department must understand their responsibilities. The OR supervisor or unit manager checks the work of housekeeping personnel and keeps in touch with the executive housekeeper concerning their performance.

The executive housekeeper must have a thorough knowledge of the job. He or she evaluates and chooses the proper solutions for effective cleaning, sets up a program and standard of performance for employees, and sees that they are properly oriented and taught the procedures and standards. Using a checklist helps to cover all areas to be cleaned and inspected on a routine basis, whether it is daily, weekly, or monthly. A weekly or monthly cleaning routine is set up that includes walls and ceilings, in addition to the daily cleaning schedule within the OR suite (see Chap. 8).

The executive housekeeper impresses upon the personnel the importance of the work and the important part they play in enabling the OR personnel to carry out aseptic technique. The housekeeping personnel do indeed function as members of the OR team when working with the scrub and circulating nurses between operations.

Maintenance Department

The maintenance department personnel also work in close cooperation with the OR department. All operations must be supported by a continuous preventive maintenance program. This includes routine monitoring of ventilation and heating, electrical and lighting systems, emergency warning systems, and water supply. Humidity is recorded every hour in the maintenance department. All electrical equipment is checked monthly by maintenance department personnel. In addition, they regularly test the autonomous emergency power source and maintain a written record of inspection and performance.

Conductive flooring is a means of electrically connecting people and objects to prevent the accumulation of electrical charges and to equalize potentials. The maintenance department checks the conductivity of the flooring and furniture in the OR suite at least once a month and keeps a permanent record of the levels.

The hospital water supply system should not be connected with other piping systems, or with fixtures that could allow contamination of the water supply. The hot water supply and steam lines have temperature control devices regulated by the maintenance department personnel. They are cleaned on a routine schedule, usually weekly, to prevent accumulation of mineral deposits.

Central Service Department

A myriad of sterile supplies are used in the OR. Many of these are commercially prepackaged, presterilized, disposable, one-time use products. Some are prepared in the OR suite. Other items used in the OR are processed for reuse by central service department personnel. These items are cleaned, packaged, and sterilized. Central service department personnel may package and sterilize linen packs unless this is done in the laundry or disposable packs are used. In many hospitals, central service department personnel replenish supplies on the nursing units daily, according to standard inventories. A similar system may be established for the OR suite or supplies may be requisitioned as needed.

Laundry

Many hospitals use disposable linen packs. In others, the laundry packages the linens used in the OR. Then the linens are either sterilized in the laundry, central service department, or in the OR suite depending on where the sterilizing equipment is located. Even if the use of disposables negates this need, some linen is processed for the OR suite. Hospitals that do not have laundry facilities as part of their physical plant use a commercial laundry. Linen supplies are usually requisitioned on a daily basis to maintain inventory level. The *laundry manager* may assist in determining appropriate inventories.

Central Storeroom and Purchasing

A limited stock of supplies is kept in the OR suite. However, storage is generally a problem in every OR suite. Therefore, bulk inventories of many supplies are stocked in the central storeroom for requisition as needed. Usually these supplies are requisitioned on a weekly basis.

Items that are too expensive to stock in large quantities or that are used infrequently are ordered through the purchasing department as needed. As the central storeroom is a part of this department, the purchasing agent determines the supplies to be stocked for requisition and those for direct purchase as needed.

Personnel Department

Even though the availability of supplies and equipment and the physical facilities are important, these are secondary to the functioning of the OR department. The efficiency of any department depends on the persons employed in it. Therefore, the careful selection of capable, highly motivated people contributes to the efficiency and effectiveness of interdepartmental relationships. The personnel department helps screen applicants. Those seen with potential for available positions are referred to the appropriate department head. If the OR supervisor reports through nursing service, potential employees may be processed through nursing service before an interview with the OR supervisor is scheduled, or the OR supervisor may be contacted directly by the personnel department to arrange an interview with an applicant. In either situation, the personnel department assists in the hiring and terminating of all employees.

COORDINATION THROUGH COMMITTEES

Nursing Supervisors

The supervisors of all the nursing units usually meet weekly, or at least monthly, to discuss problem situations. This is an excellent mechanism for resolving conflicts between the units and for working out procedures that are mutually beneficial. The OR supervisor should attend all these meetings so that he or she is fully aware of staffing problems on other units, breakdowns in communication between the OR department and the units if these exist, etc. Only through the identification of problems can solutions be sought, and decisions made.

Infection Control Committee

The infection control committee investigates hospital-acquired infections and seeks to prevent or control them. Membership may vary in different hospitals but generally includes the chief of surgery or his or her representative, the chief surgical resident, the operating room supervisor, the director of nursing or another representative of nursing service, the infection control coordinator, a bacteriologist and/or pathologist, and the executive housekeeper. Representatives from other departments may be invited to attend a meeting when the agenda is relevant to their particular concerns.

The committee meets at least once a month. Members form a defense against hospital-acquired infections by reviewing environmental factors and by determining if the hospital is providing a safe environment for patient care. They review reports and investigate postoperative infections. Committee members also review the procedures and entire chain of asepsis in an effort to determine and then eliminate possible sources of infection.

This committee has the authority to carry out any changes necessary and to enforce strict rules to eliminate any hazardous practices. Included in its jurisdiction is the education of personnel so that they can provide a high standard of patient care. The hospital has a moral duty to provide a safe environment for its patients. The infection control committee aids the hospital in fulfilling this duty.

Disaster Planning Committee

Hospitals have an organized plan for caring for many casualties if a mass disaster occurs within the community. Planning by the intrahospital committee includes consultation with local civil authorities and representatives of other medical agencies to establish an effective chain of command and to make appropriate jurisdictional provisions. This planning results in disaster-site triage to separate and distribute patients in order to ensure the most efficient use of available facilities and services.

Disaster drills are held at least twice a year to try out the plan developed by the committee, to seek to improve it, and to acquaint personnel with it. Disaster plans include:

1 An information center at the hospital to facilitate a unified medical command and the movement of patients.

2 A receiving area for the severely wounded. Casualties are given emergency care according to their needs and are sent at once to the OR or to other units as indicated.

3 Arrangements for sending ambulatory patients to a special area. These patients are treated in the emergency department for slight injuries and are sent home, or are admitted to the hospital as indicated.

4 A plan of organization of personnel. As soon as word of disaster comes to a hospital, if it is during the evening or night, several key persons are called. These in turn phone others previously assigned to them, and these call still others, until the full staff has been notified. If the disaster occurs during the day, the full staff is usually on duty, although any off-duty personnel may be called.

Other departments are alerted and come on duty as needed; these include personnel for the blood bank, central service department, pharmacy, central storeroom, x-ray, and the various nursing units. If disposable linen packs are not in use, it may be necessary to alert some laundry personnel. Some key maintenance personnel must be available, especially electricians.

Personnel are periodically given drills so that each member knows where to report, what to do, and where extra supplies are kept in case of an emergency. Extra supplies are stored in reserve in sufficient quantities to fill possible needs.

Staff Development Committee

Representatives from all clinical areas of nursing service plan the staff educational program for nursing personnel. This program must include orientation and inservice education. Acceptance and support of the program are fostered when all units have a representative on the staff development committee because coworkers then feel that they have indirectly contributed to the input. Ideas are initially generated by the committee members. Specific plans are put into effect by the instructors with the approval of the committee.

A program is planned to ensure a thorough orientation for each new nursing service employee. Many hospitals have established a hiring policy so that all new employees begin their first day of employment on designated days of each month, i.e., the first and third Monday. For at least the first week or two of employment, all employees attend the orientation classes. All new personnel must become familiar with the philosophy, objectives, policies, and procedures of the hospital and nursing service. This general orientation program assists the new employee to adjust to the organization and environment. It is coordinated with an orientation to the duties in the unit to which the employee is assigned.

An inservice educational program must also be planned to keep the nursing staff up-to-date on new techniques, equipment, facilities, and concepts of nursing care. Programs focusing on fire prevention, electrical hazards, security measures, community health resources, and resuscitation training are important to ensure personnel and patient safety.

Professional and technical programs designed to develop specialized job knowledge, skills, and/or attitudes affecting patient care are planned and presented for the appropriate segment of the nursing service department. The OR staff development committee plans these programs for the OR staff. Staff nurses and technicians serve on this committee as well as administrative personnel.

Operating Room Committee

The OR committee is a committee of the medical staff. One surgeon is appointed chief of the department of surgery by the members of the surgical staff. In teaching hospitals, each surgical specialty also appoints a chief of the service, e.g., chief of orthopaedics. The anesthesia department also designates a chief as director of this department. These individuals are responsible for professional practice and administrative activities within their respective departments. They must maintain continuing surveillance of the professional performance of all members of the medical staff granted privileges in their specialty. They also serve as liaison representatives between the medical staff and hospital administration.

Vital to the management of the OR suite is an active OR committee. The chief of surgery, the chiefs or representatives of the specialty services, the chief of the anesthesia department, the OR nursing supervisor, the assistant ORS and/or the OR unit manager meet at regular intervals to review and formulate policies and procedures concerning OR suite activities. The hospital administrator and director of nursing service may also be members of this committee or may be invited to attend meetings relevant to their concerns.

The OR committee must consider policies and procedures pertaining to utilization of facilities, schedule of operations, maintenance of a safe environment, evaluation of techniques, and selection of new products. This may require the review of reports from other departments or committees in addition to those prepared by OR personnel. The ORS usually plans the agenda.

Since this committee determines policy and procedures for efficient functioning within the OR suite, persistent problems are brought before the committee where recommendations for corrective action are made. For example, if temperature and humidity controls are not being effectively monitored or maintained, the committee may recommend to the hospital administration that procedures be reviewed and revised by the maintenance department or that new equipment be installed. If surgeons are repeatedly late in arriving, thus delaying the OR schedule, stronger policy may be indicated for the control and better utilization of facilities. If a new product is purchased, a new procedure may need to be written to specify its use and care.

Through utilization of the problem-solving approach to decision making, the OR committee seeks to improve the working relationships of all members of the OR team and the supportive services concerned with activities within the OR suite.

Operating room activities related to procedures and techniques are supervised indirectly by the OR committee, which is responsible for enunciating policy. Policy and associated directives formulated and approved by the committee serve as guides for governing the actions of surgeons, anesthesiologists, and the OR nursing staff while in the OR suite. The ORS shares with the OR committee, hospital administration, and nursing service responsibility for clarification, implementation, and day-by-day enforcement of approved policy and procedures.

TEAMWORK TO MEET OBJECTIVES

Several factors contribute to the restoration of optimal patient health. Optimal patient health is restored:

1 Through interdisciplinary communication, mutual cooperation, consideration, and smooth, efficient collaboration.

a Unit, operating room, recovery room, and intensive care unit nurses and physicians share pertinent information concerning patients. Collected data are documented by accurate recording, thereby protecting the patient, the medical personnel, and the health care institution.

b Personnel work together in a congenial atmosphere of equality with knowledge of and respect and appreciation for each other's unique skills and contribution to patient safety and well-being. Team members benefit from the expertise of each other. Team nursing is at its finest in the OR. In some hospitals, a multidisciplinary team meets regularly to share information and exchange ideas. This enables each member to support the goals of other team members.

c Personnel are considerate of each other as well as of the patient. For example:

(1) Surgeons inform their teammates ahead of time of any anticipated potential deviation from their regular routine or the scheduled procedure. They respond to questions courteously, and show appreciation for thoughtful preparation and assistance.

(2) Nurses do all in their power to provide the best possible atmosphere to ensure the surgeon's uninterrupted concentration during the procedure. The surgeon is not to be interrupted with messages that are not of immediate urgency (particularly when he or she is about to place an aneurysm clip or deliver a cataractous lens). Neither should loud, irrelevant messages come over the intercom system to startle the surgeon. If the surgeon becomes tense, he or she may develop a tremor or cause inadvertent tissue trauma. It is always a risk to interrupt an ongoing team's concerted effort even during a relatively safe procedure.

(3) The anesthesiologist and circulating nurse assist each other with certain procedures, such as starting and checking intravenous infusions. The circulating nurse stands beside the patient during induction to be ready to assist as necessary. The anesthesiologist, while concentrating on physiologic modalities, must watch the progression of the procedure. There are appropriate and inappropriate times to inflate a blood pressure cuff, for example.

NOTE. Adequate preparation and familiarity with the operation and the surgeon's individual preferences are fundamental. If the nurses are unfamiliar with the routine and equipment it distracts the surgeon from his work, his chain of thought, or his checking on the patient's status. The dedicated surgeon's plea is for nursing personnel and other assistants to know more and care more for only then can the surgeon, who needs their expertise and cooperation, help the patient. He wants them to work *with* him, not for or against him. By not being properly oriented, assigned, prepared (both patient and the OR), or attentive (to patient and team), one puts both the patient and the surgeon's skill in jeopardy. An adequately experienced and attentive OR team is mandatory!

2 By assigning adequately oriented and competent personnel to avoid delays and keep anesthesia time to a minimum. The potential for complications increases proportionately with the length of anesthesia time and of the operation. Calm, experienced personnel greatly reduce all hazards, especially in critical situations such as correct identification of various clear solutions in syringes and prevention of electrical hazards in the use of equipment. Lack of knowledge, personnel shortage, and inadequate rest pose a serious threat to the patient and to the expected outcome of the operation. Both patient and surgeon are entitled to an adequate number of qualified nurses and technicians in the OR. Everyone must care about what happens to their patient. The need for communication and cooperation cannot be overemphasized!

3 Through constant attention to the patient's welfare. The patient on the operating table has an unconditional right to the team's complete concentration and attention at all times. The members of the team are constantly concerned with meeting that patient's needs, regarding him or her as a unique individual completely dependent on them for survival. The patient is, however, also a planner and participant in decision making and in his or her own health care.

Chapter 3

The Patient: The Reason for Your Existence

Surgery today, as defined in Chapter 1, encompasses all of the elements in the scientific care of surgical patients. The operation is the focal point for these patients. It is imperative that the patient comes to the OR optimally prepared physically and emotionally before performance of an operative procedure. The persons concerned with and/or contributing to surgical patient care are many, referred to specifically as the perioperative team. We shall discuss the responsibilities of the team, an integral member of which is the nurse who fulfills the patient's various needs. However, let us first consider the patient as an individual.

THE PATIENT

A *patient* may be defined as an individual seeking medical care. To effectively meet the patient's requirements and wants, personnel must have knowledge of his or her needs, understanding of individuality, and realization of what an operation means to a patient.

Certain beliefs exist concerning a human being. In our society, human beings:

1 Are worthwhile and unique; they are singular beings.

2 Respond to their environment psychosocially.

3 Have the capacity to adapt to both their internal and external environments.

4 Have certain basic needs that must be met in order to maintain homeostasis.

Homeostasis may be defined as the maintenance of steady or stable states (in the organism) between its different but interdependent elements. In short, it is the body's striving to maintain equilibrium within normal limits. This stability depends partly on the intactness of the body and the consistency of its functions. Change in intactness requires adjustment.

THE PATIENT'S BASIC NEEDS

Needs are factors that must be controlled or redirected to restore altered function. Nursing judgments are based on knowledge of patient needs. It is therefore essential for nurses to understand basic human needs of all persons (well or ill) because fulfilling them is an integral part of the nursing process. The surgical patient faces a grave threat to the basic needs of a human being. For convenience, these needs can be classified as physical, emotional or psychosocial, and spiritual.

Physical Needs

Physical needs are the life-sustaining necessities such as food, water, oxygen, sleep, warmth. In illness, the patient becomes acutely aware of these needs. However, patient care does not focus entirely on bodily needs.

Psychosocial Needs

The nurse's concern for the patient's emotional well-being should be as intense as it is for his or her physical health for the two are inseparably intertwined. The society the patient lives in is an integral factor in developing feelings of identity, self-worth, and satisfaction. Thwarted feelings can lead to a state of helplessness or inferiority. Development of self-actualization, what the patient can be and the best he or she is capable of, is the highest level of human development. Examples of *psychosocial* needs that also require fulfillment are:

1 *Security.* People need to be secure, feel safe, and trust those around them. They also need to feel comforted, reassured, protected, and cared about.
2 *Belonging, inclusion, affection.* Individuals need to receive empathetic understanding and response to the self-expression of their feelings and attitudes, both negative as well as positive.
3 *Recognition.* People need to be accepted as worthy individuals.
4 *Self-esteem, identity, control.* People need to be productive, make their own choices and decisions, and control one's self and environment. They also need to have their confidentiality respected.

People are social beings who need to establish satisfying meaningful interpersonal relationships, mutual interest in each other, and to know that someone cares. Risk is involved in sharing feelings with others, however, and emotional stress develops if individuals do not feel secure. If they are treated with love and kindness they feel worthy and can respond to others in the same way. Human beings also need a sense of order in their lives, as well as recreational diversion.

Spiritual Needs

Spiritual needs differ from emotional needs and include support of a person's religious views or belief in a supreme being(s), whose guidance influences life. There is inherent in people a drive for spirituality, a desire to achieve a sense of oneness with the total universe. Especially in times of stress and fear, a person reaches out or turns to religious convictions for spiritual sustenance, since fear of death has a spiritual as well as a physical dimension. Uncertainty about one's relationship with one's God can enhance patient anxiety as the operative procedure draws nearer. The inner strength derived from a strong religious faith can be a bulwark of hope for the patient facing an operation.

The hospital chaplain, available to patients of all faiths, or the patient's personal cleric provides the anxious, suffering patient with a physical contact with the familiar outside world. A spiritual advisor offers the patient a human element of comfort, warmth, and strength. The giving of sacraments to the ill does not necessarily mean that the patient is dying. Rather, through an understanding of life's subjective aspects, the clergy can be a source of great support, giving patients courage as they feel free to share their fears. The spiritual advisor, available as the patient needs him or her, fulfills a basic need by utilizing the reassuring symbols of the patient's religious experiences.

Hierarchy of Needs

In following Maslow's concept of hierarchy of needs and in setting priorities, basic lower-level or physiologic needs, those essential for survival, must be met first, followed by satisfaction of the higher-level needs such as those for safety, security, belonging and love, esteem and self-actualization. Health care personnel must be concerned with a total picture of the patient's needs and consider all of them. In illness, factors such as the location of pathology, type of operation, and effectiveness of therapy can influence needs. Also, priorities may change with changing situations. Preoperatively, anxiety and nutritional status are two factors that must be dealt with; intraoperatively, the team must concentrate on basic physiological needs such as oxygenation, circulation, prevention of shock or infection; postoperatively, team members must work to prevent complications and encourage patient self-actualization. If one's needs are not satisfactorily met, undesirable consequences can occur.

PATIENT REACTIONS TO ILLNESS

To meet patient needs, the health care team must be sensitive to patients' feelings about their illnesses. Patients' reactions influence their behavior and the staff's behavioral responses also.

Behavior

Health and human behavior are interdependent. Individuals with physiological problems, regardless of age, experience some emotional change that influences behavior. Patients react to a new interpersonal environment according to their learned behavioral patterns. The following are facts about behavior.

1 Perception of interaction within the environment creates individualized differences in personality, behavior, and needs. No two individuals are alike.
2 A person's physical and psychosocial behavior is a response to stimuli; it keeps him or her functioning and is an attempt to maintain homeostasis.
3 Behavior is complex. Behavioral acts have multiple causes in addition to a major precipitating one.
4 A person functions on many levels simultaneously. Many factors determine an individual's reaction in a given situation.
5 Behavior must be evaluated in light of the person's specific situation and of pertinent social forces such as family, culture, and environment. To understand the meaning of behavior, one must know about the individual and his or her life situation.

Patients respond to crises or personal threats in different ways. Some persons face suffering and surgical intervention with extreme courage, dignity, and fortitude while others may revert to extreme fear or helplessness when faced by even a relatively safe procedure. Overt behavior is not necessarily consistent with one's feelings but often reflects them most accurately. Patients often express their frustration and fear behaviorally in an effort to cope with stimuli.

Adaptation

Any deviation from a person's normal daily pattern of living necessitates adaptation through innate or acquired defenses. Adaptation may involve physiological or psychological changes in the individual.

Personality includes a patient's characteristic responses to anxiety (either calm acceptance or disorganization, depression, and resistance) as well as to self-image. *Self-image,* an individual's concept or ideas about self and personal philosophy of life, is often affected by other people's reactions. It may also involve constantly changing and evolving perceptions of self. These perceptions may be on both the conscious and unconscious levels. Interpersonal relationships in early childhood are among the most important social determinants of personality formation. A person's adaptive and defense structures are a basic part of personality and heredity. Therefore, individuals vary in their adaptive abilities, which is demonstrated by varied behavioral responses to illness.

Illness disrupts a person's normal living and equilibrium. It also alters self-image. One may worry about what others thinks, especially if the illness involves disfigurement as from severe burns or a communicable disease such as syphilis. A patient's initial reaction to illness may be irrational, impulsive behavior requiring patience and understanding from others. He or she may have difficulty thinking clearly, concentrating, or making intelligent, rational decisions. Both mind and body must adapt successfully in order for the patient to recover. The enormity of society's mental health problem attests to this fact. Adaptation requires energy, ingenuity, and persistence.

The coping mechanism that creates physiological or psychological changes constitutes an attempt to counteract stimuli by limiting the site, lessening the impact, or neutralizing effects so that the individual can continue to function. If adaptation is interfered with, the effects can be detrimental. Adaptation to illness includes the following three stages:

1 Transition from health: development of symptoms
2 Acceptance: coping and making decisions
3 Convalescence or resolution

Adaptation may be rapid or slow depending on the nature of the stimuli and of the individual's heredity, learned responses, and developmental needs. At any level, adaptations may be sensory, motor, or sensorimotor. The extent of adjustment required is contingent on the type of illness, the magnitude of disability, and the patient's personality.

Stress

Stress can be defined as a physical, chemical, or emotional factor that causes tension and may be a factor in disease causation. It is the result of threat perception and is manifested by changes in physiological and psychosocial behavior. Tolerance of stress depends on the individual and on the intensity of stress, its duration, and type—either localized or generalized, as pain.

Inescapable in the process of daily living, a certain degree of stress can be beneficial if it motivates an individual to increased productivity. Conversely, it can be harmful if increased or simultaneous stresses occur, straining the individual's coping ability. If the individual's adaptive powers are inadequate or malfunctioning, the stress may become overwhelming. In the latter situation, new secondary stresses more incapacitating than the initial one develop, creating a continuous stress-adaptation cycle. Adaptive reserve may become depleted as a result.

Stressful factors can originate from within the individual or from the external environment. *Intrinsic factors,* those originating from within, that affect a patient include:

1 Hereditary or genetic factors, such as hormonic or enzymic system competency.
2 Nature of the illness or disease process. This may be influenced by nutritional status.
3 Severity of the illness or presence of a stigma.
4 Previous personal experiences with illnesses. Chronic illness has a disruptive effect on lifestyle.
5 Age. Children feel threatened. Adolescents resent an interruption of activities and are painfully aware of body changes. Older people think about infirmity and death.
6 Intellectual capacity.
7 Disturbed sensorium. Hearing or sight loss intensifies a stressful experience.
8 General state of personal well-being.

Extrinsic factors originating from external sources include those dependent on:

1 Environment. The physical and social environment of the hospital is not the same as that of the home.
2 Family role and status. Expectations and authoritative relationships affect lifestyle, modesty, attitudes.
3 Economic, financial situation.
4 Religion. Beliefs influence attitudes and values toward life, illness, and death. The fatalistic attitudes derived from some religious beliefs give a person little control over his or her environment; they can render a patient passive and apathetic. For example, Jehovah's Witnesses will not permit transfusion of whole blood or blood components. Orthodox Jews must follow dietary laws in any environment.
5 Cultural background, education, and social class. These are closely related to the patient's emotional response and living habits. Self and society are intricately interwoven. This affects interpersonal relationships and behavior. Significant elements such as food habits, daily living patterns, hygiene, family organization, child care, orientation to past, present, and future time should be analyzed in relationship to culture. An ethnic community is really a larger family. Roles taught by the cultural group influence the mores, beliefs, and social interactions of individuals. Also, responses to pain may vary according to one's cultural or ethnic background. Some groups commonly show an exaggerated emotional response; in others it is more appropriate to conceal suffering.

Social factors such as a breakdown in the role and closeness of the family, and the emphasis on isolationism and independence increase one's need for reassurance and for a sense of being cared about. The nurse must not, however, assume or make specific predictions in regard to cultural or social influence.

Disability, illness, and hospitalization accentuate feelings of vulnerability and are stress-producing, stress-exaggerating experiences that threaten a person's security and stability. They may create a crisis state that diminishes defenses and increases an emotional response to threats. The individual patient's needs, strengths, and innate defense mechanisms create unique responses to these threats. The severity of the reaction may be unrelated to the seriousness of the illness. It is often not the problem itself that is devastating, but one's perception of it. Also, the same illness may hold different meanings for different individuals. For many persons hospitalization and surgical intervention represent a critical life experience.

To decrease the traumatic consequences of an operation, health care personnel must realize that stress and pain are both physical and psychological. These components of illness become inseparable parts of the total patient experience. Stress can affect appetite and bodily functions such as digestion, metabolism, and fluid and electrolyte balance. However, during times of markedly increased stress one's emotional needs come to the fore. In facing personal threat, a person tends to mobilize defense mechanisms for flight or fight. One's ability to adapt depends in part on the support one receives. By providing effective nursing intervention at any stage of the adaptation process, the sensitive, well-educated nurse can alter the exigencies of illness and direct the patient's emotional reactions. This will facilitate therapy and recovery through behavior modification.

SPECIFIC REACTIONS TO STRESS

Individuals vary in their ability to cope with illness and stress situations. Coping mechanisms are normal and natural to some extent but their exaggeration or overuse is cause for concern. Illness produces heightened self-awareness. Stress initiates an exaggerated response of the normal defense mechanisms for self-protection. Surgical patients are in a psychologically perilous situation. They are threatened by loss of life, body parts or function, and by unfamiliar social relationships. The strangeness of the OR itself, its noise, odors, and equipment, represents to the patient a potential hazard. Stress may be expressed in one or many of the following ways:

Anxiety (Tension)

Probably the earliest and most prevalent response, anxiety is a painful, apprehensive uneasiness, feeling of uncertainty, or solicitous concern stemming from anticipation of a real or imagined threat. It incites the body's defenses. All patients experience anxieties preoperatively whether they verbalize them or not. Physiologic manifestations of anxiety may be rapid pulse usually associated with palpitation, rapid respiration, diaphoresis, dry mouth, dilated pupils, clammy skin, and, if very severe, even paralysis. The patient may become so anxious that physiologic manifestation becomes exaggerated. For example, a controlled hypertensive patient may suddenly experience increased blood pressure and electrocardiogram changes that may cause postponement of the operation. Other indications of increasing tension are stuttering, word blockage, confusion, and distortion of events. Anxiety impairs intellectual functioning. Perception, concentration, feeling of security, and self-image are also disturbed. Anxiety from stress is experienced on both physical and emotional levels. *Psychophysiological reaction* refers to anxiety reactions in which the symptoms center around one organ system, such as the cardiovascular. Psychosomatic illness results from a combination of physiologic and emotional factors that can cause structural change, such as ulcerative colitis, which may necessitate bowel resection. A person's emotional strength influences the ability to view him- or herself objectively. The intensity of feelings is multiform. Sharing a feeling with another often reduces the intensity.

Varying degrees of anxiety are to be expected. Normally patients are worried to some extent about what will happen during the operation and consequently may be restless and unable to sleep. However, patients are accessible to meaningful communication and will ask questions, desiring to know the facts. These patients are not likely to develop emotional disturbances after stress exposure. Highly anxious patients exhibit hyperactive behavior and dwell on the dangers of the operation, apparently overwhelmed by them. They may not hear what you say or be able to accept reassurance against their magnified fears. You can help these patients only if you can calm them. Research has shown the highly anxious patient to be a high-risk patient. Extreme preoperative apprehension predisposes this patient to a more difficult anesthesia induction and intraoperative period as well as to more postoperative discomfort and complications. As poorer surgical risks, these patients are prone to shock, laryngeal spasm, or cardiac arrest. A patient's unresolved severe anxiety or premonition of death will usually alert the surgeon to delay the operation until a more favorable time.

Alteration of time perception is not an unusual aspect of anxiety. To a waiting patient a minute may seem like an hour. The patient's disability strikes at his or her sense of security. In addition, the anxious patient experiences a feeling of alienation. Surrounded by strange people and equipment in an alien environment, separated from loved ones, the patient is expected to conform to an unfamiliar routine. He or she may feel helpless and alone. For surgical patients, alterations of the body produce tremendous anxiety associated not only with the procedure but also with its potential results. The independent, secure individual can cope more easily than the insecure, inferior-feeling person who may disguise his or her underlying concern with false gaiety and independence. Anxieties originating from reality sources can have a cumulative effect and add fuel to the more emotional problems. For example, a young mother facing an operation, with no responsible person to care for her family and home, has enhanced feelings of dread. Similar anxiety-inducing factors are:

1 Confusion about present and future activity: "Will I be able to do all the things I did before?"

2 Worry by the family provider: "Will we have to go into debt?"

3 Concern for unfinished projects: "Will I be able to make up my exam?" or "Will I be able to keep my new job?"

Relieving contributory stresses helps the patient to cope with the main stress—his or her illness. The individual's specific concerns depend greatly on how illness frustrates his or her specific needs.

Denial

To protect their egos patients may reject reality and danger, thereby reducing anxiety, maintaining stability, and deterring panic. By denying their concern or joking inappropriately, they repel overwhelming threats and make their difficulties more bearable. Such patients divert meaningful conversation, are superoptimistic, and are high-risk surgical patients because they are not prepared to cope postoperatively. Often restless and difficult patients in the recovery room, they have poor tolerance for even normal discomfort. Increase in symptom intensity may cause the individual to face reality. Denial should not be mistaken for courage. This reaction can be dangerous if the patient refuses to recognize a serious illness and to accept appropriate therapy.

Shock

Shock provokes a sense of unreality that acts as protective insulation. The patient may respond in an automatic manner without thought or feeling; or he or she may be unable to answer questions or function coherently. This is a common reaction in patients when a malignancy is first revealed. Their need then is for understanding and support in their efforts to face reality.

Fear

An emotion marked by dread, apprehension, and alarm, fear is caused by anticipation or awareness of danger. Visceral manifestations of anxiety may occur when a person is afraid. The patient realizes his vulnerability and his body prepares to physiologically cope with the crisis. Many childhood fears remain with a person in various forms throughout life. In illness, anxiety causes repressed fears to resurface from the subconscious and become magnified. The patient may imagine and dread something more frightening than the actual experience. Anticipatory fears are many and varied and include:

1 *Fear of the unknown.* Research has shown this fear, with its attendant feelings of uncertainty and suspense, to be the most common and virulent type of the psychologic reactions. The expected is less traumatic than the unexpected for one can more easily deal with feelings when the factors causing them are known and recognized. Fear of what might be discovered in an exploratory operation augments the patient's anxiety. Advance warning and explanations of stress situations are important for all patients but especially for those with a low degree of predanger anxiety.

2 *Fear of death.* In many instances this is a very valid fear.

3 *Fear of anesthesia.* For some patients fear of loss of consciousness is closely aligned with fear of death. "Will I survive the operation?" "Will I wake up?" "Who will care for my family if I die?" General anesthesia invokes complete dependency on the OR team for survival.

4 *Fear of impending procedure and resultant change in body integrity* (trauma, prognosis, malignancy). An operation may be a new experience for the patient or he or she may fear it as a result of previous unpleasant experiences. Invasion of the patient's body may be frightening, especially in such procedures as spinal tap, tracheostomy, gastroscopy. "What will the surgeon find?" "Will I be able to function as before or will I have to live in a crippled state?" "Do I have cancer?" This is a universal fear. "Will the operation be successful and help me?"

5 *Fear of disfigurement, mutilation, loss of a valued body part.* Patients facing amputation of an extremity or breast, or loss of an eye, are extremely anxious. An operation on the reproductive organs may affect self-image. "Will my family and society accept me or be revolted by my altered condition?" Many persons abhor the thought of an incomplete body. This fear provokes real suffering.

6 *Fear of isolation, rejection, neglect, abandonment.* Separation anxiety is common in the elderly, children, immature persons, and those without a family. A sense of being alone and alienated from others, identified as the single most consistent fear of people, accentuates the realization that everyone truly lives life alone. Loved ones can't protect us from pain, suffering, or death. No one can face uncertainties or adversity for us. Everyone must experience stress and pain personally but, in so doing, may turn to the hospital staff for protection, comfort, and warmth. A threat to one's security reawakens earlier fears of separation or abandonment; loss of functions and fear of death may be symbolically related to separation. Some persons conceal fear in a paradoxical manner such as the patient who, when asked his name by the nurse, replied, "I forget."

7 *Fear of incompetency of medical personnel.* The patient may express such a fear by asking questions such as, "Do they know what they are

doing?" "Am I being experimented on or victimized?" "Will they remove all of the cancer?"

8 *Fear of depersonalization and loss of self-control.* In the complexity of the hospital organization, the patient fears impersonal treatment and dependence on others. Such an experience has great potential for producing emotional trauma. By taking away personal possessions, such as clothes, and by subjecting the patient to anesthesia and a multitude of tubes in his or her body, health care personnel strip the individual of identity and a sense of worth. As a result, the patient may feel insignificant and lonely.

9 *Fear of invasion of privacy.* Patients must answer personal questions about their bodies and affairs; give information about their families; expose their bodies to pain, instrumentation, and examination by strangers; accept help with their bodily functions; and be subjected to other indignities. Adolescents and aged persons are especially self-conscious about bodily change and exposure. Invasive procedures, such as sigmoidoscopy, represent a bodily assault to a patient and all must be carried out without embarrassment to him or her.

10 *Fear of outcomes regarding goals and expectations.* Vain persons, for example, grieve when radiation therapy causes permanent skin discoloration.

11 *Fear of loss of livelihood.* Illness can precipitate financial crisis, especially during chronic illness or prolonged rehabilitation.

12 *Fear of burdening others.* Patients experience this fear especially during the course of a severely debilitating condition.

13 *Fear of reliance on a mechanical object* (pacemaker) or *a transplanted organ* (kidney, or corneal transplant).

14 *Fear of restriction* of movement or activity (fracture).

15 *Fear of pain and discomfort.* Many patients dread pain more than the procedure. Aristotle, the fourth-century B.C. philosopher and psychologist, classified pain as a powerful emotion rather than a sensation. Anxiety-produced pain can be intense, and is sometimes indistinguishable from actual physical pain, both of which are physically tiring and deleterious to bodily defenses. While neurological factors and the brain play a part in perception, the psychological component is well recognized. Alteration of pain perception can be achieved by attention to psychological needs. Perception can also be influenced by circumstance and by one's attitude toward a wound or degree of disability. It is interesting to note that many war casualty amputees needed only minimal analgesic medication and were in high spirits because of their dismissal from active duty and its concomitant threat of death. In contrast, paraplegic patients required considerably more medication, support, and attention because of their prolonged severe depression and, on the part of some, a desire not to survive their disability.

Depression

Illness fosters introspection that can depress the patient who wishes to escape an intolerable situation. Depression may be manifested by agitated signs of despair, hopelessness, disinterest, or desolation. Passive depression is characterized by a sad, frowning face or one with little expression, lassitude, somatic complaints, impaired thinking and memory, retarded movement and body processes, anorexia, withdrawal from others, and neglect of appearance as well as of body hygiene. Rather than being passive and inert, the agitated person is hyperactive and talkative. Like denial, depression may be detrimental to recovery and rehabilitation. Excessive depression is cause for concern and requires understanding on the part of the nurse to motivate the patient to accept illness.

Withdrawal

This is a reaction to feeling that one's physical and emotional privacy has been violated. The patient isolates himself, withdrawing from others and from communication. Withdrawal may accompany depression. Apathetic, detached, evasive, and silent, the patient may ignore the presence of others by feigning sleep or by turning his face to the wall. The patient's actions may reveal what he cannot verbalize. He may exhibit self-deprecation or an inclusion-need as a result of mistrusting staff members or of believing that they lack interest in him. In turn, lack of feedback creates a nursing problem.

Dependency

Illness forces the patient to be dependent on others. Many patients feel inadequate because others are making decisions for them. Hospitalization may provide an overly dependent person with desired mothering as early conflicts and childhood fears resurface. The nurse may be viewed as a mother-substitute. The enforced dependency of blind persons, however, does not fall in this category. Dependent patients center attention on themselves and the present moment. They are greatly concerned about body function, and interpret others' behavior in terms of rejection or acceptance. Such patients lack motivation to help themselves, finding peace of mind and security when relieved of having to make decisions or choices. A normal degree of dependency can be beneficial in providing needed rest, especially in the case of burn patients. When you have to force patients to accept dependency, reassure them that this does not lower your opinion of them.

Regression

As a reaction to stress, regression is a path of least resistance that leads to more inertia and may accompany dependency. Patients may regress to less-mature levels of behavior as they draw back to reinforce their restoration, possibly viewing the staff with ambivalence (affection, resentment).

Grieving and Mourning

Feelings of loneliness, loss, and unhappiness are common with the loss of something valued or with any body disfigurement, be it from severe burns, amputation of a part, or an alteration in body structure. The patient mourns the change or may be grieving for his or her impending death, particularly in cases of advanced malignancy. This reaction may occur especially in "-ostomy," or "-ectomy" patients. The intensity of reaction (fatigue, depression, anxiety, altered sensorium, anger, loneliness) depends on the extent and significance of the loss. Interest in life and living is regained as one's dependence on the lost object decreases. Visits by others who have lived through the same travail and survived help patients in the period of adjustment by indicating that they are not separated from the rest of humanity.

Suspicion

Suspicious patients lack complete trust, not wholly accepting what they are told or feeling that they have not been told everything. These patients take time to adapt because of their "on guard" reaction. Hard-of-hearing patients excluded from communication may be suspicious.

Anger, Hostility

Independent self-image is damaged by the passivity caused by illness. Emotional stress may be expressed verbally through open criticism of authority figures such as physicians and nurses or nonverbally through physical expressions such as clenched fists or pursed lips. Patients respond to their feelings of insecurity and dependency by being aggressive and demanding in an attempt to control their environment. They are defensive in an effort to protect themselves. They may be reacting to a feeling of being assaulted, rebelling against enforcement of rules, or emerging from apathy.

Questioning

Anxious patients seek a reason for their illness. They ask the question, "Why me?" Some persons find an answer such as "I neglected my health for other things."

Guilt, Shame, Punishment

The patient may feel ashamed of his or her illness or may think that it is a form of punishment for prior behavior or imagined wrongdoing. Invasive procedures involving body orifices may evoke fantasies that reactivate childhood fears of multilation, deprivation, or punishment that are threatening to the patient's self-image. Consciously, this may be experienced as pain or may precede depression.

Coping with Stress Reactions

Each individual patient's natural inclination toward health or illness influences preoperative response and contributes to postoperative recovery. Psychologic reactions are significant factors affecting the outcome of surgical intervention. To give adequate support in the patient's periods of crisis, the health care team must assess the patient's ability to cope with stress. Psychological preparation is as important as physical preparation but it is all too often overlooked. Crisis intervention includes comprehensive nursing care of the patient under stress through interactions with patient, family, and staff, directed toward controlling crisis behavior in reaction to stress.

The patient looks to the hospital staff to fulfill his or her multiplicity of diversified needs, which are not presented in an orderly, categorized manner. Persons with or assessing the patient must ascertain his or her needs and share this information with others. All patients' reactions to preoperative stress should be documented, discussed with attending physicians, and reduced by appropriate interventions. Severe or prolonged reactions require psychiatric consultation. Some stress and anxiety are a natural part of surgical patient experience.

MULTIDISCIPLINARY APPROACH TO CARE

Specialization tends to separate the body into systems and parts, to fragment and categorize care.

Yet the human body is a miraculously complex creation functioning as a coordinated unit, an organized entity or person who is an interacting member of family and society. The meld of components that make up the whole person has been discussed. Modern surgery subscribes to a theory of total patient care that treats the whole person through a patient-centered approach. This concept of total patient care is not new. Hippocrates (b. 460 B.C.) advocated, "To cure the human body you must have knowledge of the whole thing." Today that concept is as valid as ever. Total surgical patient care involves meeting all the physical, psychosocial, and spiritual needs during the preoperative, intraoperative, and postoperative phases. Patients have a striving for wholeness that acts as a catalyst to healing. As noted in Chapter 2, many persons contribute to total care; each has a unique responsibility in the continuity of care process.

Traditionally led by the physician, with increasing leadership from nurses, the health care team is dedicated to maintaining optimal health and/or restoring it when altered by disease, injury, or deformity. The team components may vary with the situation and the patient. The surgical care team is concerned with a favorable outcome from surgical intervention.

In viewing the team in its broadest scope, one can consider the patient as the central part or hub of a wheel with many persons and departments as the supporting framework (see Fig. 3-1). All center their efforts at the hub, meaning that the patient is the center of attention always, not only when under the OR spotlight. The ultimate beneficiary of teamwork is the patient. Imperfection in any one part of the wheel imperils the performance and security of all.

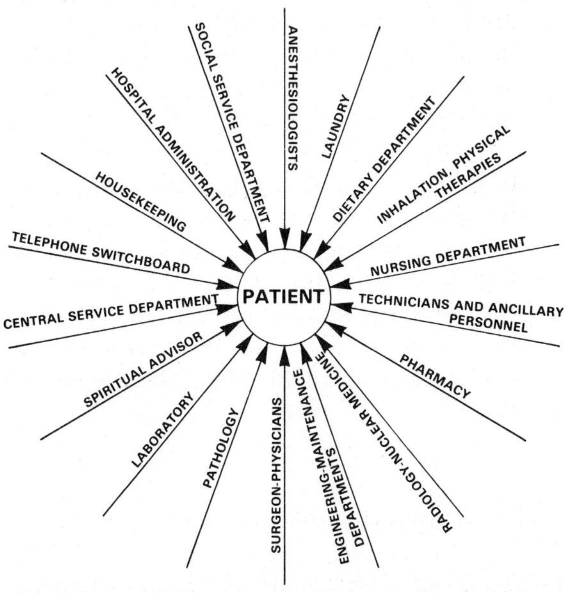

Figure 3-1 The patient is the focus of attention of the entire health care team.

While no one's contribution is minor and each is important to the whole, certified surgeons, anesthesiologists, and registered nurses are the primary directors of surgical patient care. Each has a unique contribution to make in reaching the goals.

Bill of Rights for Patients

Hospital services are a commodity that the patient as a consumer purchases to fulfill health care needs. The patient is entitled to certain rights. Access to quality care is recognized as a right, not a privilege, for every human being.

> In the interest of "more effective patient care and greater satisfaction for the patient, his physician, and the hospital organization," the American Hospital Association has adopted a Patient's Bill of Rights as a national policy statement and distributed it to its member hospitals throughout the country. Intended to give the consumer something to go by, the 12 rights, in summary, are:
>
> **1** The patient has the right to considerate and respectful care.
>
> **2** The patient has the right to obtain from his physician complete and current information concerning his diagnosis, treatment, and prognosis in terms the patient can be reasonably expected to understand.
>
> **3** The patient has the right to receive from his physician information necessary to give informed consent prior to the start of any procedure and/or treatment.
>
> **4** The patient has the right to refuse treatment to the extent permitted by law, and to be informed of the medical consequences of his action.
>
> **5** The patient has the right to every consideration of his privacy concerning his own medical care program.
>
> **6** The patient has the right to expect that all communications and records pertaining to his care should be treated as confidential.
>
> **7** The patient has the right to expect that within its capacity a hospital must make reasonable response to the request of a patient for services.
>
> **8** The patient has the right to obtain information as to any relationship of his hospital to other health care and educational institutions insofar as his care is concerned.
>
> **9** The patient has the right to be advised if the hospital proposes to engage in or perform human experimentation affecting his care or treatment.

10 The patient has the right to expect reasonable continuity of care.

11 The patient has the right to examine and receive an explanation of his bill regardless of source of payment.

12 The patient has the right to know what hospital rules and regulations apply to his conduct as a patient.*

This document gives patients the right to know what is being done to, for, and about them and their illnesses. For those patients not wishing to know the facts during a crisis, their wish should be respected with only capsule explanations or essential information given. The duty of disclosure is not absolute.

The patient's rights are correlated with the operating room team members' individual responsibilities, which were delineated in Chapter 2 as role functions. The following information expands for emphasis many facets of total patient care.

Communication

Communication is the basis for the continuum of patient care and for teamwork among the staff. Relationships between people are established through communication. Therefore, the nurse must know general principles specifically applicable to the nursing role.

Communication has been defined as a process by which meanings are exchanged between individuals, everything that one mind can use to affect another. It is an effort by one person to get close to another. In therapeutic communication, the goals are patient-directed, patient-centered. Communication is effective only when the patient, physician, and nurse understand one another. A capacity for feeling is the most effective constituent of communication.

Importance of Communication

1 Communication is necessary for successful interpersonal relationships.

2 Patients need support in adjusting to health-related problems and hospital environment.

3 We fallaciously assume that others know what we mean; communication serves to clarify our meaning.

Communication is facilitated by using the acronym EARS—listen:

*Nursing Outlook, 21(2):82, Feb 1973. Reprinted with permission.

1 Earnestly—look into the speaker's eyes

2 Actively—give the speaker your entire attention

3 Receptively—acknowledge what message the speaker is conveying

4 Sensitively—interpret the speaker's message

Briefly, some principles are as follows:

1 Communication incorporates:
  a A sender (speaker, encoder).
  b A message sent via a transmission channel.
  c A receiver (listener, decoder).

2 The sender puts thoughts into words or some other channel of communication, then transmits an idea in the form of a message to the receiver who attempts to understand the thought.

3 Goals of communication are to inform, to obtain information, to release tension, to explore problems.

4 Channels of communication are:
  a Verbal—audio-aural language and word symbols.
  b Nonverbal—(kinesthetic) facial expression, tone of voice, gesture, posture, body movements.

5 The setting for communication and the attitudes of those involved influence the degree of effectiveness. One's emotional state affects listening. An anxious patient may not hear, may misunderstand, or may draw erroneous conclusions.

6 The use of unqualified statements is avoided.

7 Communication should be source-centered rather than message-centered.

8 Prerequisites are to know what you're going to say and to say what you mean. As the speaker, verify or paraphrase until you are convinced that the receiver has the message.

9 Shadings of meanings a message can have are:
  a What the speaker means to say—what he actually says.
  b What the receiver hears—what he thinks he hears.
  c What the speaker says—what the receiver thinks the speaker said.

> NOTE. 1. Two people must have mutual understanding about the meaning of a word. Language should convey meaning. 2. The mind seems to decode messages in relationship to its own background of experiences, prejudices, moods. A person can hear and repeat what you said without believing a word of it. 3. Don't evaluate the receiver's comprehension totally on the basis of language.

10 For accurate interpretation of communication one should know the other's level of intellect.

11 Barriers to communication can be:

  a Verbal—changing the subject, having a judgmental attitude (stating one's own opinion about a patient or situation), offering false or inappropriate reassurance, jumping to conclusions or taking things for granted, using medical facts or nursing knowledge inappropriately.

  b Nonverbal—showing a lack of trust or feeling, disinterest, revulsion.

Criteria for Determining the Success of Communication

1 Feedback. Letting the sender know how you perceived the message so the sender can discover if it was understood as intended. There is a breakdown in communication when the idea of the receiver doesn't match the idea of the sender.

2 Appropriateness of reply.

3 Efficiency. Is the sender overloading the listener?

4 Flexibility. Is there no control versus too much control?

5 Specific results. Behavioral changes indicate that the goal is reached.

Through communication the nurse can influence individual behavior to encourage the patient to express feelings or redirect them toward more beneficial behavior.

Verbal communication is directed toward patient care in conference, study of patient problems, teaching, providing interdisciplinary liaison, and safeguarding the patient. It is the keynote of care planning among all personnel. *Nonverbal communication* provides clues to feeling and attitude in one's interpretation of them as signals. We often communicate through nonverbal channels without realizing it, and those forms of expression sometimes speak louder than words. When the patient is feeling sad, lonely, or isolated, touch by the nurse is a most effective means of communication.

Patients can indicate their needs by what they say or do not say. Physicians and nurses must verify that their transmissions are being internalized by the patient, incorporated within as guiding principles. They must repeatedly affirm to the patient how much he or she means to them. Patients under stress have a deep need to communicate and establish a positive relationship with their physicians and nurses.

ACCEPTANCE OF OPERATION

The patient must reconcile the need or weigh the advantages and disadvantages for surgical intervention. Every patient is entitled to receive sufficient information upon which to intelligently base a decision. The patient has the right to decide what will be done to him or her.

Patient-Physician Relationship

The attending physician must adequately explain, in clear, simple language, the nature, purpose, extent, potential hazards, and expected outcome of the procedure proposed as well as other available options of therapy. The patient usually wants to know about anticipated duration of hospitalization, absence from work, and cost of operation. Physicians, both surgeons and anesthesiologists, must inform the patient, not delegate this responsibility to a nurse or assistant.

> NOTE. Adequate translation must be provided for the patients with a language barrier.

The physician-patient relationship is a contractual one. However, the physician is under no legal obligation to accept as a patient any given person. In fact, the intensity of litigation may preclude the physician's doing so since positive guarantee of a favorable outcome of surgical intervention can never be fully given. Patients want and deserve reassurance but the key to all medical discussion is the risk versus benefit ratio. Everyone wants a black or white answer. This is not possible in medicine.

The surgeon is responsible for informing the patient about a proposed operation, its inherent risks and complications. The explanation should reasonably include discussion of removal of parts, disfigurement, disability, and what the patient may expect in the postoperative period. It should be meaningful without creating unnecessary anxiety over very rare or insignificant hazards. Preoperative discussion also should include advice to the patient regarding diet, bathing, smoking, and other factors that might affect the outcome.

The anesthesiologist also has a responsibility to inform the patient of any unfavorable reactions to a medication or anesthetic agent that may be given during the operation. The risks of anesthesia must be explained, but without causing the patient undue stress.

Explanations are given prior to the time the patient or legal guardian signs a written, informed consent document. Written, informed consent is necessary for any procedure that may possibly be injurious to the patient. The surgeon is responsible for making certain that the patient or legal guardian is adequately prepared to sign this document.

It is valuable for the physician to have a family member or relative present during his or her explanation to the patient, especially if the patient is elderly, as persons facing a proposed operation are under stress. They often do not listen to or comprehend the physician's explicit information even if it is repeated. Also, they may misconstrue what is said. Some patients go to the OR still not clear about the operative procedure to be performed in spite of a careful discussion beforehand. For this reason, many physicians will again, in a nonstressful manner, simply repeat the basic facts on a second occasion preoperatively. For legal protection physicians often record a brief progress note covering the explanatory conversation and the patient's reaction. Failure to provide full disclosure of the risks of the procedure and alternative modes of therapy have led to successful negligence suits. The physician is liable for misrepresentations, whether by affirmative statement or nondisclosure.

If the physician or patient has doubts as to the necessity of any operation, the American College of Surgeons recommends that an additional opinion be secured from a qualified specialist in the appropriate field of surgery. Such a second opinion may be particularly indicated if the procedure involves extended disability. Consultation is a common and desirable part of good surgical practice. Special consultation or consent may be required by hospital policy for procedures to terminate reproductive capability through sterilization and/or therapeutic abortion. It is common practice to have a second medical opinion in consultation before asking a patient to consent to procedures such as amputation of an extremity or removal of an eye.

The patient has a right to withdraw his written consent prior to the operation if his determination to do so is a rational one. The surgeon is notified and the patient is not taken to the OR. The operation is postponed until a more propitious time when the patient is willing. The patient makes the final decision on what treatment he will accept.

Immediately after the operation, the surgeon speaks to the patient's family and discusses with them pertinent information including procedure performed, patient's tolerance, and prognosis. On the rare occasion when a patient expires during an operation, it is the attending physician's responsibility to inform the family or next of kin. The surgeon has the ultimate responsibility of facing the patient and the family whether the outcome of surgical intervention is satisfactory or unsatisfactory. Postoperatively, the surgeon follows the patient's progress until he deems discharge from his or her care or return back to a referring physician to be indicated and safe.

Written Consent

A written consent is not an infallible legal protection for the surgeon and hospital, but it does have legal value for all concerned with patient care. Consent documents vary from hospital to hospital and state to state. Most hospitals ask the patient or legal guardian to sign a *general consent* form upon admission, usually in the hospital admitting office. This form authorizes the physician in charge and hospital staff to render such treatment or perform such procedures as the physician deems advisable. This general consent is relied on only for routine duties carried out in the hospital. Physicians and nurses must be knowledgeable about the statement on the form used in their hospital. A signed consent is legally regarded as valid for a period of about 6 months.

A consent document specifically relating to any procedure possibly injurious to the patient also should be signed before the procedure is performed. Often referred to as an *operative permit,* the patient's consent is generally required for:

1 Each operation performed such as a secondary incision and drainage
2 Any procedure for which general anesthesia is administered such as the examination of a child under anesthesia
3 Procedures involving entrance into a body cavity such as a bronchoscopy
4 Any hazardous therapy such as radiation or chemotherapy

Purposes of Consent

1 To protect the patient from unratified procedures
2 To protect the surgeon and hospital or facility from claims of an unauthorized operation or other invasive procedures

Validity of Consent The document must contain the patient's name in full (a married woman's given name), surgeon's name, procedure to be performed, patient's and authorized witness(es)' signatures, and date of signatures.

The patient giving consent must be of legal age, mentally alert, and competent. The patient must sign before premedication is given and prior to going to the OR or other treatment area, except in life-threatening, emergency situations. Before elective operation, the patient should be asked to sign at least 1 day preoperatively. This may be done in the surgeon's office, hospital admitting office, or nursing unit, but *it must be an informed consent freely given without coercion.* If the patient is:

1 A minor, a parent or legal guardian must sign.
2 An emancipated minor, married or independently earning a living, he or she may sign or a spouse of legal age may sign.
3 An illiterate, he or she may sign with an *X,* after which the witness writes "*patient's mark.*"
4 Unconscious or inebriated, a responsible relative or guardian signs.
5 Mentally incompetent, the legal guardian who may be either an individual or an agency must sign. A court of competent jurisdiction may legalize the procedure in the absence of the legal guardian.
6 A child of an unwed minor parent, consent is signed by the next of kin to the unwed parent.

Witnessing a Consent The patient's or guardian's signature must be witnessed by one or more authorized persons. They may be physicians, nurses, or other hospital employees as established by policy. By his or her signature the witness signing a consent document attests to:

1 The identification of the patient or legal substitute
2 The fact that the signing was voluntary

Consent in Emergency Situations In a dire emergency, consent is desired but not essential. While every effort should be made to contact the family, the patient's perilous physical condition takes precedence over operative permit. In such situations, the patient's condition usually prevents his or her signing. Permit for operation, especially on a minor, may be accepted from a legal guardian or responsible relative by telephone, telegram, or written communication. If by phone, two nurses monitor the call and sign the form, which is signed by the parent or guardian on arrival at the hospital. In lieu of the above-mentioned methods, a written consultation by two physicians other than the surgeon will suffice until a relative can sign a consent.

Responsibility for Permit The ultimate responsibility for obtaining consent is the surgeon's. The consent document becomes a permanent part of the patient's medical record and accompanies him or her to the OR. It is the duty of the circulating nurse (RN or charge nurse) and the anesthesiologist when checking the patient's identity and chart on arrival in the OR to be certain that:

1 The consent is on the chart and properly signed.
2 The information on the form is correct.

The attending surgeon should also check before anesthetic is administered. If the surgeon intends or wants to perform a procedure not specified on the consent form, the OR nurse has a responsibility to inform the surgeon and/or a proper administrative authority of the discrepancy.

PATIENT-NURSE RELATIONSHIP

The professional nurse shares a special experience with the patient at a time of great stress and need in his or her life. Their relationship encompasses feelings, attitudes, and behavioral approaches. It must be humanized in structure.

The nurse's first goal is to promote and establish a meaningful, therapeutic relationship so that individualized care can be given. This relationship is a face-to-face, heart-to-heart one—a most essential element of effective clinical nurse-patient interaction. It is not the length of time the nurse spends with the patient that is so important, but the quality of the association. Mutual trust and understanding are the vital components. Effective interaction involves concern for the personhood of both patient and nurse. Then patient goals can be formulated together and decisively achieved.

As the nurse and patient begin to know each other, their identities and roles become apparent, and they develop feelings for each other. To achieve a viable cooperative relationship, the patient must know that the nurse unconditionally cares about his or her life both within and outside of the hospital. Giving of yourself is something that you give someone forever. The nurse is aware that personal interaction is often predicated on attitudes and past experiences. Knowledge of the patient and the impact of surgical intervention on his or her life situation is therefore indispensable.

Operating room nursing involves patient-nurse interaction through direct patient contact and care; consequently, it is a discipline in nursing. It is not purely technical nor procedure-oriented. Both nurses and technicians work, in different capacities, toward the common goal of the safest possible care of the patient and of a favorable surgical outcome. While technical assistants provide a very real contribution to surgical patient care, nowhere in the hospital are the qualities of the registered nurse more needed or better utilized than in the OR as the RN implements a personalized, patient-oriented approach to care through his or her understanding, judgment, and skills. The nurse-patient role is an ongoing one. OR nursing care requires meticulous preplanning with goals developed through the nursing process.

Nursing Process: Problem-Oriented System

The nursing process, the dominant nursing modality, provides systematic nursing care planning and delivery. A *process* is the act of proceeding through a series of actions that contribute to an end. It provides a framework for cyclic problem solving in a logical, interrelated sequence of steps. All these steps are recorded for documentation and sharing among health care team members. These steps comprise a rational method of determining patient problems, formulating a plan for solving them, implementing the plan, and evaluating its effectiveness in resolving the problems identified. A *problem* may be defined as any condition or situation in which the patient requires help to maintain or regain physical, emotional, or social equilibrium. The scientific process of problem solving can well be applied to nursing practice. The process furnishes an organized approach to nursing care and a mode of determining patient outcomes resulting from that care, while adhering to the philosophies of nursing. An *independent nursing function* is the selection of priority needs in a given situation. Rationale for the selection and the patient's viewpoint are needed.

The problem-solving approach to patient care is comprised of the following four steps:

Assessment A purposeful nurse-patient interaction that continues through all phases of the nursing process begins by the nurse getting to know the patient and what is happening to him or her. *Assessment* consists of appraising the patient and his or her existing and potential nursing care needs. This is the basis for individualized care planning and establishment of nursing goals related to the patient's problems. From specific data collected and analyzed the nurse constructs a data base, a composite picture of the patient's condition, to serve as a basis for comparison with subsequent observations and postoperative status. The data collected through interview and observation become the *nursing history.* The nursing history includes subjective material (what the patient states he or she is experiencing such as pain or anxiety) and objective material (that which can be validated by another person such as the unit nurse, family member, social worker).

From the nursing history, a concise, easily used information source, the nurse develops a *nursing diagnosis,* which is a statement of a conclusion reached by valid deduction. It describes in specific words the patient's health problem in which the responsibility for therapeutic decisions can be assumed by the professional nurse. The diagnosis may change as new data show invalidity or resolution of the original diagnosis.

Planning From the nursing diagnosis the nurse structures a flexible, individualized nursing care plan designed to seek ways to achieve solutions to the patient's problems. This plan designates specific, necessary actions and possible nursing interventions to meet each problem listed, indicating priority of each goal and expected outcome. Plans to assist the family in helping the patient orient to reality as well as supportive, therapeutic, palliative, preventive, and rehabilitative measures to assist the patient are included. The patient's preferences are considered. Goals should be realistic. Alternative options or interventions are a necessary part of the plan. They permit modification at any phase of the process as necessary. The nursing diagnosis, nursing orders, and rationale are written on the nursing care plan. The written format of nursing interview forms or assessment guides vary from hospital to hospital, but all elicit essentially the same information.

NOTE. A *nursing order* is a specific strategy or action to help meet a patient need.

The nurse's plan is only as good as the data, the information known about the patient. The nurse's actions are never better than the plan. All factors that influence subsequent actions, utilizing the total care concept, are included. Consultation with other health professionals while planning helps ascertain how best to meet the patient's needs. In formulating a care plan, the nurse utilizes analysis, application of knowledge, interpretation, and decision making.

NOTE. The acronym SOAP applies in developing a nursing care plan. It means Subjective/Objective Assessment and Planning.

Implementation Putting the written nursing care plan into action is the third phase of the nursing process. Patient responses are recorded. Hopefully, the nursing interventions, which are the execution of the nursing regimen, will be therapeutically effective. All actions focus on the patient and are directed to the goals. Nursing actions directly affect patient outcomes. Instruction of the patient and family members aids them in coping with problems and is a nursing function.

Evaluation Comparison of actual results with expected outcome is *evaluation.* The effectiveness and appropriateness of goals, plans, and actions are measured by the interpretation of patient responses. Evaluation is a continual process of reassessing patient needs, modifying goals and priorities, and revising plans when expected outcomes are not achieved or the patient's condition and adaptive levels change. The determination of patient response and the degree of goal realization are also verified by direct observation. The patient tells the staff how care received was perceived, focusing on categories such as safety, environment, teaching, and meeting of physical and emotional needs. In addition to judicious examination of nursing management of the patient and patient response, quality of care given is reviewed in terms of objective achievement of the criteria. Were all patient needs identified? Was care planned according to needs? Was the plan instructive, practical, adaptable? Was the patient's preparation for operation adequate physically, emotionally, and spiritually? What factors influenced goal achievement or lack of it? Tools used in evaluation include charts, records, care plans, and nursing audit. The purposes of evaluation are:

1 To improve the quality of the patient's total nursing care.

2 To influence policy making and procedures. New methods are devised from evaluation and research.

3 To reveal areas where inservice is needed for nursing personnel.

4 To formulate and revise the hospital's quality assurance program. Evaluation provides an objective means for upgrading the standards of the quality of nursing care.

5 To provide data for self-evaluation. The nurse is accountable for her own actions and the actions of those under her supervision.

PRE- AND POSTOPERATIVE VISITS

While the primary area of the OR nurse's practice is within the OR suite, the broadened scope of professional OR nursing encompasses phases of pre- and postoperative care that contribute to the continuity and to the total patient care approach. Pre- and postoperative visits to patients are made by registered nurses skilled in interviewing, a technique for the development of the patient-nurse relationship. The OR nurse's interview affords the nurse an opportunity to learn about the patient and to establish rapport, using communication skills. The nurse uses this knowledge in implementing the nursing process.

Unless specified otherwise, a *preoperative visit* refers to communication between a surgical patient and an OR nurse prior to the time the patient is brought to the operating room. A *postoperative visit* is one made to the same patient, preferably by the same OR nurse, for the purpose of evaluating patient preparation and intraoperative nursing care.

Before the inception of these visits, the OR nurse had only a minimal amount of time to see and get to know the unanesthetized patient. She had only a capsule portrait of the person. Although even now the same OR nurse may not see the patient through to the resolution of the problem or crisis if during a long procedure she is reassigned or goes off duty, the preoperative visit affords a special opportunity to learn about the patient, to observe patient behavior directly and symbolically, and to establish rapport before assuming responsibility for that patient's care. The postoperative visit eliminates a short, one-time contact. Since knowledge about the patient and how he or she views the impending operative procedure are prerequisites for effective nursing intervention, the visits also foster quality patient care, providing the OR nurse with a basis for developing the nursing process and an ongoing relationship with the patient. The nurse is therefore included in all aspects of care, not only in the intraoperative phase when the patient is medicated and possibly unconscious. The nurse interviews the patient during these visits with specific objectives in mind.

Objectives of the Preoperative Visit

1 To make a nursing assessment of the physiological, psychological, and sociocultural status of the patient.

2 To increase the effectiveness, efficiency, and safety of nursing care rendered within the operating room.

3 To provide for continuity of care through direct patient contact preoperatively and postoperatively as well as during surgery.

4 To assist the patient and family members with the management of anxiety.

5 To provide information and answer questions about those aspects of hospitalization for which OR nurses are responsible.

6 To complement the roles of team members in preparing the patient for surgery, thus strengthening interdisciplinary interrelationships and enhancing patient care.

7 To provide a means whereby OR nurses can expand their role and self-insight, thereby increasing self-actualization.*

Nurse-Interviewers

Pre- and postoperative interviewing should be done by professional nurses with operating room orientation, experience, and complete knowledge of operative procedures, as well as pre- and postoperative care. Ideally, the circulating nurse who will be with the patient during the operation makes the visits, but this is not feasible in all situations due to staffing and time factors. Patient interviewing requires training and special skills in data collection and observation. OR nurses who have learned and are adept at these skills will be comfortable visiting patients. In some hospitals, a *visiting-nurse team,* working an afternoon-evening shift of duty, visits patients scheduled for operation, fills out forms, and prepares the written individualized care plans. The circulating nurses review these plans for their patients before the operative procedures and implement the plans. The visiting team may be comprised of staff nurses, master clinicians, or an OR and a recovery room nurse together. The two-nurse team approach provides nurse orientation (role model concept) and feedback as a less-experienced interviewer may accompany an experienced one. For group instruction, teams of nurses representing the operating room, recovery room, and intensive care unit are effective.

Some research studies have affirmed that surgical patients who received preoperative instruction from and interaction with the OR nurse suffer less apprehension, tolerate the procedure better, and are more secure and comfortable postoperatively since they remember what they are taught, receive more continuity of care, and react more positively to their surgical experience than other patients. Pre- and postoperative visiting is desirable and mutually beneficial to OR nurses and surgical patients.

Interviewing Skills

Interviewing, a form of verbal interaction, is a valuable tool for obtaining information. There is a great range of interviewing techniques. The interview can be *directive,* structured with predetermined questions in a fixed order that limit reponses, or *nondirective,* in which the patient is given more latitude in responding. An example of a directive question is: "Have you had an operation before?" An example of a nondirective question is: "Tell me about your previous operation." The choice of technique depends on the information desired.

A structured form of interview is valuable in learning about an individual's health and work history. The unstructured type gives one a portrait of the patient's emotional reactions, concerns, and personality. An effective preoperative interview usually includes questions about both facts and feelings with informal observation an essential component. All questions should be relevant. The setting should be conducive to communication. The interviewer must be able to handle the situation with spontaneity, judgment, and tact. The interview must be meaningful to both the patient and the nurse.

Steps to Successful Preoperative Visits

1 Carefully review the patient's chart and records so that you can quickly focus on critical issues. These data reveal medical and nursing histories, diagnosis, and operation to be performed. Collect any information rele-

*C Alexander et al., Preoperative visits: The OR nurse unmasks, AORN J 19(2):404, Feb 1974, copyright © 1974, Association of Operating Room Nurses, Inc. 10170 E. Mississippi Ave., Denver, Co. 80231. All rights reserved. Reprinted with permission.

vant to planning care in the OR. Discuss the patient and the nursing care plan with the unit nurses if possible prior to visiting the patient. Find out all you can about the patient. The nursing history, taken on admission by the unit nurse, includes the following pertinent information:

a Biographical information: name, age, ethnic background, educational level, patterns of living, previous hospitalization and operations, religion.

b Physical findings: vital signs, height, weight, skin integrity, allergies, presence of pain, drainage, bleeding, state of consciousness and orientation, sensory or physical deficits.

c Special therapy: tracheostomy, inhalation therapy, hyperalimentation.

d Emotional status: understanding, expectations and specific problems concerning comfort, safety, language barrier, etc.

These preoperative parameters are essential for accurate intra- and postoperative assessment.

2 "Introduce yourself and explain the purpose of your visit. Tell the patient that such visits are routine so that he does not feel he has been singled out because he is extremely ill."*

a Put the patient at ease; see that he is comfortable. *Sit* close to him where he can easily see and hear you. Choose an optimal time without interruptions. Early evening is usually best, after supper and before visitors, or during the morning or afternoon of the day before the operation if the patient is in the hospital. Do *not* conduct your interview the morning of the operation! If the patient is in acute physical distress, consider rescheduling the visit.

b Allow adequate time for the interview. This is usually 10 to 20 minutes, unless the patient has special needs, and thus requires more time. Give the patient time to think and express himself.

c Except in the case of children, persons needing an interpreter, or the mentally handicapped, it is advisable to first speak with the patient alone. Then, if the patient is willing, the family may be invited to participate and ask questions. This affords the patient privacy and he may feel freer to talk. The family should be present during teaching to learn how to assist the patient.

NOTE. For how to conduct preoperative visits to children see Chapter 26.

d Maintain the patient's self-respect.

e Instill confidence in the patient by your appearance and attitude. Establish rapport by demonstrating warmth and genuine interest. Avoid an authoritative manner.

f Use language at the patient's level of development, understanding and education.

3 "Tell the patient the time of surgery, approximately how long it will take, and how long he will probably be in the recovery room. This will be helpful to his family. They will know how long they will have to wait and when to plan their visits. Make sure the patient and family know where the operating room waiting room is."*

a Orient the patient to the OR environment and interpret hospital policies and routines.

b The nurse may ask the patient what family members or friend(s) will be at the hospital during the operation and should inform him how early they should be there to see him before he is medicated.

c If it is hospital policy to do so, tell the patient that the family will be informed when he arrives in the recovery room and when he is returned to the unit.

4 "Obtain information from the patient. Ask him to tell you what his understanding is of his surgical procedure."*

a Permit the patient to talk; listen attentively. Your 50 percent of the conversation is for information gathering and teaching but throughout the visit collect data that will assist the OR staff in providing care.

b Direct questions must be used with caution and are not suitable for collecting all objective data. Word questions to elicit more information than a one-word answer. Pass the initiative to the patient. However, remember the ability to view oneself objectively varies with the individual. The patient may give inaccurate information, telling you what he thinks you want to hear, to preserve his self-esteem and present himself in a favorable light.

c In assessing information the patient has, check its accuracy and what instruction he needs. Ask him a question such as, "What have your doctor and the nurses told you about your operation tomorrow?" Discuss too his conception of the OR.

*C Alexander et al., Preoperative visits: The OR nurse unmasks, AORN J 19(2):407, Feb 1974, copyright © 1974, Association of Operating Room Nurses, Inc. 10170 E. Mississippi Ave., Denver, Co., 80231. All rights reserved. Reprinted with permission.

*Ibid.

d A patient's statement that ends in a question may be either a request for more information or an expression of a feeling or attitude about the nurse's competence.

5 "Review the preoperative preparations that he will experience and instruct the patient briefly about what to expect postoperatively. Tell him the unit nurse will give him more information."*

a Familiarize the patient with whom and with what he will see in the OR and RR. If you will not be caring for the patient in the OR, tell him a colleague of yours will be there to greet him and take care of him.

NOTE. Many OR nurses wear OR attire and laboratory coat with name tag when they visit patients. This familiarizes the patient with the way they will see personnel the next day. Attire must be changed if the nurse reenters the OR suite after the visit.

b Use your discretion as to how much the patient should know and wants to know. Use well-chosen words that do not connote an anxiety-inducing situation. Do not use words with unpleasant associations such as knife, needle, or nausea.

c Postoperative recovery begins with preoperative teaching but keep explanations short and simple. Excessive detail can increase patient anxiety, which itself reduces the attention span. (Preoperative teaching will be discussed in more detail later in this chapter.)

d Give practical information about what the patient should expect such as withholding fluids, the drowsiness and/or dry mouth from preoperative medications, transportation to the OR, the holding area, and where he will be taken after the operation. Instruct him not to hesitate to ask for assistance at any time. Give any relevant special precautions.

e Give reasons for procedures and regulations; this reduces patient anxiety. With children and the elderly, one often needs to repeat information.

f Be realistic about what you can accomplish. Explain only the procedures of which the patient will be aware.

6 "Tell the patient that the anesthesiologist will visit him to discuss specific questions relative to anesthesia, if this is routine."*

7 "Answer the patient's questions regarding the surgical procedure in general terms. Encourage the patient to ask his physician any specific questions."*

a Be honest and responsible in your communications about a proposed diagnostic or operative procedure. Complement, but do not overlap, the surgeon's area of responsibility. Do not be unrealistic, falsify truth, or give false reassurance to patient or family.

b Be extremely cautious about spelling out specific details of treatment, procedure, and postoperative care unless you have been thoroughly briefed by the surgeon in charge. Surgeons' care plans are also individual and tailored to their own techniques as well as to the patients' problems. Forms of therapy may be controversial. Continual interdisciplinary communication is mandatory.

8 "Discuss the patient's and family's feelings or anxieties regarding the operation and anticipated results."*

a Motivate and assist the patient and family to gain perspective, objectivity, awareness, and insight. A skilled professional nurse will know how to discourage wishful thinking for miraculous cures while at the same time communicating understanding of their fears and wishes for an easy, fast recovery.

b Observe emotional reactions.

c As an interviewer, be emotionally objective yourself about pain, mutilative surgery, death, sexuality. Listen to what the patient is asking without feeling threatened if you have to talk about painful aspects or don't know the answers to questions such as "Why me?" Show that you care. Patients scheduled for spinal or local anesthesia and/or for operations on the face or genitalia often experience great anxiety.

d Acknowledge the impact of the procedure on the patient's sexuality, if appropriate.

e Try to help the patient solve problems for himself when possible. Ask questions that help him explore a subject or his feelings but do not probe to elicit responses. Do not destroy his coping mechanism. Encourage an appropriate one. The visit is not a structured psychiatric counseling session!

f Listen to anxieties in a realistic time frame and get others to follow through as necessary. Don't attempt too full an agenda.

*Ibid.

*Ibid.

Sort out what is legitimate. You can't solve all problems in 20 minutes. For example, say "I'll share this information with the doctor (or unit nurse) so someone else can help you with this problem." Use colleagues' expertise to assist you or to make proper referral.

g Be self-aware. Comfort the patient if indicated; give him a sense of security. Touch him if appropriate. A perceptive nurse can tell when the patient resents touch; respect his feelings. Patients with decreased visual acuity appreciate the assurance that a touch can give, but always speak first to avoid startling the patient. Reassure him that he will not be alone but that he will be *constantly* attended by competent staff.

h Alert the family as to what they will see in the intensive care unit, such as monitors and machines, if the patient is to be sent there.

i Ask the patient, "Do you have any concerns about tomorrow?" Never bring a patient's feelings into the open and then cut him off. Allow time to deal with problems. Try to increase the patient's trust in the team.

9 "If available use audiovisual materials—pamphlets, notebooks, photographs, drawings, etc.—to supplement the interview."*

a These materials are especially useful for explaining complicated procedures such as total joint replacement and some pediatric procedures.

10 "Make a note of any information which will improve nursing care in the operating room, i.e., physical problems which might affect positioning or require special setups."*

a The preoperative visit is a time for discovery and planning for problem prevention. The nursing care plan will include preparation for extra tall, obese, paralyzed, or left-handed patients to guard against a traumatic experience. For example, an intravenous infusion should be started in the right arm of a left-handed person, to minimize limitation of manual dexterity.

b Observe physical limitations such as pain on moving, loss of an extremity, or sensory loss. These tell the nurse how much cooperation to expect from the patient. A pad and pencil may be needed to communicate with a patient who is unable to speak.

*Ibid.

c Ask if the patient wears any type of prosthetic devices. Explain, per accepted hospital policy, that these must be removed prior to operation either at the bedside or in the OR.

d While talking to the patient, assess his special needs. It is important for the OR nurse to know about the presence of an implanted pacemaker, for example. Electrosurgery could cause it to malfunction, and so would be contraindicated. Preexisting medical conditions alter how the patient should be managed in the OR (for example, chronic obstructive respiratory disease).

e Know the patient's special requests.

11 "Give the patient an opportunity to ask questions."*

a If you are unable or unprepared to answer a legitimate question, tell the patient that you will find out the answer. For example, say, "I don't know but I'll get that information for you."

b *Don't:* interrupt the patient; avoid eye contact; interrogate or belittle him for his fear; avoid answering questions; introduce irrelevant topics; argue with him; use hospital jargon; conduct the visit out of curiosity; relate your own experiences in detail; moralize; joke inappropriately; contradict; offer false reassurance; avoid an uncomfortable situation—face it, resolve it.

12 "Offer reassurance when possible, especially regarding the competency of the staff. Maintain an attitude of hope."*

a Help both yourself and the patient turn negative feelings into positive useful responses.

b Offer realistic hope but do not minimize the seriousness of the operative procedure.

Preoperative Teaching

The overall nursing care plan includes directives for educating the patient and family about the illness and their part in managing it. *Teaching,* a function of nursing practice, is a process of action embracing perception, thought, feeling, and performance. During the preoperative visit, the OR nurse supplements instruction by other nursing team members and gives information unique to the patient's specific operation. The OR nurse teaches patients how to assist and encourages

*Ibid.

them to participate in their own postoperative recovery. He or she teaches patients:

1 How they will feel and the nursing actions that will provide comfort.
2 The reasons for what will happen postoperatively.
3 What is expected of them. The aim of using specific measures is to prevent a health crisis or postoperative complication.
4 What they can do to make their own postoperative period easier and hasten recovery. The nurse makes patients aware that actions can be taken that are effective.

Effective Teaching Patient teaching involves emotional energy on the part of the nurse. It can produce behavioral changes in patients, however, as they become involved in the learning experience. By learning, patients can participate in their care and be better prepared physically and emotionally for the operation. They also learn how to utilize the health care system. Learning self-help has a positive effect on the patient. Another advantage is that the patient knows what to expect and where to go for help after discharge, if needed, such as to an -ostomy or -ectomy club.

Patient teaching may be conducted in an informal, individual manner or in a formal group teaching setting adapted for patients with similar problems such as laryngectomy, colostomy, or mastectomy. The nurse-instructor should first formulate, in conjunction with other team members, attainable objectives with patient input and determine the patient's emotional receptivity and mental capacity. She also assesses the patient's acceptance of his problem, developmental level, sight, hearing, etc. Also, before beginning an explanation, the nurse should ascertain what the patient already understands about his condition and the topic to be taught. Verify what the patient knows, what he needs to know, and what he wants to know. Identify, by observation and what the patient says, where problems exist. An understanding relationship with the patient facilitates teaching.

Teaching should be slanted to the family members' particular circumstances to help these persons cope with the problem to the extent of their ability; also, success or failure of treatment is often contingent on what happens to the patient after he or she leaves the hospital. The family's knowledge and ability to cope and help are important factors.

Points to Consider

1 Arrange conditions so that learning can occur; an undisturbed environment and proper timing are important and conducive to it.
2 Language is the fundamental tool for education. Use understandable terminology and be knowledgeable. Do not equate intelligence level with educational level. The nurse is accountable for what she teaches.
3 Set priorities and teach what is significant and appropriate to the patient's particular problems.
  a Break down the instruction into manageable steps; for example, instruct the patient to deep breathe, then cough.
  b Put content in sequence of activities in order to facilitate learning.
  c Give reasons and benefits; for example, movement of legs and toes postoperatively, unless contraindicated, aids circulation and prevents venous stasis.
  d Adapt your teaching method to the specific situation. The patient may reject teaching not relevant to the immediate present. For example, a patient about to be operated on for heart valve replacement may listen but may actually be concentrating on the fact that his or her heart is going to be incised.
  e Don't overburden the patient with a multitude of facts.
4 Recognition of need, not pressure, should be the motivating factor in learning.
5 To evaluate understanding, ask the patient to repeat to you in his or her own words what you taught.
6 Legible instructions are helpful for review. Go over the material with the patient. Test his or her comprehension by asking questions, since pain, anxiety, and medication can hinder understanding.
7 As the resource person, be consistent, concise, and organized. Repeat instructions to help the patient retain them.

After the Preoperative Visit

At the end of the preoperative visit and teaching session, the OR nurse should not depart from the patient abruptly, but should leave an entree for the return postoperative visit.

Immediately after leaving the patient's bedside, the OR nurse writes a summary of the visit on the nurses' notes or progress sheet in the patient's chart to convey pertinent information to the unit nurses and surgeon. This information includes the teaching she has given as well as the patient's needs for further pre- and postoperative information and instruction. Identified family attitudes and needs are also included. This becomes a permanent part of the patient's record.

The OR nurse then prepares the written nursing care plan for the intraoperative phase of the patient's care based on the information obtained from and observations made about the patient. Some nurses save time by dictating into a tape recorder extraneous reference information that is unessential to developing the nursing diagnosis. Some written documentation is necessary, however, to correlate the visit with the nursing audit, a part of the evaluation phase of the nursing process.

NOTE. Assessment guidelines or nursing interview forms specifically designed for the OR nurse are valuable tools to organize and record data gleaned during the preoperative visit. However, it is advisable that the patient not see the nurse writing a great deal as he or she may become uncomfortable and less communicative. The nurse should concentrate on remembering pertinent data, unusual observations, and teaching to record them after the visit.

Postoperative Visit

The postoperative visit terminates the OR nurse-patient relationship. The preoperative visit is evaluated at that time:

1 Was it helpful?
2 What could have been improved?
3 Did it contribute to a positive surgical experience?
4 Was the teaching utilized, helpful, adequate?
5 Did the visit effect change in the patient postoperatively? Did it effect change on a long-term basis?

The OR nurse-interviewer confers with the rest of the nursing team, unit and RR nurses, and the physicians to evaluate patient care and make recommendations for improvement in it and in interpersonal relationships. The interdisciplinary conference is an effective medium for the accomplishment of these goals. Also, an evaluation form should be given to the patient to be filled out objectively. Excellent OR management of the patient can be nullified by inadequate pre- and/or postoperative care.

To be successful, a visiting program requires the cooperative effort and input of various personnel who should participate in structuring it at its inception. In this way, duplication of action and feelings of resentment are avoided. These personnel should include unit, RR, ICU and OR nurses, surgeons, anesthesiologists, and hospital administrators. The program should be reviewed periodically and revised as necessary.

An effective program and positive patient experience promote good public relations. The visits present a friendly, caring hospital image to the public it serves.

Pros and Cons of Pre- and Postoperative Visits

The *advantages* of such visits are self-evident; they include the following:

1 As an expert, the OR nurse is well qualified to discuss a patient's OR experience, to orient and prepare patient and family for it and for the postoperative period.
2 The OR nurse can review critical data before the procedure and assess the patient before planning nursing care.
3 Visits improve and individualize intraoperative care and efficiency; avoid needless delays in the OR.
4 Visits prolong OR nurse-patient contact. Some patients are reluctant to reveal their feelings and needs to someone in a short-term relationship.
5 Visits reduce the isolation of OR nursing from other clinical specialities.
6 Visits provide a means for evaluating total patient care. They disclose omissions in the effectiveness of the nursing process as well as errors of commission such as trauma, complications, and infection.
7 Visits make intraoperative observations more meaningful.
8 Visits contribute to patient cooperation and involvement.
9 Visits facilitate all communications.
10 Visits enhance the positive self-image of the OR nurse and contribute to job satisfaction, which in turn reduces job turnover, a benefit to the hospital. Because of increased patient contact, visits make OR nursing more attractive to those who enjoy patient proximity and teaching.

The *problems* of pre- and postoperative visits include the following:

1 Visits require additional time, energy, training and often staffing.

2 Late patient admissions and heavy OR schedules make visits difficult.
3 Visits may produce friction among different team factions if the program is not well planned and executed.
4 Repetitious interviewing may lead to a stereotyped manner and a lack of enthusiasm and spontaneity on the part of nurse-interviewers.
5 If skill is not employed, patients being interviewed may feel that their privacy is being invaded.
6 Barriers to visits may arise from the nurse's inability to
  a Verbalize.
  b Handle or accept dying.
  c Handle emotionally upset or angry persons.
  d Function efficiently outside of his or her customary environment.

Preoperative Visit by Anesthesiologist

Since the anesthesiologist is knowledgeable in the pathophysiology of disease as it pertains to anesthetic agents' actions, participation in the patient's preoperative preparation can reduce intraoperative complications as well as postoperative morbidity and mortality. The anesthesiologist therefore visits patients scheduled for anesthesia, usually the evening before the operation.

Judgment and skill are extremely important in the selection of agent and the administration of anesthesia; firsthand knowledge of the patient is extremely valuable. Like the OR nurse, the anesthesiologist discusses matters within his or her own jurisdiction, seeking information and aiming to establish rapport, inspire confidence, and alleviate fear. Preparation for anesthesia begins with this visit.

In the administration of anesthesia there is no compromise with quality. If laboratory or special test reports are not back promptly, as is sometimes the case with late admissions, decisions and the operation are delayed until all essential information is available.

Before meeting the patient, the anesthesiologist also reviews the patient's past and present hospital records and charts.

After introduction to the patient, the anesthesiologist:

1 Takes a history pertinent to the administration of anesthetic agents by questioning the patient in regard to past anesthetic experiences, adverse reactions to drugs, or habitual drug usage. Tranquilizers, cortisone, reserpin, for example, influence the course of anesthesia. Smoking habits, familial problems, for example, hemophilia, and previous blood transfusions also influence the choice of anesthesia.
2 Personally evaluates the patient's physical and emotional status.
  a Examines the patient as necessary to obtain the information desired.
  b Palpates needle insertion site and observes for skin infection if a regional anesthesia, such as a spinal, is contemplated.
3 Investigates the patient's exercise regimen, which is indicative of cardiac reserve.
  a May observe the patient for dyspnea or claudication during a short exercise tolerance test.
4 Inquires about teeth and explains that delicate dental work may be damaged inadvertently during airway insertion.
5 Inconspicuously observes the patient for anything that might present a technical difficulty, for example:
  a A short stout neck may cause respiratory problems.
  b Active athletic persons require more anesthetic than inactive persons.
6 Explains his or her preference of anesthetic in this situation, pending the surgeon's approval, and informs the patient what to expect concerning anesthesia.
  a The patient's wishes are also taken into consideration when the choice is made.
7 Warns the patient about restricted or prohibited oral intake before an anesthetic and gives the reasons for it.
8 Discusses the time and method of transportation to the OR.
9 Reassures the patient of his or her constant presence and postoperative observation in the recovery room or intensive care unit.

After leaving the patient, the anesthesiologist:

1 Estimates the effect of the necessary position during the operation on the patient's physiologic processes.
2 Records preliminary data on the anesthesia chart.
3 Writes the preanesthesia orders, including times for medication administration.
4 Writes a summary of the visit and of proposed anesthetic management of the patient on the physicians' progress note.
  a There is medicolegal value in this preoperative summary.
5 Assigns the patient a physical status category, for the purpose of anesthesia, as per

the classification adopted by the American Society of Anesthesiologists.

a For example, Class 1 theoretically includes relatively healthy patients with localized pathologic processes, and Class 5 includes moribund patients with small chance for survival who are operated on in an attempt to save life. The operation is a resuscitative measure; little or no anesthesia is required for a massive pulmonary embolus, for example.

Special considerations

1 In emergency situations, e.g., a ruptured spleen, ideal practices may be altered or disregarded to meet the exigencies of the situation.

Examples: If a patient is hemorrhaging, there is no time to wait to restore a low red blood count. A multiple trauma patient with a full stomach may have to have a nasogastric tube inserted and suction applied, spinal anesthesia if applicable, and be operated on in spite of food ingestion.

2 In other situations, the operation is necessarily postponed as anesthesia would be hazardous. Examples: acute respiratory infection, cardiac decompensation.

The anesthesiologist has other responsibilities in addition to those discussed above. The role of the anesthesiologist as a member of the OR team was referred to in Chapter 2. Specific functions related to the administration of anesthetic agents will be discussed in Chapter 9. In addition to preoperative assessment of the patient and administration and maintenance of intraoperative anesthesia, the anesthesiologist may see the patient postoperatively. He or she has a responsibility to inform the patient of any unfavorable reaction to a medication or agent given so that the patient will be forewarned in the future and report these reactions to other physicians and anesthesiologists.

INTRAOPERATIVE NURSING CARE

The professional OR nurse asks creative questions such as, "In what ways can I assure the safety and welfare of the patient?" She or he analyzes the data. What are the patient's needs? What nursing interventions will meet these needs? Points to consider in planning OR nursing care are:

1 Diagnosis and impact of surgical intervention
2 Surgical anatomy and location of operative site
3 Calculated risks of the proposed procedure on other physical needs
4 Psychosocial and spiritual needs

Based on the preoperative assessment, the OR nurse devises an intricate plan for intraoperative care to fulfill needs and expedite the operation safely for the patient.

The patient's welfare and individual needs are paramount in every facet of activity within the OR. They must not be compromised. Seemingly routine details have significant importance. For example, taking a defective hemostat out of circulation may save a patient from a fatal hemorrhage. Checking the spotlight helps to assure the surgeon of clear vision in the operative area. Since in the OR one deals continually with anxiety and stress, a sense of tension more or less prevails from the team's constant need to accommodate to a variety of intense situations within a short period of time. An OR team is always on the alert, geared and ready to respond to any eventuality. Although time is of the essence in order to keep anesthesia and procedure time to a minimum, a protective factor for the patient to provide as little disturbance to physiologic homeostasis as possible, *efficiency and safety must not be sacrificed for speed.* While the ideological differences of personnel may at times be a source of conflict, teamwork and the task at hand must overcome any disparities. Also, problems in the OR suite due to many complex procedures, heavy operating schedules, or shortages of personnel or available staff must not interfere with the delivery of efficient, individualized patient care.

Being a surgical patient oneself at some time, although not desirable, is perhaps the best way of gaining insight into knowing what it feels like to be on the other side (see Fig. 3-2). The perception of modern nursing's founder, Florence Nightingale, was especially acute. She said, "Almost any person who behaves decently well exercises more self-control every minute of his day than you will ever know until you are sick yourself." Riding horizontally in an elevator on a stretcher is an extremely different sensation from moving vertically. Although premedication dulls the senses, when the circulating nurse asks and assists the patient to move onto the operating table, the patient is jolted from his or her sedated calm by the realization that "This is it—the moment I've dreaded is now actually here." The stark sterility of the operating room is completely obvious and the patient looks to the nurse as mentor. It is then

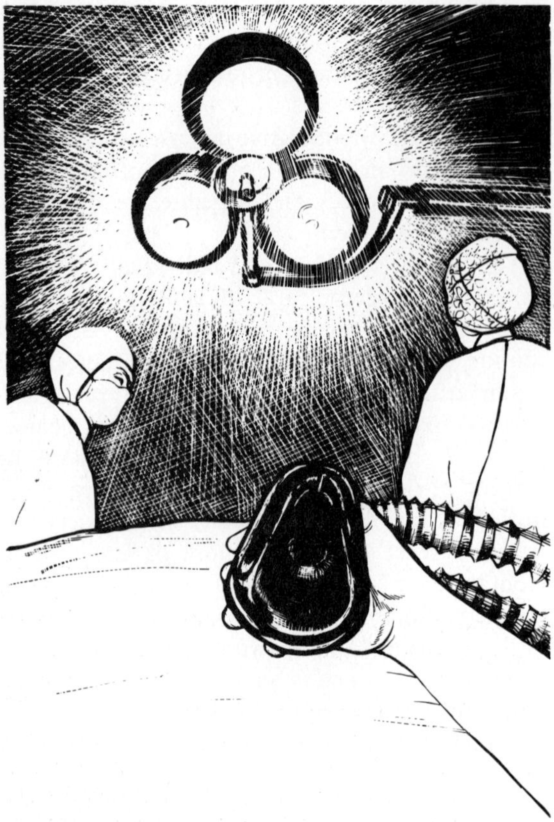

Figure 3-2 The operating room from the patient's perspective.

that the nurse-patient relationship, the basis of nursing, reveals whether the nurse stands or falls. A fundamental element in this relationship is effective communication.

In OR nursing practice, even though preoperative and postoperative visits are made, nurses' contacts with patients are limited and less than those of the unit nurses. OR nurses have a relatively short time in which to gain patients' trust and to reassure them. The risks involved in the operation are reduced when patients have hope, confidence, and are reconciled to the need or desire for the procedure. The nurse, as a central figure in patient care, can do much to relieve fear and provide security. Patients look to the OR nurse as a knowledgeable expert. In times of crisis, they want the physical presence of a trusted, competent, compassionate person. Human beings are interdependent. Patients expect the nurse to be cognizant of their problems, conditions, and willing to help them. They interpret a nurse's attitude toward them as one of acceptance or rejection and their concept influences his or her effectiveness. Behavior is related to expectation. Consequently, the nurse's behavior affects the patient in either a positive or negative way. Positive actions include spending time with and staying close to the patient as distance may be interpreted as disapproval; giving concerned attention to the patient's needs and discomfort; looking directly at the patient when he or she speaks; touching the patient with kindliness; appearing poised and confident in a professional manner. Negative actions include frowning; ignoring the patient; failure to respond to patients' feelings or needs. The way in which something is said and done is equally as important as what is said and done. Sometimes inaction is indicated. The perceptive nurse can determine such instances.

Although formal routines for care, procedures, and teaching have been set up, each patient, as a frightened human being, deserves care with a personal touch as he or she faces a disruptive life experience. The patient must not be treated as an inanimate object or anonymous person beneath the drapes, or categorized by disease or operative procedure. The patient is a living, feeling person, not "Dr. Brown's hysterectomy," "the cardiac in Room 4," "the arthritic I need help in moving," or "the case we just sent to recovery." Medical jargon such as this is depersonalizing, demoralizing, and totally unacceptable as well as offensive to the patient. The goal of OR nursing is to combine *efficiency with caring*. The nurse must never become insensitive to patients because of depersonalized hospital routine or her own prejudices.

Protection of the patient's modesty, dignity, and privacy whether he or she is conscious or unconscious is essential. Unnecessary exposure must be avoided. The gown and cotton blanket protect modesty in addition to keeping the patient warm. Also, the operating room door should be kept closed for privacy; this is a point in aseptic technique as well. Operations may be viewed only by authorized persons with a definite function and all privileged information is kept confidential.

Patients are unnerved by perceptible harmful stimuli such as strange odors; disturbing sights such as a used but uncleaned operating room, soiled linen, instruments, equipment, unconscious patients, bright lights; isolation or detachment from others or the group; hustle and bustle type of activity or unpreparedness; embarrassment from body exposure; loud noises such as voices, inappropriate conversation or whistling, staff disagreements, patient's moaning, instruments clattering, sterilizer noises.

Anxiety and preoperative sedation tend to alter the patient's ability to interpret events objectively.

He therefore makes his own interpretation of what he hears, usually relating everything to himself, although he may not actually be the subject of conversation. Lack of consideration can destroy the patient's confidence in the team. An overheard, thoughtless comment can produce a lasting traumatic memory and fear that the patient may pass on to others. Negative recall can become anxiety-inducing in similar future experiences. Think before speaking and do not converse near the patient while excluding him from the conversation. Sedation does not imply exclusion. The patient may be aware of conversation although appearing to be asleep! Out of the patient's hearing, conversation should pertain only to the work at hand, for the OR is not the place for social discourse. The patient may misinterpret or react unfavorably to what he hears. Hearing is the last sense lost as a person becomes unconscious, as in general anesthesia, and it is not known at precisely what moment a person can no longer hear and interpret what is said near him.

Implementing the Care Plan

Professional education prepares the OR nurse for fundamental functions as a clinical nursing practitioner-leader, a coprofessional with physicians in giving and promoting continuous care of surgical patients. In the OR, the surgeon is in charge of the operation but the RN circulating nurse is the guiding spirit. She is the organizer, coordinator, stabilizer, and manager of the OR to which she is assigned. Her responsibilities are so extensive as to warrant frequent reiteration and review. The surgeon relies on the circulating nurse to prepare for and keep the operation running smoothly as a result of meticulous planning and experiential expertise. She coordinates and implements the nursing care plan with and through other team members. As the circulating nurse, the RN is responsible for patient and employee safety.

Safety is a prime concern. The OR suite is generally considered to be the most critical area of the hospital complex in relation to safety. It imposes a high degree of vulnerability on the patient and the entire professional, allied technical, and ancillary staff. According to an official report,* the OR suite is the site in the hospital where most incidents alleging malpractice occur. Patients lack the power to defend and protect themselves during surgical intervention. Therefore, the nurse is their advocate, representative, and protector. She gives supportive care and safeguards them from emotional or physical harm by constant vigilance. The nurse can minimize potential hazards by:

1 Never leaving a sedated patient unguarded. In addition to causing mental anguish from a feeling of abandonment, if left unattended the patient may injure him- or herself in a fall or on equipment.

2 Using good body mechanics and adequate restraints. Injury can occur to personnel during positioning or alignment of the patient due to faulty body mechanics, or the patient can fall due to inadequate assistance, restraints, or stabilization during transport or transfer to the operating table.

3 Correctly identifying patients, operative sites, drugs, or medications. An incorrect operation on the patient or error in medication is usually the result of inadequate identification.

4 Creating, maintaining, and controlling an optimally therapeutic environment in the OR. This involves control of the physical environment, such as temperature and humidity, and personnel. Traffic flow in and out of the room should be kept to a minimum. The more movement and talking, the greater the room's microbial count. Once the patient is in the OR, it should be kept quiet so that the effects of sedation are not counteracted. A tranquil, relaxed atmosphere is conducive to team concentration and orderly functioning so all can go well. Standards of ethical conduct should be strictly enforced.

5 Assuring that mandatory aseptic principles are adhered to by the entire team at all times. There is no compromise with sterility. Proper sterilization and housekeeping practices must be followed without deviation.

6 Preventing a foreign body from remaining in the wound of the patient. All needles, sponges, and instruments are counted. Sharp items must be protected before disposal to prevent injury to personnel.

7 Careful handling and accurate labeling of all specimens and cultures. An error could mean an inaccurate diagnosis, improper therapy, or reoperation.

8 Respecting equipment. Proper care and handling assure efficient functioning, a protection for both patient and team members, and an economic benefit for the hospital. Faulty electrical or anesthesia equipment or their improper usage can cause burns, electrocution, or explosion.

9 Documenting all that occurs as part of the patient's permanent record. Writing nurses' notes or progress notes on the patient's chart and com-

*Department of Health, Education, and Welfare: Publication OS-7389, Secretary's Commission on Medical Malpractice, January 16, 1973.

pleting an intraoperative observation checklist provides a profile of what has happened to the patient. Records and forms must be accurate and specific. State what happened and why. Besides having legal value, records are of value to the postoperative care team in their assessment and interpretation of altered physiological status, i.e., pain or drainage from the trauma to living tissue occurring during operation.

10 Adhering to established standards of safety. The circulating nurse enforces these standards. A comprehensive safety educational program to supplement the work of the safety committee and full-time safety professionals is essential.

FULFILLING SPECIAL NEEDS

In general, the healthy body can tolerate the trauma of a surgical procedure without serious sequelae. However, the debilitated, chronically ill, or age-extreme patient has increased difficulty combating the stress of surgical trauma to tissues and alteration of physiology from anesthetic agents. An added hazard is the patient's possible concealment from the surgeon of pertinent facts or conditions that, if uncorrected, may predispose him or her to unnecessary complications and discomfort.

The importance of sending each patient to the operating room in the best possible physical and emotional condition must be emphasized. Adequate rest and balanced nutrition are essential factors. Diagnostic and laboratory studies not only assist in establishing diagnoses, but also pinpoint areas of deficiencies. Surgical intervention is often postponed until a cardiovascular situation is optimized, for example, lowering hypertension or correcting cardiac arrhythmias. Preoperative therapy is given as indicated to control diabetes, reduce obesity, and treat infection in order to decrease anesthesia risk.

Patients of various ages and stages of development have different needs. Ways of meeting those needs will vary. A family-centered approach is valuable; research has indicated that a person's immediate family is responsible for two-thirds of all specific influences on him or her and for one-half of the more general influences. Particularly with aged patients, family cooperation is essential for communication with, interpretation to, and assistance with the patient.

Many patients have special needs but space precludes mention of them all. The more common secondary problems associated with surgical intervention will be discussed. These may be encountered in patients coming to the OR for all types of operations.

Nutrition

Nutrition refers to the sum of the processes concerned in the growth, maintenance, and repair of the living body as a whole or of its constituent parts. Decreased intake and increased metabolic demands create nutritional problems in surgical patients.

The application of principles of aseptic technique, gentle handling of tissues, and physiological support are preeminent in modern surgery but they are not enough for patients with *protein calorie malnutrition* (PCM). *Metabolism* is the phenomenon of synthesizing foodstuffs into complex elements and complex substances into simple ones in the production of energy. It involves two opposing phases referred to as:

1 *Anabolism,* or constructive metabolism, the conversion of nutritive material into complex living matter—tissue construction

2 *Catabolism,* or destructive metabolism, concerned with the breaking down or dissolution by the body of complex compounds, often with the release of energy

Metabolic disorders can complicate the outcome of surgical intervention. Dietary deficiencies disturb the body's nutritional homeostasis and may markedly alter a patient's nutritional status and needs. Hormonal response to physical stress involves both anabolic and catabolic effects on the body with catabolism predominant. The degree of metabolic reaction may depend greatly on the body's reserve of labile protein. The type and extent of the operative procedure, the preoperative nutritional state, and the effect of the operation on the patient's ability to digest and absorb nutrients affect immediate postoperative metabolism.

Biochemical changes accompany surgical intervention. One of the major ones is *protein catabolism.* Limited food intake preoperatively, catharsis, and adrenocortical response to crisis augment a catabolic response. Trauma and blood loss also have a contributory effect. Metabolic disease, dehydration, and fever increase one's need for calories and nutritional substances. This is also true in patients with severe burns, infection, or toxemia where essential nutrients such as nitrogen are lost. Abnormalities of the gastrointestinal tract and digestive organs may produce malnutrition through incomplete digestion, absorption, or excretion of nutrients. Digestion and absorption are also affected by deviations in digestive secretions, timing of passage through gastrointestinal tract, and stomach capacity.

Biochemical tests monitor nutritional status. These include proteins, albumin/globulin determination and ratio, and blood urea nitrogen level. Body weight is significant also. If calorie intake is inadequate, protein is converted into carbohydrate for energy. Protein synthesis then suffers.

The average adult patient needs about 1500 calories daily to spare body protein. Hypermetabolic states can double that requirement to 3000 calories and 18 to 19 grams (g) of nitrogen for nitrogen retention, if liver function is normal. Depleted reserves of essential elements must be replenished to replace tissue loss and expedite wound healing. In laboratory studies, protein deficiency impairs collagen formation thereby delaying the healing process. Vitamins K and C are also important (see Chap. 12). The surgeon is justifiably concerned about the patient's nutritional status since malnutrition lowers host resistance by impairing lymphocyte and neutrophilic functioning. A definite relationship has been demonstrated between hypoproteinemia and terminal postoperative infection.

Electrolyte and metabolic disturbances other than protein catabolism may accompany surgical intervention and lead to imbalance. These disturbances can result from:

1 Cell destruction, leading to potassium depletion.

2 Changes in blood lipids; calcium and magnesium absorption are depleted in poor absorption.

3 Diminished glucose tolerance resulting from stress.

4 Gastric drainage; chlorides are lost.

5 Fluid loss from drainage tubes, diaphoresis, vomiting, or diarrhea.

6 Maxillofacial injury; inability to take oral nutrition.

7 Radiation enteritis.

8 Disease of bowel, liver, biliary tract, intestinal tract obstruction, or gastrointestinal fistula.

9 Use of drugs. Drugs may have a therapeutic or adverse affect on metabolic balance. Broad-spectrum antibiotics, for example, while limiting a disease process can, in association with dietary inadequacy, cause vitamin K deficiency in aged patients by inhibiting the intestinal bacteria that produce that vitamin. Drug detoxification and/or excretion may be altered in patients with kidney or liver damage, leading to possible drug overdosage. Metabolism is also altered by immunosuppressive drugs and antimetabolites that interfere with nutritional function. Corticosteroids, while being valuable therapeutic drugs, may increase the patient's susceptibility to infection and loss of muscle protein.

10 Loss of muscle tissue leading to increased nitrogen loss.

11 Inadequate oxygen–carbon dioxide exchange that can disrupt the patient's acid-base balance.

Nutritional Supplements Changes in fluid and electrolyte balance affect kidney function, cellular metabolism, and oxygen concentration in circulation. Tissue hydration and distribution of body electrolytes are essential. Adequacy of essential nutrients at the cellular level is crucial. Therefore, by dietary management, physicians aim to correct metabolic and nutritional abnormalities prior to the operative procedure. In some cases, special nutritional supplements are indicated to build up the patient or to compensate for a permanent metabolic handicap. A chemically defined elemental diet may be administered orally or via a nasogastric tube or a gastrostomy tube with constant infusion pump. Successful therapy is indicated by weight gain, a rise in plasma albumin, and a positive nitrogen balance.

Hyperalimentation [Total Parenteral Nutrition (TPN)] *Parenteral hyperalimentation* is another method of fulfilling nutritional requirements. Essential nutrients are delivered directly into the bloodstream intravenously via an indwelling catheter. This mode of therapy is used for patients with nutritional defects not amenable to oral therapy or nasogastric intubation, or who fail to gain weight by other means. Intravenous infusion by peripheral vein is precluded in some patients because the amount of fluid necessary to supply the adequate calories and nitrogen would exceed the body's fluid tolerance, leading to pulmonary edema and congestive heart failure. For these select patients and for those requiring long-term intravenous therapy, for example, following cerebrovascular accident, hyperalimentation provides the daily nutrition necessary for protein synthesis.

Hyperalimentation is coordinated with other aspects of therapy to establish adequate nutrition, fluid, and electrolyte balance. Increasing protein nourishment in the pre- and postoperative periods lessens protein loss and destruction of cell nuclei, muscle, and connective tissue. It also counteracts the increased catabolism resulting from the stress of surgical intervention. The therapy is beneficial to select patients but is not without danger or complications.

Basic Solution To supply the necessary calories in small volume, a concentrated hypertonic solution is administered; it usually consists of 25% glucose with synthetic amino acids to provide 1000 calories and 6 g nitrogen, for protein synthesis, per liter. The physician orders the solution contents for each patient. The serum electrolyte needs of the individual patient determine essential elements, vitamins, and minerals. The solution is a medium for bacterial and fungal growth so it must be kept refrigerated, but not frozen, until used. It is warmed to room temperature before administration and may hang at room temperature for no more than 12 hours. Solutions are prepared in the pharmacy with strict aseptic technique, under a filtered air laminar flow hood (see Chap. 4). Mixing of additives poses another sepsis risk.

NOTE. 1. Commercial solutions are available. If used, they are modified to meet individual needs. Some sensitivity reactions have been reported.
2. Each flask should be inspected and the expiration date noted before use. Also, a cloudy solution with floating particles should not be used as it may be contaminated.
3. Basic solutions can provide 2500 to 3000 calories daily.

Environment Catheter insertion should be performed in a controlled environment, an area with an air-filtering system where bacterial levels are acceptable. Strict aseptic technique is used.

NOTE. The Center for Disease Control, Atlanta, Georgia, in 1971 recommended that catheter insertion be done in the OR by a scrubbed sterile team.

Vein Selection A large-diameter vein in a region of high blood flow must be selected to instantly dilute the irritating hypertonic solution in order to prevent phlebitis or vein occlusion at the introduction site. The subclavian to the superior vena cava route is preferred in adults, the external jugular to the superior vena cava for infants.

Because the superior vena cava is situated within the thorax, contiguous to the right atrium, there is consequent cyclical variation in intracaval venous pressure. This pressure becomes negative during atrial filling and during respiratory inspiration. Therefore, any leaks in the external portion of the tubing can permit the sucking of air into the system during negative venous pressure. Precautionary measures must be taken at all times against inadvertent introduction of air into the system, which can result in air embolus. Leakage in the line must be prevented. All connections in the parenteral hyperalimentation setup should be taped to prevent accidental separation. The patient is instructed not to touch the insertion site but to report any discomfort.

During catheter insertion and subsequent essential tubing changes, the patient may be requested to bear down with his or her mouth closed—forced expiration against a closed glottis (Valsalva maneuver) to produce a positive phase in the central venous pressure.

Infusion Rate The goal is a continued constant infusion rate of the prescribed solution over a 24-hour period. The rate is calculated on the basis of the amount of fluids ordered for a 24-hour period. Slow administration is necessary because bypassing the regulatory mechanism in the gastrointestinal tract and liver places an increased burden of elimination on the cells and kidneys. The flow rate must be maintained as ordered. It should not be speeded up since an overload of hypertonic solution can cause massive dehydration of body cells. The solution should not be infused more rapidly than it can be metabolized or hyperglycemia can result. Insulin may then be prescribed. Hypoglycemia may develop from too slow an infusion rate. A decreased flow rate may result from a plugged filter or change in body position. *Constant monitoring is necessary*; the flow rate and patency of the infusion system should be checked every 30 minutes.

Precautions Strict asepsis for catheter insertion, maintenance, and infusion is mandatory. Sepsis is a very real and serious complication. Maintenance of a closed intravenous system with minimal catheter manipulation is important. The technique itself introduces a foreign body and exposes the patient's circulation to a potentially dangerous external environment at a time when he or she can least afford complications. Possibility of sepsis is the greatest deterrent to hyperalimentation therapy. Conscientious care is positively obligatory.

NOTE. Every time the line is entered there is risk of contamination. Therefore, the parenteral alimentation line should be used *only* for the delivery of nutrition. It should not be used for piggyback intravenous setups as for administration of blood constituents, medications, central venous pressure monitoring, or blood drawing for laboratory analysis.

Hyperalimentation therapy is discontinued gradually to permit adjustment to a lowered glucose level. Rebound hypoglycemia must be guarded against.

Other Considerations

1 Hyperalimentation therapy is not a contraindication to ambulation.

2 Long-term parenteral hyperalimentation, although hazardous, can be accomplished at home with adequate professional instruction, supervision, assistance, and unyielding observance of strict aseptic technique.

Obese Patients

Obesity is prevalent in our present-day society. It may be of:

1 Endocrine origin; usually associated with biliary, hepatic, or endocrine disease. Special diets are required.

2 Nonendocrine origin; usually associated with excessive caloric intake. Nonendocrine obesity is referred to as *morbid obesity* when weight exceeds 100 lb over the ideal weight for one's height.

Persons who are 10 to 30 percent overweight experience an increased incidence of morbidity and mortality from increased demand on the heart, hypertension, cerebral hemorrhage, diabetes, and diseases of the digestive system such as liver or gall bladder disease. The degree of morbidity varies with the severity of the obese condition.

The marked increase in the physical size of these persons presents problems for the OR and RR teams. Safety precautions against injury, falls, and burns must be emphasized. Problems include the following:

1 Transporting and lifting the obese patient are difficult. Mechanical patient lifters are desirable (see Chap. 8). If they are not available, extra persons are needed to ensure safety in lifting.
- **a** Tables and stretchers must be properly stabilized as always.
- **b** In moving the patient from stretcher to operating table it may be helpful to suggest that the patient feel for both sides of the table, so that he or she does not move too far and fall.

2 Positioning on the operating table is often difficult and requires special care.
- **a** Massive tissue must be carefully protected and protuberances on the operating table must be well padded to prevent bruising.
- **b** Extra personnel are often necessary to assist in proper positioning.
- **c** Ventilation and circulation must be assured.
- **d** The electrosurgical unit grounding plate must not be surrounded by overlapping skin folds; the tissue could be burned.

3 Adipose tissue retains anesthetic drugs longer because many are fat soluble, and the tissue has a poor blood supply.

4 The mechanics of operating are more difficult; operating time is lengthened.
- **a** Accessibility of organs, especially deep ones such as the gall bladder, may be a problem.
- **b** The type of instrumentation needed may contribute to operative trauma and postoperative pain.

5 Healing may be delayed because of poor vascularity and the frequent coincidence of diabetes. Obese patients have an increased incidence of postoperative wound infection and disruption. (See Chap. 12.)
- **a** A sterile closed drainage system is often used to drain accumulated fluid thereby facilitating healing.
- **b** It is harder to eliminate "dead space" in wound closure, and the tissue has a poor blood supply.

6 These patients are frequently self-conscious; your discretion is essential!

Diabetic Patients

The stress of an operation is reflected in all body systems in relatively healthy patients. For the labile diabetic patient who vacillates from the precipice of insulin shock to one of ketoacidosis, the hazards are greater yet, since surgical intervention upsets the normal regimen of caloric intake and insulin or medication program.

Stress, infection, or fever present additional problems of metabolic regulation. All three raise the blood sugar level. Stress stimulates the pituitary and adrenal glands. The former secretes an *adrenocorticotropic hormone* (ACTH), which stimulates the production of glucocorticoids. These in turn increase *gluconeogenesis,* the formation of glucose by the liver from noncarbohydrate sources. The resulting extra glucose enters the bloodstream. Coincidentally, the adrenals secrete epinephrine, which accelerates the conversion of glycogen in the liver to glucose, also raising the blood sugar. More insulin is needed. The primary goal of diabetes control is to maintain a stable internal environment thereby averting a metabolic crisis. Extreme care must be taken to *prevent:*

1 Hyperglycemia and its accompanying severe fluid loss, causing dehydration.
   a Some medications increase blood sugar level, e.g., cortisone.
2 Ketoacidosis and acetonuria.
   a These are due to insulin insufficiency from natural cause, or reduced or omitted insulin dosage.
   b They may result in coma if allowed to progress untreated.
3 Hypoglycemia and hypoglycemic shock.
   a These are due to too much insulin.
   b They are of faster onset than ketoacidosis.
   c Hypoglycemia is especially dangerous. It can occur during major procedures because of omission or delay of oral intake.

Prevention of these states is dependent on:

1 Physician's treatment of choice of diabetes
2 Severity of the disease
3 Type of onset, i.e., juvenile or adult
4 Existence of complicating conditions and type of operation

Persons with a mild form of the disease usually withstand surgical intervention without crisis. Intraoperative metabolic control is more difficult in patients with juvenile onset, who have marked unpredictability and greater extremes in blood sugar levels, as well as in severe diabetics. Lengthy major procedures with extensive tissue trauma present the greatest challenge to regulation.

Preoperative preparation includes careful laboratory testing, including fasting and postprandial blood sugar determinations, urinalysis for sugar and acetone, complete blood count, blood urea nitrogen, and serum electrolyte determinations. A chest x-ray and electrocardiogram are also advisable.

Common Complications of Diabetes

1 Inadequate circulation from premature vascular disease, causing deficient tissue perfusion. Hyperlipemia affects both coronary and peripheral arteries.
2 Susceptibility to infection, delayed healing.
3 Neuropathy; any nervous disease.
4 Nephropathy; small blood vessels in the kidney are affected.
5 Diabetic retinopathy and blindness; small vessels in the eye are affected.
6 Biliary and pancreatic diseases.

Postoperative control is also a problem, especially if the patient remains under stress from a diagnosis necessitating change in life-style or body image, for example, amputation of an extremity.

Special Considerations

1 Blood sample for serum glucose may be drawn 1 hour preoperatively.
2 Reduced preoperative insulin dose may be ordered to guard against hypoglycemia or insulin shock during the operation.
3 Preoperative medication dosage may be one-fourth to one-half of the regular dosage for a narcotic.
   a These drugs may cause nausea and vomiting, which predispose to fluid and electrolyte imbalance and can precipitate a hypoglycemic reaction from a decreased need for insulin. An adequate glucose supply is essential to central nervous system function.
4 It is difficult to detect metabolic crisis in unconscious patients, therefore, blood sugar levels are closely watched, in addition to fractional urine specimens, to ascertain necessary insulin dosage.
5 Continuous intravenous access throughout the operation is vital for insulin-dependent patients, in case of a metabolic problem.
   a Optional methods of management are available. One which may be used for severe diabetics is a continual flow infusion intra- and postoperatively to provide daily carbohydrate requirement, with subcutaneous insulin administration, until oral intake is resumed. Amounts are determined by serum glucose levels.
6 Nasogastric suction may cause acidosis, dehydration, or electrolyte imbalance.
7 Adequate hydration must be maintained because a rising blood sugar level upsets osmotic equilibrium.
8 Precautions against thrombophlebitis should be taken. Antiembolic stockings usually are worn by the patient.
9 Skin integrity must be guarded to avoid sepsis.
   a Hyposensitive tape is used on the skin.
   b Strict asepsis is especially important.

Pediatric Patients

Pediatric patients react differently than adults. Infants, especially the premature, and young children are especially susceptible to the trauma of surgical procedures, physically and emotionally. The nurse's response to the young patient in a supportive, nurturant manner can reduce trauma and prevent complications. Accurate information with explanations geared to how the child looks at things, previews of procedures through play techniques, and as much individual care as possible during critical periods pre- and postoperatively are all part of desired protocol.

Modern pediatric surgery has opened new horizons. For example, with prevailing techniques and care, newborn infants with congenital defects, who formerly lived only a few days or spent a life of restricted activity, are now in most instances able to live a normal, active life. Chapter 26 details the special needs of infants and children.

Geriatric Patients

Surgery for the over-65 age group once was considered out of reach of the surgeon's skill because the risks were too high. Now, many of these persons are successfully operated on for conditions that years ago made life barely endurable for the aged. Obviously, the number and severity of existing pathological conditions will influence the surgical risk of this ever-increasing population.

Persons are not ill simply because they are old but chronic illness and multiple pathology often are companions of the aged. Assessment of older persons differs somewhat from that of younger people. The elderly usually function best mentally and physically in a familiar setting, therefore, home visits and supportive health services are particularly helpful. For emotional health, the aged need to be involved and to retain control over their lives. A loss of physical and financial security and life-long friends can be devastating. Aged patients gain comfort from familiarity. Consequently, during hospitalization, having some personal possession with them such as a clock, calendar, or prized photograph assists the elderly in orienting to their new surroundings. Good lighting is also helpful. Many of these persons are past- rather than present-oriented so always introduce yourself to expedite their adjustment. Also, give special attention to individual living patterns and idiosyncrasies and indulge them as far as is consistent with their safety. Treating the elderly in a respectful manner is not only commendable but expected by the patient, and serves to preserve his or her self-esteem.

Conditions to which geriatric patients are prone are hypoproteinemia, and cardiovascular, renal, digestive, or pulmonary problems. Coronary artery and cerebrovascular disease are prevalent. Chronic bleeding may decrease blood volume and oxygenation of tissues. Decreased vital capacity, oxygen intake, and carbon dioxide removal reduce cardiac reserve. General debilitative changes such as atherosclerosis, deteriorated skin and muscular integrity, and weakened sensorium (hearing, sight, feeling—impaired ability to feel pressure or temperature) develop gradually over the years and present additional problems. Special precautions and patience are always indicated in caring for the geriatric patient. The following factors should be taken into account:

1 Slow adaptation, reduced cardiac reserve, and diminished blood flow throughout the body with inadequate perfusion result in the patient's inability to respond rapidly to sudden change in position.

2 Older people do not tolerate fluid and blood loss well. Hypovolemia can rapidly progress to a crisis situation.

3 Slow circulation or hypotension predispose the elderly to thrombus formation. Antiembolic stockings, leg exercises, and early ambulation are precautionary measures.

4 The aged must be well supported during diagnostic procedures as dizziness and weakness can result from slow cardiac compensation. Also, it is difficult for an orthopneic cardiac patient to lie flat as some tests require. These persons need extra pillows. Do not lay them flat until necessary. Older people also tire easily.

5 Geriatric patients are especially susceptible to infection because of immunologic changes and decreased immunoglobulin production. Extreme vigilance in technique is paramount. These patients may have hidden infection with masked symptoms.

6 Pulmonary complications often follow operations on patients with chronic pulmonary diseases. Be sure the patient is warm and does not lie for hours with a damp gown or linens.

7 Arthritis is a common affliction. Support a stiff knee or spine curvatures with pillows.

8 Drug tolerance may be poor and detoxification slow due to slow blood flow to the liver or impaired hepatic function. Usually narcotics and sedatives are given only with extreme caution; the normal dosage is reduced; the patient is observed closely for untoward reaction. Sometimes medications are administered early because of slow absorption. Drugs, altered sleeping and eating patterns, an unfamiliar environment, and the physical changes of aging all contribute to mental confusion. All drugs interact with anesthetic agents and affect physiological functioning. Therefore, a minimum number of medications is desirable. Anesthetic agents are myocardial and respiratory depressants; they must be thoughtfully selected and the patient carefully monitored (see Chap. 9).

9 Acute renal problems preclude operation. Impaired renal function or dehydration may cause renal failure.

10 Most aged patients require special attention to nutrition. Poor teeth or eating habits and limited finances may contribute to malnutrition.

11 Aged persons have difficulty swallowing due to loss of secretions, reduced esophogeal peristalsis, and neuromuscular changes. They must be watched for possible aspiration.

12 All of the responses of older people are slower than normal; for this reason the utmost patience is required. Do not rush them or confuse them with a multiplicity of orders. Give them time to respond without loss of dignity.

13 Provide for sensory deficiencies and do not distract the patient from the situation at point; at best, concentration is difficult.

14 Motivate the patient toward recovery by encouraging self-help.

In summary, geriatric patients particularly require thorough preoperative assessment, an experienced anesthesiologist, and careful postoperative management.

Catastrophic Illnesses

While the OR nurse is most frequently involved with patients who have a favorable prognosis, she or he will also care for those of all ages with a terminal illness who are operated on to relieve a specific problem. Maximum patient comfort and relief of physiological disturbances are the primary concerns. Included in this category are some of the patients with malignancies. Those who have metastatic disease are often severely debilitated. All require highly individualized care.

The manner in which the patient is told the diagnosis and prognosis naturally has a great impact. Statements to these patients must be worded cautiously to avoid weakening their hope of recovery. Significantly, patients who have been judiciously and thoughtfully informed are easier to talk to, accept therapy more readily, and have greater trust in and communicate more openly with the hospital staff. The suspense of uncertainty is frequently harmful. Each patient handles in his or her own way the pain of and the living with the diagnosis. Although it is not always so, many persons nevertheless consider the diagnosis of cancer a death warrant and react accordingly. The nurse must emphasize the present, focusing on the patient's strengths, attributes, and how he or she can best utilize the remaining ones. It is difficult to find hope when one faces a radical procedure such as a laryngectomy or radical neck dissection. The discerning nurse will use a philosophy of hope but not focus on the positive without acknowledging the negative. She may say, "I understand, but what is the advantage of this procedure? How is it going to help you?"

Listening to these patients is particularly important. In individualizing care it is wise not to be ultracheerful. Patients are not deceived. Be completely supportive. For her own effectiveness the nurse should mentally review the stages of dying: denial, isolation, anger, bargaining, depression, acceptance. These stages do not always occur in this sequence, however.

Persons caring for patients with a terminal or catastrophic illness must remember that they are interacting with people who have different priorities and values. These patients are present-oriented, for many have little future. They review their existing sense of values and the quality of their lives in hopes of living each day to the fullest since such a diagnosis alters one's perspective. They rearrange their ultimate goals for existence. Some persons appreciate living each day. Others are anxious to end their suffering.

The chronically ill patient feels especially threatened for disability requires a reorientation of self-image. Another problem is that chronic illness often creates an emotional and financial burden on the family. Consequently, family members may have ambivalent feelings toward the patient because of the necessary changes in their lives that the illness precipitates.

A few of the special problems these conditions give rise to are as follows:

1 The common therapies, e.g., radiation, chemotherapy, and steroids, frequently cause gastrointestinal disturbances and severe hematological depressions, such as leukopenia or lymphopenia (see Chap. 27).

2 Inhibition of blood supply and nourishment can result in necrotic tissue. Prolonged confinement in bed increases one's susceptibility to decubitus ulcers.

3 Inactivity promotes catabolism and muscle wasting.

4 Preoperative preparation is especially intensive for patients able to tolerate an operation. Often surgical intervention is palliative rather than curative.

5 Many operations are long and complex radical procedures, such as hemipelvectomy.

Death in the OR

Although an infrequent occurrence, when a patient expires in the OR the surgeon in charge notifies the next of kin. The circulating nurse notifies the OR supervisor immediately. This may be unnecessary as the OR supervisor should be informed of any patient's deteriorating condition and all crises or emergencies.

Individual state law and hospital policy must be adhered to in caring for the body. In some states, the body of the patient who expires in the OR automatically becomes the property of the coroner. The circulating nurse's responsibilities in the care of the body include:

1 To give after-death care to the body or to see that this is done according to hospital policy before it is taken to the hospital morgue. Some hospitals employ a mortician who assists in the disposition of the body and with the necessary details.
  - **a** Follow the procedure book. Be sure identification is correct.
  - **b** The body should be refrigerated within 1 hour of death.

2 To arrange for transportation of the body to the morgue.
  - **a** The nurse signs a form releasing the body from the OR. The nursing assistant or person taking the body also signs this form.
  - **b** Extreme care should be taken in the suite to prevent other patients from seeing the body and/or the stretcher bearing it away.

PREPARATION OF ALL PATIENTS FOR OPERATION

Emotional Preparation

By fulfilling spiritual and psychosocial needs, the hospital staff should furnish the preoperative patient with as much peace of mind as is possible. Understandably, as the time for operation approaches, the patient's tension level rises.

If the patient has not seen his or her cleric or the hospital chaplain before coming to the OR and makes such a request, the OR nurse should make every effort to get in touch with that person before anesthesia induction.

Physical Preparation

Preoperative physical preparation is designed to help the patient overcome the stresses of anesthesia, fluid and blood loss, immobilization, and tissue trauma. Preparation often begins before the patient's hospital admission, with the institution of nutritional or drug therapy and a special bathing regimen (see Chap. 11). Physical preparation on the unit is as follows:

On Admission A history and chest x-ray are taken of all patients. Certain basic laboratory tests and a physical examination are also routinely performed.

> NOTE. Patients admitted for ambulatory surgery may have tests the morning of admission or a day or two before. The results must be on records that accompany the patient to the OR.

If the patient is over 35 years old, or has a special problem such as a cardiac disease, an electrocardiogram is taken. If transfusion is anticipated, the patient's blood is typed and cross-matched. Special diagnostic procedures are performed when specifically indicated. An attempt is made to bring all patients to their best possible physical status. Finally, appropriate consultations are sought when necessary.

Evening before an Elective Operation

1 The operative site is prepared. Hair removal and skin cleansing are done according to hospital policy (see Chap. 11).

2 Nail polish is removed from the patient's fingers and toes to permit observation of nail bed color, one indication of oxygenation and circulation.

3 Special preparation is given as ordered.
  - **a** Preoperative enemas are given when it is advantageous to have the bowel and rectum empty as in the case of gastrointestinal procedures such as bowel resection or sigmoidoscopy, and operations in the pelvic, perineal, or perianal areas.

4 Ideally, both the OR nurse and anesthesiologist visit the patient.

5 A bedtime sedative is given for sleep as ordered.

6 Oral intake is discontinued as ordered, usually nothing by mouth (NPO) for 8 hours preceding the operation, to prevent regurgitation or emesis and aspiration of gastric contents. This instruction is also given to ambulatory surgery patients to follow at home.

Before Leaving for the OR At this time, the patient's physical and emotional status and vital signs should be assessed and recorded by the unit nurse. Any untoward symptoms or extreme apprehension must be reported to the surgeon as they could affect the patient's intraoperative course. The following preparations are made:

1 Bed linens are changed and the patient puts on a clean hospital gown.
2 All jewelry, except a wedding ring, and eyeglasses are removed for safekeeping. The ring, if worn, must be securely taped or tied to the finger to prevent loss.
  a In some instances of marked decrease in visual acuity, the patient may be permitted to take his or her glasses to the OR. The nurse must safeguard them.
3 Dentures and removable bridges are removed for general and local anesthesia, unless otherwise ordered, to safeguard them and prevent obstruction to respiration under anesthesia.

  NOTE. Sometimes dentures are permitted in cases of local anesthesia if the patient can breathe more easily with them in place.

4 Prostheses such as eye, extremity, breast, and contact lenses are removed for safekeeping.
5 Hairpins are removed to prevent scalp injury or a possible source of static electricity near the anesthesia machine. Long hair is braided. Wigs are removed.
6 Antiembolic stockings or an elastic bandage may be ordered applied to the lower extremities prior to the operation to prevent embolic phenomena.
  a This is often done prior to abdominal or pelvic procedures, and for patients who have varicosities, are prone to thrombus formation, or have a history of embolus, and some geriatric patients.
7 The patient voids to prevent overdistention of the bladder or incontinence during unconsciousness. This is especially important for abdominal or pelvic procedures where a large bladder may interfere with adequate exposure of abdominal contents or may be traumatized. Time of voiding is recorded.

  NOTE. Indwelling catheter insertion, when indicated, is usually done in the OR after the patient is anesthetized (see Chap. 11).

8 The patient, bed, and chart are accurately identified and identifications fastened securely in place.

  NOTE. 1. If the patient has a language barrier, an interpreter may accompany him or her to the OR and stay until anesthesia induction.
  2. A preoperative checklist will help the unit nurse to assure that the patient has been properly prepared and that all essential records are accompanying him or her to the operating room. The nurse should remind the physician to order essential medications, normally taken orally, that must be given or substituted by another route when patient is on "nothing by mouth" preoperatively.

9 Preanesthesia medications are given as ordered.

  NOTE. Patients receiving preanesthesia medication should be cautioned to remain in bed and not to smoke. Many of the drugs cause drowsiness, vertigo, or postural hypotension. Therefore, the side rails should be raised on the bed.

Transportation to the OR Suite

Patients are usually taken to the OR suite about 45 minutes before scheduled procedure time. For reasons of safety they are transported via stretcher. Elevators should be designated "For OR use only." This ensures privacy and minimizes microbial contamination. The patient must be kept comfortable, warm, and safe during transport. Side rails are raised, restraint straps applied. Intravenous solution bags or bottles are hung on poles or standards during transportation attached securely near the foot of the stretcher where there is less danger of injury to the patient if the container should fall. Gentle handling is indicated to prevent dislodging intravenous needles or indwelling catheters. A unit nurse or nursing assistant should stay with the patient until relieved by an operating room nurse or anesthesiologist, to whom the patient's chart is given.

Admission to the OR Suite

Exchange and Holding Areas Patients are brought through the outer corridor to the holding area by outside personnel. OR personnel transfer the patient to an OR stretcher where he or she remains until taken into the operating room. The patient goes to the recovery room and from there to the unit on this stretcher. It is then brought back to a stretcher-cleaning room where the entire stretcher, including the wheels, is decontaminated before being brought into the OR suite.

This procedure is ideal from the standpoint of

preventing contamination from entering the OR but there are occasions to justify bringing patients to the suite in their beds. These include patients in traction, on Stryker frames, or cardiac patients who must not be moved until transferred to the operating table.

A patient on a Stryker or similar frame should have broad muslin bands across the body and legs while being transported. These should be left in place until the patient is moved onto the operating table. Some patients may be operated on while on the frame. The surgeon chooses the course that best benefits the individual patient. The bed or frame can be decontaminated in the exchange area and made up with clean linen before being brought into the room after the operation.

Beds, stretchers, frames, and tables must be stabilized by locking the wheels and by personnel when a patient is moving from one to the other. The patient should be instructed and assisted to prevent a fall or injury.

Some hospitals have individual anesthesia induction rooms where the patient waits and is administered an anesthetic before being taken into the operating room.

A quiet, restful atmosphere enables the patient to gain full advantage of premedication. Some holding areas and operating rooms have soft, recorded music. This is conducive to relaxation, especially for patients under local anesthesia, as the music diverts their attention from the many other sounds.

Immediate Preanesthesia Preparation A line-up of stretchers with each patient gowned alike is not conducive to preserving the patient's personal identity. Nowhere may a patient feel more alone than in a holding area. By introducing herself and pleasantly greeting the patient by name, the circulating nurse can do much to dispel the patient's apprehension and assure him that he is not alone nor among disinterested people. Patients appreciate seeing a familiar face and it is advantageous if the nurse herself made the preoperative visit. A compassionate expression in her eyes and voice, a reassuring touch of the hand, and a positive statement such as, "You look rested and comfortable; is there anything I can do for you?" can convey her concern and expectance of the patient's arrival. Respect and genuine warmth rather than superficially endearing words inspire confidence. An anxious patient looks to *his* nurse for comfort, reassurance, and personal attention. He must know that the nurse will be with him constantly. Also, because of lethargy, a medicated patient needs and wants direction.

If the patient is drowsy, unnecessary conversation should be avoided. However, the nurse should answer questions and see to the patient's comfort. Keep the patient warm or turn down the cover if he is too warm. Place an extra pillow under the patient's head or under an arthritic knee. Moisten dry lips, if requested. Any delay or unusual circumstance should be explained.

The circulating nurse has a number of important duties to fulfill in a short period of time. She must:

1 Check the identity of the patient, stretcher or bed, and chart.
  - **a** When the patient comes to the hospital, an identifying wristband is put on in the admitting office. The unit nurse checks the band before the patient leaves for the OR. The circulating nurse compares the information on the wristband with the information on the chart, and with the information on the operative schedule: name, anticipated procedure, time, surgeon.
  - **b** The identification on the stretcher or bed assures the patient's return to the same one following the operation if this is the procedure. If the patient is an infant or child, the identification tag on the crib should be out of reach.

2 Check siderails, restraining straps, intravenous infusions, and indwelling catheters.

3 Observe the patient for reaction to medication.

4 Observe the patient's anxiety level.

5 Check the physical exam, medical history, laboratory tests, x-ray reports, and operative consent form in the patient's chart.
  - **a** Pay particular attention to allergies and any previous unfavorable reactions to anesthesia or blood transfusion.

6 Review the orders and nursing care plan. Ask the patient if he or she has taken anything by mouth, if NPO order was written to prevent aspiration.

Usually for physical and psychological comfort, the patient is not transferred to the operating table until time for anesthesia induction. Ideally, the main preparations for the procedure will have been completed before the patient is taken into the OR so that the circulating nurse can then devote her attention to the patient. If the nurse is more intent on equipment than on the patient, the patient may feel abandoned.

The anesthesiologist also has immediate preanesthesia duties. He or she:

1 Checks the pulse, respiration, and blood pressure to serve as a baseline for subsequent recordings under anesthesia.

2 Reviews the preoperative physical examination, history, and laboratory reports.

3 Listens to the heart and lungs.

4 Checks for denture removal or any loose teeth. The latter may be secured with thread, which is taped to the patient's cheek to prevent possible aspiration.

5 Makes certain the patient is comfortable and secure on the operating table (see Chap. 10 for a discussion of safety measures).

EVALUATION FOR QUALITY ASSURANCE

A discussion of the patient would not be complete without another mention of standards of nursing practice and quality assurance since the patient is the focus of concern for perioperative nursing care.

Each patient deserves the best possible care. Without the structure that the nursing process provides, health care services would be fragmented and accountability for the quality of services rendered made difficult. Society demands accountability of those who provide services. Patients are protected by laws and standards of acceptable practices.

Nursing practices must comply with established policies and procedures of the hospital or other health care facility and with professional standards of practice. The nurse can be held legally responsible for unethical, illegal, or unsafe practice if she fails to exercise judgment that is considered standard nursing practice. She is responsible for her own acts in the patient-physician-nurse relationship and is required to exercise skilled judgment in making her own decisions. The nurse must see that all nursing procedures and techniques are correctly executed, always keeping the outcome in mind.

Quality assurance programs (see Chap. 30) provide a means for determining the quality of care received by a patient in a particular health care setting, in this discussion, the operating room. Nursing care in the OR can be evaluated in the context of the total nursing process: assessment, planning, implementation, evaluation. Quality is determined by identifying observable characteristics, judged according to standards, for an optimum achievable degree of excellence of care. Quality assurance is important for professionalism, accountability, and cost containment. A program includes:

1 Determining standards and criteria.

2 Implementing and achieving these standards.

3 Evaluating the results. Did the program succeed? What changes need to be made to improve practice and action?

Health care professionals continually aim to improve the health/wellness outcomes for patients; alteration in health status is the end result of care. A provocative thought: The essence of quality care is in the utilization of the therapeutic potential present in each interaction in which the nurse practitioner is involved. Nurses may improve the quality of patient care by:

1 Comprehending nursing problems, providing specialized nursing interventions, and meeting the patient's physiological and psychological needs based on observation and assessment of the patient's responses

2 Helping the patient and family adapt to what happens in the OR in relation to their perceptions and expectations through teaching

3 Delivering and supervising clinical patient care with skilled planned nursing intervention and interdisciplinary collaboration

4 Coordinating all activities in the OR by planning, preparing for, and expediting the operative procedure, keeping in mind individual patient, surgeon, and team needs

To summarize, productive care and improved patient outcome result from better directed efforts as indicated by evaluation, the fourth step in the nursing process.

Chapter 4

Asepsis and the Principles of Sterile Technique

HISTORICAL INTRODUCTION

Early concepts of infection and the crude methods used to combat it seem strange indeed in the light of modern scientific knowledge, yet they were devised by the ablest minds of the times. Those minds, working on the three basic techniques—elimination of infection, control of hemorrhage, and anesthesia—have made possible the progress of modern surgery.

In ancient times, demons and evil spirits were thought to be the cause of pestilence and infection. Weird methods employed to drive them away were, of course, futile; however, purification by fire had more validity than was then realized.

In the pre-Christian era, Hippocrates (b. 460 B.C.) foreshadowed asepsis when he advocated the use of wine or boiled water for irrigating wounds. But hundreds of years were to elapse before surgeons understood the reason for irrigation.

Galen (A.D. 131–200), the Greek physician and founder of experimental physiology, was the most distinguished physician of antiquity after Hippocrates. He practiced in Rome and upheld high standards of technique for his time. There is some evidence of his having boiled the instruments that he used in caring for wounded gladiators. His anatomical investigations were unrivaled in antiquity for their accuracy and fullness. His writings, along with those of Hippocrates, were the established authority for medicine for many centuries.

Early records are extant with descriptions of epidemics, purulence, fumigation, and wound management. Sporadically, light began to be shed after the Middle Ages on methods to improve operative technique.

Andreas Vesalius, born in Brussels in the early sixteenth century, came under the influence of the great anatomy teachers of the University of Paris. He was much impressed by the Latin translation (in 1531) of Galen's *De anatomicis administrandis.* After obtaining an MD degree, Vesalius and an artist collaborated to publish six very large plates—the *Tabulae anatomicae sex,* which became a landmark in the history of anatomical nomenclature. The plates represented an attempt to standardize both the form and meaning of anatomical terms and were based on the physiology theorized by Galen. Modern anatomical nomenclature is an adaptation of that of Vesalius, a founder of the study of anatomy. Although a few surgeons from the twelfth to the nineteenth centuries felt that wounds need not suppurate, even the learned Vesalius believed and taught that "laudable pus" was an essential part of the healing process. This universally accepted thought persisted in spite of the fact that some pioneering surgeons were finding that ventilation, sanitation, and heat-treated bed linens reduced their patient infection rate.

The acceptance of scientific inquiry was slow and the inquirer subject to condemnation. Michael Sevetus (1511–1533), a Spanish physician and theologian who studied in Paris with Vesalius, was burned to death as a heretic because he attempted autopsies.

The idea of contamination by air or fomites did not surface until Girolama Francastoro, the Italian physician and poet, printed his theory of contagion in the year 1546. It held that contagion was due to the passage of minute bodies, capable of self-multiplication, from the infector to the infected. He was the first to describe typhus fever, a prevalent disease of the times. His theory opened the way to the modern concept of infection and communicable diseases of epidemic proportions.

By the seventeenth century the world had barely begun to shake itself free from superstitions. Science was just beginning to emerge. Into such a world, Antony Leeuwenhoek was born in Holland. An obscure man, not learned in Latin, which educated men spoke, he heard that if one very carefully ground very small lenses out of clear glass, one could see objects much larger than they appeared to the naked eye. His invention of the microscope, the precursor of many great discoveries, evolved from his great love for grinding lenses. His painstaking work with minutia was challenged by his contemporaries. By the middle of the century, however, European rebels were suspicious of everything that formerly had passed for knowledge and stated that they would trust only the perpetually repeated observations of their own eyes and the careful weighings of their own scales, and listen only to the answers that experiments gave them.

Leeuwenhoek's follower was Lazarro Spallanzani, a young Italian. His cruel experiments on himself involved studies of digestion, but he also experimented on the multiplication of microbes and their "spontaneous generation." He proved that microbes may live without air. Humanity owes much to these bold, persistent explorers and fighters of death.

Europe was not the only seat of interest in disease and infection in the eighteenth century. Indeed, America was struggling with epidemics as it battled to survive as a new nation. Diseases that are controlled today by inoculations and antibiotics ravaged the Revolutionary Army. Frequently, the clergy practiced medicine, attempting to save lives as well as souls. One Boston physician, Zabdiel Boylston, introduced inoculation for smallpox in 1721. Some of Washington's troops were inoculated, but many uninoculated soldiers died. Diseases that plagued the losing side frequently tipped the scales of history and were often dreaded more than the enemy.

The field of medicine interested Noah Webster throughout his long life. The pestilence of the Revolutionary War camps was embedded in his memory. In 1799, he wrote the first American work of any real worth on general epidemiology. As an editor, he also frequently reprinted British articles describing medical treatment such as that for damaged nerves. Life expectancy at birth in the colonial period was 35 years; by the turn of the century it had risen to 50 years. American medicine was developing but lacked the maturity of European medicine.

Surgical technique has advanced markedly since the nineteenth century. In the light of present-day practice, one is shocked to learn that the surgeon of that time operated in a Prince Albert coat and used the same blood- and pus-absorbing sponges for every patient he treated. During an operation, he often held the scalpel between his teeth, to protect the blade. The nineteenth-century surgeon unwound sutures from a nonsterile spool and hung them in a buttonhole of his Prince Albert. He kept a household pincushion nearby for his needles. Some instruments had beautifully carved ivory or bone handles, filled not only with bacteria but with dirt and filth.

Dr. Oliver Wendell Holmes, the renowned nineteenth-century Harvard physician, poet, and humorist, stated that "life is a fatal complaint and an eminently contagious one." While not an experimental scientist himself, nor known for any original discoveries, he employed his skill and knowledge for good causes. In 1843, Holmes wrote of the contagious nature of puerperal fever ("childbed fever") expressing the belief that it was carried from patient to patient by nurses and doctors. However, many physicians still believed that infection occurred by an act of Providence.

The true pioneer was Ignaz Semmelweis (1818–1865), an Austrian who established the etiology of puerperal fever, then a major cause of maternal mortality. He required the doctors and medical students on his wards to wash their hands in a chlorinated-lime solution before examining patients. By this method, in a year's time Semmelweis reduced the mortality rate to one-twelfth of its previous level. However, his ideas were not understood and his writing created controversy that seemed to accomplish nothing outside of his own hospital. The great value of his discovery was not recognized by other doctors of his time. Presumably because of this, he was committed to a hospital for the insane, and met with an early death.

It was Louis Pasteur, the French chemist and microbiologist, who established the validity of the germ theory of disease. He discovered that fermentation of wine is the result of minute organisms. Fermentation failed because the necessary organisms were either absent or unable to grow properly. All previous explanations had been without experimental foundation. He found that he could halt the organisms' growth by heat. Recognizing that lactic and alcohol fermentation were accelerated by exposure to air, Pasteur wondered whether the invisible organisms were always present in the atmosphere or were spontaneously generated. By experimentation in the pure air of the high Alps, he destroyed the theory of spontaneous generation of organisms, proving that they came from similar organisms with which ordinary air was impregnated. His discoveries stimulated his interest and led to his studies of infection and putrefaction in living tissue. In spite of a paralyzing stroke, he worked on, later isolating the germ causing chicken cholera epidemic and the bacillus of anthrax. He developed the Pasteur vaccine for rabies. His greatest contribution was laying the foundation for bacteriology as a science and teaching the role of bacteria in causing disease.

The German physician Robert Koch was also a founder of bacteriology and won a Nobel prize for isolating the tubercle bacillus. Every modern student of bacteriology learns Koch's postulates. Briefly they are:

1 A specific organism must be seen in all cases of an infectious disease.
2 This organism must be obtained in pure culture.
3 Organisms from pure cultures must reproduce the disease in experimental animals.
4 The organism must be recoverable from the experimental animals.

These postulates have served as guides to the discovery of the etiologic agents in many of the most important diseases of man, animals, and plants. Koch traveled extensively studying the prevalent infectious diseases. His advocacy of the use of bichloride of mercury as an antiseptic was the forerunner of interest in antisepsis.

Before and during the mid-nineteenth century, wounds or injury to an extremity invariably resulted in gangrene. Amputation was routinely performed in an attempt to prevent *septicemia,* a significant invasion of microorganisms into the bloodstream.

Joseph Lister, an English surgeon, is known as the father of modern surgery. Of all the persons who heard of Pasteur's work at the time, Lister was the one to see the value of the germ theory in relation to surgery, and to pursue its course. Since the relationship between bacteria and infection was known, he searched for a chemical to combat the bacteria and surgical infections. He first used a carbolic solution on dressings and reduced the mortality rate of his patients somewhat. Lister then felt infections were airborne and his principle was to kill them in the wound and the surrounding area. In 1865, he started the use of a carbolic spray in the operating room. Soon he was using it in the wound, on articles in contact with the wound, and on the hands of the operating team. The result was a notable decrease in mortality rate. Lister soaked sutures in carbolic, the "carbolized catgut," and arrived at the conclusion that infection did not occur if sutures were soaked in an antiseptic solution. Heretofore the belief had been that sutures themselves caused infection.

Lister's principle of antiseptic surgery, which initiated the modern era of surgery, was derided by many surgeons of the day, especially in London. Sir James Young Simpson, who discovered and first used chloroform as an anesthetic, was bitterly opposed to the principle. He did not see the relation between that principle and the mortality rate of surgical patients, even though he was greatly concerned about the high prevailing rate. He once remarked that an English soldier at Waterloo had a better chance of survival than a man on an operating table.

Even though Lister's method reduced the mortality rate, the carbolic solution caused wound necrosis and skin irritation in both patients and operators, and was said to "favour hemorrhage," making hemostasis difficult. Although unable to decide whether putrefaction was "germinal or chemical," some surgeons were convinced of the value of antiseptics, but it was not until 1879 at a medical meeting in Amsterdam that Lister's antiseptic principle of surgery was truly accepted by the medical profession.

It is interesting to note that developments in nursing accompanied advances in medicine. During the mid-nineteenth century, Florence Nightingale advocated the use of pure air, pure water, efficient drainage, cleanliness, and light for health. Her nursing experience during the Crimean War proved the efficacy of these practices. In 1876, Dr. Henry Bigelow of Massachusetts General Hospital took student nurses from the Boston Training School to the operating room for clinical instruction. In 1889, Johns Hopkins University opened its hospital. It included operating room nurse specialization.

Progress in sterile technique was slow, no doubt hindered by tradition, but with the advent of sterilization, continual progress was made.

Evolution of Sterilization

The industrious German surgeons assisted the transition from antisepsis to asepsis. Gustav Neuber was resolute about requiring the complete cleanliness of the operating room, advocating scrubbing the furniture with disinfectant solution, and requiring the wearing of gowns and caps. He eventually sterilized everything in contact with the wound.

"Sterilization" by boiling was introduced around the middle 1880s. Everything used during an operation, including linens, dressings, and gowns, were boiled. Some surgeons felt Lister's method to be adequate and spoke disparagingly of the boiling practice.

In 1876, heat-resistant bacteria were demonstrated. About 1886, Ernst von Bergmann and his associates introduced the steam sterilizer. This was a great improvement over von Bergmann's previous method of soaking surgical supplies in bichloride of mercury, which he felt was an improvement over Lister's carbolic solution. However, surgeons soon learned that steam in itself is inadequate for sterilization. Steam must be under pressure to raise the temperature sufficiently to kill heat-resistant microorganisms. Pressure steam sterilizers were then developed to kill resistant spores. Much of the sterilizing equipment used in America was designed in Europe until the 1900s. Vacuum-type pressure sterilizers and hot air sterilizers followed.

Used as a fumigant for insects in the early twentieth century, ethylene oxide was recognized as an antibacterial agent around 1929, when it was used to sterilize imported spices. It has been employed as a sterilizing agent in industry and hospitals since the 1940s.

Sterilization by irradiation developed thereafter although it remains expensive and impractical for general hospital use. It is used for commercial sterilization of surgical supplies, among other things.

Factors in Technique

Coincidentally with the development of sterilization, other factors in aseptic technique developed. These include refinement of operative technique by William Halsted (see p. 238), and use of controlled environment, modern OR attire, and precise housekeeping methods. Surgeons learned that all things that come in contact with a wound should be free from microorganisms, i.e., sterile.

SURGICAL CONSCIENCE

The key words of operating room practice are caring, conscience, discipline, and technique. Optimal patient care requires an inherent surgical conscience, self-discipline, and the application of principles of asepsis and sterile technique. All are inseparably related.

A surgical conscience may simply be stated as a surgical Golden Rule, i.e., do unto the patient as you would have others do unto you. One must consider each patient as oneself, or as a loved one. An individual develops a surgical conscience that remains inherent thereafter. In the last century, Florence Nightingale well summarized what is, in essence, its meaning. She said, "The nurse must keep a high sense of duty in her own mind, must aim at perfection in her care, and must be consistent always in herself." Surgical conscience involves a concept of self-inspection coupled with moral obligation. Involving both scientific and intellectual honesty, it is self-regulation in practice according to a deep personal commitment to the highest values. It incorporates one's own values at a conscious level and monitors one's own behavior and decision making in relation to those values. In short, a surgical conscience is one's inner voice for the conscientious practice of asepsis and sterile technique *at all times.*

A surgical conscience does not permit a person to excuse an error but rather to readily admit and rectify one. It becomes so much a part of the person that he or she can see at a glance or instinctively know if a break in technique or violation of a principle occurs. Conscience dictates that appropriate action be taken, whether the person is with others or alone and unobserved. A surgical conscience therefore is the foundation for the practice of strict aseptic and sterile techniques. Practice according to that conscience results in pride in self and in accomplishment, as well as an inner confidence that one is giving quality care.

A very important aspect in assisting the development of a surgical conscience in others is not to castigate a person for an error but to praise that person instead for admitting it, and to help him or her correct the violation. Fear of criticism is the primary deterrent in admission of fault. No one should be reluctant to admit a frank or questionable break in technique. However, any individual with an underdeveloped motivation to carry out practices as closely to perfection as is possible has no place in the operating room suite.

DEFINITIONS

To understand infection, infection control, the principles of aseptic and sterile technique, and the application of these principles in the operating room, you will need to know the meaning of the following terms.

Aerobe Microorganism that requires air or presence of oxygen for maintenance of life. Adj., aerobic.

Anaerobe Microorganism that grows best in oxygen-free environment or one that cannot tolerate oxygen, e.g., *Clostridium* species that causes gas gangrene. Adj., anaerobic.

Antibiotic Any of a variety of substances, both natural or synthetic, that inhibit growth of or destroy microorganisms; used as a therapeutic agent against infectious diseases. Some antibiotics are selective for a specific organism; some are broad-spectrum.

Antisepsis The prevention of sepsis by the exclusion, destruction, or inhibition of growth or multiplication of microorganisms from body tissues and fluids.

Antiseptics Organic or inorganic chemical compounds that combat sepsis by inhibiting growth of microorganisms without necessarily killing them. These agents are used on skin and tissue to arrest the growth of endogenous (resident flora) microorganisms. They must not be strong enough to destroy tissue, however.

Asepsis The absence of microorganisms that cause disease; freedom from infection; exclusion of microorganisms. Adj., aseptic; without infection.

Aseptic Technique The method by which contamination with microorganisms is prevented.

Bactericide An agent that destroys bacteria. Adj., bactericidal.

Bacteriostasis The inhibition of the growth of bacteria. However, the bacteria are undamaged to the extent that they will grow if placed in a favorable medium, away from the action of chemicals. Adj., bacteriostatic; most antiseptics are bacteriostatic because they do not kill bacteria.

Contaminated Soiled with microorganisms.

Cross Contamination Transmission of microorganisms from patient to patient and from contaminated inanimate objects to patients and vice versa.

Cross Infection Infection contracted by a patient from another patient or staff member, and/or contracted by a staff member from a patient.

Disease A specific entity that is the sum total of numerous expressions of one or more pathological processes; failure of the body's adaptive mechanisms to counteract adequately the stress to which it is subject, resulting in disturbance in function or structure of any part, organ, or system of the body.

Disinfectants Agents that kill all growing or vegetative forms of microorganisms, thus completely eliminating them from inanimate objects. Syn., germicide. The suffix *-cide* means to kill; adj., -cidal. Reference is made frequently to the specific action of the following disinfectants.

- **Bactericide** Kills gram-negative and gram-positive bacteria unless specifically stated to the contrary. Action against a specific species of bacteria may be elaborated; i.e., pseudomonacide kills *Pseudomonas aeruginosa,* tuberculocide kills tubercle bacillus.
- **Fungicide** Kills fungi.
- **Virucide** Kills viruses.
- **Sporicide** Kills spores.

Disinfection The chemical or physical process of destroying all pathogenic microorganisms except spore-bearing ones; it is used for inanimate objects, but not on tissue.

Epidemiology The study of occurrence and distribution of disease; the sum of all factors controlling the presence or absence of a disease.

Fomite Inanimate object that may be contaminated with infectious organisms and serves to transmit disease.

Infection Invasion of the body by pathogenic microorganisms, and the reaction of tissues to their presence and to toxins generated by the organisms. Adj., infectious.

Microaerophilic Pertaining to microorganisms that require free oxygen for growth but thrive best when oxygen is less in amount than that in the atmosphere.

Microorganisms Living organisms, invisible to the naked eye, including: bacteria, fungi, viruses, yeasts, and molds. Syn., microbe; adj., microbial.

Opportunists Microorganisms that do not normally invade the tissue. They are capable of causing infection or disease if introduced mechanically into the body through injury. The tetanus bacillus is an example.

Pathogenic Producing or capable of producing disease.

Pathogenic Microorganisms Those microorganisms that cause infectious disease. True microorganisms can invade healthy tissue through some power of their own; they can injure tissue by a toxin that they produce.

Sepsis Severe toxic febrile state resulting from infection with pyrogenic microorganisms, with or without associated septicemia.

Septicemia Clinical syndrome characterized by a significant invasion of microorganisms from a focus of infection in the tissues into the bloodstream. The microorganisms may multiply in the blood. Infection of bacterial origin carried through the bloodstream is sometimes referred to as *bacteremia.*

Spores An inactive but viable state of microorganisms in the environment. Certain bacteria and fungi will sustain themselves in this form until the environment is favorable for vegetative growth. The spore stage is highly resistant to heat, toxic chemicals, and other methods of destruction.

Sterile Free of microorganisms, including all spores.

Sterile Field The area around the site of incision into tissue or introduction of any instrumentation into a body orifice that has been prepared for use of sterile supplies and equipment. This area includes all furniture covered with sterile drapes and personnel who are properly attired.

Sterile Technique The method by which contamination with microorganisms is prevented to maintain sterility throughout the operative procedure.

Sterilization The process by which all pathogenic and nonpathogenic microorganisms, including spores, are killed. This is an absolute term used to refer *only* to a process capable of destroying *all* forms of microbial life, including spores.

Sterilizer The chamber or equipment used to attain either physical or chemical sterilization. The agent used must be capable of killing all forms of microorganisms.

Superinfection A secondary subsequent infection caused by a different microorganism as seen following antibiotic therapy.

Surgically Clean Mechanically cleansed but unsterile. Items are rendered surgically clean by the use of chemical, physical, or mechanical means that markedly reduce the number of microorganisms on them.

Terminal Sterilization and Disinfection The procedures carried out for the destruction of pathogens at the end of an operative procedure in the OR or in other areas of patient contact, i.e., recovery room, ICU, nursing unit.

INFECTION

Careful attention is given to the preoperative preparation of the patient and to the creation and maintenance of a therapeutic environment. All possible measures are utilized to prevent complications. A very serious and potentially fatal complication is postoperative infection, which may result from a single break in technique. Therefore, knowledge of causative agents and their control as well as meticulous practice of aseptic and sterile techniques are the basis of prevention.

The development of passive and active immunization, sterile and aseptic techniques, and antibiotic therapy have had revolutionary effects on surgical practice. Nevertheless, the ideal state of infection-free operative procedures may not be a reality in all situations. Wound and systemic infections continue to occur because all the facts are not understood, and individual discipline in carrying out techniques is sometimes lacking. It has been said that every operation is an experiment in applied and practical bacteriology. The worldwide problem of infection persists to plague patient and physician alike. Infection is a health hazard of great expense and significance, affecting the final outcome of operative treatment. The quality of life, both physical and psychological, can be drastically altered, sometimes permanently, by infection and the associated "d's": delayed healing, discomfort, distress, dependency, and dollars.

Not infrequently, disability, deformity, and disaster with ultimate death are the result of infection. A mild infection is potentially a severe one.

Clinically, infection is the product of entrance, growth, metabolic activities, and pathophysiological effects of microorganisms in living tissue. It can develop in the surgical patient as a preoperative complication following an injury, or as a postoperative complication of cross contamination or cross infection.

Process of Infection

Sepsis involves three stages: invasion, localization, and resolution leading to recovery. However, the progress toward recovery may revert back to extension of the infection. The characteristics, invasive qualities, and sources of the etiologic microorganism are important in prevention and treatment. Prompt identification of the infecting agent and sensitivity testing are essential so that appropriate antibiotic therapy can be instituted.

Acute bacterial infection is the most common sepsis in surgical patients. Infection usually develops as a diffuse, inflammatory process, known as *cellulitis,* characterized by pain, redness, and swelling. This inflammatory response is the body's initial defense directed toward localization and containment of the infecting agent. Red blood cells, leukocytes, and macrophages infiltrate the cells, with abscess formation (suppuration) often following. An *abscess* is the result of tissue liquefaction with pus formation, supported by bacterial proteolytic enzymes that break down protein and aid in the spread of infection. Fibrolysin, for example, an enzyme produced by hemolytic Streptococcus, may dissolve fibrin and delay localization of a streptococcal infection. However, the body attempts to wall off an abscess by means of a membrane that produces surrounding induration (hardened tissue) and heat. Localized pus should be promptly drained.

If localization is inadequate and does not contain the infectious process, spreading and extension occur, causing regional infection. Microorganisms and their metabolic products are carried from the primary invasion site into the lymphatic system, spreading along anatomic planes, causing lymphangitis. Failure of the lymph nodes to hold the infection results in uncontrolled cellulitis. Subsequently, regional and/or systemic infection may develop, characterized by chills, fever, and signs of toxicity. Septic emboli may enter the circulatory system from septic thrombophlebitis of regional veins communicating with local infections. These emboli and pathogenic microorganisms in the blood seed invasive infection and abscess formation in remote tissues.

Sepsis elevates the patient's metabolic rate 30 to 40 percent above average, imposing additional stress on the vital systems. For example, cardiac output is some 60 percent above normal resting value. The body's defenses and ability to meet the stress govern whether the infectious process progresses to septic shock (see Chap. 29) with grave prognosis, or whether resolution and recovery are the outcome. Multiple infection sites, the presence of shock, and inappropriate antibiotic therapy result in poor prognosis.

The ultimate resolution of infection depends on immunological and inflammatory responses capable of overcoming the infectious process. This is associated with drainage and removal of foreign material, including the debris of bacteria and cells, lysis (disintegration) of microorganisms, resorption of pus, and sloughing of necrotic tissue. Healing then ensues.

Classification of Infections

Surgical infections may be classified in various ways: by source or base, by anatomic location and pathophysiological changes, or by etiology.

Classification by Source This broad classification includes the following infections:

1 Home- or community-based infections. These are natural disease processes that develop or were incubating before a patient's admission to the hospital. *Spontaneous* infections requiring operative diagnosis and/or treatment for management, or as adjuvants to medical therapy, include acute appendicitis and osteomyelitis plus many others. Therapy consists of identification of infection site, etiology, excision or drainage, prevention of further contamination, and augmentation of host resistance.

2 Nosocomial infections. Infections that patients acquire during hospitalization are known as *hospital-acquired, hospital-associated,* or *nosocomial infections.* They may occur as complications of operative or other procedures performed on uninfected patients. The terms also refer to complicating infections in organs unrelated to the operative procedure, occurring with or as a result of postoperative care. Examples of various nosocomial infections are:

   a Cellulitis or abscess formation, related to the operative procedure

b Thrombophlebitis or peritonitis, regional extensions of postoperative or posttraumatic infections
c Liver or lung abscess, visceral infection resulting from operation often performed for penetrating injuries or malignant metastases
d Bacteremia or septicemia, postoperative systemic infection resulting from dissemination of microorganisms into the bloodstream from a distributing focus
e Urinary tract or respiratory tract infection, infected decubiti

Hospital acquired infections may be *exogenous,* from sources outside the body, or *endogenous,* from sources within the body. Most postoperative wound infections result from seeding by endogenous microorganisms. Disruption of the balance between potentially pathogenic organisms and host defenses permits the invasion of microorganisms for which the patient himself is the primary reservoir. For example, abdominal sepsis may result from enteric flora if the intestine is perforated or transected. However, cross contamination occurs when organisms are transferred to the patient from another individual.

Classification by Etiology This classification of infections includes:

1 Bacterial infections. These are infections caused by aerobic bacteria, microaerophilic bacteria, anaerobic bacteria, or mixed infections (aerobic and anaerobic, gram positive and gram negative, synergistic microorganisms).

2 Nonbacterial infections. These infections are caused by fungi or by viruses. Specific organisms are discussed later in this chapter.

Predisposing Factors

Incidence and types of infections that occur in surgical patients are affected by the following factors, which substantially increase the risk of infection.

1 Malnutrition. Whether primary or secondary to catabolic disease, malnutrition is a major factor influencing response to all types of infections since a number of factors, such as inflammatory response, are altered in the malnourished host. Protein deficiency is especially significant in extensive burn or multiple injury patients with greatly raised caloric requirements.

2 Age. Premature infants, newborn infants, and geriatric patients are especially prone to infection.

3 Obesity. Avascular subcutaneous fatty tissues are especially susceptible.

4 Chronic disease. Fibrocystic disease, diabetes, and malignancies upset normal physiology.

5 Remote focus of infection, especially in the respiratory or urinary tracts. Infection is a contraindication for any elective operation. Remote infection increases threefold the chance of wound infection.

6 Impaired defense mechanisms. Immunologic response is deficient because of disease, drug therapy such as steroids and immunosuppressive agents, or radiation. Patients of this status, referred to as *compromised hosts,* are often the victims of infection caused by endogenous microbial flora, which are normal but potentially pathogenic flora within their own bodies. Lack of integrity of the immune system, such as leukopenia or defective immunoglobulin synthesis, can be life-threatening.

7 Cardiovascular or respiratory determinants. Examples are tissue perfusion or structural bronchopulmonary disease.

8 Lengthy preoperative hospitalization. Some organisms maintain virulence by passing from patient to patient. The hospital environment is a concentrated reservoir of microorganisms that can colonize patients, especially those who have received antibiotics. The organisms are rapidly and easily transferred between people and equipment. A noncarrier may become a carrier of an organism that eventually causes an infection of endogenous origin.

9 Certain types of operations. Many procedures involve the genitourinary or gastrointestinal tracts. Some contamination occurs whenever these tracts are opened. Extent of contamination at operation is an important factor.

10 Duration of operation. The longer the procedure, the greater the chance for contamination and infection.

11 Operative technique. Injured ischemic tissues, denuded bone, and microbial and implanted foreign bodies or prosthetic devices have a propensity for microbial invasion. A wound heals faster if tissues are gently handled because fewer cells are destroyed. Necrotic tissue is microbial media. All invasive techniques are potential contaminants.

12 Indiscriminate use of antibiotics (see p. 85). Suppression of normal flora of the skin, bowel, and pharynx, which may play a protective role in defense against pathogenic organisms, may predispose the patient to infection. Antibiotics suppress normal flora.

13 Breakdown of isolation procedures (see p. 84).

14 Lack of knowledge on the part of hospital personnel regarding epidemiology.

In summary, many factors influence the incidence of infection. The exposure of an increasingly high number of high-risk patients to the hospital environment, inhabited by virulent antibiotic-resistant organisms, contributes to infection. High-risk patients increasingly undergo complex and/or prolonged diagnostic and operative procedures under anesthesia. The accompanying instrumentation and use of medical devices open more portals for microbial entry. Complex therapeutic or supportive procedures, such as invasive monitoring by means of indwelling, intra-arterial or intravenous catheters, may provide microorganisms with an entry to the bloodstream. Continuous urinary catheterization increases the prevalence of urinary tract infection. The concommitant administration of drugs that reduce bodily resistance is a significant factor that favors development of nosocomial infection.

Factors Contributing to Infection

It has been said that infection is the unfavorable result of the equation of the dose of microbes multiplied by virulence and divided by resistance. Simply stated, infection results from the interaction of three elements: organisms, tissues, and host defenses.

1 *Pathogenic microorganisms* must be introduced or present, survive, and propagate in the wound or other body tissue. Severity of infection depends in part on the size and virulence of the inoculum (microbe-containing substance). The infecting agent must reach the host.

2 *Local factors* play a role. The location of the operative or invasive site and condition of the tissues therein are significant. Necrotic, devitalized, avascular tissue, or presence of foreign bodies or accumulated blood, enhance infection by providing excellent media for harboring organisms. Various body tissues have different powers of resistance. The abdomen, thigh, calf, and buttocks are especially susceptible. The face, scalp, and chest are more resistant. However, severe traumatic injuries and debilitating chronic diseases can make all tissues susceptible to infection. Other local factors, such as the presence of drains, are significant.

3 *Host defense mechanisms* are extremely important. Knowledge of infectious processes and immunology has become more sophisticated. The biologic relationships between host defense, trauma of operation, and antibiotic therapy are complex. Body responses vary with the type of infecting microorganism, the immune response of the patient, severity of infection, and effectiveness of treatment. The general condition of the patient affects resistance to microbial invasion.

Etiologic Microorganisms

Infections may be caused by one or several types of organisms. The types are numerous and vary in regard to incidence and significance of infection produced. The reader is referred to a standard textbook of microbiology for details.

Bacteria are classified as gram positive or negative and by the environment that sustains their life. The most common pathogens are:

1 Aerobic bacteria
   - a Gram-positive cocci, such as *Staphylococci* and *Streptococci* species
   - b Gram-negative cocci, such as *Neisseria gonorrhoeae*
   - c Gram-negative bacilli, such as *Escherichia coli, Klebsiella* species, *Pseudomonas aeruginosa, Proteus* species, Providence species, *Serratia marcescens, Citrobacter* species, *Salmonella* species, *Alcaligenes fecalis, Hemophilus influenzae, Enterobacter aerogenes, Flavobacteria*
   - d Gram-positive bacilli, such as *Bacillus* species, *Mycobacterium* species

2 Microaerophilic bacteria
   - a Gram-positive cocci, such as hemolytic and nonhemolytic streptococci

3 Anaerobic bacteria
   - a Gram-positive cocci, such as peptostreptococcus, peptococcus
   - b Gram-positive bacilli, such as *Clostridium tetani* and *Clostridium welchii*
   - c Gram-negative bacilli, such as *Bacteroides* species, *B. fragilis*

4 Nonbacterial microorganisms
   - a Viruses, such as *Herpesvirus, Hepatitis virus* (infectious and serum)
   - b Fungi, such as *Candida albicans, Histoplasmosis capsulatum, Phycomycosis* species

NOTE. This list is incomplete but includes *the organisms that most frequently cause nosocomial infections.* Some of the organisms are primary invaders; others are opportunists that secondarily invade or superimpose upon an already infected host with inhibited resistance. Identification of causative organisms will direct investigation, e.g.: streptococcus from personnel, mycobacterium from inanimate objects.

Viability of Organisms Organisms need moisture, food, proper temperature, and time to reproduce. When they are transferred from one place to another, they pass through a dormant or lag phase of about 5 hours. Then each organism divides itself every 20 minutes. Air or objects containing live microorganisms contaminate on contact. Viable microorganisms are killed by the processes of sterilization (see Chap. 5).

Toxins of Microbial Origin Pathogenic microorganisms produce substances that adversely affect the host locally and/or systemically upon invasion. Toxic substances affecting tissues, cells, and possibly enzyme systems are formed by microorganisms incidental to their metabolic activities. These substances diffuse from the microbial cell. The cellular substance of a wide variety of organisms is toxic also. In addition, harmful effects may be produced indirectly by the activation of tissue enzymes by the bacteria. Such toxic substances include the following:

1 *Exotoxins,* classic bacterial toxins, are the most potent toxins known. As little as 7 oz (200 cc) of crystalline botulism type A toxin is said to be able to kill the world's entire population. Exotoxins appear to be proteins, are denatured by heat, and are destroyed by proteolytic enzymes, those which break down protein. The formation of exotoxins is relatively uncommon but their actions are multiple.
2 *Endotoxins* are contained within the cell wall of bacteria. The nature of their toxicity is not clear. Endotoxins are heat stable and are not digested by proteolytic enzymes. On parenteral inoculation they cause a rise in body temperature and are known as *bacterial pyrogens.* They increase capillary permeability with resultant production of local hemorrhage. Although causing injury to body cells at the site of infection, endotoxins more importantly cause serious, often lethal, effects by dissemination and widespread injury to many tissues throughout the body. Endotoxic shock, may occur in bacteremia due to gram-negative bacteria.
3 Microorganisms also form a variety of other heterogeneous toxic substances, often enzymatic in nature, which may contribute to the disease process directly or facilitate the establishment of foci of infection. The toxins, which diffuse from the intact microbial cell, have the following various effects:
   a *Cytotoxic effect* affects red and white blood cells, causing leukopenia (reduction of leukocytes below normal), for example.
   b *Clotting effect* interferes with the clotting mechanism of the blood.
   c *Enzyme effect* causes bacterial hemolysins to dissolve red blood cells or fibrin, thereby inhibiting clot formation. *Coagulase,* a substance of bacterial origin, is causally related to thrombus formation. Coagulase-positive staphylococcus, *B. subtilis, E. coli, S. marcescens,* accelerate clotting of blood and induce intravascular clotting.
4 Toxic substances are also associated with viruses.
5 Some bacteria are encapsulated, a defense mechanism against phagocytic activity of leukocytes. These bacteria may be ingested by white blood cells but instead of being killed and digested they remain within the phagocyte for a time, then are extruded in a viable condition. The presence of a capsule is associated with virulence among pathogenic bacteria.

Wound Infections

Wound infections warrant special attention since they may be acquired in the operating room. The nature and severity of these infections vary because of the myriad of factors involved. These factors may be technical, systemic, local, or environmental. It is difficult to isolate and measure the effect of any one variable since there is no assurance that the other factors have remained constant during the test period. Each factor is important; all are interrelated in clinical infection. The phases of wound healing can be interrupted by infection at almost any level. A wound infection results from the introduction of virulent organisms into the receptive wound of a susceptible host. Response may be local or systemic. Moisture and warmth of wounds create an environment conducive to bacterial growth.

Classification of Operative Wounds Operative wounds may be specifically classified by:

1 Clinical significance
   a *Uninfected.* Heal without discharge.
   b *Possibly infected.* Inflamed, with no discharge, or culture-positive serous fluid.
   c *Infected.* Suppuration present.
2 Contamination-infection risk
   a *Clean.* Gastrointestinal, respiratory, or urinary tract is not entered; no inflamma-

tion is present; no break in technique occurred. May be mechanically drained.

b *Clean-contaminated.* Gastrointestinal, respiratory, or urinary tract is entered without significant spillage. Break in technique occurred. Wound is mechanically drained.

c *Contaminated.* Gross spillage or acute inflammation is encountered. Break in technique occurred. Fresh traumatic wounds.

d *Dirty and infected.* Pus or perforated viscus encountered. Old traumatic wounds from a dirty source, or with necrotic tissue, foreign body (bullet), or fecal contamination.

The infection rate in clean wounds is naturally considerably lower than in contaminated or dirty wounds. The critical issue is elimination of infection in clean wounds, for overt tissue destruction may result from infection. Wound sepsis remains one of the prime problems in the surgeon's daily practice (see Chaps. 12 and 29).

SOURCES OF CONTAMINATION

In spite of the fact that there are many variables associated with sepsis, people remain the major source of microorganisms that continually contaminate an environment. Everything on or about a human being is contaminated by him or her in some way. Additionally, the action and interaction of personnel and patients contribute to the prevalance of organisms.

Operating room personnel are primarily concerned with protecting the environment of the operating room suite. The Committee on Operating Room Environment (CORE), a standing committee of the American College of Surgeons (ACS), functions to oversee and improve this environment. Use of the OR should ensure that operative procedures will be performed under optimal conditions within the limits of professional capability. Carl Walter, MD, has identified the three most salient areas of sources for the introduction and spread of microorganisms. They are:

1 The outer interchange area, which is opened to personnel generally

2 The restricted intermediate zone open to properly attired authorized personnel

3 The sterile work area or inner zone, occupied by the operating teams and patients, including the operating rooms, scrub rooms, and induction areas (see Chap. 6)

Many sources contaminate the OR environment. These are:

Skin

Skin of patients, operating team members, and visitors constitutes a hazard. Hair follicles, sebaceous and sweat glands (sudoriferous) contain abundant resident microbial flora. An estimated 4000 to 10,000 viable particles are shed by an average individual's skin per minute. Some people disperse up to 30,000 particles per minute. *Shedders* are persons who present an additional hazard in that they are densely populated with virulent organisms that they shed with skin cells into the environment. The organisms usually are *Staphylococcus aureus.* Shedders have a much higher incidence of wound infection. True shedders are estimated to be 1 in 50 persons. Cosmetic detritus is also laden with skin bacteria. Major areas of microbial population on all persons are the head, neck, axilla, hands, groin, perineum, and feet. Microbial shedding is contained most effectively by maximum skin coverage.

Hair

Hair is a gross contaminant and major source of Staphylococcus. The microbial population attracted to and shed from hair is directly related to length and cleanliness. Hair follicles and filaments harbor resident and transient flora.

Nasopharynx

Organisms forcibly expelled by talking, coughing, or sneezing give rise to bacteria-laden dust and lint as droplets settle on surfaces and skin. Persons known as *carriers* harbor many organisms, notably *Group A Streptococcus,* which may be carried pharyngeally or rectally. These organisms usually are transmitted by direct contact. More surgeons and anesthesiologists are carriers than nurses because of their intimate contact with patients' respiratory tracts. Carriers do not usually present a real threat in the absence of an overt lesion. However, when clusters of infection break out postoperatively, shedders and carriers who disseminate organisms and whose organism matches that of infected patients are sought.

Fomites

Contaminated particles are present on inanimate objects such as furniture, operating room surfaces (walls, floors, cabinet shelves), equipment, supplies, linens. Stringent measures, to be discussed, are used to control contact contamination from such sources. Covert contamination may result, however, from improper handling of equipment such as anesthesia apparatus, or intravenous lines and fluids. Contamination may result from the administration of unsterile medications or use of unsterile water to rinse sterile items.

Air

Thousands of submicron size particles per cubic foot of air are present in the OR. During a long operative procedure, the particle count can rise to over a million particles per cubic foot. From the refuse in ventilation filters observed in one study, an estimated 10 to 20 milligrams (mg) of debris may be shed by each individual in the room during the course of an operation. Air and dust are vehicles for transporting microorganism-laden particles. Air movement and thermal currents entrain dust and microbial particulates that remain airborne and can then settle onto open wounds, burns, or other susceptible tissue. Since airborne contamination is generated by personnel, every movement increases the chance of wound infection.

Microorganisms have an affinity for horizontal surfaces, the largest of which is the floor. From it, they are projected into the air. Floor cultures are a good index of the infectivity of the environment since they are a qualitative and quantitative reflection of the microorganisms in the area.

Endogenous as well as exogenous microbial flora carriage is significant. The patient's skin, oropharynx, tracheobronchial tree, and gastrointestinal tract support the growth of innumerable organisms, which reflects the amount and kind of infection in the hospital population. Microorganisms from infected patients or carriers settle on equipment and flat surfaces, then become airborne.

An effective ventilation system is essential to avoid patients and staff breathing contaminated air that predisposes them to respiratory infection and that increases the incidence of microbial carriers among OR personnel. It is generally believed, however, that objects, not air, are the major vehicles for the transmission of pathogens and that person-to-person contact remains the most frequent means by which infection is spread.

Human Error

An exogenous source of contamination not to be underestimated is human error. Lives are at stake, no less so if breaks in technique occur through lack of knowledge or lack of adherence to principles of technique and their applications. Errors must be readily admitted and corrected.

INFECTION CONTROL

Infection control translates knowledge into action. It incorporates development and maintenance of an attitude of awareness of infection with acceptance of individual and collective responsibility to prevent infection. It has been said, unfortunately, that a professional staff is the only thing more adaptable than microorganisms in circumventing controls. Although the scope of infection control encompasses the entire hospital, the focus of this text is infection control in the surgical patient, primarily control of wound infection that can obviate the benefits of surgical intervention.

Purposes

The purposes of infection control are to:

1 Minimize infection, and hopefully to eventually obliterate it
2 Improve wound healing
3 Minimize disability, morbidity, and mortality
4 Reduce the cost of hospital care

The many aspects of infection control include:

1 Establishment and utilization of an effective infection control program
2 Recognition of hazards and consistent adherence to established control practices
3 Provision of maximum protection to patients by means of physical barriers to microorganisms and functional measures of control
4 Limitation of the use of antibiotics apt to result in resistant strains of microorganisms

Infection Control Program

An effective infection control program aims to reduce the incidence of infections and to control sources. Information collected through surveillance serves as a basis for corrective action. This information includes written records and reports of known or potential infections among patients and personnel.

Guidelines and standards for a comprehensive

infection control program and surveillance have been published by the Joint Commission on the Accreditation of Hospitals (JCAH), a voluntary agency of professional surveyors that formulates national standards for accreditation. *The reader is referred to the JCAH Accreditation Manual for Hospitals for complete details.* In general, these standards and guidelines include:

1 The establishment of an effective hospital infection control program monitored by a multidisciplinary committee (infection control committee)
2 The development of specific written infection control policies and procedures for all services throughout the hospital
3 Preventive surveillance and control procedures relating to the hospital environment
4 Provision for essential laboratory support
5 Written policies defining indications for isolation and necessary provisions for it
6 Definitions of nosocomial infections for surveillance purposes to provide for early uniform identification and reporting of infections
7 Determination of hospital infection rates
8 Coordination with the medical staff on action regarding findings from the staff's review of clinical use of antibiotics
9 Ongoing review and evaluation of all aseptic, isolation, and environmental control techniques of the hospital
10 Orientation of new employees in regard to personal hygiene and the importance of infection control while caring for patients
11 Input into content and scope of employee health service
12 Reporting, evaluating, and maintaining records of infections that occur in patients and personnel

Infection Control Coordinator

An infection control program utilizes the services of a key person and agent of the infection control committee, the *infection control coordinator.* Since this person is often a registered nurse with special training in epidemiology, microbiology, statistics, and research methodology, he or she may be referred to as an *infection control nurse* (ICN) or *nurse epidemiologist.* The infection control coordinator keeps his or her finger on the pulse of the infection situation in the hospital by monitoring the hospital environment for infections. While in close collaboration with the infection control committee, the ICN's duties include all aspects of control activities such as:

1 Prompt investigation of outbreaks of disease or infection above expected levels.
2 Prompt identification of the origin and etiology of such outbreaks by epidemiologic study.
3 Acquisition, correlation, analysis, and evaluation of surveillance data and bacterial colony counts for infection control.
4 Tracing factors that contribute to infection problems.
5 Consultation with supervisors of critical areas, such as the OR. In the case of clusters of wound infections, the ICN confers with the ORS and reviews the OR log to see if the infected patients had the same procedure, same operating team, or operative problem.
6 Conduction of educational programs for personnel who influence infection control. The ICN is a consultant to all hospital personnel.
7 Assistance in employee health programs in regard to screening, immunizing, and monitoring personal health of OR personnel.
8 Assistance in development and implementation of improved patient care procedures.
9 Comparison of monthly statistics. There is cause for concern if the monthly reported operative wound infection rate rises significantly. Reports and data can help improve aseptic technique, if brought to attention of personnel.
10 Supervision of reporting appropriate diseases to public health authorities.
11 Comparison of products for effectiveness.

In short, the infection control coordinator identifies problems, collects data to find the causes, investigates solutions, and makes recommendations for determining hospital policies and procedures relative to infection control. In working with infection problems, the ICN's main aim is to find a common denominator. This often leads to the source of the problem. For example, an outbreak of postoperative respiratory infections would lead to investigation of cleaning and sterilization of anesthesia equipment and respirators. If the patient develops signs and symptoms of infection within the immediate postoperative period, a causative factor in the OR is suspect. A ratio of one coordinator for every 250 beds in the hospital has been recommended. The success of the control program depends in part on the information provided by a conscientious coordinator.

Surveillance

The Center for Disease Control (CDC) in Atlanta is an agency of the Department of Health, Education and Welfare. It is also the third largest section of the United States Public Health Service. Functioning on both national and international levels, its activities are multifaceted. It carries out a national surveillance of disease incidence and a broad national program against disease, including health education, especially in regard to communicable diseases. Through liaison with state and local health departments, assistance and consultation from the Center are available to local hospitals when there is need for specific problem solving, analysis of surveillance data, or on-site investigation of a serious infection outbreak. As part of its commitment to the prevention of nosocomial infections, the Center conducts a National Nosocomial Infections Study, a nationwide surveillance program in cooperation with participating hospitals.

The agency also furnishes to hospitals information on how to structure an infection control program. In addition, CDC renders aid to local or state health departments in times of epidemics.

Utilization of the Center's facilities is optimized in the training course that the Center sponsors for nurses who wish to work in infection control. This unique course includes basic microbiology, principles and methodology of epidemiology, role of the infection control nurse, and guidance in setting up a hospital infection control program. Follow-up support is given the trainees in their subsequent work situations, as needed.

The CDC provides a worldwide service as a valuable resource for information. Its many publications include: *Outline for Surveillance and Control of Nosocomial Infections; Isolation Techniques for Use in Hospitals; Guidelines for Prevention of TB Transmission in Hospitals;* and *Morbidity and Mortality Weekly Report.* In conjunction with continuous research, the Center's established guidelines for intravenous therapy, respiratory therapy, urinary catheterization, and other at-risk procedures present further evidence of CDC's concern with infection control measures.

Effective action results from adequate background information. An important aspect of infection control, *surveillance* involves input or data collection, analysis, and action or regulatory activities. Quality control, establishment of and conformance to standards, is a prerequisite for rational infection control. The value of a surveillance program is the establishment of a statistical data base that can be subsequently correlated with testing to locate a problem or pinpoint changes in infection rates over a period of time. This is accomplished by a comprehensive culturing program or careful periodic checks on the effectiveness of essential equipment, for example, of sterilizers and anesthesia equipment. However, extensive random bacteriologic sampling of personnel and environment when no problem exists is not recommended by the CDC.

Effective surveillance, predicated on an understanding of epidemiology, requires:

1 Investigation of every instance where a patient becomes infected to ascertain if the infection is nosocomial or community-acquired.
2 Prompt reporting of infection in any patient to define incidence and type of infection in the hospital.
3 Monitoring of hospital patients, personnel, and environment according to written standards.
4 Identification of factors that place a patient at risk.
5 Clear definitions of infections, an infection control coordinator, computerized records. Storage and programming provide comparisons.
6 Monitoring of wound infection rate to alert the staff to deviations from normal and to permit assessment of the value of changes in procedures. Standards continually change because of technological developments.
7 Protection of the patient from reasonable risk for which reasonable control is available. Alerting the surgeon to symptoms of an infection. These measures help to avoid litigation.

Surveillance data are studied to ascertain trends of infection, high rates associated with specific surgical services or operative procedures, or clustering in certain areas. Microbiological surveys are important in evaluating procedures. For example, sampling of floors indicates if the cleaning procedure is effective. Surveys help to answer the question, "What is the problem?" Surveillance, therefore, provides a basis for improving conditions, procedures, and the quality of patient care.

ENVIRONMENTAL CONTROL

The *operating room environment* is the area of the hospital in which operative procedures are performed. Environmental control is a necessary part of an infection control program because of involvement of the inanimate environment, as well as the animate, in the transmission of infection and disease. Concentration is on high-risk areas and procedures. The aim of a microbiologically controlled environment is to keep contamination to an irreducible minimum and to maintain balance in favor of the patient, not of the microorganisms.

OR suites are designed with optimal function and safety in mind and to protect patients from sources of contamination and to provide the least travel distance for them. The suite includes specific areas for traffic, support systems, administration, communication, and storage. There should be a distinct separation of clean and soiled activities, areas, and personnel as well as of sterile and unsterile supplies. Traffic patterns are designed to flow smoothly and to prevent backtrack or cross-over traffic (see Chap. 6).

Barriers

The establishment of barriers is for the purpose of isolating the operative wound from infectious contaminants. *Barriers* retard or prevent the transfer of microorganisms. Various types include:

1 Barriers to skin
  - **a** Preoperative skin preparation of the patient (see Chap. 11) and operating team (see Chap. 7).
  - **b** Special OR attire worn only within the OR suite (see Chap. 7).
  - **c** Sterile drapes to cover the patient and sterile field (see Chap. 11).
  - **d** Occlusion of incised skin edges from the operative wound (see Chap. 11).

2 Barriers to nasopharyngeal flora and hair
  - **a** Wearing of masks and hoods, part of attire.
  - **b** Removal of hair from operative site (see Chap. 11).
  - **c** Exclusion from the OR of personnel with acute infection or skin lesion.
  - **d** Use of anesthesia screen to separate anesthesia area from sterile field.

3 Barrier to fomites
  - **a** Proper packaging of supplies, and sterilizing procedures (see Chap. 5).
  - **b** Dust covers placed over cool, dry sterile items in storage.
  - **c** Disinfection of OR surfaces, although no residual environmental disinfectant exists.
  - **d** Clean, preoperative bed linen.

4 Barriers to airborne contamination
  - **a** *Conventional air-conditioning systems,* when properly designed, installed, and maintained, effectively reduce the number of airborne bacteria by removing dust and aerosol particles. As fresh clean outside air is supplied, lint- and dust-contaminated air is removed. Recirculation of filtered air at a rate of no less than 25 air exchanges per hour is considered safe and economical. The system reduces organisms to 1 to 3 per cubic foot. The dilution principle is used. Air enters from the ceiling, is diluted, and passes out through the lower portion of the room. Filters should be located downstream of air-processing equipment so microorganisms will not be drawn into the room. Warming and cooling fresh air to totally resupply the OR air is an expensive procedure.
  - **b** *Laminar airflow* is a special air-handling system for improving the filtration, dilution, and distribution of air. It is used during high-risk procedures such as total hip replacement or other procedures in high-risk patients. Laminar airflow is a controlled unidirectional, positive pressure stream of air that moves either horizontally or vertically across the operative area and room. The controlled airstream entrains particulate matter and microorganisms, thereby preventing their drifting with uncontrolled movement; it sweeps up dormant particles as well. The flow returns to the system, passes through a prefilter to remove gross particles, and then passes through a high-efficiency particulate air (HEPA) filter in each module that traps and eliminates over 99 percent of all particles larger than 0.3 micron. This includes virtually all bacteria and most viruses. A rate of 100 to 400 air changes per hour is possible, with most systems delivering about 240 an hour. While the system provides microbial-free air (0 to 1 organism per cubic foot), *it is not a substitute for meticulous aseptic technique.* There is no substantial evidence to date that the decrease in particle count results in a significantly reduced rate of operative wound infection.

    The system is available in horizontal or vertical flow, and comes with a vacuum hose inlet for use with multiple negative pressure masks and gowns. This unique attire of a bodysuit and hood vacuum system, resembling a spacesuit, prevents bacteria shed by the team from reaching the patient. The entire body is covered. Air, piped into the headpiece, is removed through filtered tubes. The hood or helmet is wired for hearing and speaking. Negative pressure gowns are impervious to moisture and microorganisms. No mask is needed with the helmet. The system provides for the appropriate body cooling of the wearer.

    Unidirectional clean-air systems are a valuable adjunct to controlling airborne contamination. They reliably reduce bacterial contamination at the wound site.

NOTE. A bioclean room, a special enclosure within an OR, referred to as a *greenhouse,* is used in some locales in conjunction with laminar airflow.

c Traffic in and out of the OR, necessitating opening and closing doors, must be kept to a minimum, as well as the number of persons within an OR during preparation and operation. Cabinet doors should also remain closed.

d The application of a textile lubricant to the final rinse during laundering minimizes lint resulting from friction of fibers against each other. Disintegrated paper from disposable products is a source of lint on fabrics. Therefore, paper products should not be discarded with soiled linen.

Housekeeping

Excellent housekeeping practices using the most effective supplies, techniques, and equipment available are a most important aspect of infection control. *Housekeeping* procedures include cleaning and disinfecting the operating rooms and suite, handling soiled laundry, and disposing of solid wastes. They are carried out according to established practices, policies, and schedules. These procedures are performed by environmental service personnel under supervision. Good housekeeping cleaning techniques should reduce microbial flora by about 90 percent. *Detergent-disinfectants alone are no substitute for thorough mechanical cleansing,* the proverbial elbow grease. Locations that by design or construction are difficult to clean, and areas that may be touched by patients or personnel are of primary concern.

Any equipment or procedure requiring water in its operation presents a hazard, especially if water is not continually changed or sinks cleaned. Unsterile water, the universal solvent and transporter, can support, maintain, and protect almost every contaminant produced by human beings. The numbers, types, and species of microorganisms in a water supply are limited only by the attention paid the equipment containing it. Water especially supports the growth of certain gram-negative bacilli, including *Pseudomonas, Alcaligenes, Flavobacterium* genus. Aerosols produced during the hand scrub of the team become airborne, and contaminate. Disinfectants reduce the contamination of cleaning water.

Some points in housekeeping especially relevant to infection control and prevention of cross infection are listed below to emphasize the importance of OR environmental control.

1 Faucet heads should be a type that does not hold water. They should be removed for sterilization. Handwash antiseptic containers should be sterilized before refill.

2 No surface should remain wet, thereby supporting microbial growth.

3 Organic debris should be promptly removed from walls and OR surfaces with a germicide to prevent drying and airborne contamination.

4 Lights and overhead tracks should be cleaned at least twice daily.

5 The entrance to the OR suite as well as other floors in corridors and rooms should be cleaned with the wet-vacuum system; i.e., dry debris is removed with dry vacuum, the floor is sprayed with detergent-disinfectant solution and wet-vacuumed.

6 Housekeeping equipment should be kept clean and dry, and never stored moist in a dark area conducive to microbial growth.

7 Disposable waste should be put in covered receptacles lined with plastic liners.

8 Service elevators rather than chutes should be used to remove soiled laundry and waste disposal from the OR suite. Chutes become grossly contaminated and are both an airborne contamination and a fire hazard.

9 Waste should be contained at the source of origin to prevent aerosol generation during handling. Contaminated waste must be decontaminated and/or sterilized before compaction or disposal in the general environment. Incineration is the most effective means of waste disposal, especially of infectious wastes.

10 *Adequate time must be allowed between patients for proper terminal disinfection of the room and sterilization of supplies at the conclusion of the operation.*

NOTE. The OR supervisor must not assign a patient to any OR of questionable environment from which the patient might acquire a wound infection.

Isolation

Isolation of patients by diagnosis or prognosis is another means of infection control. The specific technique is related to the mode of transmission of pathogenic microorganisms, i.e., contact, air, or fomites. The two general types of isolation are:

1 Isolation of known infected patients to prevent colonization of organisms in personnel and other patients.

2 Protective or reverse isolation to protect patients with impaired immune defenses, especially organ transplant and burn patients, from extraneous microbial contamination. The isolated patient exists in a self-contained environment.

Isolation precautions and guidelines are detailed in hospital procedure books, and in a CDC manual, *Isolation Techniques for Use in Hospitals.* Variations in availability of and demands for isolation facilities affect their utilization. Common categories of isolation are strict isolation, respiratory precautions, wound or skin precautions, enteric precautions. Isolation techniques must not be implemented in a way that would cause the patient to feel victimized. The patient should be educated to accept the regimen.

Cross Infection in the OR Specific isolation precautions are observed in the OR, as indicated, in addition to routine aseptic techniques. While each patient in the OR should be considered a potentially infected one, terminal cleaning and disinfection are especially important following operation on a patient with established infection or communicable disease.

Care, caution, and competence contribute greatly to the prevention of *cross infection,* which stems mainly from lack of proper technique by involved personnel. Aseptic technique is an important factor. The more microorganisms are prevented from entering an environment, the greater the chance of lowering the cross-infection rate. *The importance of thorough handwashing cannot be overemphasized.*

Tuberculosis Tuberculosis is caused by *Mycobacterium tuberculosis,* an aerobic gram-positive bacillus. While the incidence of the disease in the general population has decreased, treatment takes place in the general hospital, increasing the risk of transmission. In the hospital, the disease must be monitored and controlled to prevent cross infection. Unsuspected active cases represent a particular hazard. Patients with acute disease are isolated for at least 2 weeks following initiation of chemotherapy. For care of surgical patients, recommendation has been made to:

1 Postpone elective operation in active cases until the patient shows response to chemotherapy.
2 Use disposable anesthesia equipment as much as is feasible. Reusable equipment must be immediately sterilized after use.
3 Use respiratory isolation precautions for suspected patients and those with positive sputum.

Hepatitis The OR and hemodialysis unit are high-risk areas for contracting hepatitis because of the team's intimate contact with the patient's blood, blood products, and with equipment such as needles and intravenous lines. While hepatitis is acquired by oral or parenteral routes, the transmission route of a hospital-acquired disease is not entirely clear. A significant proportion of cases of infectious hepatitis results from exposure other than parenteral injection of blood. Personnel safeguards include:

1 Impeccable handwashing and decontamination of equipment and materials
2 Avoidance of parenteral exposure such as accidental self-puncture with a contaminated needle
3 Possibly enteric precautions of isolation as per hospital routine

Operative Technique Mentioned repeatedly, operative technique is one of the most important factors influencing wound healing (see Chap. 12). The acronym GEM should apply to the surgeon: gentle, expeditious, and meticulous.

An important factor in technique is the use of a sterile instrument tray for wound closure in infectious procedures to reduce inoculum delivered to the wound. If infection is obvious at the time of operation, implantation of organisms into susceptible tissue must be avoided. Tissue traumatized during operation, such as that of the chest or abdominal wall, can be protected by the use of fresh sterile instruments for wound closure. In fact, it is advisable to isolate wound closure materials and equipment on the instrument table so that every wound may be closed with previously unused instruments.

Antibiotic Therapy

Antibiotics, sometimes referred to as *antimicrobial drugs,* are a prominent part of the surgeon's armamentarium. They act by killing or inhibiting the growth of bacteria. *Antibiotics are adjuvants to, not substitutes for, strict adherence to aseptic principles and careful operative technique.* A major problem developed when indiscriminate use of these drugs led to the development of resistant strains of organisms that concentrate in patients and the environment. Also, the efficacy of antibiotics is greatly reduced when multiple organisms are involved in the infection. Sufficient risk of infection should warrant their use. Patients should be questioned as to allergy before the drug is administered and closely watched for signs of toxicity, as evidenced by skin rash, gastrointestinal disturbance, renal disorder, fever, or blood dyscrasia. Antibiotics are utilized in the following two ways:

1 *Therapeutically,* to eliminate sensitive, viable organisms during a period with clinical evidence

of infection. A broad-spectrum drug may be given while awaiting results of cultures and sensitivity tests.

2 *Prophylactically,* to prevent development of infection. A preventive antibiotic is one that is given prior to surgical intervention, bacterial invasion, or clinically evident infection. Preoperative antibiotics are effective as supplements to host defense mechanisms in selected patients. The question does not seem to be whether to use prophylactic antibiotics, but rather the dosage and duration of administration. The outcome of infection is determined in the first few hours after bacterial invasion. This is due to the fact that capillary permeability and host response are at a peak immediately after bacterial contamination. Therefore, timing of drug administration is crucial. The antibiotic must be present before bacterial inoculation because response is more intense as the dose of bacteria increases. Selection of an appropriate drug and early use are pertinent factors in preventing infection.

The organisms must be sensitive to the drug. Susceptibility of microorganisms to antibiotics varies widely depending on multiple factors. Period of administration should avoid potential side effects and conversion to resistance. An effective blood level should be attained before the patient comes to the OR or the bacteria invade. Systemic administration is recommended, since the antibiotic must reach the site of potential infection to be effective. The action of the drug must not be inhibited at the site of bacterial activity. To be effective, a prophylactic antibiotic should be present in adequate concentration at or prior to the time of contamination or bacterial invasion.

Drug selection is governed by considerations such as the site of operation, the potential pathogens to be found there, and the patient's history of sensitivity. The antibiotic is administered preoperatively, intraoperatively, and for a short period postoperatively. The use of prophylactic antibiotics is indicated in:

1 Clean wounds, only in instances of known carriers or insertion of prosthetic implants

2 Clean-contaminated wounds, in specific procedures such as transection of the large intestine, biliary tract procedure, or penetrating trauma

3 Contaminated or dirty wounds, with gross contamination

4 Traumatic wounds, with incomplete debridement or delayed closure

5 Extensive procedures for metastatic malignancies (compromised host)

Trend in Infection There has been a drastic change in the pattern of life-threatening infections since the advent of broad-spectrum antibiotics and penicillinase-resistant penicillins. *Penicillinase* is an enzyme found in many bacteria, which antagonizes the action of penicillin. While gram-positive bacteria (staphylococci, pneumococci, and beta-hemolytic streptococci) continue their pathogenic activity, it is the resistant gram-negative bacilli, aerobic and anaerobic, which deeply concern clinicians. Gram-negative infections have increased fourteenfold in 15 years. Another grave concern is the increasing incidence of gram-negative infections by bacteria of supposedly low virulence (*Serratia*), capable of causing deep, latent infections. These organisms all rapidly colonize hospitalized patients, and are transferred to other individuals by hands or equipment.

NEED FOR STERILE TECHNIQUE

Strict aseptic and sterile techniques are needed at all times in the operating room. Freshly incised or traumatized tissue easily can become infected. Intact skin is the body's first line of defense against infection. Infraction of the integrity of the skin creates a portal of entry for microorganisms. Therefore, anything unsterile in contact with the patient is potentially dangerous. All operative procedures are performed under sterile conditions. Conversely, terminal decontamination and sterilization of all material and equipment used during an operation is performed with the assumption that *every patient is a potential source of infection for other persons.*

It is essential that all members of the operating team know the common sources of contamination by microorganisms in the operating room, and the means by which they reach the sterile field and operative wound. Sterile technique is the responsibility of everyone caring for the patient in the OR. *All members of the operating team must be ever vigilant in safeguarding the sterility of the operative field.*

PRINCIPLES OF STERILE TECHNIQUE AND ILLUSTRATIONS OF APPLICATION

Strict adherence to sound principles of sterile technique is mandatory for the safety of the patient. This adherence reflects one's surgical conscience. *Principles remain the same; it is the degree of adherence to them that varies.* The principles of sterile technique are applied:

1 In preparation for operation, by sterilization of necessary materials and supplies
2 In preparation of the operating team to handle sterile supplies and to intimately contact the wound
3 In creation and maintenance of a sterile field, including preparation and drape of the patient, in order to prevent contamination of the wound
4 In maintenance of sterility and asepsis throughout the operative procedure
5 In terminal sterilization and disinfection at conclusion of operation

If the principles are understood, the need for their application becomes obvious. Sterile technique is the basis of modern surgery.

Principles

Only Sterile Items Are Used within a Sterile Field Some items such as linen, sponges, or basins may be obtained from the stock supply of sterile packages. Others, such as instruments, may be sterilized immediately preceding the operation and removed directly from the sterilizer to the sterile tables. Every person who dispenses a sterile article must be sure of its sterility and of its remaining sterile until used. Proper packaging, sterilizing, and handling should provide such assurance. *If you are in doubt about the sterility of anything, consider it not sterile.* Known or potentially contaminated items must not be transferred to the sterile field, for example:

1 If a sterilized package is found in a nonsterile workroom.
2 If you are uncertain about actual timing or operation of a sterilizer.
3 If an unsterile person comes into close contact with a sterile table and vice versa.
4 If a sterile table or unwrapped sterile items are not under constant observation.
5 If a sterile package falls to the floor, it must be discarded (see Chap. 8, p. 142).

Gowns Are Considered Sterile Only from the Waist to Shoulder Level in Front, and the Sleeves The following practices must be observed:

1 Sterile persons keep hands in sight and at or above waist level (see Fig. 4-1).
2 Hands are kept away from the face and elbows close to one's sides. Arms are never folded because there may be perspiration in the axillary region.
3 Changing table levels is avoided. If a sterile person must stand on a platform to reach the operative field, the area of the gown below the waist must not brush against sterile tables or draped areas.
4 Items dropped below waist level are considered unsterile, and must be discarded.

Tables Are Sterile Only at Table Level The result is that:

1 Only the top of a sterile draped table is considered sterile. The edges and sides of the drape extending below table level are considered unsterile.
2 Anything falling over or extending over the table edge, such as a piece of suture, is unsterile. The scrub nurse or technician does not touch the part hanging below table level.
3 In unfolding a sterile drape, care is taken that the part that drops below table surface is not brought back up to table level.

Persons Who Are Sterile Touch Only Sterile Items or Areas; Persons Who Are Not Sterile Touch Only Unsterile Items or Areas For example:

1 The sterile team members maintain contact with the sterile field by means of sterile gowns and gloves.
2 The nonsterile circulating nurse does not directly contact the sterile field.
3 Supplies for sterile team members reach them by means of the circulating nurse opening the wrappers on sterile packages.

Unsterile Persons Avoid Reaching over a Sterile Field; Sterile Persons Avoid Leaning over an Unsterile Area For example:

1 The unsterile circulating nurse *never* reaches over a sterile field to transfer sterile items.

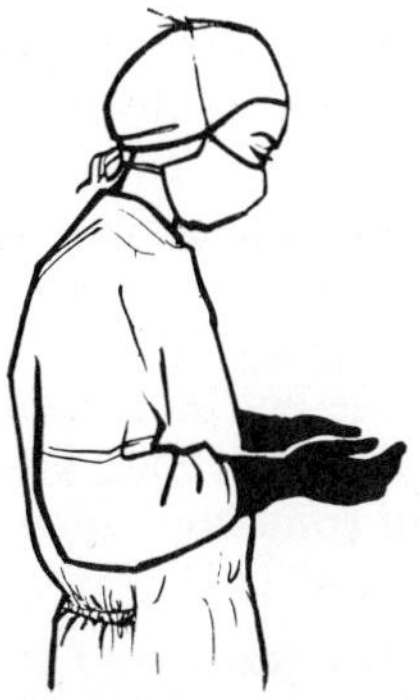

Figure 4-1 Sterile person keeps the hands in sight and at or above waist level. Gowns are considered sterile only from waist to shoulder level in front.

2 In pouring solution into a sterile basin, the circulating nurse holds only the lip of the bottle over the basin to avoid reaching over a sterile area (see Fig. 4-2).

3 The scrub nurse sets basins or glasses to be filled at the edge of the sterile table; the circulating nurse stands near this edge of the table to fill them.

4 The circulating nurse stands at a distance from the sterile field to adjust the light over it to avoid microbial fallout over the field.

5 The surgeon turns away from the sterile field to have perspiration removed from his or her brow.

6 The scrub nurse drapes a nonsterile table toward her first to protect her gown (see Fig. 4-3).

7 The scrub nurse stands back from a nonsterile table when draping it to avoid leaning over an unsterile area (see Figs. 4-4, 4-5, 4-6).

The Edges of Anything That Encloses Sterile Contents Are Considered Unsterile Boundaries between sterile and unsterile are not always rigidly defined, for example, the edges of the wrappers on sterile packages and the caps on solution bottles. The following precautions should be taken:

1 In opening sterile packages, a margin of safety is always maintained. The ends of flaps are secured in the hand so they do not dangle loosely. The last flap is pulled toward the person opening the package thereby exposing package contents away from the nonsterile hand.

2 Sterile persons lift contents from packages by reaching down and lifting them straight up, holding elbows high.

3 Steam reaches only the area within the gasket of a sterilizer. Instrument trays should not touch the edge of the sterilizer outside the gasket.

4 Flaps on peel-open packages should be pulled back, not torn, to expose sterile contents. Contents should be flipped or lifted upward and not permitted to slide over the edges. The inner edge of the heat seal is considered to be the line of demarcation between sterile and unsterile.

5 If a sterile wrapper is used as a table cover, it should amply cover the entire table surface. Only the interior and surface level of the cover are considered sterile.

6 After a sterile bottle is opened, the contents must be used or discarded. The cap cannot be replaced without contamination of pouring edges.

A Sterile Field Is Created as Close as Possible to the Time of Use The degree of contamination is proportionate to the length of time sterile items are uncovered and exposed to the environment. Precautions must be taken as follows.

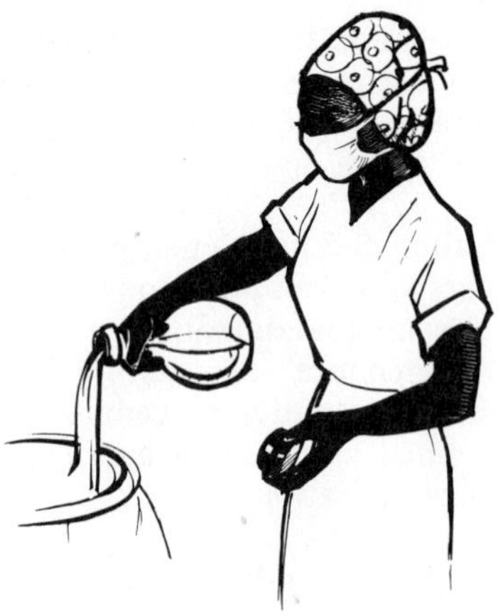

Figure 4-2 Circulating nurse pouring sterile solution into a sterile basin. Note that only the lip of the bottle is over the basin. A nonsterile person avoids reaching over a sterile field.

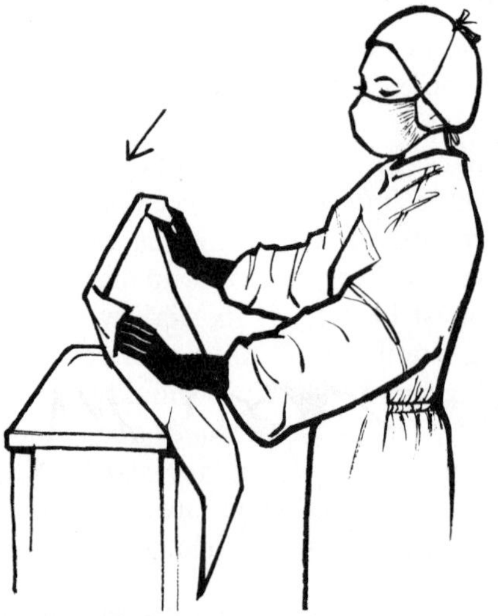

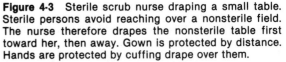

Figure 4-3 Sterile scrub nurse draping a small table. Sterile persons avoid reaching over a nonsterile field. The nurse therefore drapes the nonsterile table first toward her, then away. Gown is protected by distance. Hands are protected by cuffing drape over them.

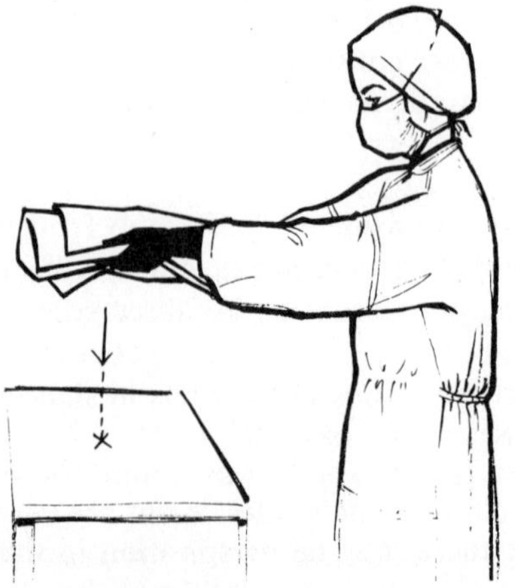

Figure 4-4 Draping a large nonsterile table. Scrub nurse holds the sterile fan-folded table drape high and drops it onto the center of the table, standing back from the table to protect her gown.

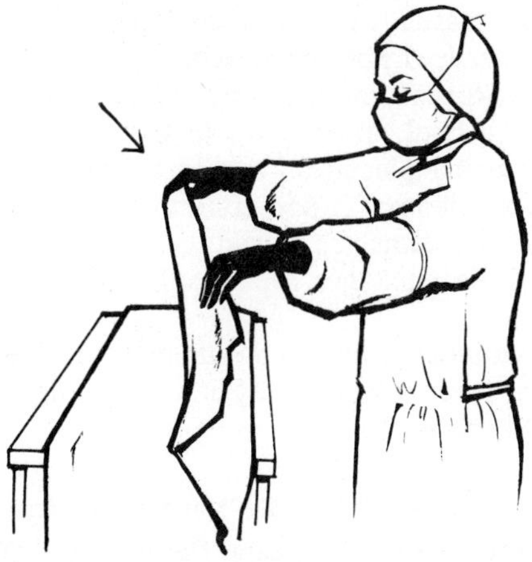

Figure 4-5 Scrub nurse unfolding sterile table drape. She stands back from the nonsterile table and unfolds the drape first toward her. Note that hands are inside the sterile cover to protect them.

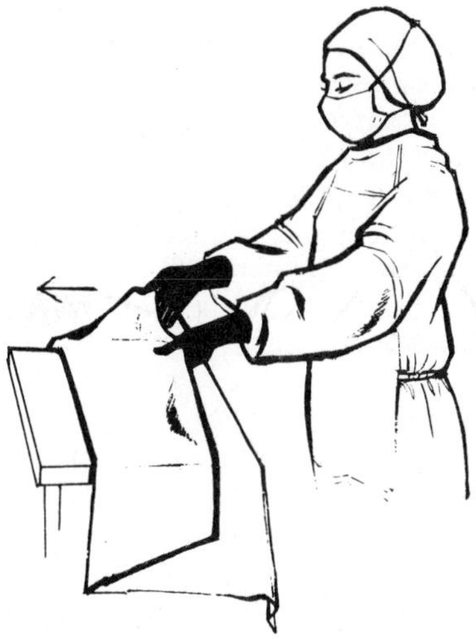

Figure 4-6 Nurse continuing to unfold the sterile table drape. Hands are inside the sterile cover for protection. She may now move closer to the table, since the first part of the unfolded drape now protects her gown.

1 Sterile tables are set up just prior to the operation (see Chap. 8, p. 135).

2 It is difficult to uncover a table of sterile contents without contamination. Covering sterile tables for later use is not recommended. Care must be taken to avoid the edges of the table cover touching the table contents. Two people, one at each end, simultaneously peel back the cover.

Sterile Areas Are Continuously Kept in View Inadvertent contamination of sterile areas must be readily visible. In order to ensure this principle:

1 Sterile persons face sterile areas.

2 Once sterile packs are open in a room, or a sterile field set up, someone must remain in the room to maintain vigilance.

Sterile Persons Keep Well within the Sterile Area They allow a wide margin of safety when passing unsterile areas and follow these rules for passing:

1 Sterile persons stand back at a safe distance from the operating table when draping the patient.

2 Sterile persons pass each other back to back (see Fig. 4-7).

3 A sterile person turns his or her back to a nonsterile person or area when passing.

4 A sterile person faces a sterile area when passing it.

5 A sterile person asks a nonsterile individual to step aside rather than risk contamination.

6 Sterile persons stay within the sterile field. They *do not wander* around or go outside the room.

7 Movement within and around a sterile area is kept to a minimum to avoid contamination of sterile items or persons.

Sterile Persons Keep Contact with Sterile Areas to a Minimum The following rules are observed:

1 Sterile persons do not lean on sterile tables and on the draped patient.

2 Sitting or leaning against a nonsterile surface is a break in technique. If the sterile team sits to operate, they do so without proximity to nonsterile areas.

Unsterile Persons Avoid Sterile Areas A wide margin of safety must be maintained when passing sterile areas. Follow the rule for passing: unsterile persons face and observe a sterile area when passing it to be sure they do not touch it. The circulating nurse restricts all activity to a minimum near sterile areas.

Destruction of the Integrity of Microbial Barriers Results in Contamination The integrity of a sterile package or sterile drape is destroyed by perforation, puncture, or strike-through. *Strike-through* is the soaking of moisture through unsterile layers to sterile layers or vice versa. Ideal barrier materials are abrasion resistant, impervious to permeation by fluids or dust that transport microorganisms. The integrity of a sterile package and its expiration date for sterility must be checked just prior to opening it (see Chap. 5, p. 106). To ensure sterility:

1 Sterile packages are laid on dry surfaces.

2 If a sterile package becomes damp or wet, it is resterilized or discarded. Any part of a package that comes in contact with moisture is considered nonsterile.

3 Drapes are placed on a dry field.

4 If a solution soaks through a sterile drape to a nonsterile area, the wet area is covered with additional sterile drapes or towels.

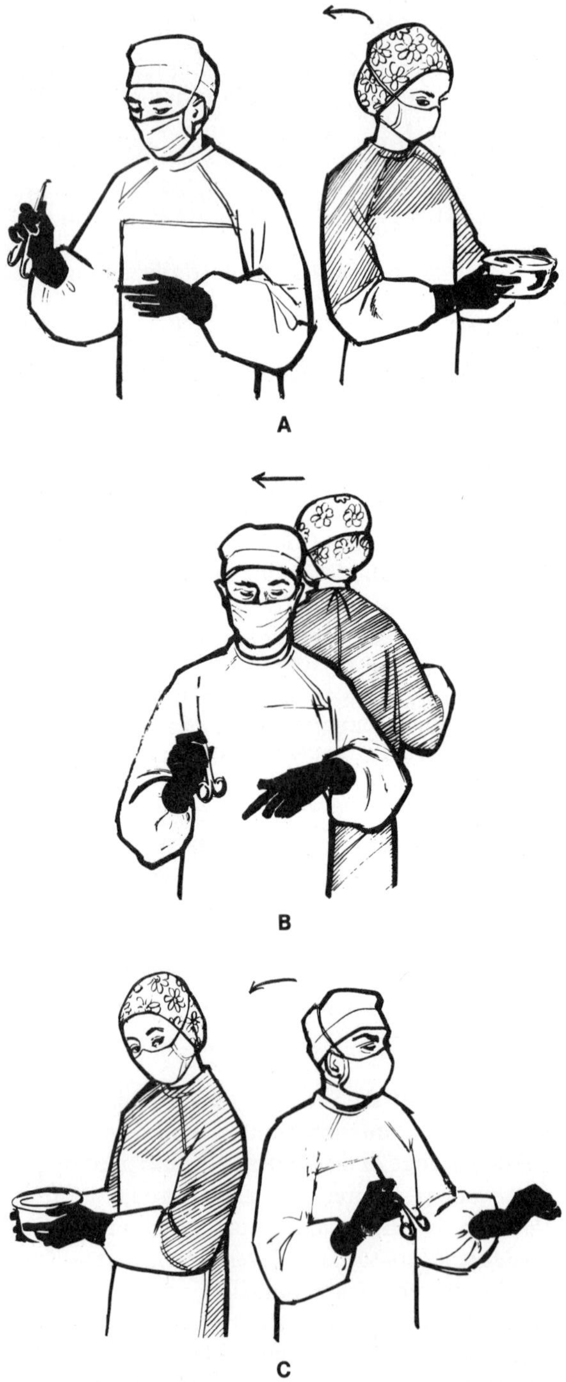

Figure 4-7 (A, B, and C) Sequence of one sterile person going around another. They pass each other back to back, keeping well within the sterile area and allowing a margin of safety between themselves.

5 Packages wrapped in muslin or paper are permitted to cool, after removal from the sterilizer, before being placed on a cold surface to prevent steam condensation and resultant contamination.

6 Sterile items are stored in clean dry areas.

7 Sterile packages are handled with clean dry hands.

8 Undue pressure on sterile packs is avoided to prevent forcing sterile air out and pulling unsterile air into the pack.

Microorganisms Must Be Kept to an Irreducible Minimum It is recognized that perfect asepsis in an operative field is an ideal to be approached; it is not absolute. All microorganisms cannot be eliminated. However, this does not obviate the necessity for strict sterile technique. There is general agreement that:

1 *Skin cannot be sterilized.* Therefore, skin is a potential source of contamination in every operation. Defenses within the body usually can overcome the relatively few organisms remaining after the patient's skin preparation. The organisms on the hands and arms of the operating team are a hazard. All possible means are used to prevent entrance of microorganisms into the wound. Such preventive measures include:
   a Gowning and gloving of the operating team without contamination of the sterile exterior of gowns and gloves.
   b Sterile gloved hands do not directly touch skin and then deeper tissues. Instruments used in contact with skin are discarded and not reused.
   c If a glove is pricked or punctured by a needle or instrument, the glove is changed immediately. The needle or instrument is discarded from the sterile field.

2 *Some areas cannot be scrubbed.* When the operative field includes the mouth, nose, throat, or anus, the number of microorganisms present is great. Various parts of the body, such as the gastrointestinal tract and vagina, usually are able to prevent infection from flora that normally inhabit these parts. However, the following steps may be taken to reduce the number of microorganisms present in these areas and to prevent scattering them:
   a The surgeon makes an effort to use a sponge only once, then discards it.
   b The gastrointestinal tract, especially the colon, is contaminated. Measures are used to prevent spreading this contamination (see Chap. 17, p. 316 and p. 325).

3 *Infected areas are grossly contaminated.* The team avoids disseminating the contamination.
4 *Air is contaminated by dust and droplets.* Environmental control measures are used.

NO COMPROMISE WITH STERILITY

Sterility is never taken for granted. It must be maintained and checked. Chapter 5 details the procedures for sterilization and for ensuring sterility.

Basically, there is no compromise with sterility, which is an absolute state. An item is either sterile or unsterile. Always be as certain of sterility as it is possible to be. That certainty rests on the fact that the necessary conditions have been met, that all factors in sterilization have been observed. Obviously it is impossible to prove that every package is free from bacteria, but a single break in technique can cost the life of a patient. Operating room personnel must maintain the high standards of sterile technique that they know are essential.

PREVENTION OF WOUND INFECTION

All the factors previously discussed are relevant and therefore it may be helpful to summarize them, since prevention of wound infection in the surgical patient is essential. Preventive measures should concentrate on:

1 Control of endogenous infection
2 Use of strict sterile technique
3 Careful operative technique and wound closure
4 Reduction of exogenous or environmental sources of contamination such as airborne microorganisms
5 Thorough, prompt cleansing and debridement of traumatic wounds
6 Prevention of intraoperative contamination of wound
7 Judicious use of prophylactic antibiotics in selected patients
8 Meticulous handwashing
9 Sterile technique for dressing change
10 Dissemination of wound infection statistics to surgeons

Serious sequelae, such as wound disruption or septicemia, may follow wound infection. Therefore, it must be assiduously prevented.

Chapter 5

Sterilization and Disinfection

Pathogenic microorganisms and those that do not normally invade healthy tissue are capable of causing infection if introduced mechanically into the body. Therefore, hospitals must have specific standardized procedures, based upon accepted principles and practices, for the sterilization or disinfection of all supplies and equipment used in the operating room. Sterilization renders items safe for contact with tissue without transmission of infection, as long as sterility is maintained. Disinfectants are used to kill as many microorganisms in the environment as possible on items and materials that cannot be sterilized.

METHODS OF STERILIZATION

Bacterial spores are the most resistant of all living organisms because of their capacity to withstand external destructive agents. The physical or chemical process by which all pathogenic and nonpathogenic microorganisms, *including spores,* are destroyed is absolute. Either supplies and equipment are sterile or they are not. That certainty rests upon the fact that all factors and necessary conditions have been met in the sterilization process. Selection of the agent to achieve sterility depends primarily upon the nature of the item to be sterilized. The time required to kill spores in the equipment available for the process then becomes critical. Each method of sterilization has its advantages and disadvantages. Sterilizing agents are:

1 Steam under pressure—moist heat (physical)
2 Ethylene oxide gas (chemical)
3 Activated glutaraldehyde (chemical)
4 Hot air—dry heat (physical)
5 Ionizing radiation (physical)

Steam under Pressure—Moist Heat

Moist heat in the form of saturated steam under pressure is a dependable physical agent for the destruction of all forms of microbial life, including spores. Heat destroys microorganisms, but this process is hastened by the addition of moisture. Steam in itself is inadequate for sterilization. Pressure, greater than atmospheric, is necessary to increase the temperature of the steam for thermal destruction of microbial life. Death by moist heat is caused by the denaturation and coagulation of protein or the enzyme-protein system within the cells. These reactions are catalyzed by the presence of water. Steam is water vapor. It is saturated when the steam contains the maximum amount of water vapor.

Direct saturated steam contact is the basis of the steam sterilization process. Steam at the proper temperature and for the proper time must penetrate every fiber and reach every surface of the items to be sterilized. When steam enters the sterilizer chamber under pressure, it condenses upon contact with cold items. This condensation liberates heat, simultaneously heating and wetting all items in the load, thereby providing the two requisites: moisture and heat. *This sterilization process is spoken of in terms of degrees of temperature and time of exposure,* not in terms of pounds of pressure. Pressure increases the boiling temperature of water, but has no significant effect on microorganisms or steam penetration.

Vegetative forms of most microorganisms are killed in a few minutes at temperatures ranging from 130 to 150°F (54 to 65°C); however, certain bacterial spores will withstand a temperature of 240°F (115°C) for more than 3 hours. No living thing can survive direct exposure to saturated steam at 250°F (121°C) longer than 15 minutes. As the temperature is increased, the time may be decreased. A minimum temperature-time relationship must be maintained throughout all portions of the load to accomplish effective sterilization. Exposure time depends upon the size and contents of the load, and the temperature within the sterilizer.

Advantages

1 Steam sterilization is the easiest, safest, and surest method of sterilization. Items that can be steam-sterilized without damage should be processed with this method.

2 Steam is the fastest method. The total time cycle is shortest.

3 Steam is the least expensive and most easily supplied. Steam is usually piped in from the hospital boiler room. An automatic, electrically powered steam generator can be mounted beneath the sterilizer for emergency stand-by when steam pressure is low, or in situations where steam lines are not available.

4 Most of the sterilizers in use have automatic controls and recording devices to eliminate the human factor from the sterilization process as much as possible when operated and cared for according to the recommendations of the manufacturer.

5 Many items, such as stainless steel instruments, withstand repeated processing without damage. It leaves no harmful residue.

Disadvantages

1 Precaution must be used in preparing and packaging items, loading and operating the sterilizer, and drying the load.

2 Items must be clean, free from grease and oil, and nonheat sensitive.

3 Steam must have direct contact with all areas of an item.

4 Timing of cycle must be adjusted for differences in materials and size of load; these variables are subject to human error.

Types of Steam Sterilizers Sterilizers designed to use steam under pressure as the sterilizing agent frequently are referred to as *autoclaves* to distinguish them from sterilizers employing other agents. *References in this text to an autoclave mean steam sterilizer.* Personnel charged with the responsibility of operating an autoclave must fully understand the principles and operation of each type. They must be aware of problems that cause malfunction, such as attaining sterilization temperature and maintaining it for the required period of time, trapped air, and dirty traps.

Gravity Displacement Sterilizers The metal construction contains two shells, either round or rectangular, to form a jacket and a chamber. Steam fills the jacket that surrounds the chamber. After the door is tightly closed, steam enters the chamber at the back, near the top, and is deflected upward. Air is more than twice as heavy as steam. Thus, by gravity, air goes to the bottom and steam floats on the top. Steam, entering under pressure and remaining above the air, displaces the air both in the chamber and in wrapped items downward, and forces it out through the discharge outlet at the bottom front. The air passes through a filtering screen to the waste line. The thermometer, located at this outlet below the screen, measures the temperature in the chamber. When steam has filled the chamber it begins to flow past the thermometer. Timing of the sterilizing period starts only when the thermometer reaches the desired temperature.

When air is trapped in the chamber or in wrapped items, the killing power of the steam is decreased in direct proportion to the amount of air present. It is important to remember that the vital discharge of air from the load always occurs in a downward direction, never sidewise. Therefore, all supplies must be prepared and arranged to present the least possible resistance to the passage of steam through the load from the top of the chamber downward. Also, air- and steam-discharge lines must be kept free of dirt, sediment, or lint. The filtering screen should be cleaned daily. The discharge lines are flushed with trisodium phosphate weekly (see below).

Most gravity displacement autoclaves operate on a standard cycle of 250 to 254°F (121 to 123°C) at a pressure of 15 to 17 lb per square inch (lb/in²). Size of the chamber and contents will determine exposure period; the minimum is 15 minutes.

High-Speed Pressure Sterilizer Often called a *flash sterilizer,* this autoclave operates by gravity displacement, but is designed to function rapidly at a higher temperature. It can be adjusted to operate at 27 lb pressure per square inch to increase the temperature to 270°F (132°C). *The minimum exposure time at this temperature is 3 minutes, but only for unwrapped items.* With this cycle, the entire time for starting, sterilizing, and opening the autoclave is 6 to 7 minutes. The temperature can be set for operation at 250°F (121°C) for standard cycles at 25 lb pressure.

High-Vacuum Sterilizer In this type of autoclave the air is almost completely evacuated from the chamber before the sterilizing steam is admitted. This is accomplished to the desired degree of vacuum by means of a pump and a steam-injector system. The prevacuum period of 8 to 10 minutes effectively removes the air to minimize steam penetration time. The steam injector preconditions the load and also helps eliminate air from the packages. When the sterilizing steam is admitted to the chamber, almost instantly the steam penetrates to the center of the packages. Provided the items making up the load are easily penetrable and the sterilizer is functioning properly, there is no demonstrable time differential between complete steam penetration of large or small, tight or loose packages. Air is not displaced by steam. Therefore maximum capacity can be utilized. A postvacuum cycle draws moisture from the load to shorten drying time.

Temperatures are controlled at 272 to 276°F (133 to 136°C). A complete cycle takes approximately 15 minutes. Temperature, time, and degree of vacuum are recorded on a graphic chart. Although equipped with automatic controls, cycles can be operated manually or by gravity displacement of air.

Washer-Sterilizer This type of sterilizer is designed to wash and terminally sterilize instruments and some other items immediately after the operation is completed. Cold water fills the chamber and mixes with detergent to dissolve and loosen blood and debris. Steam and air, injected through powerful jet streams located near the bottom of the chamber, create turbulence of the water is heated, it rises and carries debris to the water line. Steam then enters at the top of the chamber to force wash water out through the bottom drain. Steam under pressure floods the chamber to sterilize the items at 270°F (132°C).

Although designed specifically for the combination of washing and sterilizing cycles, some units can be programmed for use as a flash sterilizer.

Precautions With all four types of steam sterilizers, the following precautions must be taken to ensure safe operation:

1 Turn valve on for steam in the jacket prior to use. Steam may be kept in the jacket throughout the day. (It may be turned off at the end of the operating schedule.) This maintains heat, so do not touch the inside of the chamber when loading. (Check sterilizer; not all have a steam jacket.)

2 Never put heat-sensitive items in a steam sterilizer of any type; they will be destroyed.

3 Close the door tightly before activating either automatic or manual controls.

4 Do not set a manually operated timer, unless it is an automatically controlled device, until the desired temperature registers on the thermometer and recording graphic chart. *Thermometers, not pressure gauges, are the guides for sterilization.*

5 Open the door only when the exhaust valve registers zero. Stand behind the door and open slowly to avoid steam escaping around the door. the door.

6 Daily wash the inside of the chamber with trisodium phosphate solution, rinse with tap water, and dry with lint-free cloth.

7 Remove and clean filtering screen daily.

8 Flush the discharge lines weekly with hot solution of trisodium phosphate: 1 oz (30 ml) to 1 qt (1000 ml) of hot water. Follow flush with rinse of 1 qt (1000 ml) of tap water.

Preparing Items for Steam Sterilization

Surgical Instruments Special attention must be given to cleaning surgical instruments prior to sterilization. An *ultrasonic cleaner* should be available for cleaning instruments that the washer-sterilizer has not adequately cleaned during terminal sterilization. High-frequency sound is a source of energy used for cleaning. It is not a method of sterilization. *An ultrasonic cleaner is not a sterilizer.* Therefore, instruments must be terminally sterilized before being placed in an ultrasonic cleaner.

Surgical instruments vary in configuration from plane surfaces, which respond to most types of cleaning, to complicated devices that contain box locks, serrations, blind holes, and interstices. Ultrasonic energy, high-frequency sound waves, thoroughly cleans the latter type by the process of cavitation. The tiny bubbles, generated in the cleaner solution by high-frequency sound waves, expand until they are unstable, then collapse. The *implosion* (exact opposite of explosion) of these bubbles generates minute vacuum areas that dislodge, dissolve, or disperse soil. These bubbles are small enough to get into the serrations, box locks, and crevices of instruments that are impossible to clean by other methods.

Instruments should be completely immersed in cleaning solution. The tank should be filled to a level 1 in. (2.5 cm) above the top of the instrument tray. Suitable detergent, as specified by the manufacturer, is added. Temperature of the water should be 80 to 110°F (26.6 to 43°C) to enhance effectiveness of the detergent, but it should not coagulate protein on the instruments. Instrument trays must be designed for the maximum transmission of sonic energy. An important relationship exists between wire gauge, opening size, and the sonic frequency. A large mesh of small wire size transmits more energy than heavy wire with narrow spacing.

Solution is degassed by turning on the ultrasonic energy. Gas, present in most tap water, impedes the transmission of sonic energy. An electric generator supplies electrical energy to a transducer. The transducer converts the electrical energy into mechanical energy in the form of vibrating sound waves that are not audible to the human ear because they are of such high frequency. If excess gas is present, it prevents the cleaning process from being fully effective because the cavitation bubbles fill with gas and the energy released during implosion is reduced. Tap water should be degassed for 5 minutes or longer each time it is changed.

After cleaning, instruments must be thoroughly rinsed and dried. Glassware, rubber goods, and thermoplastics also can be cleaned by this method. Instruments that are well cleaned in a detergent solution in a washer-sterilizer may not need ultrasonic cleaning after every use.

Instruments Sets Standardized basic sets of instruments or trays of instruments selected for specific operations are prepared for sterilization after thorough cleaning. Instruments must be placed in *perforated* trays to allow steam penetration around the instruments and to prevent trapping air in the tray.

Stainless steel instruments should be arranged in the tray in a definite pattern to protect them from damage and to facilitate their removal for use. Heavy instruments are placed in the bottom of the tray. All detachable parts must be disassembled. Hinged instruments must be open with box locks unlocked to permit steam contact on all surfaces. They can be strung on a pin or rack. Sharp and delicate instruments are placed on top. (See Chaps. 8 and 14 for further discussion of the care and handling of instruments.)

The size and density of wrapped instrument sets should not exceed a maximum weight of 17 lb (7.6 kg), or approximately 100 instruments. This is necessary to ensure adequate drying.

Basin Sets Basins and solid utensils must be separated by a porous material, if they are nested, to permit permeation of steam around all surfaces and condensation of steam from the inside during sterilization. Sponges or linen are not packaged in basins; steam could be deflected from penetration through fabrics.

Linen Packs Freshly laundered linen drapes and gowns must be fanfolded or rolled loosely to provide the least possible resistance to penetration of steam through each layer of the material.

Linen packs must not exceed a maximum size of 12 by 12 by 20 in. (30 by 30 by 50 cm), and not weigh more than 12 lb (5.5 kg). Linens are loosely crisscrossed so that they do not form a dense impermeable mass. The outside wrapper becomes the table drape when the pack is opened. The wrapper should not be drawn up too tightly, but must hold securely.

Rubber Goods and Thermoplastics A rubber sheet or any other impervious material should not be folded for sterilization as steam cannot penetrate it nor displace air from folds. It should be covered with a piece of linen of the same size, both loosely rolled and then wrapped.

The mechanical cleaning of tubing, including catheters and drains, is a factor in reducing microbial count inside the lumen. A residual of distilled water should be left in the lumen of any tubing to be steam-sterilized. This becomes steam as the temperature rises and helps to displace the air in the lumen and to increase the temperature within it. Tubing should be laid out so that there are no kinks in it.

Suction tips must be removed from tubing. Detachable rubber or plastic parts should be removed from instruments and syringes for cleaning and sterilizing. Rubber surfaces should not touch each other, metal, or glassware during sterilization to avoid melting or sticking and to permit steam to reach all surfaces. Rubber bands must not be used around solid items as steam cannot penetrate through or under rubber.

Wood Products During sterilization, lignocellulose resin (lignin) is driven out of wood by heat. This resin may condense onto other items in the autoclave and cause reactions if it gets into the tissues of a patient. Therefore, wooden items must be individually wrapped and separated from other items in the autoclave.

> NOTE. Repeated autoclaving dries wood so that during sterilization it will adsorb moisture from the saturated steam. As the water content of saturated steam decreases, the steam becomes superheated and loses some of its sterilizing power. Because of these problems, the use of wood products that require steam sterilization should be minimized and their repeated sterilization avoided.

All Items Whether washed by hand, in a washer-sterilizer, or in an ultrasonic cleaner, all items with detachable parts or parts that can be separated must be disassembled for cleaning, packaging, and sterilizing. Items must be clean and dry, except lumen of tubing, prior to sterilization. Manuals, often with photographs, or index file cards are available in the room in which supplies are packaged for ready reference during preparation and wrapping of single items, packs, or trays. Instructions must be strictly followed to assure safety in sterilizing items.

Packaging The packaging materials for *all* methods of sterilization must:

1 Permit penetration of the sterilizing agent to achieve absolute sterilization of all items in the package.

2 Allow release of sterilizing agent at the end of the exposure period.

3 Cover items completely and easily, and fasten securely with tape or heat seal that cannot be resealed after opening.

> NOTE. Pins, staples, paper clips, or other penetrating objects must never be used to seal packages. These cannot be removed without destroying the integrity of the package and contaminating the contents. If a staple, for example, is used to secure the end of a package, it is impossible to remove it without tearing the package. Scissors cannot be used to cut off the end of a package and the contents drawn out over this cut end. The item would be contaminated by the edge of the packaging material. For the same reason, packages are never torn open below a seal.

4 Permit identification of the contents and evidence of exposure to a sterilizing agent.

> NOTE. Indicator tapes or strips on the outside of packages change color during exposure to a sterilization process. They do not indicate sterility, only that the package has been sufficiently exposed to a given parameter to turn the color. Other factors that guarantee sterility must be fulfilled (see biological testing, p. 105).

5 Provide an impermeable barrier to microorganisms, dust particles, and moisture. Items must remain sterile from time removed from the sterilizer until used.

6 Resist tears and punctures in handling. If accidental tears and holes do occur, they must be visible.

7 Maintain integrity of package at varying atmospheric and humidity levels.

> NOTE. In geographic areas of high altitude or dry climates, some packaging materials are susceptible to rupture during sterilization or will dry out and crack in storage.

8 Permit easy removal of the contents with transfer to the sterile field without contamination or delamination (separation into layers).

9 Be economical.

The wrapping of packages should be done in a room far enough removed from sterile storage areas so that mixing sterile and nonsterile packages is not possible. Nonsterile cabinets should be labeled conspicuously. The procedure for sending items to the sterilizer and receiving them from it should be set up so that sterile and nonsterile packages can never be confused en route. The procedure must be understood by everyone.

The following materials may be safely used for wrapping items for *steam sterilization:*

Muslin Although often spoken of as linen, 140-thread count unbleached muslin usually is used for wrappers. These are of double thickness; they are sewn together on the edges only so that they are free from holes. Packages are wrapped in two layers of double-thickness muslin (four thicknesses) to serve as a sufficient dust filter and microbial barrier. This muslin wrapper is not moisture resistant. A 288-thread count muslin allows a single-thickness wrapper that is moisture retardant and is an improved barrier to microbial penetration.

Items are easily enclosed in muslin with all corners of the wrapper folded in. A small cuff turned back on the first fold over the contents provides a margin of safety to avoid contamination when opening after sterilization. Packages can be securely fastened with pressure-sensitive indicator tape.

The *advantages* of muslin as a wrapper are:

1 Muslin may be the most economical material, after the initial investment, because it can be used many times.
2 A package wrapped in muslin may be opened on a table so that the wrapper becomes a sterile field drape. Muslin is memory-free so will lie flat.

NOTE. *Memory* is the ability of a material to retain a specific shape or configuration.

3 Danger of tearing or gouging holes in muslin is minimal. Small holes (not rips) can be heat-sealed with double-vulcanized patches; they should never be stitched. A sewing machine will leave needle holes in muslin. Wrappers should be discarded after four to six patchings.
4 Muslin is flexible and easy to handle.

The *disadvantages* of muslin wrapper are:

1 Muslin must be laundered to rehydrate, inspected on an illuminated table, patched if necessary, delinted, and folded after each use.
2 It may create free-floating lint in the OR.
3 Muslin's opacity prevents its contents from being seen.
4 Muslin has limited storage life after sterilization: 30 days maximum in closed cabinets, 21 days or less on open shelving. Sterility is not maintained for prolonged periods unless muslin-wrapped package is hermetically sealed in plastic overwrap.
5 Muslin wets easily and dries quickly so that water stains may not be obvious. A 288-thread count muslin may overcome this disadvantage.

NOTE. Heavy, tightly woven fabrics, such as canvas, duck, or twill, will retard the penetration of steam so that sterility cannot be assured.

Nonwoven Fabric A combination of cellulose and rayon with strands of nylon randomly oriented through it has the flexibility and handling qualities of muslin. Nonwoven fabric is available in three weights. Lightweight is used in four thicknesses like muslin; medium is most economical for wrapping items in two thicknesses; and heavy-duty is desirable for wrapping linen packs and basin sets when the wrapper will become the table drape. Packages are wrapped in the same manner as with muslin.

The *advantages* of nonwoven fabric wrapper are:

1 It is disposable, eliminating the need for inspection and repair.
2 It provides an excellent barrier against microorganisms and moisture during storage after sterilization.
3 It is strong enough to be tear-resistant, yet easy to handle with very little memory.
4 It is lint free.

The *disadvantages* of nonwoven fabric wrapper are:

1 It is expensive because it is a one-use item. Breaks in fibers that are difficult to detect in the folds may occur after more than one sterilization cycle. Therefore, wrapper should be disposed of after use.
2 Its opacity prevents its contents from being seen.
3 The heavy-duty type may retain droplets of water caused by steam condensing on the surface of instruments during the initial phase of high-vacuum sterilization. Damp or wet packages may result, but may not be noticed until the package is opened. An absorbent towel placed in the bottom of the instrument tray and another under the tray during the wrapping procedure will help absorb moisture for thorough drying of instruments.

Paper If paper products are used, acceptability for steam penetration must be proven. Most craft, parchment, crepe, and glassine papers are acceptable. Available in sheets or envelopes, paper is sealed with pressure-sensitive tape.

The *advantages* of paper wrapper are:

1 It is disposable and inexpensive as a one-use item. Reuse is unsafe because quality may not be consistent with repeated exposure to heat.
2 It provides a good, long-term, poststerilization contamination barrier.

The *disadvantages* of paper wrapper are:

1 It is difficult to spread open so that contents can be removed; it has memory and flips back easily and may not open flat to provide a sterile field.
2 Paper is relatively easy to puncture or tear; it is impossible to see small holes and cracks.
3 Paper wets easily and dries quickly making contamination difficult to detect.
4 Paper's opacity prevents its contents from being seen.

Plastic Polypropylene film of 1 to 3 mil thickness is the only plastic acceptable for steam sterilization. It is usually used in the form of pouches presealed on two or three sides. The open sides must be heat-sealed after the item is placed in the pouch.

NOTE. Polyethylene melts in steam. Nylon (polyamide) will not permit adequate escape of condensate when package is cooling, thereby creating moisture within contents of the package. Nylon may adhere itself to contents in high-vacuum sterilization so that aseptic transfer is impossible after sterilization.

The *advantages* of polypropylene pouch are:

1 Its transparency allows its contents to be seen.
2 Polypropylene provides an excellent barrier against microorganisms and moisture for prolonged poststerilization storage.

The *disadvantages* of polypropylene pouch are:

1 It may be difficult to seal to avoid rupture during sterilization; it requires a high heat-sealing temperature.
2 Its limited flexibility makes it difficult to handle.

Combination of Paper and Plastic Pouches and tubes made of a combination of paper on one side and plastic film on the other are satisfactory for wrapping single instruments, catheters, drains, and small items. A peel-open seal, for aseptic presentation, may be preformed on one end. The other end is either heat-sealed or closed with tape after the item is inserted in the pouch or tube.

NOTE. If package does not have a preformed, peel-open seal and a heat-sealing machine is not used, ends must be folded to create a sterile edge for presentation of the sterile contents, and sealed with a closure tape that is easily removed without tearing the package.

The *advantages* of paper and plastic package are:

1 Good permeability on paper side with good visibility of contents on plastic side.
2 It is generally easy to seal with peel-open access for sterile presentation.
3 It is economical and durable.
4 It provides an excellent barrier against microorganisms for poststerilization storage.

The *disadvantages* of paper and plastic package are:

1 Heat seals may rupture during sterilization.

NOTE. A double heat seal should be applied to ensure against accidental opening. A *double peel-open package* (an item packaged inside a peel-open package that is placed into a slightly larger outer peel-open pack) gives extra protection. The seal must not reseal itself if opened.

2 Materials may delaminate during sterilizing or opening procedures.

Loading the Autoclave When using a high-vacuum autoclave, follow the recommendations of the manufacturer for packaging, loading, and sterilizing time. A gravity displacement autoclave must be loaded in such a way that steam can displace the air downward and out through the discharge line. Wire mesh or perforated metal shelves separate layers of packages. The following directions apply to this type of autoclave:

1 Flat packages are placed on the shelf on edge so that flat surfaces are vertical as shown in Figure 5-1.
2 Large packages are placed in one layer only on a shelf without touching each other. Small packages may be placed on the shelf above.

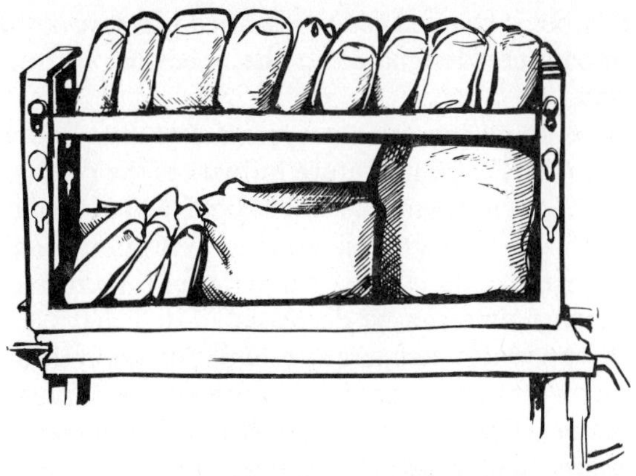

Figure 5-1 Proper loading of autoclave; place packs on edge and do not overload the rack. Steam must completely surround and penetrate every package.

3 If small packages are placed one on top of another, they should be crisscrossed.

4 Gloves and rubber goods are placed on edge, loosely arranged, one layer to a shelf, to allow free steam circulation and penetration. No other articles should be with them.

5 Basins or any solid containers are placed on their sides to allow air to flow out of them. They should be placed so that if they contained water, it would all flow out.

6 Solutions are sterilized alone. At the completion of the sterilization cycle, the steam should be turned off and the temperature allowed to drop to 212°F (100°C) before opening the exhaust; set the selector to "slow exhaust." Otherwise the solutions will boil over. Allow the pressure gauge to reach zero before opening the door so that the caps will not pop off.

Timing the Load Timing of a sterilization cycle begins when the desired temperature is reached throughout the autoclave chamber. If the autoclave does not have an automatic timing device with a buzzer that sounds at the end of the cycle, an oven timer can be set after the proper temperature has been reached to time the load and to alert personnel when the cycle is completed.

Materials that need exposure for different lengths of time to assure sterilization in a gravity-displacement autoclave should not be combined in the same load if the maximum time needed will be destructive to some items. Items may be sterilized wrapped or unwrapped, alone or combined with other items. Time of exposure varies depending on these factors and on the temperature of the steam. Minimum time standards, calculated after effective steam penetration of porous materials and the rate of heat transfer through wrapping materials, are listed.

Materials	250°F (121°C)	270°F (132°C)
Basin sets, wrapped	20 min	10 min
Basins, glassware, and utensils, unwrapped	15 min	3 min
Instruments, with or without other items, wrapped as a set in double thickness wrappers	30 min	15 min
Instruments, unwrapped but with other items including a towel in the bottom of tray or a cover over them	20 min	10 min
Instruments, completely unwrapped	15 min	3 min
Linen packs, 12 by 12 by 20 in. (30 by 30 by 50 cm) maximum size, 12 lb (5.5 kg) maximum weight	30 min	Not recommended except in high-vacuum sterilizer. Fabrics and rubber deteriorate more rapidly with repeated sterilization at higher temperature for prolonged periods in gravity displacement autoclaves.
Linen, single items wrapped	30 min	
Rubber and thermoplastics, including small items and gloves, but excluding tubing, wrapped	20 min	
Tubing, wrapped	30 min	15 min
Tubing, unwrapped	20 min	10 min
Sponges and dressings, wrapped	30 min	15 min
Solutions, flasked	(Slow exhaust)	(In the high-vacuum, the automatic selector determines correct temperature and exposure period.)
75-ml flask	20 min	
250-ml flask	25 min	
500-ml flask	30 min	
1000-ml flask	35 min	
1500-ml flask	45 min	
2000ml flask	45 min	

Most autoclaves are equipped with automatic time-temperature controls and a graphic recorder. Time and temperature for each load are recorded for a 24-hour period. Check the record of each load before unloading it to be certain that the desired temperature was achieved. Also, daily the temperature being recorded should be checked with the thermometer to see that the recording arm is working properly.

Drying the Load After the autoclave door is opened, a load of wrapped packages is left untouched to dry for 10 to 30 minutes. The time required depends upon the type of supplies in a load; large packages require a longer time than small ones. Packages are then unloaded onto a table padded with a piece of linen or onto a wooden cart with shelves of widely spaced slats. Warm packages laid on a solid, cold surface become damp from steam condensation, and thus contaminated.

Much time is saved in loading and unloading the autoclave if the rack of wire shelves can be rolled onto a transfer carriage. The shelves are loaded and rolled into the autoclave. After sterilization, the rack can be rolled out onto the carriage again without handling the individual packages while they cool.

Ethylene Oxide Gas

Ethylene oxide gas is used to sterilize items that are heat- or moisture-sensitive. *Ethylene oxide* (EO) is a chemical agent that kills microorganisms, including spores, by interfering with the normal metabolism of protein and reproductive processes, resulting in death of the cells. Used in the gaseous state, ethylene oxide gas must have direct contact with the microorganisms in or on items to be sterilized. Because pure ethylene oxide gas is highly flammable and explosive in air, it is diluted with an inert gas such as a fluorinated hydrocarbon or carbon dioxide for use in most sterilizers. These mixtures provide a safe, nonflammable agent for EO gas sterilization.

Ethylene oxide sterilization is dependent upon EO gas concentration, temperature, humidity, and exposure time. Gas is supplied in high-pressure metal cylinder tanks or disposable cans. Mixtures contain 10 to 12 percent ethylene oxide. In the sterilization process, air is withdrawn from the sterilizing chamber and the gas mixture enters under pressure. In general, the EO gas concentration in the sterilizer ranges between 450 to 800 mg per liter of chamber space. Gas sterilizers normally are not equipped with gas analyzer devices. The only means for controlling EO concentration is to operate the sterilizer according to the manufacturer's instructions, making certain that the chamber is charged to the specified pressure at the temperature designated in the operating instructions.

Gas sterilizers usually operate at 120 to 140°F (49 to 60°C). Temperature influences the destruction of microorganisms and affects the permeability of EO through cell walls as well as through packaging materials. As temperature is increased, exposure time can be decreased. 140°F (60°C) is the uppermost temperature limit for many heat-sensitive plastic materials, however. Sterilization may be achieved at room temperature, but the exposure time must increase as the temperature decreases to effectively kill spores.

Moisture is an essential element in achieving sterility with EO gas. Desiccated or highly dried bacterial spores are resistant to EO gas. They must be hydrated. The moisture content of the atmosphere immediately surrounding the organisms and the water content of the organisms themselves are important to the action of EO gas. Consequently, the relative humidity of the room atmosphere where items are packaged and held for sterilization should be at least 50 percent, and not less than 30 percent, to hydrate them during preparation. Humidity of 40 to 80 percent is maintained throughout the sterilization cycle.

Time required for complete destruction of microorganisms is primarily related to gas concentration and temperature. However, cleanliness of the items, type of materials, arrangement of the load, and rate of penetration also influence exposure time. Drawing an initial vacuum at the start of the cycle aids in the penetration of the gas. Generally, sterilization cycles of 3 to 6 hours are utilized. The cycle is totally automatic once the sterilizer is closed and the controls are activated.

Advantages of EO Gas

1 It is an effective substitute agent for most items that cannot be sterilized by heat.

2 It provides an effective method of sterilization for items that steam and moisture may erode; it is noncorrosive and does not damage items.

3 It completely permeates all porous materials.

> NOTE. EO gas does not penetrate metal, glass, and petroleum-based lubricants. Whether or not it penetrates oils, liquids, or powder depends upon the amount in the containers. If the material is spread thin, the gas will penetrate, but it will not go through bulk. EO gas sterilization is *not* recommended for these products.

Glass ampuls can be sterilized in ethylene oxide as the gas does not penetrate glass. But a glass vial with a rubber stopper must not be put in the sterilizer as the gas will penetrate the rubber and may react with the drugs in solution and cause a potentially harmful chemical reaction.

4 Automatic controls preclude human error by establishing proper levels of pressure, temperature, humidity, and gas concentration. Sterilizer must be operated according to manufacturer's instructions.

5 It leaves no film on items.

6 EO gas sterilization is used extensively in preparation of packaged, presterilized items commercially available because packaging materials that prolong storage life can be used.

Disadvantages of EO Gas

1 EO gas sterilization is a complicated process so biologic indicators should be used to verify the adequacy of every cycle.

NOTE. Never gas-sterilize any article that can be appropriately steam-sterilized.*

2 Items that absorb EO gas during sterilization, such as rubber, polyethylene, or silicone, require an aeration period (see p. 103). Air admitted to the sterilizer at the end of the cycle only partially aerates the load.

3 Toxic by-products can be formed in the presence of droplets of moisture during exposure of some plastics, particularly polyvinyl chloride.

4 Repeated sterilization can increase the concentration of the total EO residues in porous items. These increased levels can be hazardous unless gas can be dissipated.

5 EO is a vesicant if it comes in contact with the skin, and may cause serious burns if not immediately removed.

6 If inhaled, EO gas can be irritating to mucous membranes. Its presence is easily detectable by odor. Overexposure to the gas causes eye and nose irritation, and long exposure may result in nausea, vomiting, and dizziness. It is not cumulative in the body. At room temperature EO is a colorless gas.

NOTE. Continuous daily exposure of up to 7 hours duration to no more than 50 parts per million (ppm) probably is safe. Higher concentrations can be tolerated for shorter periods to a maximum of 3000 ppm for 1 hour daily. EO gas at 50,000 or more ppm can be fatal within a few minutes. It must be vented from the sterilizer to the outside atmosphere to avoid personnel exposure. Leave the sterilizer door open for at least 5 minutes before unloading to allow residual ethylene oxide gas to dissipate.

7 EO sterilization takes longer than steam sterilization; it is a long, slow process.

8 EO gas requires special, expensive equipment. Gas is somewhat expensive per cycle.

Types of Gas Sterilizers Stationary EO chambers range in size from 16 by 16 by 29 in. (40 by 40 by 73 cm) to very large units that will accommodate several mattresses. These chambers can be automatically or manually operated to achieve sterilization because the factors of gas concentration, temperature, humidity, and time are controlled. They operate at elevated temperatures and not only inject moisture to optimally control humidity, but also create a vacuum of 25 to 27 in. (625 to 675mm) Hg to aid the penetration of the gas. At the end of the time exposure, a postvacuum helps exhaust the gas from the load.

Portable, small units are also available. Some of these chambers operate for a standardized time cycle at the temperature and relative humidity level of the room. To compensate for room temperature, a higher concentration of gas is used. The gas flows through the chamber from an ampul broken within the chamber or from a cartridge affixed outside the chamber. Other small units are manually controlled and equipped with a heating element and a vacuum system.

Preparing Items for Gas Sterilization

All Items All items must be thoroughly cleaned and dried, as for steam sterilization. Disassemble detachable parts. Separate syringes. Remove impermeable caps, plugs, stylets, etc.

Lumens Any tubing or other item with a lumen should be blown out with air to force dry before packaging as the water combines with the EO gas to form a harmful acid, ethylene glycol.

Lensed Instruments Endoscopes (see Chap. 15, p. 301) with cemented optical lenses require special cement for EO gas sterilization.

Lubricated Instruments Remove all traces of lubricant, especially a petroleum-based lubricant. EO cannot permeate the film. Air-powered instruments can be lubricated with sterile lubricant after sterilization, just prior to use.

*Recommendation approved by the Association for Advancement of Medical Instrumentation Subcommittee on Ethylene Oxide Sterilization, July 30, 1976.

Camera Some cameras and film can be EO gas-sterilized. As a permanent record or a teaching aid, photographs are sometimes taken with a sterile camera at the operative site. An especially constructed camera is used. The film is loaded before packaging for sterilization.

Packaging for Gas Sterilization Type and thickness of wrapper used influences the time it takes for gas to penetrate. Size and shape of package and porosity of the contents also influence penetration time. Acceptable materials for wrapping items for EO gas sterilization include:

Muslin Double-thickness muslin is used as for steam with the same advantages and disadvantages.

Nonwoven Fabric Spunbonded olefin (polyethylene) is highly permeable to EO and moisture. It offers the same advantages as the nonwoven fabric described for steam sterilization although the two are not interchangeable; the cellulose/nylon/rayon combination should be confined to steam sterilization.

Paper Double-thickness paper is used as for steam with the same advantages and disadvantages.

Plastic Both polypropylene and low-density polyethylene of 3 mil or less thickness, film or pouches, may be used. Polyethylene is easier to handle than polypropylene and EO gas penetrates it more rapidly. Express as much air as possible from pouches before heat sealing to avoid rupture when vacuum is drawn in the sterilizer.

> NOTE. Materials *not* to be used for EO sterilization because of inadequate permeability include nylon, polyvinyl chloride film, Saran, polyester, polyvinyl alcohol, cellophane, and aluminum foil.

Combination of Paper and Plastic Pouches and tubes can be used as described for steam, except that double wrapping may not allow adequate permeation of the EO gas and moisture. Avoid combinations of materials that make a nonpermeable package for adequate humidification and gas penetration.

Items wrapped for gas sterilization should be tagged, "for gas," to avoid their inadvertently being steam-sterilized and damaged.

Loading the Sterilizer Procedures and precautions used for loading the gas sterilizer do not differ from those used for loading the autoclave. Overloading creates conditions whereby EO, moisture, and heat penetration can be retarded. Air space should be provided between the chamber ceiling and the topmost packages in the load. Also packages should not touch the walls of the chamber. Do not stack packages tightly; allow air space between packages for circulation of EO gas and moisture.

Timing the Cycle Closely follow the instructions provided by the manufacturer of the sterilizer.

Aerating Items Sterilized in Ethylene Oxide Gas Adequate aeration for all absorbent materials that will come in contact with the human body, either directly or indirectly, is absolutely essential. EO exerts toxic effects on living tissue. Residual products after sterilization can include:

1 *Ethylene oxide.* Porous materials, such as plastic, silicone, rubber, wood, and leather, absorb a certain amount of the gas that must be removed. The thicker the walls of the items, the longer the aeration time must be. Residual EO in plastic tubing or parts of a heart-lung pump oxygenator machine causes hemolysis of blood. Rubber gloves or shoes worn immediately after exposure can cause irritation or burns on the skin. Acceptable limits for residual EO are:*
   a 25 ppm for blood dialysis units, blood oxygenators, heart-lung machines, and all implants.
   b 250 ppm for all topical medical devices.
2 *Ethylene glycol.* This is formed by a reaction of EO with water or moisture that leaves a clear or brownish oily film on exposed surfaces of items. This film on plastic or rubber endotracheal tubes or airways can cause irritation to mucous membranes. Acceptable limits of ethylene glycol are:*
   a 250 ppm for blood dialysis units, blood oxygenators, heart-lung machines, and all implants.
   b 1000 ppm for all topical medical devices.
3 *Ethylene chlorohydrin.* This by-product is formed when a chloride ion is present to combine with EO, such as in polyvinyl chloride plastic. Rubber, soft nylon, and polyethylene items that have been in contact with saline solution or blood can retain enough chloride ion to

*Bureau of Medical Devices and Diagnostics, "Ethylene Oxide Sterilization: A Guide for Hospital Personnel," Food and Drug Administration, Public Health Service, U.S. Department of Health, Education and Welfare, Oct. 1, 1975; and the Association for Advancement of Medical Instrumentation Subcommittee on Ethylene Oxide Sterilization, revised July 30, 1976.

cause this reaction in the presence of moisture. Disposable products should be discarded after use to avoid this hazard. Acceptable limits of ethylene chlorohydrin are:*

a 25 ppm for blood dialysis units, blood oxygenators, heart-lung machines, and all implants.

b 250 ppm for all topical medical devices.

Aeration after sterilization to diffuse any residual products from porous items may be accomplished with ambient (room) air or in an aerator chamber designed for this purpose. Manufacturers of products suitable for EO sterilization should provide written instructions regarding sterilization exposure time and ambient or mechanical aeration time. These recommendations must be followed.

The nature of the item, the material in which it is packaged, the intended use of the item, and the temperature and air flow in the area influence aeration time.

Packages may be removed from the sterilizer and placed in a clean, well-ventilated storage area. Intravenous or irrigation fluids in plastic bags must not be stored in this aeration area as residual diffusing gas could be absorbed through the plastic. At room temperature the following *aeration times* for various materials are recommended:*

1 Nonporous items of metal and glass may be used immediately.

2 24 hours—paper, and thin rubber products.

3 48 hours—gum rubber thicker than $\frac{1}{4}$ in. (6.35 mm) and polyethylene items.

4 96 hours (4 days)—all other plastics except polyvinyl chloride items.

5 168 hours (7 days)—polyvinyl chloride and other plastic and rubber items that are sealed in plastic packages; will come in direct contact with blood; will be implanted, inserted, or applied to body tissues; or will be used for assisted respiration.

Aeration of exposed items at an elevated temperature enhances the dissipation rate of absorbed gases, resulting in faster removal. The entire load on the sterilizer carriage can be transferred into an *aerator*. A heater is in the upper part of the chamber. A blower system draws in air from the outside and heats it to 120 to 140°F (49 to 60°C). All materials remain in the aerator for 8 to 12 hours or longer, depending on the elevated temperature and instructions of the manufacturer of the aerator.

*Bureau of Medical Devices and Diagnostics, "Ethylene Oxide Sterilization: A Guide for Hospital Personnel," Food and Drug Administration, Public Health Service, U.S. Department of Health, Education and Welfare, Oct. 1, 1975; and the Association for Advancement of Medical Instrumentation Subcommittee on Ethylene Oxide Sterilization, revised July 30, 1976.

Activated Glutaraldehyde

Activated glutaraldehyde solution (aqueous Cidex activated dialdehyde solution) is the method of choice for sterilizing heat-sensitive items that cannot be steam-sterilized if an ethylene oxide gas sterilizer is not available or the aeration period makes EO sterilization impractical. Immersion in a 2% aqueous solution of activated, buffered alkaline glutaraldehyde is *sporicidal* (kills spores) within 10 hours. An acid glutaraldehyde solution (Sonacide) is also available.

Advantages

1 Activated glutaraldehyde solution has a low surface tension; it thus penetrates into crevices and is readily rinsed from items.

2 It is noncorrosive, nonstaining, and completely safe for all instruments that can be immersed in a chemical solution.

3 It does not damage lenses or the cement on lensed instruments.

4 It is not absorbed by rubber or plastic.

5 It has low volatility so solution can be reused throughout the effective activation period.

6 It is effective at room temperature.

Disadvantages

1 Solution must be activated by adding powdered buffer to liquid. Shake to dissolve activator.

2 Alkalinized glutaraldehyde solution changes pH and gradually loses effectiveness after date of activation. Mark expiration date on container when activated. Solution is reusable until this date, according to manufacturer's instructions.

3 Even though chemical has low toxicity and irritation, rinse items thoroughly in sterile water prior to use.

4 Activated glutaraldehyde solution has a mild odor.

Preparing Items for Sterilization by Immersion With this agent, as with all others, items should be clean and free of organic debris and blood. This agent will attack some organic materials. It remains highly active in the presence of protein matter in serum, mucous, and soap films. The human hepatitis virus cannot be isolated so removal of blood is critical. Items should be washed thoroughly in a nonfilming solution, rinsed, and dried prior to immersion.

Items to be sterilized should be placed in a container deep enough to completely immerse them. Be certain that items are dry before submerging so that the solution will not be diluted. Lumen of instruments or tubing must be completely filled with solution.

Timing the Immersion Cycle Activated glutaraldehyde solution is bactericidal, pseudomonacidal, tuberculocidal, fungicidal, and virucidal in 10 minutes for disinfection. Ten hours are required for sterilization.

Rinsing Following Immersion Items must be thoroughly rinsed in sterile water before use.

Hot Air—Dry Heat

Dry heat in the form of hot air is used primarily to sterilize anhydrous oils, petroleum products, and bulk powders that steam and ethylene oxide gas cannot penetrate. Death of microbial life by dry heat is a physical oxidation or slow burning-up process of coagulating the protein in the cells. In the absence of moisture, higher temperatures are required than when moisture is present because microorganisms are destroyed through a very slow process of heat absorption. Dry heat is the most infrequently used method of sterilization.

Advantages

1 Hot air penetrates certain substances that cannot be autoclaved.
2 Dry heat can be used in laboratories to sterilize glassware.
3 Dry heat is a protective method of sterilizing some delicate, sharp, or cutting edge instruments. Steam may erode or corrode cutting edges.
4 Instruments that cannot be disassembled may be sterilized in hot air.
5 Carbon steel does not become corroded or discolored in dry heat as it may in steam.

Disadvantages

1 A long exposure period is required because hot air penetrates slowly and possibly unevenly.
2 Time and temperature vary for different substances.
3 Overexposure may ruin some substances.
4 It is destructive to fabrics and rubber goods.

Types of Dry Heat Sterilizers

Hot Air Oven The most efficient and reliable sterilizer is an electrically heated mechanical convection hot air oven. It has a blower within it that forces air in motion around the load to hasten heating of substances and ensure an even temperature in all areas of the oven.

Autoclave The autoclave with steam only in the jacket can be used as a substitute for a hot air oven. However, this is not as reliable and demands a lengthy exposure because the maximum temperature that can be attained in the chamber is 250 °F (121 °C). The exposure period must be a minimum of 6 hours and preferably overnight.

Preparing Items for Dry Heat Sterilization

Oils The amount of mineral oil, lubricating oil for electric or air-powered instruments, etc., put in a container should not exceed 1 oz (30 ml). Preferably the layer depth of the oil is not more than $\frac{1}{4}$ in. (6.35 mm). The greater the depth, the longer the exposure period must be.

Impregnated Gauze Strips of gauze bandage covered with no more than 4 oz (120 ml) of melted petroleum jelly or other oil-base liquid should be arranged in a stainless steel container to provide a maximum layer depth of $\frac{1}{2}$ in. (12.5 mm).

> NOTE. Most hospitals purchase sterile packages of impregnated gauze products to eliminate the hazards inherent in preparation and sterilization of these products within the hospital.

Powders An ounce (30 cc) of powder should be spread out in the container so the layer depth does not exceed $\frac{1}{4}$ in. (6.25 mm).

Packaging Materials for Dry Heat

Glass Petri dishes, ointment jars, flasks, or test tubes can be used. Cotton plugs or muslin are used to cover tops of flasks and tubes.

Stainless Steel Boats or Trays Covers must fit tightly. They can be held in place with indicator tape.

Muslin and Paper These materials can be used for wrapping instruments. Powders can be put in double glassine envelopes.

Loading the Sterilizer Allow space between items and along the chamber walls so that the hot air can circulate freely. Never load the chamber to full capacity.

Timing the Load Time of exposure varies depending on the characteristics of the individual items, the layer depth in containers, and the temperature in the sterilizer. If the amount in each container is kept to the minimum and the sterilizer loaded according to manufacturer's recommendations, items are exposed for a minimum period of:

1 One hour at 340 °F (171 °C)
2 Two hours at 320 °F (160 °C)
3 Three hours at 285 °F (140 °C)
4 Six hours at 250 °F (121 °C)

Ionizing Radiation

Some of the sterile products commercially available are sterilized by *irradiation.* Ionizing radiation produces ions by knocking electrons out of atoms. These electrons are knocked out so violently that they strike an adjacent atom and either attach themselves to it, or dislodge an electron from the second atom. The ionic energy that results becomes converted to thermal and chemical energy. This energy causes the death of microorganisms.

The principal sources of ionizing radiation are beta particles and gamma rays. Beta particles, free electrons, are transmitted through a high-voltage electron beam from a linear accelerator. These free electrons have a high energy. The higher the energy, the further the electrons will penetrate into matter before being stopped by collisions with other atoms. Thus, their usefulness in sterilizing an object is limited by the density and thickness of the object and by the energy of the electrons. However, they produce their effect by ionizing the atoms they hit, producing secondary electrons that, in turn, produce lethal effects on microorganisms.

Cobalt 60 is a radioactive isotope capable of disintegrating to produce gamma rays. Gamma rays are electromagnetic waves. They have the capability of penetrating to a much greater distance than beta rays before losing their energy from collisions. Because they travel with the speed of light, they must pass through a thickness measuring several feet before making sufficient collisions to lose all of their energy. Cobalt 60 is the most commonly used source for irradiation sterilization.

Advantages

1 Ionizing radiation penetrates most materials to sterilize reliably.

2 Gamma rays can penetrate large bulky objects, so cartons ready for shipment can be sterilized in the cobalt 60 irradiator. Irradiation sterilization presently is limited to commercial use.

CONTROL MEASURES

Biological Testing

Positive assurance that sterilization conditions were achieved by either steam under pressure, ethylene oxide gas, or dry heat can be obtained only through a biological control test. The most dependable form of biological control is a preparation of living spores resistant to the sterilizing agent. *Bacillus stearothermophilus* spores are used to test steam under pressure; *Bacillus subtilis var niger strain globigi* are used for ethylene oxide and dry heat.

Ampuls of spores in suspension may be used. Biological spore strips are also commercially available in especially prepared envelopes or capsule units. These are stored at room temperature and kept dry prior to use. Each of these units contains a strip to be sterilized and a control strip that is not sterilized.

An ampul or biological spore strip is placed inside, in the center, of the largest and most dense pack or packaged item that is routinely processed in a given sterilizer. This test pack is placed near the bottom at the front of the sterilizer and sterilized in a routine cycle. When the cycle is completed, the test ampul or strip is removed from the pack and sent with a control ampul or the control strip to the bacteriology laboratory. If spore strips in envelopes are used, the test and control strips are aseptically transferred into a culture medium and incubated for 7 days. With the closed capsule system, the incubation period is shortened to 24 hours for *B. stearothermophilis* and 48 hours for *B. subtilis.*

Biological tests of all steam sterilizers and hot air ovens are conducted on a regular schedule, at least weekly. Every ethylene oxide gas sterilization cycle should be tested. Where feasible, the test results should be ascertained prior to use of EO gas-sterilized items. All laboratory reports are filed as a permanent record.

Process Monitors

Process monitors are designed to indicate that packages were exposed to sterilization conditions. These controls include such devices as special tapes, chemically impregnated discs, tablets or solutions sealed in glass tubes or plastic bags, etc., that change color. These devices can be placed on the outside or inside of packages. Since they do not test sterility, it is advantageous to have an indicator on the outside of every package to differentiate sterilized from unsterilized items. If the indicator does not change color, it alerts personnel that the sterilization cycle may have been inadequate. Process monitors should be used with every package sterilized.

To readily check for air entrapment in the high-vacuum steam sterilizer, the Bowie-Dick test can be used daily. Three pieces of indicator tape, about 8 in. (20 cm) long, are crisscrossed on a record sheet placed between layers of fabric in the center of a pack of towels. This test pack must be exposed to the sterilizing cycle alone in an otherwise empty chamber. If residual air remained in the pack, which inhibited steam penetration during the cycle, the tape does not change color.

Sterilization Date

A date on each package sets a limit on the number of days an item will be considered sterile. The date the package was sterilized may be stamped on the package as it is removed from the sterilizer; thus an undated package is not sterile. Some hospitals write the date on the package when it is wrapped. Others use a monthly, color-coded, machine-labeling system. Where possible, load control numbers should be used to designate the sterilization equipment used, cycle, and sterilization date.

SHELF LIFE

Determination of maximum *shelf life,* the time a sterile package may be kept in storage, depends on the following factors:

1 Conditions of storage
  - **a** Storage areas must be clean; free of dust, dirt, and vermin.
  - **b** Closed cabinets prolong storage of muslin- and paper-wrapped items to 30 days, as opposed to open shelving with a storage life of 21 days.
  - **c** All sterile items should be stored under conditions that protect them from extremes of temperature and humidity. Prolonged storage in a warm environment at a very high humidity can cause moisture to condense inside packages and allow microorganisms to grow into and through the packaging material. Ventilating and air-conditioning systems with filtered air should maintain temperature below 80°F (27°C) and relative humidity between 30 and 60 percent.
  - **d** Sterile storage areas should have controlled traffic patterns.

2 Material used for packaging
  - **a** Muslin- and paper-wrapped items may be stored for 21 to 30 days, then resterilization is required. However, if these items are sealed in an airtight plastic bag immediately after sterilization, following cooling or aerating, their shelf life can be prolonged from 6 to 12 months, if this dust cover does not have cracks or holes in it. The dust cover is removed before the sterile package is taken from a storage area into the OR.

3 Seal of the package
  - **a** Tape-sealed packages wrapped in nonwoven fabrics or plastic film can be stored for 3 to 4 months.
  - **b** Heat-sealed or hermetically sealed items can be stored for 6 months to a year.

4 Integrity of the package
  - **a** Commercially packaged, sterilized items are usually considered sterile until the package is opened or damaged, or becomes outdated.
  - **b** The item is no longer considered sterile after accidental puncture, tear, or rupture due to crushing of a package.
  - **c** Accidental wetting of a package, except hermetically sealed plastic, contaminates the contents.

Sterile supplies must be checked daily for outdated items. Any packages that become outdated or contaminated must be resterilized. Shelf life can be minimized by inventory control and rotation of sterile supplies. By adjusting the standard number of packages kept sterile to daily needs, packages seldom become outdated. In the interest of economy and good management, the stock supply of day-to-day items should be regulated so that there are enough for the busiest day with used items replenished daily. In this way the need for resterilization of most items is eliminated. Some items deteriorate with repeated sterilization. Many items are seldom used yet several must be kept sterile at all times. These supplies should be sterilized, or commercially sterilized items ordered, only in quantities sufficient to ensure prompt use and rapid turnover. Older supplies are always used first so that they do not become outdated. Commercially sterilized packages can be date-stamped as they go into inventory. Some have manufacturer's expiration dates on the package.

DISINFECTION

Surfaces and items that cannot be sterilized must be disinfected to eliminate as many microorganisms from the environment as possible. Disinfection differs from sterilization by its lack of sporicidal power. It is utilized in the OR suite for two major purposes, which are:

1 To kill pathogenic microorganisms on inanimate surfaces and objects that cannot be sterilized.
2 To prevent or arrest growth of microorganisms on body surfaces. (This application, referred to as *antisepsis,* for preparation of the skin of personnel and patients prior to operation is discussed in Chapters 7 and 11.)

Disinfection of inanimate surfaces can be accomplished with chemical or physical agents. These agents have two types of applications:

1 Housekeeping disinfection, which deals with floors, walls, furniture, large equipment, etc.
2 Instrument and small equipment disinfection.

NOTE. Critical items that come in contact with body tissue below the skin or mucous membranes, either directly or indirectly, *must be sterile.* Semicritical items that contact only unbroken skin or mucous membranes may be disinfected. Sterilization is *always* preferable for items that come in contact with the patient.

The best housekeeping agents are not the best instrument disinfectants and vice versa. An all-purpose disinfectant does not exist.

Chemical Disinfectants

Chemical agents, including ethylene oxide, must be registered with the Pesticide Regulation Division of the Environmental Protection Agency (EPA) to be sold in interstate commerce. An EPA registration number is granted only when all the requirements of laboratory test data, toxicity data, product formula, and label copy are approved. The product must do what the label says it does. To be labeled for hospital use, a chemical disinfectant must be proven effective against *Staphylococcus aureus* (gram-positive), *Salmonella choleraesuis* (gram-negative) and *Pseudomonas aeruginosa* (gram-negative), the most resistant gram-positive and -negative organisms. The agent can be classified as a hospital disinfectant without being pseudomonacidal, but it must be labeled whether it is or is not effective against this organism.

The EPA defines a *disinfectant* as an agent that kills growing or vegetative forms of bacteria. The terms *germicide* and *bactericide* may be used synonymously with disinfectant according to this definition. However, the tubercle bacillus has a waxy envelope that makes it comparatively resistant to aqueous germicides. Effective agents against the tubercle bacillus should be labeled *tuberculocidal.* Agents also are labeled if they kill fungi *(fungicide),* viruses *(virucide),* and/or spores *(sporicide).*

The safest products for use in the OR suite include all categories of "-cidal" action. With few exceptions, chemicals are not sporicides, however. Analysis of the label statements helps determine whether a product is appropriate for a specific purpose in the OR. Factors to be considered in the selection of an agent include:

1 Microorganisms differ markedly in their resistance to chemicals.
   a. *Low-level*: most vegetative bacteria, fungi, and lipoprotein (lipid- and protein-coated) viruses are susceptible to chemicals.
   b *Intermediate*: tubercle bacilli and nonlipid viruses are significantly more resistant.
   c *High-level*: bacterial spores are tremendously resistant.
2 Disinfectants differ widely in level of cidal action they produce and the mechanisms involved. All are protoplasmic poisons that either coagulate or denature cell protein, oxidate or bind enzymes, or alter cell membranes. In-use culture testing must determine the number of viable microorganisms after an agent is used for the intended purpose.
3 Nature of microbial contamination influences results of chemical disinfection. Bacteria, spores, fungi, and viruses are present in the air and on surfaces throughout the environment. However, organic soil, such as blood, plasma, feces, and tissue, absorbs germicidal molecules and inactivates some chemicals. Therefore, good physical cleaning prior to disinfection helps reduce numbers of microorganisms present and enhances cidal action.
4 Requirements of the chemical agent vary.
   a Housekeeping products should be detergent-disinfectants that meet the requirements for cleaning and disinfection:
      (1) Effective against a broad spectrum of microorganisms, including *Pseudomonas aeruginosa* and the tubercle bacillus, preferably in the presence of organic soil.

(2) Must be compatible with tap water used for use-dilution.
(3) Must not leave a residual insulating film that will affect electrical conductivity.
(4) Should be nontoxic and nonirritating to patients and personnel.
(5) Should be virtually odorless.

b Instrument and equipment disinfectants should kill as many species of microorganisms as possible to effectively decontaminate items for handling by personnel or in preparation of semicritical items for patient use, such as stethoscopes and monitors.

5 Kill time is correlated with concentration of the agent and the number of microorganisms present. Most chemicals are used in aqueous solution. Water brings chemical and microorganisms together. Without this water reaction the process stops. Increasing the concentration of the chemical may shorten the exposure time, but not necessarily. Disinfectants should be premixed in the required concentration and stored in properly labeled containers to ensure that personnel utilize the product in the correct concentration. *Instruments must be completely submerged for the maximum time recommended by the manufacturer of the product used, or used as recommended for housekeeping purposes.* All instruments should be clean and dry when put into solution. Drippy, wet items will dilute the solution and change the concentration of the chemical agent.

6 Composition of items to be disinfected varies. Nonporous items such as metal instruments, are more easily disinfected than porous materials.

NOTE. Seepage of the disinfectant solution into an ampul can occur if the ampul has a microscopic hole or crack in it. If this material is injected or implanted, serious reactions can result. If ampuls cannot be sterilized in steam or ethylene oxide gas, a color dye must be added to the disinfectant solution. If color seeps into the ampul or the solution becomes cloudy, discard. Do not use any suspicious ampul.

7 Method of application influences effectiveness of chemical agent.

a Direct application of a liquid disinfectant, either by mechanical action for housekeeping purposes or by immersion for instrument disinfection, is the most effective method of applying chemicals to the surface of inanimate objects.

b Aerosol spray, from a pressurized container, is an effective method of spot disinfection on smooth surfaces and into crevices not otherwise accessible.

c *Fogging* is the process of filling the air in a room with an aerosolized disinfectant solution in an attempt to control microbial contamination. Action on airborne contaminants is temporary because the agent dispersed through the air settles on surfaces or is exhausted through the ventilating system. This method is potentially toxic to personnel and patients. Unless all surfaces are completely covered by a layer of the disinfectant solution for the minimum exposure period, disinfection is incomplete. Fogging is impractical and too ineffective to be an acceptable method of disinfection in OR suites.

Chemical agents used for disinfection include:

Alcohol 70 to 95% ethyl or isopropyl alcohol kills microorganisms by coagulation of cell proteins.

Effectiveness

1 It may be used as a housekeeping disinfectant for spot cleaning, such as damp-dusting furniture and lights or wiping electrical cords, without leaving residue on treated surfaces.

2 It can disinfect semicritical instruments. To prevent corrosion of metal, 0.2% sodium nitrite must be added.

3 It is bactericidal, pseudomonacidal, and fungicidal in minimum of 10 minutes exposure.

4 It is tuberculocidal and virucidal for all viruses in minimum of 15 minutes exposure.

Hazards

1 It is volatile; it will act only as long as in solution. Alcohol becomes ineffective as soon as it evaporates and loses cidal activity below 50 percent concentration; therefore, discard at frequent intervals.

2 It is inactive in the presence of organic soil. It does not penetrate skin oil that lodges on instruments through handling.

3 It will blanch asphalt tiles of floors.

4 It can never be used on lensed instruments with cement mountings because it dissolves cement.

5 With long exposure, it will harden and swell plastic tubing and items, including polyethylene.

Chlorine Compounds Inorganic chlorine is valuable for disinfection of water, but it has limited use in the hospital. Chlorine compounds kill microorganisms by oxidation of enzymes. Sodium hypochlorite, 1 to 5%, has limited use.

Effectiveness

1 It is a housekeeping disinfectant for spot cleaning of floors and furniture.
2 It is bactericidal, fungicidal, tuberculocidal, and virucidal.

Hazards

1 It is unstable and dissipates rapidly in presence of organic soil.
2 Its odor may be objectionable.
3 It is corrosive to metal; cannot be used for instrument disinfection.

Formaldehyde In either solution or gas, formaldehyde kills microorganisms by coagulation of protein in cells. Solution may be 37% formaldehyde in water, or 8% formaldehyde in 70% isopropyl alcohol.

Effectiveness

1 It is an instrument disinfectant. To prevent corrosion of metal, 0.2% sodium nitrite must be present.
2 It is bactericidal, pseudomonacidal, and fungicidal in minimum of 5 minutes exposure.
3 It is tuberculocidal and virucidal in minimum of 10 minutes in alcohol solution; in minimum of 15 minutes in aqueous solution.
4 It is sporicidal in minimum of 12 hours.

Hazards

1 Its fumes are too irritating for housekeeping use.
2 It is toxic to tissues, so instruments must be thoroughly rinsed with sterile water before use.
3 Rubber and porous materials may absorb formaldehyde so they should not be disinfected in this agent.
4 As a gas, it must have 70 percent relative humidity in the chamber for use as a fumigant.

Glutaraldehyde An aqueous solution of 2% activated, buffered glutaraldehyde (Cidex solution), kills microorganisms by denaturation of protein. This is the agent of choice for sterilizing instruments that cannot be steam-sterilized when an ethylene oxide gas sterilizer is not available, or for disinfecting semicritical instruments between patient uses. (Glutaraldehyde was discussed in detail under "Methods of Sterilization" in this chapter, see p. 000). Glutaraldehyde is not recommended for housekeeping purposes. Both alkaline and acid glutaraldehyde solutions are available for instrument disinfection.

Iodophors A complex of iodine with detergent kills microorganisms through the process of oxidation of essential enzymes. Iodine, when properly used, is an effective disinfectant. The iodine-detergent complex enhances the "-cidal" activity of iodine and renders the iodine nontoxic, nonirritating, and nonstaining when used as directed. A minimum concentration of 100 ppm of available iodine is needed; however, concentration varies in the products available. The manufacturer's instructions for use must be followed.

Effectiveness

1 Iodophors are used as housekeeping disinfectants for floors, furniture, walls, etc. Iodine is effective as long as it is wet. It is more effective in an aqueous rather than alcoholic solution for cleaning purposes because an aqueous solution dries more slowly.
2 An iodophor may be used as an instrument disinfectant. To prevent corrosion of metal, 0.2% sodium nitrite must be added.
3 Iodophors are bactericidal, pseudomonacidal, and fungicidal in minimum of 10 minutes exposure.
4 They are tuberculocidal and virucidal in minimum of 20 minutes exposure, with a minimum concentration of 450 ppm of iodine.

Hazards

1 Some iodophors are unstable in the presence of hard water or heat, or subject to inactivation by organic soil.
2 Iodine stains fabrics and tissue, however, this is reduced or is temporary when used as an iodophor.

Mercurial Compounds Mercurial compounds bind enzymes of bacteria, but inhibit growth rather than kill the organisms. Therefore these agents are bacteriostatic, not germicidal. They have little, if any, value in hospital disinfection.

Phenolic Compounds Derivatives of pure phenol kill microorganisms mainly by coagulation of protein. Depending upon the phenol coefficient and species of organisms, phenolic compounds may cause rapid lysis of cells, leakage of cell constituents without lysis, or death by denaturing enzymes. Pure phenol, obtained from coal tar, is an extremely caustic agent and dangerous to tissue. Derivatives are used as disinfectants, usually with a minimum of a 2% phenolic compound in an aqueous solution.

Effectiveness

1 Phenolic compounds may be used as housekeeping disinfectants for cleaning floors, furniture, walls, etc. Phenolics retain a safe level of activity in the presence of heavy organic soil. They are the disinfectants of choice when dealing with fecal contamination. They have good stability and remain active after mild heating and prolonged drying. Subsequent application of moisture to dry surfaces can redissolve the chemical so it again becomes bactericidal.

2 As an instrument disinfectant, 0.5% sodium bicarbonate must be added to prevent corrosion.

3 They are bactericidal, pseudomonacidal, fungicidal, and lipid virucidal in minimum of 10 minutes exposure.

4 They are tuberculocidal in minimum of 20 minutes exposure.

Hazards

1 Tissue irritation precludes use for instruments that will come in contact with skin and mucous membranes, e.g., anesthesia equipment.

2 Personnel should wear gloves when cleaning with these products to avoid skin irritation.

3 Phenol derivatives may be absorbed by rubber.

4 Product may have an unpleasant odor.

Quaternary Ammonium Compounds *Quats,* as these compounds often are called, cause gradual alteration of cell membranes to produce leakage of protoplasm of some microorganisms, primarily vegetative bacteria. These compounds possess detergent properties. Benzalkonium chloride, one of the most widely used of these compounds, should be used in a concentration of 1 to 750.

Effectiveness

1 They are rarely used as a housekeeping disinfectant for floors, furniture, walls, etc.

2 For instrument disinfection, 0.2% sodium nitrite must be added to solution to prevent corrosion.

3 They are bactericidal, pseudomonacidal, fungicidal, and lipid virucidal in minimum of 10 minutes exposure.

Hazards

1 Cidal effect can be reversed by adding a neutralizer, such as soap.

2 Hard water used for dilution reduces active concentration.

3 Active agent can be selectively absorbed by fabrics, thus reducing the strength perhaps to an ineffective low level. Gauze or a towel must not be put in basin used for immersing instruments.

4 Compounds are subject to inactivation in presence of organic soil.

NOTE. Mercurial compounds and quaternary ammonium compounds are not recommended for hospital use because the hazards outweigh their effectiveness in the hospital environment. Other agents discussed are more efficacious.

Physical Disinfectants

Boiling Water Boiling water cannot be depended upon to kill spores. Heat-resistant bacterial spores will withstand water boiling at 212°F (100°C) for many hours of continuous exposure. Inactivation of some viruses, such as those associated with serum or infectious hepatitus, is uncertain.

If no other method of sterilization or disinfection is available, boiling water can be rendered more effective by adding sodium carbonate to the water to make a 2% solution, which reduces the hydrogen-ion concentration. At sea level the recommended boiling time for disinfection is 15 minutes. Rubber goods and glassware must not be boiled in sodium carbonate as it is destructive to both. If sodium carbonate is not used, the minimum boiling period is 30 minutes. At high altitudes the boiling time must be increased to compensate for lower temperature of boiling water.

Ultraviolet irradiation Ultraviolet rays can kill microorganisms upon contact in air or water, and on surfaces of inanimate objects. Ultraviolet lights produce radiant energy in sufficient wavelengths and intensity for disinfection. The practical usefulness of ultraviolet irradiation in hospitals is very limited, however, because direct contact with the organisms must be made for this agent to be an effective disinfectant. Microorganisms are in a constant state of motion in the air currents of the ventilating system. Moving across the ray of ultraviolet light, pathogens may be exposed for only a fraction of a second or too minimal a time for effective contact with the radiant energy.

Ultraviolet rays can cause skin burns, similar to sunburn, and conjunctivitis of the eyes. Therefore, when working under exposure to ultraviolet irradiation, protective skin coverings and a visor over the eyes must be worn.

Chapter 6

Physical Facilities

PHYSICAL LAYOUT OF THE O.R. SUITE

Utilization of the physical facilities is important; however, it is secondary to the functioning of the people within a department. The design of an OR suite offers a challenge to the planning team to optimize efficiency by creating realistic traffic and work flow patterns for patients, personnel, and supplies. Design should also allow for flexibility and for future expansion. Architects consult surgeons and OR nursing administrative personnel before allocating space.

No one plan suits all hospitals; each is designed on an individual basis to meet projected, specific future needs. The number of rooms required is a function of:

1 The number and length of operations to be performed
2 The type and distribution by specialties of the surgical staff
3 The proportion of elective inpatient and ambulatory patients to emergency operations
4 The scheduling policies related to the number of hours per day and days per week the suite will be in use
5 The systems and procedures established for the flow of patients, personnel, and supplies

Location

The OR suite is usually located in an area accessible to the critical care surgical patient areas and the supporting service departments, i.e., central service department, pathology, and radiology. The size of the hospital is a determining factor as it is impossible to locate every desirable unit or department immediately adjacent to the OR suite. A terminal location is necessary to prevent unrelated traffic from passing through the suite. A location on a top floor is not necessary for microbial control since all air is filtered to control dust. Traffic noises may be less evident above the ground floor. Artificial lighting is controllable so that outside daylight is not a factor; in fact, it may be a distraction. Many OR suites are underground or have solid walls without windows.

Principles in Design

The universal problem of environmental control to prevent wound infection exerts a great influence upon the design of the OR suite. As much as the floor plan will permit, clean and contaminated areas are differentiated. Architects follow two principles in planning the physical layout of an OR suite:

1 Exclusion of contamination from outside the suite with sensible traffic patterns within the suite

2 Separation of clean from contaminated areas within the suite

Physical planning of an OR suite, which separates clean from contaminated areas, makes it easier to carry out good aseptic technique. The clean area is often referred to as the *restricted area.*

Type of Design

The hospital where you are working probably was constructed according to a variation of one of four basic designs:

1 A central corridor, or hotel plan
2 A double central corridor, or clean core plan
3 A peripheral corridor, or race track plan
4 A grouping, or cluster plan

Each design has its advantages and disadvantages. Efficiency does become affected if corridor distances are too long in proportion to other space, if illogical relationships exist between space and function, or if inadequate consideration was given to storage space, materiel handling, and personnel areas.

Space Allocation

Space is allocated within the OR suite to provide for the work to be done there with consideration of the efficiency with which it can be accomplished. The OR suite should be large enough to allow for correct technique yet small enough to minimize the movement of patients, personnel, and supplies. Provision must be made for:

Traffic Control Offices for administrative personnel are best located so that they have access to both the outer corridor and inner area, as these persons frequently need to confer with persons from outside as well as to keep informed of the activities within the OR suite.

A corridor on the periphery is planned to handle all traffic from the outside. A pass-through window from the outside corridor may stop traffic there. It may be used by the pathologist who is to do a frozen section in the laboratory or by any one whose errand to the OR suite may be quickly done. Pass-through windows also may be used to receive drugs, linen, and various small supplies.

Conveyors or monorails may move bags of soiled linen and trash out of the suite. Conveyors may also connect the OR suite with a central processing area on another floor of the hospital. If efficient materiel flow can be accomplished, support functions can be removed from the OR suite. Effective communications and a reliable transportation system must be established, however. Some hospitals send all their instruments and supplies to the central service department for cleaning, packaging, sterilizing, and storing. This system eliminates the need for work and storage areas within the OR suite.

Processing

Utility Room Some hospitals use a closed-cart system and take contaminated instruments to a central area outside the OR suite for cleanup. Many do their cleanup procedures in the substerile room. Some, by virtue of the limitations of the physical facilities, bring the instruments to a utility room. This room contains washer-sterilizer, sinks, cabinets, and all necessary aids to cleaning. If the washer-sterilizer is a pass-through one, it opens also into the general workroom. This eliminates the task of physically moving instruments from one room to another.

General Workroom The general work area should be as centrally located in the OR suite as possible to keep contamination to a minimum. The work area may be divided into a cleaning area and a preparation area. If instruments and equipment from the utility room are received from the pass-through washer-sterilizer into this room, an ultrasonic cleaner should be available here for cleaning instruments that the washer-sterilizer has not adequately cleaned. Otherwise, the ultrasonic cleaner may be in the utility room.

Instrument sets, basin sets, trays, and other supplies are wrapped for sterilization here. The preparation of instrument trays and sets in a central room ensures better control.

This room also contains the stock supply of other items that are packaged for sterilization. The sterilizers that are used in this room may open also into the next room—the sterile supply room. This helps to eliminate the possibility of mixing sterile and nonsterile items.

Storage

Sterile Supply Room Most hospitals keep a stock supply of sterile linen, sponges, gloves, and other sterile items ready for use in a sterile supply room within the OR suite. As many shelves as possible should be freestanding from the walls, which permit supplies to be put into one side and removed from the other; thus, older packages are always used first.

The use of disposable products may necessitate a change in physical facilities. Less space is needed for cleaning equipment, wrapping packages, etc. The need for sterilization equipment may ultimately be reduced. More sterile storage space may be needed. These factors influence the design of new hospitals or the renovation of old ones for greater efficiency.

Instrument Room Most hospitals have a separate room, or section of the general workroom, for storing nonsterile instruments. The instrument room contains cupboards in which all clean instruments are stored when not in use. Instruments usually are segregated on shelves according to surgical specialty services.

Sets of basic instruments are usually cleaned, assembled, and sterilized after each use. However, special instruments designed for specific use, such as intestinal clamps, kidney forceps, bone instruments, etc., may be stored after cleaning. Sets are then made up according to each day's schedule of operations.

Storage Room Some large, portable equipment must also be stored within the OR suite, readily accessible for use. A storage room for this equipment, such as the orthopaedic table that may not be used daily, keeps equipment out of corridors when not in use.

Architects sometimes plan for extra space to be used presently for storage but later for expansion. Rapidly changing needs, and increased efficiency in meeting them, will call for new equipment. Operating rooms become outdated due to the problem of keeping up-to-date on technological changes, and to the increasing numbers of patients operated on because of trauma or illnesses that yield to surgical intervention.

THE OPERATING ROOM ITSELF

Size

The size of individual operating rooms vary. In the interest of economy and operational flexibility, it is desirable to have all operating rooms the same size, so that they can be used interchangeably to accommodate elective and emergency operations. Adequate size for multipurposes is 20 by 20 by 10 or 400 square feet (ft^2) or approximately 37 square meters (m^2) of floor space; the maximum beyond which efficiency is lost is 20 by 30 by 10 or 600 ft^2 (approximately 60 m^2). Specialized rooms, such as those equipped for cardiopulmonary bypass, may require as much as 600 ft^2 (approximately 60 m^2) of useful space.

Substerile Room

A group of two, three, or four operating rooms may be located around a central scrub area and a small substerile room. *Only if this latter room is immediately adjacent to the OR and separated from the scrub area will it be considered the substerile room throughout this text.*

A substerile room adjacent to the OR contains a sink, autoclave, and/or washer-sterilizer. Although some hospitals centralize their cleaning and sterilizing facilities, either inside or outside of the OR suite, a substerile room with this equipment offers the following advantages:

1 It saves time and steps. Emergency cleaning and flash sterilization of items can be done here by the circulating nurse. This reduces waiting time for the surgeon, anesthesia time for the patient, and saves steps for the circulating nurse. The circulating nurse, or scrub nurse if necessary, can lift sterile articles directly from the autoclave onto the sterile instrument table without transporting them through a hallway or another area.

2 It reduces the need for a messenger service to obtain sterile instruments and allows the circulating nurse to stay within the room.

3 It keeps instrument and equipment inventory lower because instruments needed for subsequent operations are not tied up in another processing area.

4 It allows for better care of instruments and equipment that require special handling. Certain delicate or sensitive instruments, or perhaps a surgeon's personally owned set of instruments, usually are not sent out of the OR suite. They are handled only by the personnel directly responsible for their use and care, i.e., the circulating and scrub nurses.

5 It avoids spread of contamination, which can occur by removing instruments and equipment to a central cleanup area. Nurses already involved in the operation can clean up within the confines of the OR and this adjacent room.

The substerile room also usually contains a combination blanket and solution warmer, cabinets for storage, and perhaps a refrigerator for blood and medications. Specimen containers with labels may be conveniently stored in this room.

Slips for charges or other records may be kept here. Individual hospitals may find it convenient to keep other items in this room to save the time of the circulating nurse and to allow him or her to remain in or immediately adjacent to the OR during the operation.

Doors

Ideally, sliding doors should be used in the OR. They eliminate the air currents caused by swinging doors. Microorganisms that have previously settled in the room are disturbed with each swing of the door. The microbial count is usually at its peak at the time of the skin incision because this follows disturbance of air by gowning, draping, movement of personnel, and swinging doors. During the operation, the microbial count rises every time doors swing open from either direction. Also, swinging doors may touch a sterile table or person.

Sliding doors should not recede into the wall but should be of the surface-sliding type. Fire regulations require that sliding doors for ORs be of the type that can be swung open if necessary. *Doors do not remain open either during or between operations.*

Ventilation

The ventilating system in the OR must ensure a controlled filtered-air supply. Air changes and circulation provide fresh air and prevent accumulation of anesthetic gases in the room. The concentration of gases is dependent solely on the proportion of pure air entering through the air system. Twenty-five air exchanges per hour is recommended. The microbial filters in the ducts do not remove anesthetic waste gases. They do filter the air to practically eliminate dust particles.

Positive air pressure in each OR is greater than that outside in corridors, scrub areas, and substerile rooms. Positive pressure forces air out of the room. The inlet is at the ceiling. Air leaves through the outlets at floor level. If the reverse is true, air is drawn into the room around the doors and through open doors. Microorganisms in the air can enter the room unless positive pressure is maintained.

An air-conditioning system is ideal and valuable. It controls humidity to help reduce the possibility of explosion. High relative humidity (weight of water vapor present) should be maintained; 60 percent is preferable, and 50 percent is mandatory in anesthetizing locations. Moisture provides a relatively conductive medium, allowing static to leak to earth as fast as it is generated. Sparks form more readily with low humidity.

Room temperature is maintained within a range of 68 to 80 °F (20 to 26 °C). Even with controls of humidity and temperature, air-conditioning units may be a source of microorganisms that come through the filters. These must be changed at regular intervals to prevent this and the ducts must be cleaned regularly.

Floors

Floors should be conductive enough to dissipate static from equipment and personnel but not conductive enough to endanger personnel from shock. Through its inherent conductive properties, the floor must fulfill the resistance provisions of the National Fire Protection Association Standard 56A. The surface of the floor shall provide a path of moderate electrical conductivity between all persons and equipment making contact with the floor to prevent the accumulation of dangerous electrostatic charges.*

Conductive floors are available in many materials including asphalt tile, linoleum, stone terrazzo, and vinyl terrazzo. The surface must not be porous, but rather suitably hard for cleaning by the flooding, wet-vacuuming technique.

Walls and Ceiling

Requisites of all surface materials are that they be hard, nonporous, fire resistant, waterproof, stainproof, seamless, and easy to clean. In addition, walls should be free from glare. The ceiling may have acoustical (sound-proof) tiles.

Wall paneling of hard vinyl materials, such as Formica, is easily cleaned and maintained. The seams can be sealed by a plastic filler. Laminated polyester or smooth, painted plaster provides a seamless wall. Epoxy paint has a tendency to flake or chip, however. Tiled walls collect dust and microorganisms between the tiles. The mortar between them is not smooth, and most grout lines are porous enough to harbor microorganisms even after cleaning. Tiles can crack and break. A material able to withstand considerable impact without affecting the surface also may have some value in noise control. Stainless steel cuffs at collision corners help avoid damage.

*Quoted from NFPA 56A, "Standard for the Use of Inhalation Anesthetics (Flammable and Nonflammable)," p. 55, copyright © 1973. National Fire Protection Association, Boston, Mass. (See Chap. 14, p. 283, for further details of this standard.)

The walls and ceiling often are used to mount devices, utilities, and equipment in an effort to reduce clutter on the floor. In addition to the overhead operating light, the ceiling may be used for mounting an anesthesia service core, operating microscope, cryosurgery device, x-ray tube and image intensifier, electronic monitor, closed-circuit television, and a variety of hooks, poles, and tubes. Demands for ceiling-mounted equipment are diversified. However, suspended track mounts are not recommended because they engender fallout of dust-carrying microorganisms each time they are moved. If movable or track-ceiling devices are installed, they should not be mounted directly over the operating table, but away from the center of the room and preferably recessed into the ceiling to minimize the possibility of dust accumulation and fallout.

Piped-In and Electrical Systems

Vacuum, compressed air, oxygen, and/or nitrous oxide may be piped into the OR. The outlets may be located on the wall, on the ceiling, or suspended from the ceiling. As a protection to other rooms, the supply of oxygen and nitrous oxide in any room can be shut off at panels for that purpose in the corridor should trouble occur in a particular line. A panel light comes on. A buzzer rings in the room and in the maintenance department. The buzzer can be turned off but the "abnormal" panel light stays on until the problem is corrected. The anesthesiologist can switch to the tanks of gases on the anesthesia machine.

Because all flammable gases and vapors except ethylene are heavier than air and settle to the floor when released, electrical outlets and fixtures located less than 5 ft (1.5 m) above the floor must meet rigid, explosion-proof code requirements. Explosion-proof electrical plugs are widely used. An alternative is to install grounded plugs above the 5-ft (1.5-m) level and to lead cords down the wall and across the floor to the equipment. Electrical cords on the floor are hazardous to personnel. Straight or curved ceiling-mounted tracks are satisfactory for bringing piped-in gases, vacuum, and electrical outlets close to the operating table. They eliminate the hazard of tripping over cords, but they can also produce a hazard. Insulation materials around electrical power sources from mobile, ceiling mounted tracks must be protected from repeated flexing when moved along the tracks to prevent cracks and damage to wires. Rigid or retractable ceiling service columns eliminate these hazards.

Multiple electrical outlets should be available from separate circuits. This minimizes the possibility of a blown fuse or a faulty circuit shutting off all electricity at a critical moment.

All personnel must be aware that the use of electricity introduces the hazards of electric shock, power failure, and fire. Faulty electrical equipment may cause a short circuit or the electrocution of patients or personnel (see Chap. 14 for detailed discussion). This hazard can be prevented by:

1 Using only electrical equipment designed for use in the OR. Equipment must have cords of adequate length and adequate current-carrying capacity to avoid overloading.

2 Testing portable equipment immediately before use and grounding correctly.

3 Discontinuing use immediately and reporting any faulty electrical equipment.

Should *fire* ever occur in a room during an operation, the burning article must be moved immediately from proximity to the oxygen source and the anesthesia machine or outlet of piped-in gases to prevent explosion. The fire should be extinguished in the room, if possible, but the patient must be immediately removed from any danger area. Fire safety systems are installed throughout the hospital. All personnel must know the fire rules. They must be familiar with the location of the alarm box and the use of fire extinguishers.

Lighting

General illumination is furnished by ceiling lights. Most room lights are white fluorescent, but may be incandescent. Recessed lights do not collect dust. Lighting should be evenly distributed throughout the room. The anesthesiologist must have sufficient light, at least 100 footcandles, to adequately evaluate the patient's color.

Illumination of the operative site is dependent upon the quality of light from an overhead source and the reflection from the tissues. White, glistening tissues need less light than dull, dark tissues. Light must be of such quality that the pathologic conditions are recognizable. The overhead operating light must:

1 Be near daylight in color and shadowless. Multiple sources and/or reflectors achieve reduction of shadows. In some units the relationship is fixed; others have separately maneuverable sources.

2 Make an intense light, within a range of 1000 to 10,000 footcandles, into the incision without glare on the surface. It must give contrast to the depth and relationship of all anatomic structures. The light may be equipped with an intensity control. The surgeon will ask for more light when needed. A reserve of light should be available.

3 Provide the diameter light pattern and focus appropriate for the size of the incision. These are adjusted with controls mounted on the light fixture.

4 Be freely adjustable to any position or angle. Most overhead operating lights are ceiling-mounted on mobile fixtures. Some have dual lights or dual tracks with sources on each track. These can be positioned so that light is directed into a single incision or two concurrent operative sites. Many fixtures are adapted so that the surgeon can direct the beam by manipulation of sterile handles.

5 Be spark-proof where anesthetic gases are used.

6 Produce a minimum of heat to prevent injury to exposed tissues, to ensure the comfort of the sterile team, and to minimize airborne microorganisms. As the lights heat up, convection currents tend to disturb settled microorganisms and cause them to become airborne.

7 Be easily cleaned. Tracks recessed within the ceiling virtually eliminate dust accumulation. Suspension-mounted tracks or a centrally mounted fixture must have smooth surfaces easily accessible for cleaning.

A source of light from a circuit separate from the usual supply must be available for use in case of power failure. This may require a separate emergency spotlight. It is best if the operating light is equipped so that an automatic switch can be made to the emergency source of lighting when the usual power fails.

Some surgeons prefer to work in a darkened room with only stark illumination of the operative site. This is particularly true of surgeons working with endoscopic instruments and the operating microscope. (This equipment will be discussed in Chapters 15 and 16, respectively.) If the room has windows, light-proof shades may be drawn to darken the room when this equipment is in use. Because of the hazard of dust fallout from shades, many hospitals have painted the windows in the rooms where this equipment is used. Even though the surgeon prefers the room darkened, the circulating nurse or anesthesiologist must be able to see adequately to observe the patient's color and to monitor his or her condition.

Some surgeons wear a headlight designed to focus a light beam on a specific small area, usually in a recessed body cavity such as the nasopharynx. Or a light source that is an integral part of a sterile instrument such as a lighted retractor may be used to illuminate deep cavities or tissues difficult to see with only the overhead operating light.

X-Ray Viewing Boxes

X-ray viewing boxes must be installed on the wall 5 ft (1.5 m) above the floor unless they are explosion-proof. The viewing surface should accommodate standard-size films. The best location is in the line of vision of the surgeon standing at the operating table. Lights for x-ray viewers should be of high intensity.

Clock with a Second Hand

A time-elapsed clock, which incorporates a warning signal, is useful for indicating that one or more predetermined periods of time has passed. This may be used during operations for total arterial occlusion, when using perfusion techniques or a pneumatic tourniquet, or during cardiac arrest.

Cabinets or Carts

Each OR is supplied with cabinets unless a cart system is used. Supplies for the types of operations done in that room are stocked or every OR may be stocked with a standard number and type of supplies. These supplies save steps for the circulating nurse and help eliminate traffic in and out of the OR. Glass shelves and sliding doors provide ease in finding and taking out items. Many cabinets are stainless steel, however. One cabinet in the room may have a pegboard at the back upon which to hang items, such as table appliances.

In lieu of or as an adjunct to cabinets, some hospitals stock carts with special sutures, instruments, drugs, etc., for some or all of the surgical specialties. The appropriate cart is brought to the room for a specific operation.

Other hospitals stock an individual cart with those items necessary for each operation. This cart usually is prepared in the central service department and is sent to the operating room suite by clean dumbwaiter or an overhead monorail system. The cart is covered or enclosed during transport. With the monorail system, the wheels of the cart never touch the floor until ejected into the clean corridor of the OR suite. From the delivery point, the cart may be taken into the OR or substerile room, or remain in the clean corridor until needed.

With the individual cart system, each cart is adequate in size to hold the supplies, both sterile and nonsterile, for one operation. These are selected according to standard routines and the individual surgeon's preferences. Some carts are designed for both storage of supplies needed throughout the operation and to serve as the instrument table during the operation.

Furniture and Other Equipment

All furniture and equipment, permanent or portable, should contact the conductive floor by means of conductive materials. Dry graphite or graphited oil is preferred as lubricant for conductive rubber or metal caster wheels. Conductive rubber is used on feet of furniture without wheels. Furniture and equipment should be metal or some equally conductive material. Shelves and top surfaces of furniture also should be conductive. Stainless steel furniture is plain, durable, and easily cleaned. Each OR is equipped with:

1 Operating table with a mattress covered with conductive rubber, attachments for positioning patient (see Chap. 10), and armboards.
2 Instrument tables.
3 Mayo stand. The *Mayo stand* is a frame, with a removable rectangular stainless steel tray, that slides under the operating table. It is placed just above and across the patient, below the operative field. It serves to bring near the operative field a supply of instruments in constant use during the operation.
4 Small tables for gowns and gloves and/or patient's preparation equipment.
5 Ring stand for basin(s).
6 Anesthesia machine and table for anesthesiologist's equipment.
7 Sitting stools and standing platforms.
8 Standards or hangers for intravenous solution bottles or bags.
9 Suction bottle and tubing, either wall mounted or portable in a low-wheeled base.
10 Linen hamper frame.
11 Kick buckets in wheeled bases.
12 Wastebasket.
13 Writing surface. This may be a wall-mounted, stainless steel desk or an area built into a cabinet for the circulating nurse to keep and write records.

Communication Systems

A communication system is a vital link to summon routine or emergency assistance or to relay information to and from the OR team.

Many OR suites are equipped with either monodirectional or bidirectional voice communication systems connecting each room with the clerk-receptionist's desk, the OR supervisor's office, pathology and radiology departments, blood bank, and recovery room. These systems make possible instantaneous consultation through direct communication. They are useful devices for the OR team, but are potentially hazardous for the patient.

Sounds are distorted by the patient in the early stages of general anesthesia. Incoming calls over a voice intercommunication (intercom) system should not be permitted to disturb the patient at this time. Also, an awake patient should not receive traumatic information about a pathologic diagnosis, for example, from a strange voice coming through an intercom speaker box after a biopsy has been performed. Installation of any type of intercom equipment in either the adjacent substerile room or scrub area, rather than in the OR, helps eliminate disturbance for both the patient and the surgeon.

In addition to or instead of a voice system, a call-light system can summon assistance from the anesthesia staff, ORS, pathologist, nursing assistant, and/or housekeeping personnel. Activated in the OR by a foot switch or hand switches, a light alerts personnel at a central point in the suite or displays varied needs at several receiving points simultaneously.

Closed-Circuit Television

Television surveillance provides an easy method for the ORS to keep abreast of activities in each OR. By means of a black-and-white television camera with a wide-angle lens mounted high in the corner of each OR, the ORS may make rounds simply by switching from one room to another by means of push buttons at his or her desk and a screen in the office.

More commonly, television serves a number of useful purposes for the surgeon in the OR. It is widely used for teaching operative techniques. This keeps visitors out of the OR, which, in the interest of sterile technique, is advantageous. In addition, television provides a better view and more persons can see the same operation from a remote area. It can provide not only an excellent vehicle for teaching, but can also provide record keeping and documentation for legal purposes for the surgeon.

As an aid to diagnosis, an audiovideo hookup between the OR and the x-ray department permits x-rays to be viewed on the television screen in the OR without transporting the films into the OR and mounting them on viewing boxes. With an audiovideo connection between the OR and x-ray department, the surgeon gains the advantage of remote interpretive consultation when it is desired.

A two-way audiovideo system between the frozen-section laboratory and the OR enables the surgeon to examine the microscopic slide by video in consultation with the pathologist without leaving the operating table. The pathologist can view the site of the pathologic lesion without entering the OR.

For these purposes, the color television camera may be mounted over the operating table in one of a number of ways. Usually it is attached to the stem of the operating light and outfitted with detachable sterilizable handles. An operating light with a television camera mounted in the center is available.

Video screens usually are adapted television sets and may be wall-mounted or placed on floor stands that can be moved readily. All pieces of television equipment must be labeled to indicate that they comply with applicable electrical safety regulations for use in the OR. They also must be encased in nonporous materials that can be easily cleaned.

Monitoring Equipment

Monitors and computers are designed to keep the OR team aware of the physiologic functions of the patient throughout the operation and to record patient data. The anesthesiologist uses monitoring devices as an added means to ensure safety for the patient during the operation (see Chap. 9, p. 187).

In some hospitals a central room may be set up to monitor all patients undergoing operations. More frequently, the monitors are housed in a room immediately adjacent to the OR, separated by a glass partition. These rooms are staffed by well-trained personnel familiar with the types of monitoring or computerized equipment in use.

EXCHANGE AREAS

Both patients and personnel enter the OR suite through an exchange area. Transportation of patients to a holding area was discussed in Chapter 3. Personnel must be properly attired to enter the OR suite and to enter the sterile field. These procedures are discussed in Chapter 7.

Chapter 7

Surgical Scrub, Gowning, and Gloving

HISTORICAL INTRODUCTION

The evolution of special operating room attire as an adjunct to asepsis paralleled the realization of need for and the development of aseptic techniques in the latter half of the nineteenth century. Operating room nursing became a specialty of surgical nursing in the 1890s. As the nurse assumed her place in the operating theatre, her attire changed through the years, as did the surgeon's.

One of the earliest mentions of specific OR attire appeared in that era in a nurse's training handbook that advised the nurse to bathe before operations, to take a carbolic bath before laparotomy, and to wear long sleeves and a clean apron for the operation. In the late 1800s, a Scottish surgeon relied on his nurse for more than the usual assignment of holding an emesis basin, wringing sponges out of cold water or carbolic solution, and helping with dressings. He also required his nurse to hold a child in order to steady the head and neck during a tracheotomy while having the necessary instruments in her apron pocket. Whereas the apron has long since given way to the present scrub attire of scrub dresses, pantsuits, and jumpsuits, long sleeves are again recommended for anesthesiologists and circulating nurses to reduce the shedding of microorganisms.

The first use of caps and sterile gowns seems to have taken place in Germany while the value of Lister's principle of antiseptic surgery to exclude putrefactive bacteria from wounds was still being debated on the continent and in America. In some operating theatres, the bacteria-laden, infection-causing woolen suits and Prince Alberts were replaced by OR garb of sterilizable material to lessen the introduction of pathogenic organisms into the wound. Innovators in aseptic technique were the German surgeon Gustav Neuber and Hunter Robb, a gynecologist at Johns Hopkins Hospital in Baltimore, who insisted on operating room cleanliness and on the wearing of caps and sterile gowns in the OR. In 1894, Dr. Robb published a book concerning aseptic surgical technique. In spite of the advances in technique and the professions, many surgeons of that time still operated in street clothes under a pus- and blood-encrusted apron. The famous Dr. William Halsted, chief of surgery of Johns Hopkins, in 1897 designed a semicircular instrument table to separate himself, in sterile gown and gloves, from observers in street clothes who watched him operate.

Also in the 1890s, while attention was being directed to the advantage of sterile gowns, Dr. William Lane developed a technique of asepsis in which only instruments, not hands, contacted tissue. Nurses trained in the Lane technique used sponge forceps for draping and even for gowning the surgeons. Special forceps were used to attach sterile towels to wound edges to occlude skin, a technique widely adopted by orthopaedic surgeons.

The use of sterile gowns antedated the routine use of caps, gloves, and masks, although in 1883 Neuber insisted on personnel wearing caps also. Emphasis on personal cleanliness expedited acceptance of special OR attire, but these standards were not rigidly practiced in all hospitals. Various styles of turbans and showercap-style head coverings were worn from about 1908 to the 1930s, when hair was generally acknowledged to be an attraction for and shedder of bacteria. But there were no universal standards of attire at that time.

Some photographs taken in the early twentieth century show only the surgeon and instrument nurse wearing special head covering, although hair had been recognized as a contaminant years before. A 1900 photograph revealed surgeon Charles McBurney and team operating in short surgical gowns and rubber gloves but without caps or masks. Charles Mayo and team in 1913 in Minnesota were photographed operating in surgical gowns, caps, and masks. The onlookers, however, wore only a white coat over street attire. Another photo of 1918 showed the surgeon in gown, cap, gloves, and a mask below his nose, the instrument nurse in gown and head cover but no mask, and the anesthetist and other nurses in gowns but regular nurses' caps.

In 1924, one of the first operating room nursing texts described the OR nurses: the circulating nurse wears OR cap, but no mask, and a gown with a pocket for pad and pencil; the scrub nurse wears both mask and gown. By the 1930s and 1940s, scrub dresses began to replace nurses' regular uniforms that had heretofore been worn under the sterile gown. Observers in the OR were gowned, capped, and masked. In the 1960s, full skirts were replaced by close-fitting scrub dresses and pantsuits that reduced the hazard of brushing against a sterile table when near or passing by it.

Rubber surgical gloves were introduced, not to protect the patient, but to protect the wearer's hands from harsh, irritating antiseptic solutions and hand soaks of the 1870s and 1880s. Their use was not popularized until the 1890s when Halsted's nurse complained of dermatitis. One of Halsted's assistants began to routinely wear gloves for clean operative procedures in 1896 although Halsted himself is known for popularizing the use of gloves, which proved to protect patients from the bacteria of ungloved hands. Mikulicz, the pioneering German surgeon who made numerous contributions to surgery, advocated the wearing of cotton gloves in 1896 also, but these were soon found to lack the qualities of impermeable rubber gloves for infection control. Disposable latex gloves, introduced about 1958, were a welcome innovation that saved countless hours of daily glove reprocessing, repairing, and sterilizing. Today, the universal use of disposable gloves is well established.

Gauze masks were advocated by Mikulicz in 1896 when the droplet theory of infection (see Chap. 4) was demonstrated. Numerous types of masks were developed. Although routinely worn, gauze masks lacked high efficiency and often the nose was not properly covered. The efficiency of gauze masks decreases rapidly with use from saturation with saliva. Modern protocol demands that both mouth and nose be completely covered to exclude bacterial spray. Used masks are a potent source of contamination. The most efficient masks are disposable ones containing a high-efficiency filter of fiberglass or polyprofeline.

In 1950, as restrictions became more rigid, OR personnel were required to change shoes when entering the OR suite and to wear only those shoes when within the suite. Disposable shoe covers with grounding tabs are recommended and worn.

In 1975 the Association of Operating Room Nurses published Standards for OR Attire.

OPERATING ROOM ATTIRE

Purpose

The purpose of operating room attire is to provide effective barriers that prevent the dissemination of microorganisms to the patient. However, these barriers coincidentally protect personnel from infected patients. The barriers prohibit contamination of the operative wound and sterile field by direct body contact. OR attire has been shown to reduce particle count of shedding from the body from over 10,000 particles per minute to 3000 per minute, or from 50,000 microorganisms per cubic foot to 500.

Definition

Operating room attire consists of body covers, such as scrub dress, jumpsuit, pantsuit, or shirt and trouser, head cover, mask, and shoe covers. Each has an appropriate purpose to combat sources of contamination *exogenous* (external) to the patient. Sterile gown and gloves are added to this basic attire for scrubbed team members. Proper attire is one facet of environmental control.

General Considerations

1 Each OR department should have a specific complete written policy on proper wearing apparel that is known to all persons. Protocol must be strictly monitored so that everyone conforms to established policies.

2 Only approved, clean OR attire is *worn within* the restricted area of the operating room suite. Street clothes are *never* worn within the restricted area. The attire is laundered only within the hospital's laundry facilities. This policy applies to *anyone* entering the restricted area, both professional and nonprofessional personnel.

3 OR attire is *not worn outside* of the operating room suite. This protects the OR environment from microorganisms inherent in the general hospital environment and protects other persons from contamination normally associated with the OR. Also, blood-stained garb is unattractive as well as a source of cross infection. Before leaving the OR suite, everyone should change to other clothing. The OR attire should be discarded and not hung in a locker with street clothes. Clean attire is donned on reentrance to the suite.

- **a** On occasion, such as preoperative visits to patients, clean laboratory coats are worn over OR attire outside the suite. This practice is not encouraged and is acceptable only when a clean, closed, knee-length lab coat is worn only once, and scrub attire is changed upon return to the suite. These coats do not protect the clothing beneath from contamination.
- **b** An adequate supply of clean attire should always be available so that there is no infraction of the rules.

4 Dressing rooms located adjacent to the OR suite are reached through the outer corridor. Clothes and shoes must be changed before entering, or reentering the suite. This regulation applies to *all* personnel.

5 Eyeglasses should be wiped with a tissue wet with antiseptic solution before each operation to prevent cross contamination.

6 Comfortable supportive shoes should be worn to relieve fatigue. Clogs, sandals, and tennis shoes are prohibited for reason of safety.

7 Impeccable personal hygiene must be reemphasized.

8 No person with an acute infection, such as a cold or sore throat, or skin lesion, such as a furuncle or any contagious condition, should be permitted within the OR suite. Persons with cuts, burns, or skin abrasions should not scrub or handle sterile equipment as serum, a bacterial medium, may seep from the eroded area.

Components of Attire

Each item of OR attire is a specific means of protecting the patient from the sources of contamination listed in Chapter 4, such as skin flora, nasopharyngeal flora, microorganisms on hair, fomites, and microorganisms in the air.

Body Cover A large variety of scrub suits and dresses are available. All must fit the body closely. Dresses should be a wraparound style to facilitate removal. Pantsuits and trousers should have snug-fitting ankle cuffs of rib-knit or be secured with snaps or drawstrings at the ankle to contain organisms shed from the perineal region and legs. Scrub shirts and waistline drawstrings should be tucked inside pants to avoid their touching sterile areas and to reduce fallout of skin debris shed from thoracic and abdominal areas. Microorganisms multiply more rapidly beneath a covered area. One-piece jumpsuites with attached hoods and boots are convenient garb for visitors whose presence in the OR is brief, for example, pathologists.

Mask A mask is worn to contain and filter out droplets containing microorganisms expelled from the oro- and nasopharynx. One is worn at all times within the operating room. Because talking, sneezing, and coughing disperse organism-laden droplet nuclei, some authorities recommend that a mask should be worn at all times by all people in the restricted area to protect the environment. This area includes inner corridors. Reusable cotton masks are obsolete. Disposable masks are far more efficient in filtering ability (up to 99 percent). Contemporary masks of soft, clothlike material, in very fine synthetic fiber mats, fulfill essential criteria. These masks are:

1 Over 95 percent efficient in filtering microbes.

2 Cool, comfortable, and nonobstructive to respiration.

3 Nonirritating, generally. If a person is sensitive to one type, he or she should try another brand. A totally nonfiberglass one is available.

To be effective, a mask must catch all of a person's exhalations; therefore it must be worn over both nose and mouth. Air must pass only through the filtering system, so the mask must conform to facial contours to prevent leakage of expired air. Ejected droplets must not escape the filter action.

Masks are designed for close fit but improper application can negate their efficiency. Always tie the strings tightly, if that is the method of securing the mask, to prevent the strings coming loose during an operation and contaminating the sterile gown. Tie upper strings at back of head; tie lower strings behind neck. Strings are never crossed over head because this distorts contours of mask along cheeks. Some types of masks have an exterior pliable strip or noseband that can be bent to contour mask over the bridge of the nose. A close-fitting mask also helps to avoid steaming of eyeglasses. To prevent cross infection, masks should:

1 Be handled only by the strings, thereby keeping the facial area of a fresh mask clean, and hands uncontaminated by a soiled mask. Do not handle the mask excessively.

2 Never be lowered to hang loosely around the neck or be placed on top of cap. Avoid disseminating microorganisms.

3 Be promptly discarded into the proper receptacle on removal. Remask with a fresh mask between patients.

4 Be changed frequently. Do not permit one to become wet. Talking should be kept to a minimum.

Head Cover All facial and head hair must be covered in the restricted area. Various types of lightweight caps, helmets, and hoods are available for this purpose. Practically all are disposable and made of lint-free, nonporous, soft, clothlike fabric. Reusable head covers must be of a densely woven material. If hair is long, a helmet or hood must be worn to cover the neck area. Headgear should fit well to prevent any escape of hair and to confine microorganisms. A cap or hood is put on *before* a scrub suit or dress. This is done to protect the garment from contamination by hair. Also, hair should not be combed while in scrub (basic OR) attire. Persons with scalp infection should be excluded from the OR and treated.

Hair, in addition to being a gross contaminant, is also a source of electrostatic spark.

Shoe Covers Disposable or canvas shoe covers also must be worn at all times in the restricted area. They must be safe as well as impervious to moisture. Conductive shoe covers must be worn in hazardous locations or where electrical equipment is used. The black strip on conductive shoe covers must be inside of the shoe, in contact with the sole of the foot. Conductive covers provide electrical grounding for the wearer. In contact with conductive flooring, accumulated static electricity is harmlessly drained to the ground. After donning OR attire, personnel should test personal conductivity by use of a conductometer located at the entrance to any hazardous location.

Shoe covers should be worn on a single-use basis. They must be removed on leaving the restricted area and a fresh pair put on prior to reentrance to that area. Shoe soles are a source of gross contamination and of cross infection from one area of the hospital to another. Supportive footwear should be worn beneath the shoe covers.

Gowns Sterile gowns are worn over scrub attire (dress or suit) to permit the wearer to create and to come within the sterile field, in order to carry out sterile technique during an operative procedure. Sterile gowns provide an effective barrier for personnel between sterile and nonsterile areas.

Both reusable and disposable gowns, in a variety of styles, are in use. Although the entire gown is sterilized, the back is not considered sterile nor is any area below waist level, once the gown is donned. Wraparound gowns that provide sterile coverage to the back by a generous overlap are recommended. These gowns are secured at the neck and waist before the sterile flap is brought over the back and secured by ties or grips at the side or front. If the gown is closed merely by ties along the back, a sterile vest is put on over the gown to cover any exposed back area of scrub attire. The cuffs of gowns are stockinet (rib-knit) to tightly fit the wrist. Sterile gloves cover the wrists of the gown.

Gowns are made of either disposable, nonwoven, water-repellent material or densely woven cotton. Repellent materials avoid strike-through of moisture and microorganisms under normal use. Some reusable gowns have waterproof sleeves and insert over the chest area extending below the waist. Textile gowns should be reinforced at the front and forearms. Tests for permeability and strength of gown materials simulate realistic conditions with attention also to stress areas such as the elbow.

Gloves Sterile gloves complete the attire for scrubbed team members. They are worn to permit the wearer to handle sterile supplies or tissues of the operative wound. Surgical gloves are made of natural latex or synthetic rubber. Light latex disposable gloves are the most frequently used.

Gloves are packaged in pairs with an everted cuff on each to protect the outside of the sterile glove during donning. The inner paper wrap of the disposable glove package protects the sterility of the gloves when they are removed from the outer wrap. Glove packages are generally the peel-apart type. Prior to opening the package, the circulating nurse should inspect it for damage or wetness, which would indicate contamination. When the inner paper is unfolded, the wearer finds the right glove to the right, the left glove to the left, palm side up.

Both inner and outer surfaces are prelubricated with an absorbable dry powder before the sterilization process to facilitate donning, to decrease loose powder in the OR air, and to prevent adhesion of glove surfaces. Although considered absorbable and inert in tissue, this lubricant may at times cause serious complications such as granulomas or peritonitis if it is introduced into wounds. Consequently, it is important to remove the lubricant on the outside of the gloves. To do this, gloves should be thoroughly wiped with a sterile damp towel or terry washcloth after donning.

If a sterile glove is punctured or torn it must be changed immediately to prevent escape of microorganisms from the skin beneath. Some authorities estimate the incidence of glove puncture to be as high as 30 percent of unworn gloves tested. Shedders present a special threat from these imperfections.

Criteria for OR Attire

Attire should be:

1 Effective barrier to microorganisms under normal, in-use conditions. Both reusable woven and disposable nonwoven materials are used.
2 Closely woven material void of dangerous electrostatic properties. The garment must meet National Fire Protection Association Standards (NFPA-56A), including resistance to flame.
   a Undergarments of synthetic material such as nylon are permissible when in close contact with the skin, such as hosiery.
   b Nylon and other static spark-producing materials are forbidden as outer garments.
3 Resistant to blood, aqueous fluids, and abrasion to prevent penetration by organisms.
4 Designed for maximal skin coverage.
5 Hypoallergenic, cool, and comfortable.
6 Nongenerative of lint. Lint can increase the particle count of contaminants in the OR.
7 Pliable material to permit freedom of movement for the practice of sterile technique.
8 Able to transmit heat and water vapor, to protect the wearer.
9 Colored to reduce glare under lights. Various types of clothes in colorful prints that fulfill the necessary criteria are both attractive and functional.
10 Easy to don and remove.

Proper Attire

Clean, fresh attire is donned each time on arrival at the OR suite and as necessary at other times, if it is wet or grossly soiled.

NOTE. Showers should be available to personnel in case of gross contamination during a procedure.

Masks and head covers should be changed between patients. As extra precautions, known carriers who participate as sterile team members should:

1 Routinely bathe and scrub with an appropriate skin antiseptic agent; shampoo hair daily.
2 Change clothing frequently.
3 Wear two masks; use antimicrobial nasal ointment.
4 Use two scrub agents successively, double gown and double glove.
5 Use "no touch" technique; avoid touching any part of an instrument in direct contact with tissue.
6 Wash hands frequently and thoroughly.

Special attire is worn with laminar airflow systems in high-risk operations (see p. 83). Attire varies from hospital to hospital but may consist of a presterilized jumpsuit as basic attire, covered by sterile gown and gloves. A vacuum helmet is worn.

THE SURGICAL SCRUB

Definition

The *surgical scrub* is the process of removing as many microorganisms as possible from the hands and arms by mechanical washing and chemical antisepsis before participating in an operative procedure.

Microorganisms

The skin is inhabited by:

1 *Transient organisms* acquired by direct contact. Usually loosely attached to the skin surface, these organisms are almost completely removed by thorough washing with soap or detergent and water.
2 *Resident organisms* below the skin surface in hair follicles, and in sebaceous and sweat glands. They are more adherent, therefore more resistant to removal. Their growth is inhibited by the chemical phase of the surgical scrub. Resident skin flora represent the microorganisms present in the hospital environment. Many are coagulase-positive staphylococci. Prolonged exposure of skin to contaminants yields a more pathogenic resident population.

In freeing the skin of as many organisms as possible, two processes are utilized:

1 *Mechanical:* removes soil and transient organisms with friction
2 *Chemical:* reduces resident flora and inactivates microorganisms with a microbicidal or antiseptic agent

Purpose

The purpose of the surgical scrub is to remove soil, debris, natural skin oils, hand lotions, and microorganisms from the hands and forearms of sterile team members. More specifically, the purpose is:

1 To decrease the number of microorganisms on skin to an irreducible minimum
2 To keep the population of microorganisms minimal during the operative procedure by suppression of growth
3 To reduce the hazard of microbial contamination of the operative wound by skin flora

The surgical scrub is done just prior to gowning and gloving for each operation.

Sink

Adequate scrubbing and handwashing facilities should be provided for all operating team members. The scrub room is adjacent to the operating room for safety and convenience. Individually enclosed scrub sinks with knee-operated faucets are preferred to eliminate the hazard of contaminating hands after cleansing.

The sink should be designed deep and wide enough to prevent splash. A sterile gown cannot be put on over damp scrub attire without resultant contamination of the gown by strike-through of moisture.

Scrub sinks should be used *only* for scrubbing or handwashing. They should not be used to clean or rinse contaminated instruments or equipment.

Equipment

Sterilized reusable scrub brushes or disposable sponges may be used. Single-use disposable products may be a brush-sponge combination. Some are impregnated with antiseptic-detergent agents. Disposable products are individually packaged. If reusable brushes are taken from the dispenser in which they were sterilized, each brush must be removed without contaminating the others. Brushes may be wrapped to provide sterile individual packages. The brush should not cause skin abrasion. The scrubbing solution is dispensed onto the brush or sponge by foot pedal from a container attached or adjacent to the sink. Six drops, about 2 cc or 2 to 3 ml, of solution is sufficient to generate a lather for the scrub procedure. Avoid waste of antiseptic solution.

Debris must be removed from the subungual area under nail of each finger. Metal or plastic single-use disposable products are available. Reusable nail cleaners must be sterilized between uses.

NOTE. Orangewood sticks are not used to clean under fingernails because the wood may splinter and harbor Pseudomonas.

Agents for Antisepsis

Various antimicrobial (antiseptic) detergents are used for the surgical scrub. The agent must be:

1 A broad-spectrum antimicrobial agent
2 Fast-acting and effective
3 Nonirritating and nonsensitizing
4 Prolonged-acting, i.e., leaves an antimicrobial residue on the skin to temporarily prevent growth of microorganisms
5 Independent of cumulative action

While the action of the agent is important in relation to its efficacy, mechanical friction and effort while scrubbing are equally influential. Most hospitals have more than one agent available in the scrub room for personnel allergic to one agent.

NOTE. 1. Frequent scrubbing tends to prevent rapid, complete reestablishment of resident flora.

2. Variables in skin antisepsis are mechanical factors, chemical factors, and individual differences in skin flora.

The most frequently used agents are:

1 *Povidone-iodine.* An iodine-complex detergent, frequently referred to as an *iodophor,* this agent fulfills all of the criteria for the surgical scrub. Effective cleansers, iodophors also slowly release iodine for residual effect. They are cidal with every use and effective against gram-negative as well as gram-positive microorganisms. The cidal action may be sustained for up to 8 hours.

2 *Chlorhexidine gluconate.* A 4% concentration of this agent exerts an antimicrobial effect against gram-positive and gram-negative microorganisms. Residues tend to accumulate on the skin with repeated use and produce a prolonged effect. This agent is a good alternative for persons allergic to povidone-iodine, which is more effective against gram-negative organisms.

3 *Hexachlorophene.* This type of agent is most effective after buildup of cumulative suppressive action caused by regular use. The residual film is effective in keeping gram-positive organisms from proliferating, but is not effective against proliferation of gram-negative bacilli. Action of the agent is negated by alcohol.

Preparation for Surgical Scrub

General Preparations

1 Fingernails should not reach beyond the fingertip to avoid glove puncture.

2 Skin and nails should be kept clean and in good condition, and cuticles uncut. If hand lotion is used to protect skin, a non-oil base product is recommended.

3 Individual hospital dictates policy on use of nail polish. The lacquer may chip and peel thereby providing a harbor for microorganisms in crevices. No polish is preferred.

Preparations Prior to Scrub

1 Inspect hands for cuts and abrasions.

2 Remove *all* finger jewelry. (Pierced-ear studs *must* be contained by the head cover.) Jewelry harbors microorganisms. It is also a potential foreign body in the operative wound.

3 Be sure *all* hair is covered by headgear.

4 Adjust disposable mask snugly and comfortably over nose and mouth.

5 Adjust eyeglasses comfortably in relation to mask.

6 Adjust water to a comfortable temperature.

Length of Scrub

The length of the surgical scrub varies from one institution to another, as does the scrub procedure. Results of one study led to the estimate that microorganisms are decreased 50 percent by each 6 minutes of scrubbing. However, other studies have shown a vigorous, 5-minute scrub with a reliable agent to be as effective as a 10-minute scrub. *Variations in length may depend on frequency of scrubbing and the agent used.* The individual should scrub according to the written policy of the hospital and the manufacturer's recommendations for the agent used. A copy of the exact procedure should be posted in every scrub room. Skill improves with practice.

Surgical Scrub Procedure

The procedure for surgical scrub differs from one hospital to another but the recommended methods are applications of the principles of aseptic technique. These may be either the *time method* or counted *brush-stroke method.* If properly executed, they are both effective and each exposes all surfaces of the hands and forearms to mechanical cleansing and chemical antisepsis. One should think of the fingers, hands, and arms as having four sides or surfaces. Both methods follow an *anatomical pattern of scrub:* four surfaces of each finger, beginning with the thumb and moving from one finger to the next, down the outer edge of the fifth finger, over the dorsal (back) surface of the hand, the palmer (palm) surface of the hand, or vice versa, from small finger to thumb, over the wrists and up the arm, in thirds, ending 2 in. (5 cm) above the elbow. Since the hands are in most direct contact with the sterile field, all steps of the scrub procedure begin with the hands and end with the elbows.

Time Method Fingers, hands, and arms are scrubbed by allotting a prescribed amount of time to each anatomical area or each step of the procedure.

Five-Minute Scrub

1 Wet hands and forearms.

2 Apply six drops of antiseptic agent from dispenser to the hands.

3 Wash the hands and arms several times thoroughly to 2 in. (5 cm) above the elbow. Rinse thoroughly under running water, with the hand upward, allowing water to drip from the flexed elbow.

4 Take a sterile brush (from a package or dispenser), apply antimicrobial agent if it is not impregnated in the brush. Scrub nails and hands, $\frac{1}{2}$ minute for each hand.

5 With brush in hand, clean under the fingernails under running water with a metal or disposable plastic nail cleaner. Discard after use.

6 Again scrub nails and hands with the brush $\frac{1}{2}$ minute for each hand, maintaining lather.

7 Rinse the hands and brush and discard the brush or sponge.

8 Reapply antimicrobial detergent and wash hands and arms with friction to the elbow for 3 minutes. Interlace the fingers to cleanse between them.

9 Rinse hands and arms as before.

Brush-Stroke Method A prescribed number of brush strokes, applied lengthwise of the brush or sponge, is used for each surface of the fingers, hands, and arms. A short, prescrub wash loosens surface debris and transient organisms. Scrub by brush or sponge removes resident flora.

1 Wet hands and arms.

2 Wash hands and arms thoroughly to 2 in. (5 cm) above the elbow with antiseptic agent.

3 Clean under fingernails carefully under running water with reusable metal file or disposable plastic cleaner. Discard the file.

4 Rinse hands and arms thoroughly under running water, keeping the hands up and allowing water to drip from the elbows.

5 Take a sterile brush or sponge from a dispenser or package. Apply antiseptic agent to the brush or sponge if not previously impregnated.

6 Scrub the nails of the left hand 50 strokes, all sides of each finger 40 strokes, the back of the hand 10 strokes, the palm of the hand 10 strokes, the arms 40 strokes for each third of the arm, to 2 in. (5 cm) above the elbow.

7 Repeat step 6 for the right hand.

8 Rinse hands and arms thoroughly.

NOTE. 1. During and after scrubbing, keep the hands higher than the elbows to allow water to flow from the cleanest area, the hands, to the marginal area of the upper arms.

2. If a person scrubs frequently, some hospitals reduce the number of strokes per scrub in the brush-stroke method.

3. If policy dictates a 10-minute initial scrub, the 5-minute scrub may be used for subsequent operations. Once gloves are removed, hands become contaminated from contact with inanimate items.

GOWNING AND GLOVING

The sterile gown is put on immediately after the surgical scrub. The sterile gloves are put on immediately after gowning.

Purpose

Sterile gown and gloves are worn to exclude skin as a possible contaminant and to create a barrier between sterile and unsterile areas.

General Considerations

1 The scrub nurse gowns and gloves herself. She gowns and gloves the surgeon and assistants.

2 Gown packages preferably are opened on a separate table from other packages to avoid any chance of contamination from dripping water.

Drying Hands and Arms

After scrubbing, hands and arms must be thoroughly dried before the sterile gown is donned to prevent contamination of the gown by strike-through of organisms from skin and scrub attire.

The gown package for the scrub nurse contains one sterile gown, folded before sterilization, with the inside out, so that the bare scrubbed hands will not contaminate the sterile outside of the gown. A towel for drying hands is placed on top of the gown during packaging. The hands are dried as follows:

1 Reach down to the opened sterile package and pick up the towel. Be careful not to drip water onto the pack. Be sure no one is within arm's reach (see Fig. 7-1).

Figure 7-1 Scrub nurse (or technician) preparing to gown removes the hand towel on top of the gown from the opened gown package. Note that mask covers both nose and mouth and skirt of scrub dress is narrow.

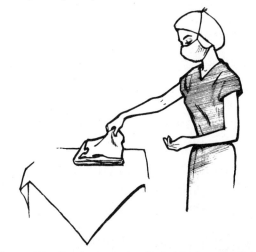

2 Open the towel full-length, holding one end. Hold it away from nonsterile scrub attire (see Fig. 7-2).

3 Dry both hands thoroughly but independently. To dry one arm, hold the towel in the opposite hand and, using an oscillating motion of the arm, draw the towel up to the elbow.

4 Carefully reverse the towel, still holding it away from the body. Dry the opposite arm on the unused (now uppermost) end of the towel.

NOTE. Often the towel is an absorbent, disposal one. Some hospitals package two absorbent washcloths in lieu of the towel. They are crisscrossed on top of the gown, to separate them. To use them, reach down to the sterile package and pick up one washcloth, being careful not to drip water. Holding the arms away from the washcloth, dry one hand, then the arm, as with the towel. Discard the washcloth. Use the second washcloth to dry the other hand and arm in the same manner.

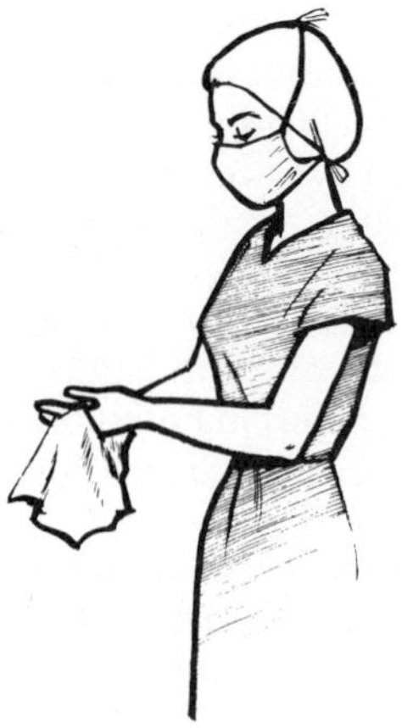

Figure 7-2 Scrub nurse drying hands holds the towel out away from body. She dries only well-scrubbed areas, hands first, and avoids contaminating hands on the areas proximal to elbows. She then discards the towel.

Gowning and Gloving Techniques

Sterile gloves may be put on in two ways: by *closed glove technique,* or by *open glove technique.* The closed glove method is preferred except when changing a glove during an operation or when donning gloves for procedures not requiring gowns. Properly executed, the closed glove method affords assurance against contamination, when gloving oneself, since no bare skin is exposed in the process. If properly done, however, gloves can be put on safely either way. *The method of gloving determines how the gown is donned.*

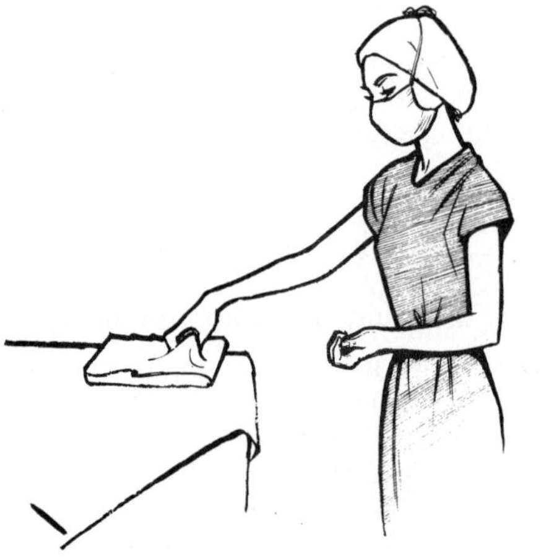

Figure 7-3 Scrub nurse, picking up gown below neck edge, lifts it directly upward and steps away to avoid touching an edge of the wrapper. Note that the sterile inside of the wrapper covers the table. Gown is folded inside out.

Closed Glove Technique

Gowning for Closed Glove Technique

1 Reach down to the sterile package and lift the folded gown directly upward (see Fig. 7-3).

2 Step back away from the table, into an unobstructed area, to provide a wide margin of safety while gowning.

3 Holding the folded gown, carefully locate the neckband.

4 Holding the inside front of the gown just below the neckband with both hands, let the gown unfold, keeping the inside of the gown toward the body. Do not touch the outside of the gown with bare hands.

5 Holding the hands at shoulder level, slip both arms into the armholes simultaneously (see Fig. 7-4).

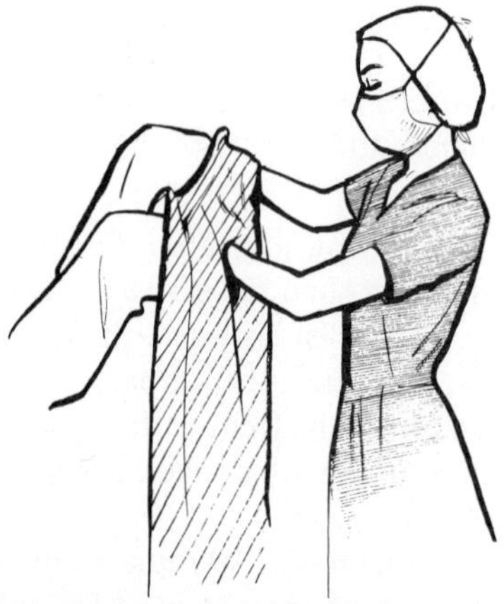

Figure 7-4 Scrub nurse, putting on gown, gently shakes out the folds, then slips arms into the sleeves without touching the sterile outside of the gown with bare hands.

6 The *circulating nurse* brings the gown over the shoulders by reaching inside to the shoulder and arm seams. She *pulls the gown on, leaving the sleeves extended over the hands.* She securely ties or fastens the back of the gown at the neck and waist, touching the outside of the gown at the line of ties or fasteners, in back only (see Figs. 7-5 and 7-6).

NOTE. 1. If the gown is wraparound style, the sterile flap to cover the back is not touched until the person has gowned and gloved. The sterile gown may be wrapped around in various ways:

a. With gloved hands, release the fastener or untie the ties at the front or right side of the gown. Hand the tie on the right to a sterile team member who remains stationary. Allowing a margin of safety, turn around to the left, thereby completely covering the back with the extended flap of the gown. Accept the tie from the assistant and secure the ties at the left side of the gown.

b. If you are the first person to gown and glove and other sterile team members are not available to assist, snap a sterile instrument such as an Allis's forceps, never a hemostat or clamps for hemostasis, to the tie on the right. Carefully hand the instrument to the circulating nurse. While she remains stationary, turn to the left, thereby covering the back. Take the tie in hand. The circulating nurse then releases and discards the instrument. Tie the ties at the left side.

c. Some disposable gowns have the end of one tie covered by a disposable strip. Hand the strip to the circulating nurse, taking care to protect the hands. Turn around toward the opposite side, thereby closing the gown. Grasp the tie at a distance from the end. The circulating nurse pulls the strip, releasing it from the still-sterile end of the tie, and discards it. Tie the ties at the front or side of the gown as indicated.

2. If the top of the gown drops downward inadvertently, discard the gown as contaminated. Never reverse a piece of sterile linen, if the wrong end is dropped toward the floor.

Gloving by Closed Glove Technique

1 Using the left hand, and keeping it within the cuff of the left sleeve, pick up the right glove, from the inner wrap of the glove package, by grasping the folded cuff.

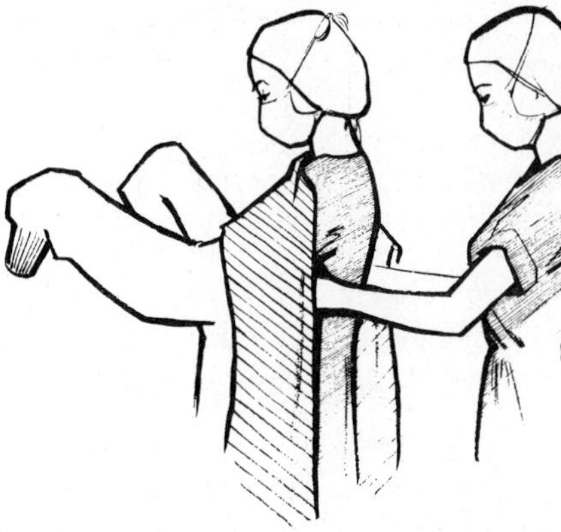

Figure 7-5 Circulating nurse, pulling the gown on for closed gloving technique, reaches inside the gown to the sleeve seams and pulls the gown on, leaving the cuffs of the sleeves extended over the hands.

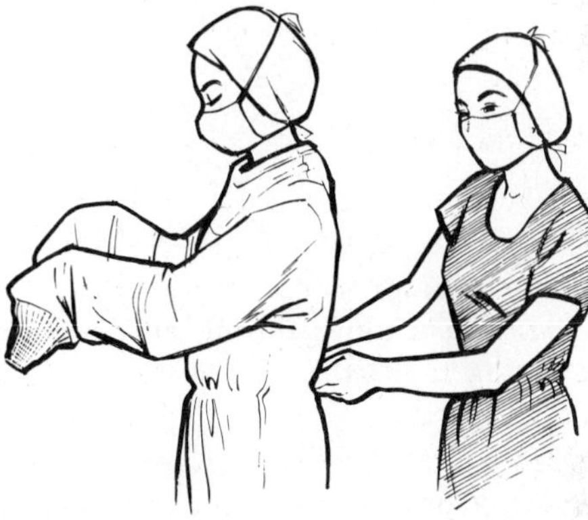

Figure 7-6 Circulating nurse completes pulling on the nurse's gown. She ties the tapes on the inside of the back and closes the fastener at the neck.

2 Extend the right forearm with palm upward. Place the palm of the glove against the palm of the right hand, grasping in the right hand the top edge of the cuff, above the palm. In correct position, glove fingers are pointing toward you and the thumb of the glove is to the right. The thumb side of the glove is down (see Fig. 7-7).

3 Grasp the back of the cuff in the left hand and turn it over the end of the right sleeve and hand. The cuff of the glove is now over the stockinet cuff of the gown, with the hand still inside the sleeve (see Figs. 7-8 and 7-9).

4 Grasp the top of the right glove and underlying gown sleeve with covered left hand. Pull the glove on over extended right fingers until the glove completely covers the stockinet cuff (see Fig. 7-10).

5 Glove the left hand in the same manner, reversing hands. Use the gloved right hand to pull on the left glove (see Figs. 7-11 to 7-13).

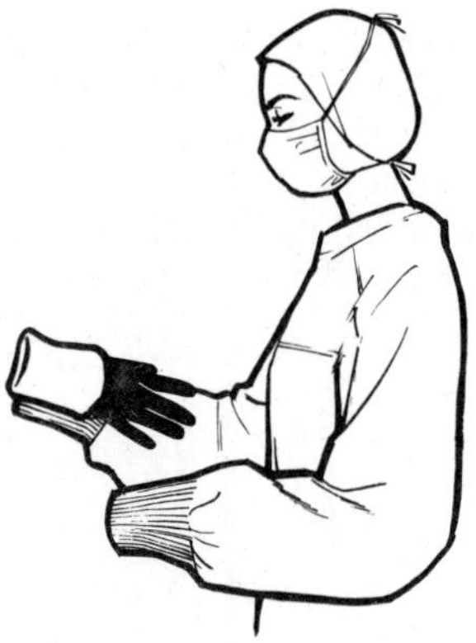

Figure 7-7 For closed gloving technique, using the left hand and keeping it within the cuff of the sleeve, the gowned scrub nurse picks up the right glove. She places the palm of the glove against the palm of the right hand, grasping the top edge of the glove cuff, above the palm, in the right hand.

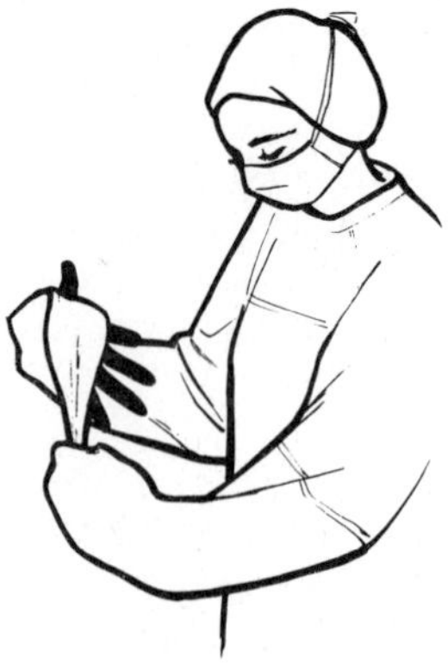

Figure 7-8 She grasps the back of the cuff in the left hand and turns it over the right sleeve and hand.

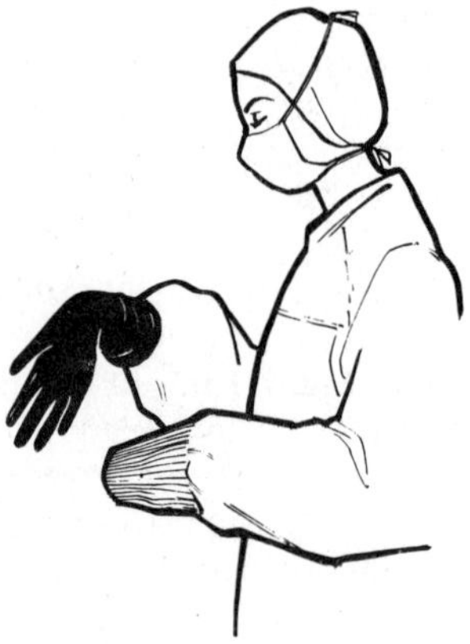

Figure 7-9 Cuff of the glove is now over the stockinet cuff of the sleeve, with the hand still inside the sleeve.

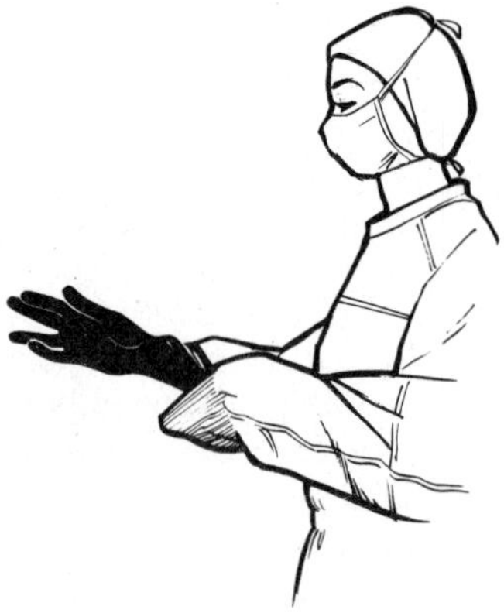

Figure 7-10 She grasps the top of the right glove and the underlying sleeve of the gown with left hand and, as she pulls the sleeve up, pulls the glove onto hand.

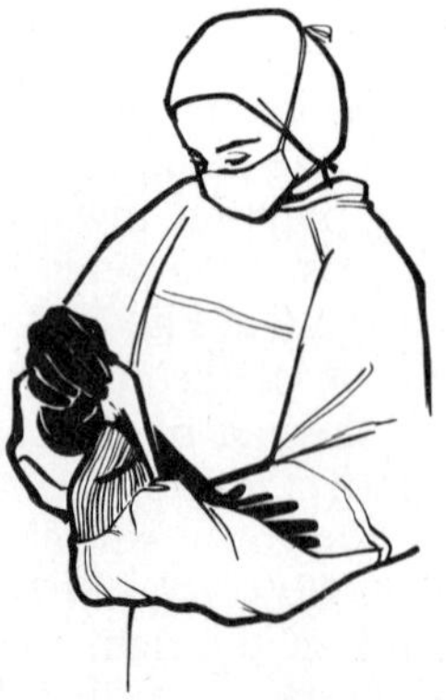

Figure 7-11 Using gloved right hand, she picks up the left glove and places the palm of the glove against the palm of the left hand. She grasps the back of the cuff, above the palm, in the right hand and turns it over the left sleeve and hand.

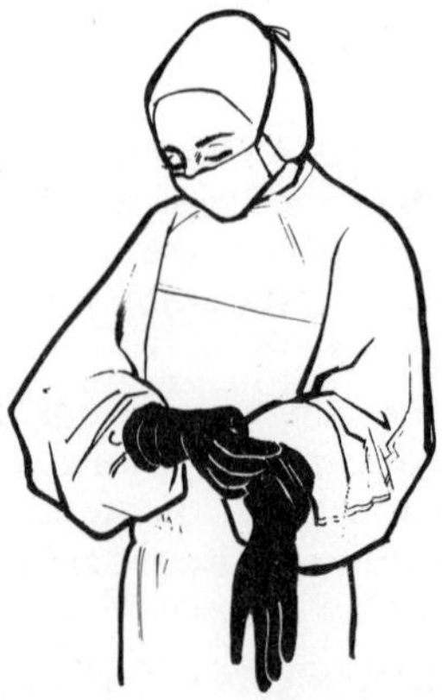

Figure 7-12 The cuff of the left glove is now over the stockinet cuff of the sleeve, with the hand still inside the sleeve.

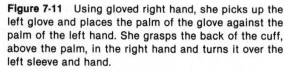

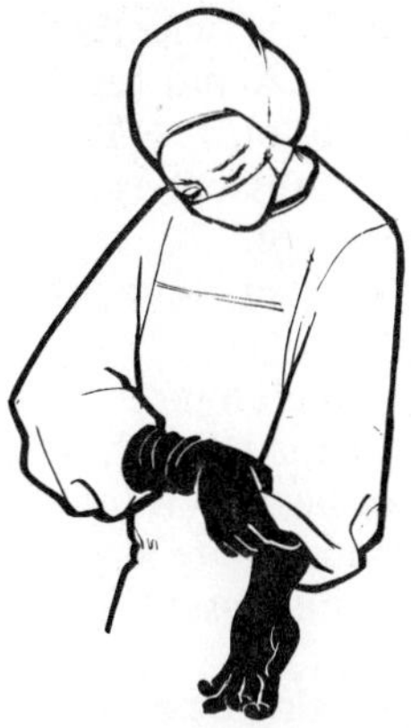

Figure 7-13 She grasps the top of the left glove and underlying gown sleeve with right hand and, as she pulls the sleeve up, pulls the glove onto hand.

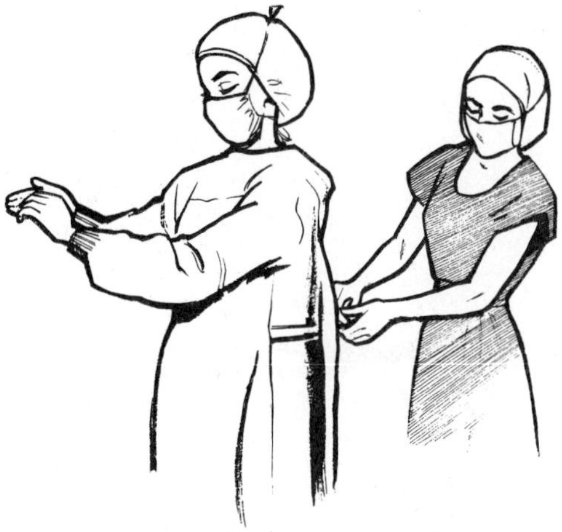

Figure 7-14 Circulating nurse fastens the back of the scrub nurse's gown for open-gloving technique. Note that hands extend through the stockinet cuffs.

Open Glove Technique

Gowning for Open Glove Technique

1 Reach down to the sterile package and lift the folded gown directly upward.

2 Step back away from the table, into a clear area, to provide a wide margin of safety while gowning.

3 Holding the folded gown, carefully locate the neckband.

4 Holding the inside front of the gown just below the neckband with both hands, let the gown unfold, keeping the inside of the gown toward the body.

5 Holding the hands at shoulder level, slip both hands into the armholes simultaneously, without touching the sterile exterior of the gown with bare hands.

6 The *circulating nurse* reaches inside the gown to the sleeve seams, and *pulls the sleeves over the hands* to the wrists. She securely closes the back of the gown at the neck and waist, with ties or fasteners, as indicated. She touches the outside of the gown at the line of ties or fasteners in the back only (see Fig. 7-14).

Gloving by Open Glove Technique This method of gloving uses a skin-to-skin, glove-to-glove technique. The hand, although scrubbed, is not sterile and must not contact the exterior of sterile gloves. The everted cuff on the gloves exposes the inner surfaces. The first glove is put on with skin-to-skin technique, bare hand to inside cuff. The sterile fingers of that gloved hand then may touch sterile exterior of the second glove, i.e., glove-to-glove technique.

1 With the left hand, grasp the cuff of the right glove on the fold. Pick up the glove and step back from the table. Look behind you before moving.

2 Insert the right hand into the glove and pull it on, leaving the cuff turned well down over the hand (see Fig. 7-15).

3 Slip the fingers of the gloved right hand *under* the everted cuff of the left glove. Pick up the glove and step back (see Fig. 7-16).

4 Insert the hand into the left glove and pull it on, leaving the cuff turned down over the hand.

5 With the fingers of the right hand, pull the cuff of the left glove over the cuff of the left sleeve. If the stockinet is not tight, fold a pleat, holding it with the right thumb while pulling the glove over the cuff. Avoid touching the bare wrist (see Fig. 7-17).

6 Repeat step 5 for the right cuff, using the left hand, and thereby completely gloving the right hand (see Fig. 7-18).

NOTE. Open glove technique is used when only sterile gloves are worn, such as for intravenous cutdown or administration of spinal anesthesia. It is also used in emergency departments when donning sterile gloves for suturing lacerations, for example. It also is used for changing a glove during an operation.

Gowning Another Person

A team member in sterile gown and gloves may assist another team member in gowning and gloving by taking the following steps:

1 Open the hand towel and lay it on the surgeon's hand, being careful not to touch the hand.

2 Unfold the gown carefully, holding it at the neckband.

3 Keeping hands on the outside of the gown under a protective cuff of the neck and shoulder area, offer the *inside* of the gown to the surgeon. He or she slips the arms into the sleeves.

4 Release the gown. The surgeon holds arms outstretched while the circulating nurse pulls the gown onto the shoulders and adjusts the sleeves so that the cuffs are properly placed. In doing so, she touches only the inside of the gown at the seams.

Gloving Another Person

1 Pick up the right glove, grasp it firmly, with fingers under the everted cuff. Hold the *palm* of the glove toward the surgeon.

2 Stretch the cuff sufficiently for the surgeon to introduce the hand. Avoid touching the hand by holding your thumbs out (see Fig. 7-19).

3 Exert upward pressure as the surgeon plunges the hand into the glove.

4 Unfold the everted glove cuff over the cuff of the sleeve.

5 Repeat for the left hand.

6 If a sterile vest is needed, hold it for the surgeon to slip his or her hands into the armholes. Be careful not to contaminate gloves at neck level. If gown is a wraparound, assist the surgeon.

Changing Gown during Operation

Occasionally a contaminated gown must be changed during an operation. The circulating

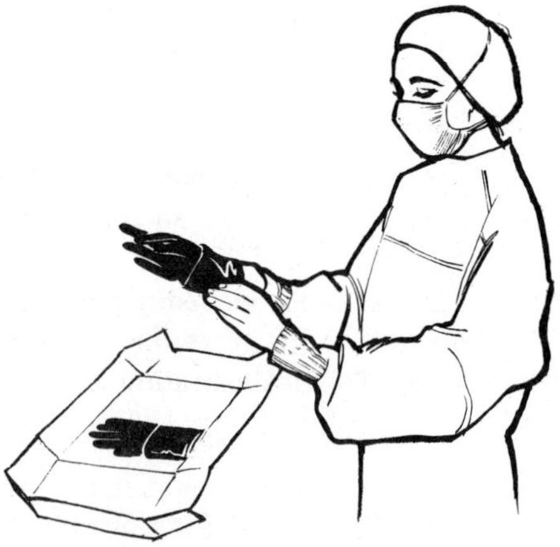

Figure 7-15 Scrub nurse gloving right hand with open gloving technique. With the left hand, she grasps the right glove on the folded-back cuff and lifts it directly up and away from the wrapper. Right hand is inserted in the glove. Note that left hand touches only the cuff or inside of the glove, skin-to-skin technique.

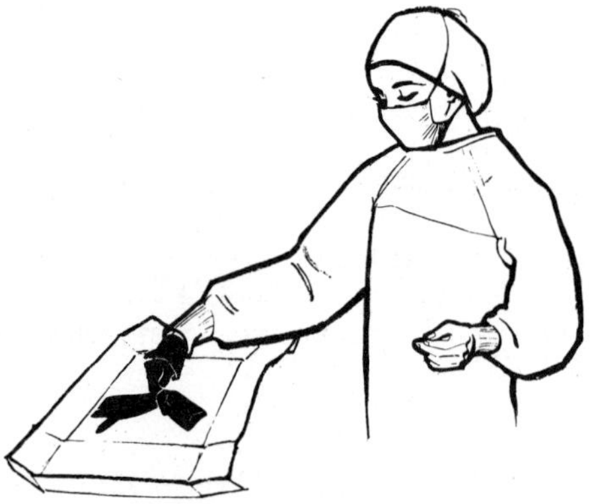

Figure 7-16 Picking up the left glove, scrub nurse lifts the glove from the wrapper by slipping gloved right fingers under the protective cuff, glove-to-glove technique. Bare hand does not touch the outside of the glove.

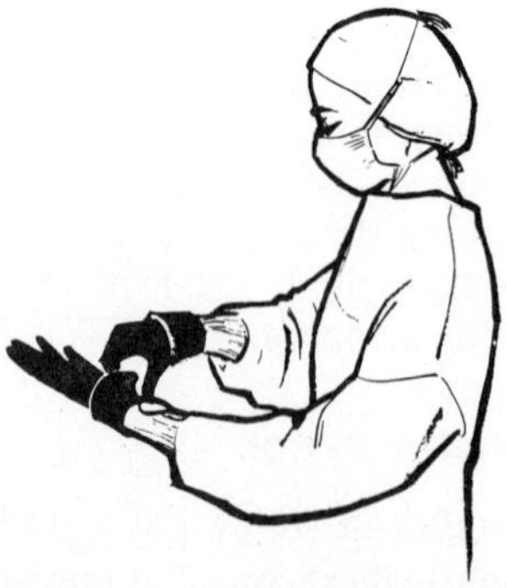

Figure 7-17 Pulling the cuff of the left glove up over the cuff of the sleeve. Gloved fingers of the right hand touch only the outside of the left glove, near the wrist. If the stockinet is not tight, nurse folds a pleat, holding it with right thumb as she pulls the glove over the cuff. Contact with exposed skin would contaminate the right glove.

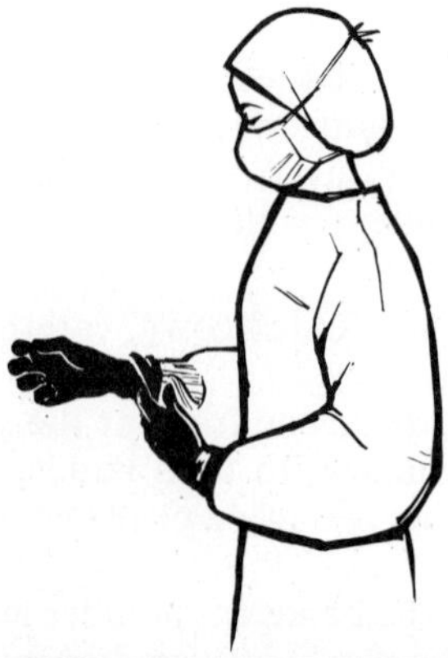

Figure 7-18 Using now completely gloved left hand, she inserts left fingers under the folded-back cuff of the right glove and pulls the glove cuff up over the right-sleeve cuff, glove-to-glove technique.

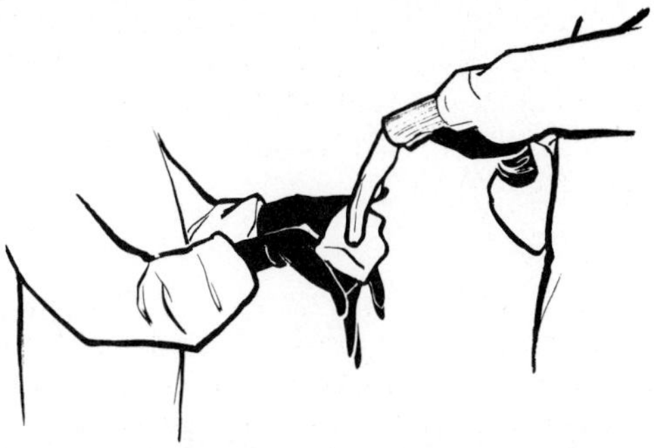

Figure 7-19 Nurse gloving doctor or another person. She holds his glove with the palm toward him. She holds her thumbs out to avoid his touching them with his bare hands.

nurse unfastens neck and waist. Grasping gown at shoulder, she pulls the gown off inside out. The gown is always removed first. The gloves are removed using glove-to-glove then skin-to-skin technique. If only the sleeve is contaminated, a sterile sleeve may be put on over the contaminated one.

Changing Glove during Operation

If a glove becomes contaminated for any reason during an operative procedure, it must be changed immediately. If you cannot step away at the moment, hold the contaminated hand away from the sterile area. To change the glove:

1 Turn away from the sterile field.
2 Extend the contaminated hand to the circulating nurse who grasps the outside of the glove cuff about 2 in. (5 cm) below the top of the glove and pulls the glove off inside out.
3 Preferably a sterile team member gloves another. If this is not possible, step aside and glove the hand using the open glove technique.

NOTE. The closed glove technique cannot be used for glove change during an operation without contamination of the new glove by the sleeve of the gown or without contamination of the hand by the cuff of the gown. The cuff must not be pulled down over hand. If this method is used, gloves and gown must be removed and another sterile gown donned before gloves.

Removing Gown and Gloves

The gown is always removed before the gloves. It is pulled downward from the shoulders, turning the sleeves inside out as it is pulled off the arms. Gloves are turned inside out, using glove-to-glove then skin-to-skin technique, as they are removed (see Chap. 8, p. 157, for illustrations).

Chapter 8

Division of Duties: Setup, Procedure, Cleanup

PRELIMINARY PREPARATIONS

Preliminary preparations of the OR are done before each patient enters by the circulating and scrub nurses together, sometimes assisted by a nursing assistant or housekeeping personnel. It is a cooperative effort. Clean surroundings are part of the skill and care that are the patient's rights. Cleaning the room is part of total patient care. (The cleanup procedure following each operation is detailed in the last section of this chapter.)

Before the First Operation of the Day

The following housekeeping duties should be done at least 1 hour before the scheduled incision time:

1 Remove unnecessary tables and equipment from the room.

2 Damp-dust the overhead operating light, furniture, flat surfaces, and all portable or mounted equipment with a germicidal solution.

3 Damp-dust the tops and rims of the autoclave and/or washer-sterilizer and counter tops in the substerile room adjacent to the OR.

4 Wet-vacuum the floors with detergent disinfectant.

Before Each Operation

After the room is clean and all surfaces are dry:

1 Put a clean sheet, arm band, and conductive strap on the operating table.

2 Position operating table under overhead operating light fixture.

3 Turn on the operating light to check focus and intensity, and preposition it as much as possible. The light should be positioned in relationship to the location of the surgeon at the operating table and to that part of the patient's anatomy that will be encountered during the operation.

4 Obtain and check electrical equipment that will be needed.

5 Connect and check suction between receptacle and wall outlet to be certain suction functions at maximum vacuum.

6 Put a waterproof linen bag or antistatic plastic bag for disposal of linen or disposable drapes in the linen hamper frame.

7 Line each kick bucket and wastebasket with an *antistatic* plastic bag with a cuff turned over the edge. These bags are not considered an explosion hazard so it is not necessary to put water in the bucket. Plastic waste disposal bags are nonconductors on which electrostatic charges may accumulate. Use care in handling them.

8 Arrange furniture with those pieces that will be draped to become part of the sterile field at least 18 in. (45 cm) away from walls or cabinets. They should be kept side by side, away from the linen hamper, anesthesia equipment, doors, and paths of traffic.

9 Put the sterile linen pack on the instrument table in place so that when opened the wrapper will adequately drape the table and the linen will be in its proper place. It is convenient to have the pack of linen wrapped in the sheets that constitute the table drape.

NOTE. Although the term *linen pack* will be used, it is recognized that many hospitals use packs of disposable fabrics (see Chap. 11).

10 Put a sterile basin set into the ring stand.
11 Obtain a basic set of sterile instruments or place tray of unsterile instruments in the steam sterilizer in the substerile room and sterilize them.
12 Select the correct size gloves for each member of the sterile team.
13 Collect additional instruments and supplies, according to the procedure book and surgeon's preference card, from cabinets in the room or other supply area within the OR suite.
14 Obtain special equipment, such as table appliances or pillows, needed for positioning the patient.

Individual Patient Setups

Each patient has a right to individual supplies prepared just for him or her. Sterile supplies should not be opened until they are ready to be used. Tables should *not* be prepared and covered for use at a later time. The scrub nurse, working with an efficient circulating nurse, has time to set up the instrument table before each operation.

The routine practice of covering sterile setups is not in the best interest of the patient. Unless under constant surveillance, sterility cannot be guaranteed. However, should a scheduled operation be canceled or delayed, and *a sterile setup not contaminated by the patient's presence in the room,* the setup may be covered with sterile drapes. It must remain in the room with the doors kept closed, and should be used preferably within an hour from the time prepared.

NOTE. If a patient is taken into the OR and for some reason the operation is canceled, the tables should be torn down and the room cleaned as if the operation had taken place.

Open Sterile Supplies

Before any sterile supplies are opened, the integrity of each package must be checked for tears and watermarks. If either are present, the package is unsafe to use. Also check expiration date and process monitor. To open packages:

1 Remove tape from packages wrapped in muslin. Check the indicator tape to be certain that the item has been exposed to a sterilization process.

2 Open linen pack, instrument set, gown pack, and basin set so that the inside of each inner wrapper becomes the sterile table cover.

NOTE. With hands on the outside of the wrapper in a folded cuff, lift the wrapper toward you to avoid contaminating the contents of the pack. The area touched falls below table level, and the inside of the wrapper remains sterile. Neither reach over the inside of the sterile table cover or the contents of the pack. Always lift the wrapper toward you (see Fig. 8-1).

3 Open other packages, such as sponges, gloves, sutures, etc., maintaining a sterile transfer to the appropriate sterile table. Touch only the outside of the outer wrapper. Avoid reaching over sterile contents.
4 Open the gown and gloves for the scrub nurse on the Mayo stand or small table.

DIVISION OF DUTIES

The circulating and scrub nurses must plan their duties so that, through coordination of their efforts, the sterile and nonsterile parts of the operation move along simultaneously. From the time the scrub nurse starts the surgical scrub until the operation is completed and the dressings applied, there is a demarcation line between the duties of the scrub and circulating nurses that neither nurse may cross. The duties of the two nursing positions are listed separately, but a spirit of mutual cooper-

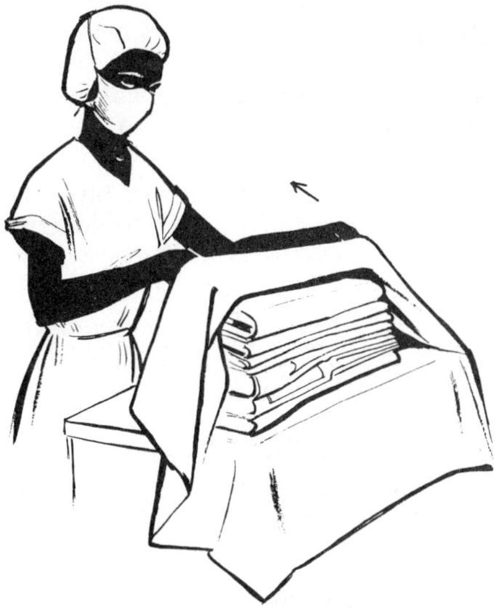

Figure 8-1 Circulating nurse opening sterile laparotomy pack. The nurse lifts wrapper back while keeping hands on the outside. Hands are in a folded cuff to avoid contaminating contents of pack. The area touched falls below unsterile table level and sterile inside of wrapper (now table cover) remains sterile.

ation is essential to move the schedule of operations efficiently and to serve the patients' best interests.

THE SCRUB NURSE

When all is in readiness for the arrival of the patient, the scrub nurse prepares for the arrival of the surgeon.

Before Surgeon Arrives

1 Do a complete scrub according to accepted practice (refer to Chap. 7).
2 Gown and glove.
3 Drape tables as necessary according to standard procedure.
  a Sometimes a second instrument table is needed for extensive operations or special types of instrumentation.
  b The scrub nurse may drape and set a small table for the patient's skin preparation. More commonly the circulating nurse opens and prepares a disposable or prepackaged prep tray (see Chap. 11).
  c The surgeon and assistant(s) may gown and glove from a small table used only for this purpose. The scrub nurse arranges the gloves for them.

NOTE. In draping a nonsterile table, always cuff the drape over the gloved hands in preparation for opening it. Lift the table drape toward you to cover the nonsterile front edge of the table first and to minimize the possibility of contaminating the front of your gown. Then place the drape over the back of the table. After the ends of the drape are unfolded over the sides of the table, be careful not to lift them to table level again as you open the crosswise folds (see Figs. 4-3 through 4-6, pp. 88 and 89).

4 Move the remaining contents of the linen pack to a corner of the instrument table if they are not preset on the table drape in a convenient place. Before being wrapped for sterilization, the contents of the pack can be set on the table drape in the spot where they should be on the table. Then when the pack is opened, the contents do not need to be handled or moved. The pack contains, from top to bottom, at least:
  a One Mayo stand cover.
  b Six to eight towels.
  c One fenestrated sheet. (The types of fenestrated sheets are discussed in Chapter 11.)
5 Drape the Mayo stand. Both the frame and the tray are draped unless the tray is wrapped and sterilized separately.

The Mayo stand cover is like a long pillowcase. It is fanfolded with a wide cuff to protect the gloved hands. With hands in the cuff, the folds of the drape are supported on the arms, in the bend of the elbows, to prevent its falling below waist level. While sliding the cover on, place your foot on the base of the stand to stabilize it (see Figs. 8-2 and 8-3).

A snugly wrapped sterile tray is placed on top of the draped Mayo frame. Or a waterproof barrier, such as a nonabsorbent disposable towel or antistatic plastic film, is placed over the cover on the tray and tucked in along the edges.
6 Leave the large solution basin in the ring stand and take the remainder of the basins to the instrument table. The wrapper on the basin set serves as the cover for the ring stand in which the large basin is left. The surgeon and assistants may need to wash their gloves during the operation. This is no hazard in an operation devoid of frank sepsis or malignancy. The solution must be nontoxic and benign in tissues, however. Sterile normal saline or water is usually used in this "splash" basin. Splash basins are not used in some ORs.

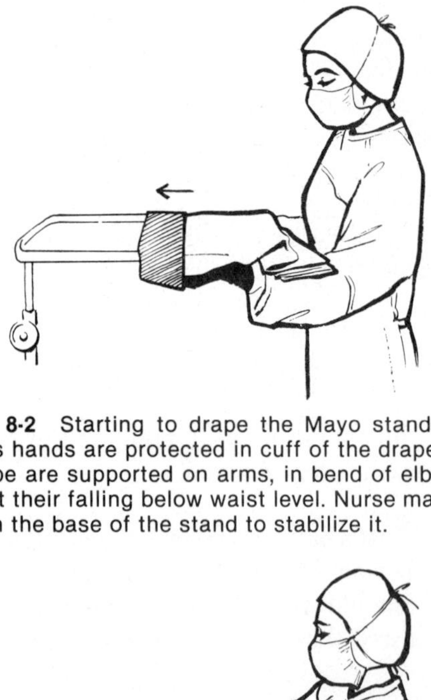

Figure 8-2 Starting to drape the Mayo stand. Scrub nurse's hands are protected in cuff of the drape. Folds of drape are supported on arms, in bend of elbows, to prevent their falling below waist level. Nurse may place foot on the base of the stand to stabilize it.

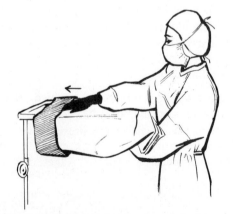

Figure 8-3 Completing the draping of the Mayo stand. The nurse's hands are protected in the cuff.

The kidney basin is left on the instrument table until needed for the specimen.

A round basin will be used for moistening sponges. Place an absorbent towel on the instrument table under it.

In addition to these basins, the basin set may also contain solution cups for the skin preparation table and a basin specifically intended for trash disposal. In lieu of this extra basin, a small paper bag may be included in the basin or instrument set for trash. The bag is left standing open on the instrument table or attached with a nonperforating clip in a convenient place on the side of the table or Mayo stand.

7 Arrange instruments on the instrument table and count them if this is the accepted practice (see p. 151 later in this chapter).

Instruments for each operation are selected according to the standard basic sets or the instrument book list for a given operation and the surgeon's preferences. They usually are prepared, wrapped, and sterilized several hours prior to the operation so that they are dry and cool for safe handling. In addition to basic sets, separate single packages of special instruments also may be sterile to be opened as indicated.

Sometimes instruments must be steam-sterilized just prior to use. If so, a towel is placed in the bottom of the tray under the instruments to absorb the moisture from condensation on them. (see Chap. 5, p. 99 for timing of the load.) Either the scrub nurse or the circulating nurse may lift the tray from the autoclave, depending on the physical location of the autoclave in relationship to the OR. The scrub nurse should not go beyond the confines of the room, but this is the practice in some suites where the autoclave is immediately adjacent to the door to the substerile room. In lifting a tray from the autoclave, the scrub nurse must be careful not to brush the sleeves or front of her gown against the autoclave. If the circulating nurse lifts the tray, she must not reach over the sterile instruments or the sterile table when placing it.

Box locks of hinged instruments must be held open during steam sterilization. Therefore, remove them from instrument pins, racks, or holders designed for this purpose and close the instruments on the first ratchet. The handles may be hung over the edge of the tray. Or take a towel from the linen pack, roll it lengthwise to form a long, narrow cushion, and place the hemostats and other instruments with ringed handles over it. Retractors and other heavy instruments can be left in the instrument tray or laid out on the table.

8 Arrange instruments on the Mayo stand for making and opening the initial incision. For each basic maneuver, a definite class of instruments of suitable size, shape, strength, and function is needed. Instruments may be classified as follows:

a Cutting or dissecting: knives and scissors
b Grasping and holding: tissue forceps
c Clamping and occluding: hemostatic forceps and clamps
d Exposing: retractors
e Suturing: needleholders

Variation in the style and number of instruments will be dictated by the type of operation. In addition to these basic instruments, the following accessory items may be added to the Mayo stand after the supplies are prepared for use:

a Sutures and needles
b Sponges

Do not overload the Mayo stand initially. Additional instruments and supplies can be added as the operation progresses (see Fig. 8-4).

9 Put blades on knife handles. To avoid injury, always use an instrument, never your fingers alone. Holding the cutting edge down and away from your eyes, grasp the blade at its widest, strongest part with a needleholder and slip the blade into the groove on the knife handle. A click indicates that the blade is in place. To prevent damage to the blade, the instrument must not touch the cutting edge (see Fig. 8-5).

10 Prepare sutures in the sequence in which the surgeon will use them. The surgeon *ligates* (ties off) blood vessels shortly after the incision is made, unless he or she prefers to use electrosurgery to seal the vessels. Therefore, prepare *ligatures* (free hand ties) first, since they are used first.

Tear foil packets across the notch near the hermetically sealed edge. Plastic packets may be torn or cut open with nurse's scissors. Re-

Figure 8-4 Contents of the Mayo stand, in preparation for an operation: (1) scalpels, (2) straight and curved scissors, (3) smooth and toothed tissue forceps, (4) retractors, (5) straight hemostats, (6) Kelly clamps, (7) Allis's forceps, (8) sponges, (9) suture towel and needleholders.

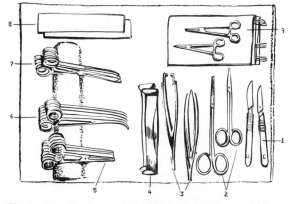

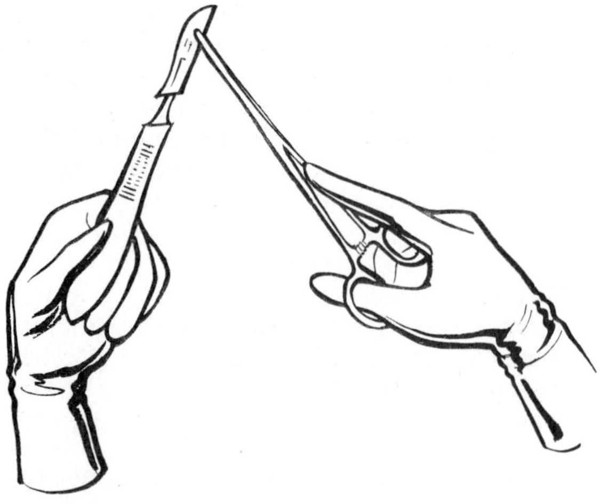

Figure 8-5 Putting the blade on a knife handle (scalpel). To avoid injury, always use an instrument, never use your hands alone. Holding it down and away from your eyes, with a strong needleholder (not a hemostat), grasp the blade at its widest, strongest part, and slip the blade into the groove on the knife. To prevent damage to the blade, the needleholder must not touch the cutting edge.

move the suture material from the packet, unless the packet is designed for single-strand dispensing. Work over the instrument table and hold onto the ends to prevent strands from dropping over the edge of the table, and thus becoming contaminated.

Place dispensing packets or strands of ligating material in a *suture book,* a fanfolded towel, with the ends extended far enough for rapid extraction. Place the largest size in the bottom layer along the fold that will be furthest away when placed on the Mayo stand. The next smaller size is placed in the next layer but not as far in so that the ends are not overriding those below; i.e., if three sizes are prepared, the medium size can be placed midway between the other two. The smallest size will be along the closest fold.

The suture book should be placed on the Mayo stand with the ends on it, *not over the edges,* and toward the sterile field. The strands are pulled out toward the operative field, *never away from it,* to prevent possible contamination.

After the ligatures are prepared, a *few* other packets may be opened and prepared for *suturing* (sewing or stitching). Seldom is it necessary to prepare large amounts of suture material in advance. Suture material, preparation, and handling are discussed in detail in Chapter 13.

11 Count surgical needles with the circulating nurse if this is the accepted practice (see p. 151).

Most hospitals use needles *swaged* (attached) to the suture material. These can be left in the inner folder of the suture packet, after counting, until the surgeon is ready to use them. The folder can be placed in a fold of the suture book.

A needle rack is prepared in advance for each operation if reusable, eyed needles are used (see Fig. 13-6, p. 264). This is sterilized with the instruments. Inspect each needle before threading for cleanliness, burrs, and integrity of the eye.

If disposable eyed needles are used, they can be threaded into the top layer of the suture book. *Needles should never be loose on the Mayo stand* as they inadvertently could be dragged into the incision or knocked onto the floor.

Surgical needles are discussed in detail in Chapter 13.

12 Count *all* sponges with the circulating nurse before doing anything else with them. Many different kinds of sponges are available. Those placed on the sterile field should have indicator radiopaque to x-ray. They are referred to as *x-ray detectable.* The following are representative of the types used:

a 3 by 3 in. (7.6 by 7.6 cm) sponges are used in small incisions.

b 4 by 4 in. (10 by 10 cm) sponges are the most common in use. They may be folded into a 2 by 2 in. (5 by 5 cm) square and used on sponge forceps.

c 4 by 8 in. (10 by 20 cm) sponges may be used for sponging or as a moist pack in a large exposed area such as in radical mastectomy.

d *Tapes,* also called *lap pads* or *packs,* are used for walling off the viscera and keeping them moist and warm. Either square or oblong, they have a loop of twilled tape sewed on one corner over which a metal ring, about $1\frac{1}{2}$ in. (3.8 cm) in diameter, can be fastened. If rings are used, they remain outside the edges of the incision while the tape is inside. Tapes are usually used moist.

e Dissecting sponges:

(1) *Peanut sponges* are very small gauze sponges used to dissect or absorb fluid in delicate procedures. They must be clamped into a forceps.

(2) *Kitner dissecting sponges* are small rolls of heavy cotton tape. These are held in forceps.

(3) *Tonsil sponges* are cotton-filled gauze with a cotton thread attached.

f Cottonoid patties, compressed rayon or cotton, are used moist on delicate structures such as nerves, brain, and spinal cord.

After the sponge count is completed (see p. 150), place on the Mayo stand a few of the appropriate-size sponges for the initial incision. These sponges are usually opened to their full length. Fix two or three sponges on sponge forceps, but leave forceps on instrument table. Put rings on tapes, if used.

13 Fill a syringe with the correct agent if a local infiltration anesthetic is to be used. Attach an appropriate-size needle and put it on the Mayo stand. This will be the first thing the surgeon will use after the patient is draped. State the kind and percentage of the solution when handing the syringe to the surgeon. The solution label must be checked by a registered nurse when it is poured and verified when it is given.

Syringes with needles are used for injection and aspiration, and syringes without needles are used for irrigation. Most hospitals use sterile disposable syringes and needles, but glass syringes and reusable needles in the same models and sizes may be used.

Syringes commonly used for injection or aspiration are:

a *Luer-Lok tip.* This has a tip that locks over the needle hub. It is used whenever pressure is exerted to inject or aspirate fluid. Sizes are available from 2 to 100 cc.

b *Ring control.* This has a Luer-Lok tip. The barrel has one fingerhold and thumbhold, which give the surgeon a secure grip when injecting with only one hand. Sizes run from 3 to 10 cc.

c *Luer slip tip.* This has a plain tip that may not give a secure connection on a needle hub. It is necessary when using some catheter adapters or a rubber connection for aspiration. Sizes vary from 1 to 100 cc.

NOTE. When using a sterile syringe be very careful not to touch the plunger except at the end, even with gloves on. Contamination of the plunger contaminates the inner wall of the barrel and thus the solution that is drawn into it. Glove powder can act as a contaminant.

Syringes used for irrigation are:

a *Bulb with barrel.* A plastic or rubber bulb is attached to the neck of the barrel. The barrel has a tapered or blunt end. This is used with one-hand control for irrigation during many types of operations. Sizes have a solution capacity of $\frac{1}{4}$ to 4 oz (7.6 to 118 cc).

b *Bulb without barrel.* This is a one-piece bulb that tapers to a blunt end. It is used to irrigate small structures.

NOTE. To fill the barrel or bulb, depress the bulb, submerge the end in solution, and release. The bulb will reinflate, thus drawing the solution into it. Warm, not hot, solution is usually used for irrigation, so check its temperature before giving the syringe to the surgeon.

Needles for injection or aspiration:
The size of needles with a lumen is designated by length and gauge. *Gauge* is the outside diameter of the needle. Although an abundance of needles are available, only a few representative sizes and their uses are mentioned.

a $\frac{1}{2}$ in. (12.7 mm) by 30 gauge, for local anesthetic in plastic surgery.

b $\frac{3}{4}$ in. (19 mm) by 24 or 25 gauge, the usual needle for any subcutaneous injection.

c $1\frac{1}{2}$ in. (3.8 cm) by 22 gauge, for subcutaneous or intramuscular injection.

d 2 in. (5 cm) by 16 or 18 gauge, for aspiration, or transfusion of blood products.

e 4 in. (10 cm) by 20 or 22 gauge, for deep injections of local anesthetic, or for intracardial injections.

After Surgeon and Assistant(s) Scrub

1 Gown and glove the surgeon and assistants as soon after they enter the room as possible. This should take precedence over other things you may be doing. However, *do not interrupt* a sponge, needle, or instrument count to do so. Such interruptions lead to incorrect counts. The surgeons take their gowns and gloves from a separate table set up for this purpose in some hospitals.

2 Assist in draping the patient, according to the routine procedure (see Chap. 11).

Many surgeons use self-adhering plastic sheeting as the first drape. Stand on the opposite side of the operating table from the surgeon to apply this drape.

Some surgeons use towels and clips with or instead of the plastic drape. Go to the same side of the table as the surgeon to hand him or her towels and clips, to prevent your reaching over the nonsterile operating table. Skin towels may be held in place with sutures rather than clips. The needle and needleholders are discarded from the sterile field after skin towels are secured in this manner.

3 Bring the Mayo stand into position over the patient after the draping is completed. Be sure that it does not rest on the patient. Position the instrument table at a right angle to the operating table.

4 Lay a towel or magnetic pad for instruments below the *fenestration* (opening) in the drape. Lay two to four sponges on this.

5 Attach the suction tubing and electrosurgical cord, if either or both are to be used, to the drapes with a nonperforating clamp. Allow ample length to reach both the incision area and the equipment. Drop the ends off the side of the table nearest the unit to which the circulating nurse will attach them.

NOTE. Once a clip or hook has been fastened through a drape, do not remove it; the points are contaminated. If it is necessary to remove one, discard it from the field and cover the area with a piece of sterile linen.

During the Operation

1 Hand the skin knife to the surgeon and a hemostat to the assistant. Some surgeons do not want the knife handed to them. Lay the knife on the instrument towel or magnetic pad for them to pick up.

NOTE. When passing a knife always hold the handle with the blade down and pointed toward your wrist, never toward the surgeon. Hold the hand pronated with the thumb apposed against the tip of the index finger and flex the wrist.

As soon as the surgeon makes the skin incision, put the knife into the specimen basin. The inside of this basin is hereafter considered contaminated. Refrain from touching anything else that is put in it. Because skin cannot be sterilized, the skin knife is always considered contaminated whether the surgeon has cut through an adhering plastic drape or not. The skin incision exposes deep skin flora of hair follicles and sebaceous gland ducts.

2 Hand up towels and hooks for fastening them to the skin, if a plastic drape has not been applied as the first drape, as soon as the subcutaneous bleeders have been ligated. These towels are placed at each side of the incision and secured to cover the skin completely during the operation. If skin towels are used, rearrange the instrument towel to make a smooth field.

3 Watch the field and try to anticipate the surgeon's needs. Keep one step ahead of him or her in passing instruments, sutures, sponges, handing up the specimen basin, etc. Notify the circulating nurse if you need additional supplies or if the surgeon asks for something not on the table. Ask quietly for supplies to avoid distracting the surgeon.

4 Pass instruments in a decisive and positive manner. When an instrument is passed properly, the surgeon knows that he has it; his eyes do not have to leave the operative site. When the surgeon extends his hand, the instrument should be slapped firmly in his palm in proper position for him to use it (see Fig. 8-6). In passing an instrument to the surgeon:

a If the surgeon is on the opposite side of the table, pass with your right hand.

b If the surgeon is on the same side of the table and to the left, use your right hand.

c If the surgeon is on the same side of the table and to the right, use your left hand.

Many surgeons use hand signals to indicate the type of instrument needed. These signals eliminate the need for talking, but such signs must be clearly understood. An understanding of what is taking place at the operative site makes them meaningful. When bleeding is obvious, the surgeon needs a hemostatic forceps. When a suture needs cutting, the need is for scissors.

Keep instruments as clean as possible. Wipe blood and organic debris from them with a moist sponge. Flush suction with saline periodically to keep tip and tubing patent. Remove debris from electrosurgical tips.

Return instruments to the Mayo stand or instrument table promptly after use. Their weight could injure the patient.

5 Place a ligature in the surgeon's hand. The surgeon keeps his eyes on the field and does not reach for the ligature except to hold his hand out to receive it. Draw a strand out of the suture book, toward the sterile field, grasp both ends, and place securely in the surgeon's outstretched hand.

Have ready, at all times during the operation, a fine and a heavy suture on needles placed in needleholders. After handing a suture to the surgeon, prepare another just like it at once. The needle or suture may break. *Account for each needle as the surgeon finishes with it.* Check its integrity. Tell the surgeon immediately if a needle is broken so that both pieces can be retrieved.

Repeat the size of a suture or ligature when handing it to the surgeon. Obviously, if the surgeon is using a long series of interrupted sutures or many ligatures in rapid succession, this repetition is not necessary. Use good judgment; be logical.

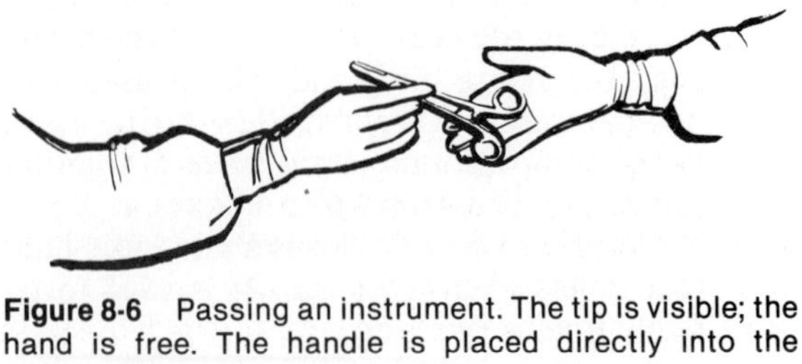

Figure 8-6 Passing an instrument. The tip is visible; the hand is free. The handle is placed directly into the waiting hand.

Also be logical in selecting instruments used for suturing. Give the surgeon long needleholders when he or she is working deep in a cavity. Short ones may be used for surface work. Give the assistant a needleholder to pull the needle through tissue for the surgeon. Then, have scissors ready when the knot is tied.

Remove waste ends of suture material from the field, Mayo stand, and instrument table. Place them in trash disposal container. Put used needles on a magnet, needle rack, or into the suture book or other container for this purpose until the needle count is completed.

6 Keep two clean sponges or tapes on the field. Put up clean ones before removing soiled ones on an exchange basis. Discard soiled sponges into the kick bucket. If a basin on the field is used to accumulate soiled sponges, touch only the outside of it. Sponges are either potentially contaminated or grossly so. Keep basin at waist level when emptying it into the kick bucket.

If sponges or tapes are added during the operation, count them with the circulating nurse before moistening or using them. Do not mix types of sponges and tapes, either on the table or in the basin of solution. Normal saline is usually used to moisten sponges and tapes because it is an isotonic solution.

7 Save all specimens of tissue according to hospital policy. Many hospitals' policies stipulate that all tissue be sent to the laboratory, even though a piece of tissue may appear to be of no value for examination or diagnostic purposes.

Take care of the tissue specimen according to hospital procedure. Specimens are put in a specimen basin or attached to an instrument until put into a specimen jar. Never put a large clamp on a small specimen; you may crush the cells, making tissue identification difficult. Disposable glove wrappers, marked right and left, can be used for holding bilateral specimens, e.g., right and left breast biopsies. Hand a specimen from the field in the basin, wrapper, or on a towel; *never place it on a sponge.* Keep the specimen basin on the field until you are certain all tissue has been removed or all contaminated items are in it. Tell the circulating nurse exactly what the specimen is. If you do not know, ask the surgeon to identify it.

8 Maintain sterile technique. Watch for any breaks. Observe the following points in technique:

a Step away from the sterile field if contaminated. Ask the circulating nurse for another glove, gown, or sleeve—whatever is needed for yourself or another member of the sterile team. If the lower arm of the gown becomes contaminated, a sterile gown sleeve can be drawn over it to cover the area.

b Change glove at once and discard the needle or instrument if a glove is pricked by a needle or snagged by an instrument.

c Discard a piece of suture material, tubing, or a sponge that falls over the edge of the sterile field without touching the contaminated part of it.

d Keep hands at waist level when at rest; they should never be below the waist.

e Keep contact with the sterile field to a minimum. No one should lean on or against the operating table, Mayo stand, instrument table, and especially not on the patient. Remember that the patient under the drapes is unable to complain!

f Leave a wide margin of safety in moving about the room. A gown bulges, and more space is necessary than you are accustomed to needing. In passing nonsterile objects, turn your back to them.

g Do not turn your back to the sterile field or to members of the sterile team. Face sterile areas in passing them.

h Do not reach behind a member of the sterile team; go around him or her. Pass another member of the sterile team back to back (refer to Fig. 4-7, p. 90).

i Keep the table and sterile field as dry as possible. Spread extra towels as needed. Keep the strings and rings on tapes in the basin, not dangling over the side of it and dripping on the instrument table.

j Discard soiled sponges from the sterile field. A basin may be placed on the drapes near the operative site to receive the soiled sponges. This is handy for the surgeon and avoids the need to turn from the field to discard sponges. It eliminates frequent turning away from the sterile field by the scrub nurse also. It prevents the need for rehandling soiled sponges. They can be emptied from this basin into the kick bucket. Be sure to touch only the outside of the basin and keep it at waist level.

k Keep talking to a minimum. Avoid coughing and sneezing.

During the Closure

1 Count sponges, needles, and instruments with the circulating nurse when the surgeon begins closure of the wound, in accordance with established count procedures.

2 Clear off Mayo stand, as time permits, leaving a knife handle with blade, tissue forceps, scissors, four hemostats, and two Allis's forceps.

NOTE. Policy in many hospitals requires that the Mayo stand remain sterile until the patient has left the room. Cardiac arrest, tracheal collapse, hemorrhage, or other emergency can occur in the immediate postoperative-postanesthesia period. Even though sterile instrument sets are nearby, valuable time can be lost opening sterile supplies when every second counts in an emergency situation. Sterile instruments on the Mayo stand, regardless of their previous use, can be used for emergency intervention. These can be lifesaving until other ones become available.

3 Have a damp sponge ready to wash the blood from the area surrounding the incision as soon as the skin closure is completed.
4 Have dressings ready. Sterile dressings are regarded as part of the operation. Their purposes are:
   a To keep the incision free from microorganisms. However, some surgeons prefer to leave the wound exposed in the belief that the coagulum that forms at the well-approximated edges in the first few minutes after the wound is sutured strengthens the wound and gives protection against microorganisms. Dressings are considered essential, aesthetically at least, by most surgeons.
   b To protect incision from outside injury, especially in children.
   c To absorb drainage.
   d To give some support to incision and surrounding skin.

   In considering which components to assemble for a particular dressing, keep in mind the needs of that particular wound. Some wounds require the opposite performance from a dressing than others do. The manner in which a dressing functions is determined by its structure. A complete dressing must consist of at least three components:
   a The *contact layer* acts either as a passageway for the secretion that emanates from a draining wound or as a barrier to protect the nondraining wound from its environment. It must conform to all body contours regardless of the site and extent of the wound, and must stay in intimate contact with the wound surface yet be nonadherent for painless removal.
   b The *intermediate layer,* which is absorbent, serves as the storage area for the secretion passing through the contact layer from a draining wound, or as a cushion to protect a nondraining wound from further trauma. To provide adequate absorbency capacity or protection, it should be layered over the contact material to the thickness required by the particular wound.
   c The *outer wrap* or *binder* holds the assembled components in proper position to serve their particular purpose.

   Pressure dressings are used frequently following extensive operations, especially in plastic surgery, in operations on the knee, and in radical mastectomies. These bulky dressings are added to the intermediate layer:
   a To eliminate dead space and to prevent edema or hematoma (see Chap. 12).
   b To distribute pressure evenly.
   c To absorb extensive drainage.
   d To immobilize a body area or to support soft tissues when the muscles are moved.
   e To help provide comfort to the patient postoperatively.

   Materials used for pressure dressings include:
   a Fluffed gauze.
   b Abdominal pads. These are gauze-covered, absorbent cellulose.
   c Single-piece, bulk dressings. These are available for use on trunk and extremities and save time in application.
   d Cotton rolls. These are used to apply gentle pressure on each side of a knee following operation on this joint, for example.
   f Foam rubber.

THE CIRCULATING NURSE

Circulating nurses wash hands and arms for 5 minutes at beginning of the day before entering the OR, but do not don sterile gowns and gloves. Persons who wear sterile attire touch only sterile items; persons who are not sterile touch only unsterile items. Therefore, the circulating nurse must assist the sterile scrub nurse by providing the sterile supplies needed to prepare for the arrival of the surgeon.

After the Scrub Nurse Scrubs

1 Fasten the back of the scrub nurse's gown.

2 If the tray of instruments is in the autoclave in the substerile room, sterile lifting handles must be used to bring the tray from the autoclave to a sterile surface. Never reach over the sterile instruments or the sterile surface when placing the tray. The tray may be set on the basin in the ring stand to avoid the danger of contaminating the instrument table with moisture.

3 Open packages of sterile supplies, such as syringes, suction tubing, sutures, sponges, gloves, etc. Many of these items are prepackaged, presterilized, disposable products. Others are wrapped and sterilized by hospital personnel. Care must be taken in opening all sterile packages to avoid contamination.

NOTE. If a sterile package drops to the floor, discard it. Compression resulting from the fall can cause air and dust to enter the package, and it can no longer be considered sterile.

Some packages are designed so that the circulating nurse can flip a rigid item onto the sterile field without reaching over it. *Many soft items do not flip.* If it does not flip easily, put the item on the edge of the table with the inside of the wrapper everted over the hand. *Never reach over the sterile field and shake an item from the package.* An alternative method is for the scrub nurse to pick the item from the package as the circulating nurse opens it and holds the contents exposed (see Figs. 8-7, 8-8, and 8-9).

NOTE. The routine use of transfer forceps is considered obsolete. Should a need arise, such as for removing a single instrument from a flash sterilizer, a sterile transfer forceps may be used. At this time, a package containing a forceps is opened and used for a single transfer or placed in a sterile container for use as needed during the remainder of *that* operation. The circulating nurse touches only the handles. Always carry a forceps high and in sight; never swing it at your side. Avoid touching the tip to the instrument table when placing items.

If the forceps is placed in a container of disinfectant solution to maintain sterility during the operation, when using or holding the forceps, keep the tip horizontal to the handle or below it. Never hold it above the horizontal level; the solution will run to the nonsterile handle, then contaminate the tip when it is lowered again. Forceps and container are cleaned with the instruments at the end of the operation and resterilized.

4 Flip suture packets onto the instrument table. Check the list of materials and sizes on the surgeon's preference card and check with the surgeon.

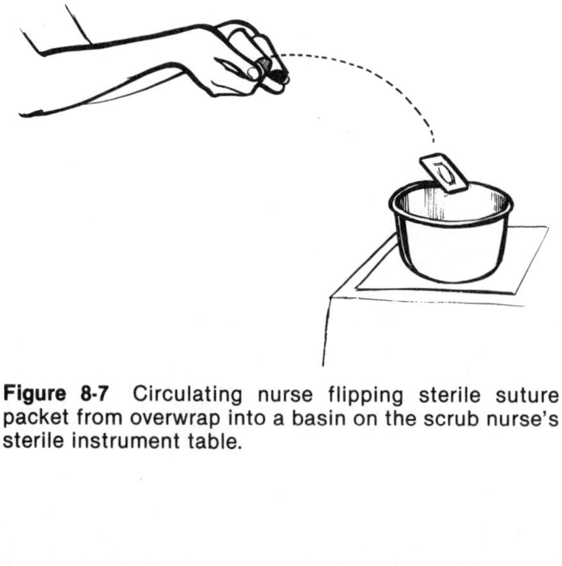

Figure 8-7 Circulating nurse flipping sterile suture packet from overwrap into a basin on the scrub nurse's sterile instrument table.

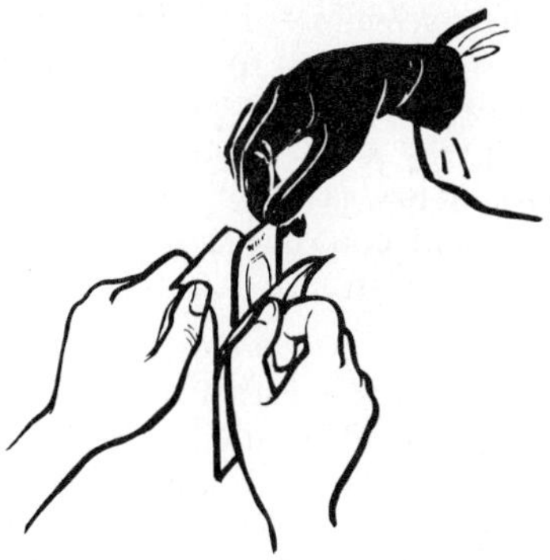

Figure 8-8 Scrub nurse taking the contents from the suture packet opened and held by the circulating nurse. The scrub nurse avoids touching the unsterile outer wrapper.

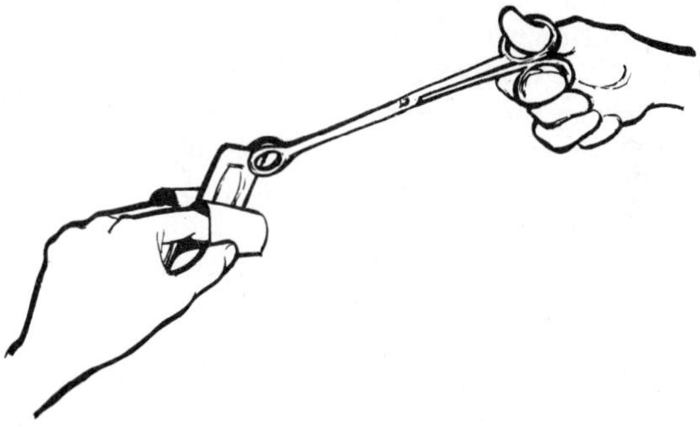

Figure 8-9 Circulating nurse removing sterile suture inner packet from overwrap with sterile forceps.

NOTE. Avoid opening suture packets that will not be used. Wait until the patient is in the OR before opening any packets. The operation might be canceled and then they would be wasted. Be conservative in opening packets. If you cannot anticipate the surgeon's need for sutures and do not receive instructions, you can generally keep just a packet or two ahead of actual need during the operation and thus avoid waste.

5 Pour solution (usually normal saline) into the splash basin in the ring stand and the round basin for sponges on the instrument table. Pour a small amount of antiseptic agent for skin preparation in the solution cups to be used for this purpose.

6 Count sponges, needles, and instruments with the scrub nurse as required by hospital policy and procedure. Record immediately (see section on counts later in this chapter, p. 150).

After the Patient Arrives

1 Greet and identify the patient. Introduce yourself to the patient if you have not made the preoperative visit. Check wristband for identification.

2 Check the nursing care plan and patient's chart for pertinent information.

3 Cover the patient's hair with a cap. (The patient's hair is covered to prevent dissemination of microorganisms, to protect it from being soiled, and to prevent a static spark near the anesthesia machine.)
4 Take the patient into the OR after the surgeon sees him or her and the anesthesiologist is ready for induction. (The patient should see the surgeon before being anesthetized.)
5 Assist the patient in moving from the stretcher to operating table. Both the stretcher and table must be stabilized by locking the wheels when a patient is moving from one to the other. During transfer, avoid unnecessary exposure of the patient. Remember that the cotton blanket and gown protect modesty as well as provide warmth. Handle the blanket and gown gently to avoid dispersing lint and microorganisms into the air; they can settle on the sterile tables. In moving the patient, also give special caution to catheters, drainage tubes, intravenous infusions, and traction apparatus. Do not dislodge them.
6 Check to be certain the conductive strap under the patient is in contact with skin, with one end of the strap fastened to the metal frame of the operating table. This assures an electrical connection of the patient to the conductive floor.
7 Apply restraints comfortably. Place a safety strap loosely 2 in. (5 cm) above the knees. The patient's legs must not be crossed (see Chap. 10, p. 212). Place the patient's arms at his or her sides on the table and tuck the arm band around them. If an intravenous infusion is running or will be started, place that arm on a padded armboard at a right angle to the table. Secure the arm with a wrist strap. The arm must be immobilized to prevent peripheral extravasation of solution, which can cause local tissue necrosis.

NOTE. The angle of abduction of the arm should never be greater than 90°, a right angle with the body. The brachial nerve plexus can be damaged by lengthy, too-severe abduction of the arm.

8 Help the anesthesiologist, as needed, to apply and connect necessary monitoring devices.
9 Assist the anesthesiologist, surgeon, or assistant to start intravenous (IV) fluids. Unless this is taken care of entirely by the anesthesiologist, obtain the following equipment:
a Tourniquet.
b Sponges saturated with antiseptic solution for skin preparation. Thorough skin antisepsis is imperative.
c Intravenous administration set of sterile tubing with air filter and needle, cannula, or catheter.

NOTE. $1\frac{1}{2}$ in. (3.8 cm) by 20 or 21 gauge needles usually are used for intravenous fluids when blood transfusion is not anticipated; $1\frac{1}{2}$ in. (3.8 cm) by 16 or 18 gauge needles are used when blood transfusion is anticipated. When prolonged postoperative fluid therapy or hyperalimentation is anticipated, an inert, nontoxic, radiopaque plastic catheter is inserted through either a venipuncture through the skin or a cutdown through a skin incision to expose the vein.

A venous cutdown is done in other selected situations: for central venous pressure monitoring, thrombosed superficial veins, or superficially collapsed veins due to shock or prolonged preoperative IV therapy. The cutdown site is an open wound and insertion of the catheter should be considered a minor operative procedure. Sterile gloves, drapes, and a tray of sterile instruments and sutures are needed. Have assorted sizes of intravenous catheters available so that the surgeon can choose the size best suited to the vein. A soft, pliant catheter takes the contour of the anatomy and is not easily dislodged by movement of the patient.

d Plastic or glass container of parenteral infusion solution. Intravenous solutions frequently used in the OR include:
(1) Normal saline.
(2) Dextrose, 5 or 10%, in water.
(3) Dextrose in saline.
(4) *Dextran,* an artificial plasma-volume expander, acts by drawing fluid from the tissues. It remains in the circulation for several hours. It interferes with cross-matching of blood.
(5) *Mannitol,* an osmotic diuretic agent, has an effect on renal vascular resistance. Depending on the percentage of drug in solution, it can produce either an increase or decrease in renal blood flow. It may be given prophylactically to prevent renal failure. It is also used to decrease intracranial and intraocular pressure. It is rapidly excreted by the kidneys.
(6) *Ringer's solution,* a physiologic salt solution, is infused in patients in whom the body's supply of sodium, calcium, and potassium has been depleted or for improvement of circulation and stimulation of renal activity.

Usually, normal saline or dextrose solution is started initially.

NOTE. Gently squeeze plastic bag to detect leaks; check glass for cracks. Check solution for clarity or discoloration. A cloudy solution is contaminated. If the circulating nurse hangs the solution, a second registered nurse or doctor must check the label on the container before it is administered. All solutions given are charted and monitored to see that they are running at the proper speed. Usually this is the responsibility of the anesthesiologist.

e Adhesive strips to firmly secure needle or catheter and tubing to the patient's skin to prevent motion that may cause entry of microorganisms into the skin wound or traumatize the vein.

f Stopcock to regulate or stop flow of solution through the tubing into the vein.

During Induction of General Anesthesia

1 Stay in the room and near the patient to comfort him or her and assist the anesthesiologist in the event that excitement or any other contingency occurs. The patient must be guarded during induction to prevent possible injury or fall from the operating table. Further restrain or hold the patient if necessary. The circulating nurse must not leave the room until the anesthesiologist says the patient no longer needs to be guarded.

2 Be as quiet as possible. Excitement may occur during induction from tactile or auditory stimulation. It occurs more commonly in alcoholics. A strong startle reaction to sound can provoke life-threatening cardiac arrhythmias in any patient, however. Hearing is the last sense lost. *The room must be kept completely quiet until the patient is anesthetized.* Any stimulation while the patient is under light anesthesia is highly dangerous and must be avoided. A quiet, undisturbed induction makes for a much safer and easier maintenance of and recovery from anesthesia.

After the Patient Is Anesthetized

1 Reposition the patient only after the anesthesiologist says that the patient is anesthetized to the extent that he or she will not be disturbed by being moved or touched. (Positioning of the patient is discussed in Chapter 10.)

2 Attach anesthesia screen and other table attachments as needed. These always are placed after the patient is anesthetized and positioned to prevent injury to the patient.

3 Note the patient's position to be certain all measures for his or her safety have been observed.

4 Place indifferent electrode plate in contact with the patient's skin, if electrosurgical unit is to be used, to ground the patient properly. Avoid scar tissue, and hairy or bony areas (see Chaps. 12 and 14 for further discussion of electrosurgical units).

5 Expose the appropriate area for skin preparation. Turn the blanket downward and the gown upward neatly to make a smooth area around the operative site.

6 Turn on the overhead spotlight over the site of incision. Bright light should not be focused on the patient before he or she is asleep or eyes are covered. Preoperative medication affects pupils. Dim light is restful and not irritating.

7 Arrange the sterile prep tray and pour solutions if this has not already been done. Don sterile gloves and prepare the operative site. (Patient skin preparation is discussed in Chapter 11.)

> NOTE. The first assistant may be the person who preps the patient. This person first scrubs his or her own hands and arms, then puts on sterile gloves.

8 Cover or bag the prep tray immediately after use. The sponges are not included in the sponge count so they must not be discarded in the kick bucket. A disposable tray may be bagged for disposal with the trash after the operation is completed.

After Surgeon and Assistant(s) Scrub

1 Assist with gowning. Reach inside the gown to the shoulder seam to do so. If closed glove technique is used, pull gown sleeves only so far that the hands remain covered. If open technique is used, pull each sleeve over the hands so that the gown cuffs are at the wrists. Fasten the back of the gown.

2 Observe for any breaks in technique during draping (see Chap. 11). Stand near the head end of the operating table to assist the anesthesiologist in fastening drape over the anesthesia screen or around IV standard next to the armboard.

3 Assist the scrub nurse in moving Mayo stand and instrument table into position, being careful not to touch the drapes.

4 Focus the overhead operating light on the site of incision, unless sterile handles will be used. The beam of light should pass the surgeon's right ear and center at the tip of his or her right index finger (or left for left-handed surgeon).

5 Set platforms for team members who need them, or place stools in position for surgeon who prefers to operate seated.

6 Position kick buckets on each side of the operating table and the splash basin, if used, near the surgeon.

7 Connect suction if necessary. Suction caps are designed so that the inlet for fluid is below the outlet for vacuum. These connections must not be reversed. If they are, the contents of the container are picked up and carried into the vacuum system, clogging it and making it nonoperational. Most hospitals use disposable suction collection units to facilitate disposal.

8 Connect electrosurgical electrode cord or any other electrical equipment to be used. Place footpedals within easy reach of the surgeon's foot. Tell the surgeon the settings on all machines.

During the Operation

1 Be alert to anticipate needs of the sterile team such as adjusting the operating light, removing perspiration from brows, and keeping the scrub nurse supplied with sponges, sutures, hot saline, etc. Ideally, the circulating nurse watches the operation closely enough to see when routine supplies are needed and gives them to the sterile team without their having to ask for them. You must know all supplies, instruments, and equipment and be able to get them quickly. You must know their use and care. This is particularly important in emergency situations such as cardiac arrest.

2 Stay in the room as much as possible. *Inform the scrub nurse if you must leave.* Be available to answer questions or offer helpful suggestions to the scrub nurse. Kindly help builds up a learner's confidence.

3 Keep discarded sponges carefully collected, separated by sizes, and counted. The method used depends upon provision made for the care of soiled sponges in each hospital. (Refer to suggested methods of guarding sponges on p. 152 of this chapter.) It is convenient to keep them in submultiples of the total number of each type of sponge in each package.

Soiled sponges should be placed in an area of the room away from traffic, cabinets, and doorways, but in full view of the scrub nurse and anesthesiologist. Sponges that have been used should be kept at a level well below the sterile field on a moistureproof surface. Do not place them on absorbent linen as it soaks through. Lint, dust, and trapped organisms will be dispersed into the air as the sponges dry and are handled for counting or disposal. Sponge forceps or gloves, *never bare hands,* are used to handle and count sponges because of the danger of hepatitis transmission. Gathering them directly into plastic bags eliminates extra handling and the hazards that accompany the transfer of dry, soiled sponges. Before placing them in bags, both the circulating and scrub nurses should count them.

4 Weigh sponges for blood loss as requested. Some anesthesiologists and surgeons prefer to have sponges weighed for blood loss rather than visually estimating it. A scale calibrated in grams usually is used to weigh bloody sponges during the operation before they dry out.

The weight of each dry sponge must be known. Usually a chart of the dry weight for one of each type of sponge is attached to the the scale. This weight is multiplied by the number of sponges of each type to be weighed. The scale platform is covered with waxed paper or plastic sheeting to protect it from contamination. Allowing for the dry weights of the number of sponges to be weighed and the cover, adjust the scale to register at zero. When the blood-soaked sponges are weighed, the reading on the scale equals the blood loss; 1 g equals 1 cc. The scale must be checked frequently for accuracy.

Record the total blood loss each time sponges are weighed, always adding the new weight to the preceding weight. Keep a current total. A tally board for this purpose may be mounted on the wall where the anesthesiologist and surgeon can read it easily.

Total blood volume monitoring determinations may be used for estimation of operating blood loss (see Chap. 9, p. 189).

5 Obtain blood products for transfusion as necessary. Transfusions of whole blood, plasma, or packed cells must be carried out according to policy of the hospital. Basic rules usually include the following:

a Blood products are obtained from the blood bank by a person responsible for signing them out to the proper patient. Usually a nursing assistant from the OR staff can do this.

b Blood products are started by an MD or RN after a careful comparison of the label on the bag or bottle with the identity of the patient. A second professional person confirms these data. The label stays on the container while the blood product is transfused.

c Another solution may be infused immediately prior to hanging a blood product. In changing from this solution to a blood product, avoid the possibility of air entering the tubing. A blood-transfusion filter must be used. Filter should be changed after second or third unit of whole blood because the filter can become clogged with microaggregates.

d The anesthesiologist records on the anesthesia record the following information:

(1) Name of the person who started the transfusion of whole blood, plasma, or packed cells.

(2) Time started and drops per minute.

(3) Amount and information on the label: group, Rh factor, and number.

e Cold, refrigerated blood may induce hypothermia. Blood may be warmed as it is transfused by immersion of the administration tubing in a controlled water bath or infused through sterile coils in a temperature-modifying device. Temperature must be controlled between 89 to 105 °F (32 to 41 °C).

f To have blood near the patient during operation, a refrigerator with controlled temperature may be installed in the OR suite. It has a recording thermometer. An alarm bell rings if a dangerous temperature is reached. Fluctuations in temperature cause red blood cells to deteriorate. Microorganisms can multiply in blood when outside a refrigerator. If blood is brought to the OR and not needed, it should be returned to the refrigerator in the suite or the blood bank immediately. Do not allow blood or its derivatives to stand unrefrigerated in the OR.

g A transfusion of wrong blood can be fatal. All established measures must be strictly observed for the safety of the patient. The patient is observed closely for any type of reaction. This probability increases in direct proportion to the number of units transfused. The most common type of reaction is *allergic*; *febrile* is almost as common; and *hemolytic* reactions are possible. Transfusion reactions under anesthesia may be accompanied by profound hypotension and temperature change. However, the common physical reactions and chills are not seen in the anesthetized patient. If any suspicious reactions occur:

(1) Stop the transfusion.
(2) Report the reaction to the surgeon and the blood bank.
(3) Return the unused blood to the blood bank along with a sample of the patient's blood.
(4) Send a urine sample to the laboratory as soon as possible.
(5) Take vital signs frequently.
(6) Complete an incident report covering the details of the reaction to be kept on file.

Compatible bank blood is not always immediately available. Even when it is, posttransfusion serum hepatitis is a potential danger for the patient. *Autotransfusion,* the reinfusion of the patient's own blood, may be used either during elective or emergency operations. This blood may be collected days or weeks preoperatively and stored in the blood bank, or drawn just prior to or during the operation. Recovery of blood as it is lost and reinfusion during the operation is *intraoperative autotransfusion.* This requires sterile equipment that simultaneously suctions blood from the operative site, filters, anticoagulates, defoams, and returns it to the patient with minimal blood-cell damage. An autotransfusion unit for this purpose must be easily and quickly assembled as it may be lifesaving in an emergency situation. Autotransfusions can be used for a patient who will not allow blood transfusion for religious reasons but will accept his or her own blood if it is returned immediately.

6 Know the condition of the patient at all times. Keep the OR supervisor informed of any marked change in the patient's condition or unanticipated procedure. Also tell the ORS if the operation will not finish at the scheduled time. This is important in a busy department as it may be necessary to rearrange the schedule.

7 Prepare and label specimens for transportation to the laboratory. Wrong patient identification on a specimen can result in the wrong diagnosis for two patients. Each container is labeled with the name of the patient, hospital and room numbers. A requisition specifying the laboratory test that the surgeon desires accompanies the specimen. This includes date, name of surgeon, pre- and postoperative diagnoses, operative procedure, and tissue to be examined including its source.

Containers for storing specimens may be plastic bags, waxed cardboard cartons, or glass jars with preservative solutions. Preservative solutions vary. All must be handled with care to avoid spillage. Handling of specimens should be held to a minimum and *never done with bare hands.* If instruments are used for handling, be careful not to tear or damage tissue. The routine for each type of tissue specimen may vary as follows:

a Pathological specimens should not be allowed to dry out. A solution of aqueous formaldehyde most often is used as the fixative until the specimen is processed further in the laboratory.

b Cultures should be refrigerated or sent to the laboratory immediately. When placed immediately into media, they can be stored in an incubator indefinitely.

Cultures are obtained under sterile conditions. The tips of the swabs must not be contaminated by any other source. The circulating nurse may hold the tube; however, swabs are handled only by sterile team members. OR and laboratory personnel must be protected from contamination. The circulating nurse can hold open a small paper or plastic bag for the scrub nurse to drop the tube into if it is handled on the sterile field. This technique eliminates the need for the circulating nurse to handle the tube, and alerts laboratory personnel to be cautious in handling to prevent spread of microorganisms and to protect themselves.

c Smears and fluids should be taken to the laboratory as soon as possible. These may be placed on glass slides or drawn into evacuation tubes.

d Stones are placed in a dry container so that they will not dissolve.

e Foreign bodies should be disposed of according to hospital policy and a record kept for legal purposes. A description of the object is recorded. The foreign body may be given to the police, surgeon, or patient, depending on the legal implications, the hospital's policy, or the surgeon's wishes.

f Amputated extremities are wrapped before sending them to a refrigerator, which is usually in the morgue.

8 Complete the patient's chart, the permanent operating room records, and requisitions for laboratory tests or chargeable items, as required. Requisitions are made out as a record of:

a Charges to patients for supplies, according to hospital routine.

b A piece of equipment sent from the OR with the patient to the unit, e.g., an instrument such as an intestinal clamp left on the patient following a colostomy, a tracheotomy set that accompanies the patient following thyroidectomy, wire scissors if the patient has had teeth wired together. These items are to be returned. The requisition usually is made out in duplicate; the carbon copy accompanies the item, and the original is filed by the lender until the item is returned.

9 Remember and be alert to any breaks in sterile technique.

a Do not touch or reach over the sterile field. When placing sterile items, transfer should be made to the edge of the instrument table to avoid exposing it to contamination with microorganisms in dust or lint shed from a sleeve, arm, or wrapper.

b Face sterile areas when passing. Just as no unsterile equipment should be placed between two sterile surfaces, no unsterile person should pass between two sterile surfaces or two sterile team members. All unsterile personnel should face and remain at least 1 ft (30 cm) from any sterile surface.

c Do not touch unwrapped items to the nonsterile rim or door when removing them from the autoclave.

d Do not touch the edge of the cap or lid to the lip of the container before or after pouring sterile solution. The outside of the cap is not sterile.

e Wash hands vigorously for at least 15 seconds after each patient contact or handling contaminated items. Hasty handwashing is better than not washing at all. Friction and water alone will remove most surface organisms from the hands. However, wash hands frequently with an antiseptic agent. If you do not work up a good lather and use friction, your hands will still be contaminated. Be sure to clean under fingernails; microorganisms can grow under them. Turn the faucet handles off with a paper towel, if a knee or foot control is not available.

f Keep conversation to a minimum. Do not handle mask and cap unnecessarily. Keep hair covered and mask in place.

g Decontaminate floor and walls promptly during the operation if contaminated by organic debris such as blood and sputum. A phenolic, iodophor, or other broad-spectrum detergent-disinfectant can be applied from a squeeze bottle to the soilage. This prompt decontamination helps prevent microorganisms from drying and becoming airborne.

During the Closure

1 Count sponges, needles, and instruments with the scrub nurse. Report the counts as correct or incorrect to the surgeon. Complete the count records (for details of count procedures, see p. 151). Collect soiled sponges and put into plastic-lined kick bucket.

2 If another patient is scheduled to follow (TF):

a Phone, or ask the clerk-receptionist to call the unit at least 45 minutes before the scheduled time of operation to request that the preoperative medication be given. This usually is not necessary for the first scheduled patient of the day, but is the procedure for subsequent patients when the exact time of operation is uncertain. For these patients, the anesthesiologist usually orders medication "on call."

b Send a nursing assistant for the patient or notify the unit to transport the patient. The patient should be in the OR suite 30 minutes before the time of anticipated incision. If a holding area is included in the OR suite, the patient may arrive earlier to receive preoperative medication there.

c Check the surgeon's preference card and the procedure book. Collect supplies that will be needed; get them organized to the extent possible. These can be assembled in the substerile room or left in a cabinet. They cannot be put on furniture in the room until it is cleaned after this operation is completed. Advance preparation is not necessary if a cart system is used.

3 Prepare for room cleanup so minimal time will be expended between operations, but check with scrub nurse before leaving the room.
   a Remove x-rays from the viewbox, place them in the envelope, and take them to the designated area to be returned to the x-ray department.
   b Return blood not needed for transfusion to the refrigerator or have it taken to the blood bank by a nursing assistant.
   c Obtain washer-sterilizer tray, instrument tray, and other items necessary for the cleanup procedure (see details of procedure in last section of this chapter).
4 Send for a recovery room stretcher, ICU bed, or prepare the patient's stretcher or bed with a clean sheet, whatever is the accepted practice. Also alert nursing assistants and housekeeping personnel that the operation is nearing completion, so that they can be ready to assist as needed. This helps to shorten the time between operations.

After the Operation Is Completed

1 Open the neck and back closures of gowns of surgeon and assistants so that they can remove them without contaminating themselves.
2 Assist with outer layer of the dressing. Ideally, this outer layer should be conforming, stretchable to avoid constriction if edema develops, and capable of clinging to itself so that it will stay in position without telescoping if mobility is desired. *Adhesive tape* is used most frequently. Benzoin may be sprayed on the skin around the intermediate layer, before applying adhesive tape, to increase its adhesion. Apply the tape firmly but not tightly, to avoid traction on the skin and wrinkling of it. Traction and wrinkling, rather than sensitivity to the tape, may cause skin irritation.

   NOTE. If the patient has a known sensitivity to regular adhesive tape, hypoallergenic tape should be used. It causes little or no reaction. It is lightweight yet strong, sticks well, is porous, and allows skin to breathe.

   Slightly elastic bandage provides gentle, even pressure to hold bulky dressings in place. This bandage also may be used to hold other kinds of dressings or to bind a splint onto an extremity. It stretches to conform to body contours, does not constrict, yet gives firm support. The types available include:
   a Four-ply crinkled-gauze bandage.
   b Cotton-elastic bandage.
   c Cotton-elastic bandage with adhesive on one side. This is especially useful in holding dressings on the chest, as it is firm yet permits chest expansion.

   Montgomery straps are used to hold bulky dressings in place that require frequent changes or wound inspections. They are made in pairs, in assorted widths, with strings. One strap is put on each side of the dressing and the strings are tied across the dressing.

   An *abdominal binder* may be needed to hold large abdominal dressings. If necessary, it usually is applied after the patient is moved from the operating table.
3 See that the patient is clean. Wash off blood, feces, or plaster. Put on a clean gown and blanket.
4 Have the nursing assistant bring in a clean recovery room stretcher or ICU bed. Check the name on the patient's stretcher or bed to be sure that he or she is returned to the proper one if this is the procedure. Lock the wheels before moving the patient.
5 Help move the patient to the stretcher or bed. Before moving a patient from the operating table, be sure all arm and leg restraints and table appliances have been removed. A lifting frame or Davis patient roller is a great help in moving unconscious and obese patients. The Davis patient roller consists of a series of rollers, mounted in a frame long enough to accommodate an adult patient. The edge of the roller is placed under the arm band and the patient's side. With the patient's head and feet supported, pull on the arm band and roll the patient onto stretcher or bed. The following precautions must be taken in lifting or rolling the unconscious patient:
   a Splint the arm if an intravenous is running to protect the needle.
   b Support the arms at the sides with the arm band, so that they do not dangle.
   c The anesthesiologist guards the head and neck from injury.
   d Lift or roll the patient gently and slowly to avoid circulatory depression. At least four people are needed; one to lift the head, one to lift the feet, one beside the stretcher or bed to pull, and one beside the patient to lift him or her from the operating table. The action of all must be synchronized.
   e Remove the arm band, which has been used as a lifting sheet, by rolling the patient gently from side to side. Brush burns result if linen is pulled from under the patient.
   f Place the patient in a comfortable position most conducive to maintenance of respiration and circulation. This may vary with the type of operation; for example, the patient should usually:

(1) Be semilateral following laparotomy.
(2) Be semiprone following tonsillectomy, for drainage.
(3) Be lateral, on affected side, following transthoracic operations, to splint the side.
(4) Have an operated extremity supported on a pillow.

g Raise the siderails before the patient is transported out of the OR.

6 Hang IV solution bags or bottles on a standard attached near the foot end of the stretcher or bed, where there is less danger of injury to the patient if it should fall or break.
7 Connect all drainage systems as indicated. This must be done at once to prevent extravasation of urine, bile, or other fluid with consequent irritation or infection. Attach the tubing to the bottom sheet, leaving a loop next to the patient. Drainage tubing should be positioned so that downward flow is aided by the force of gravity. The drainage bag should be kept below the level of the tubing to prevent retrograde flow.
8 Be sure that the chart and proper records including the nursing care plan accompany the patient. Send extra units of blood as needed. Send other supplies as indicated.
9 Have the nursing assistant assist the anesthesiologist in taking the patient to recovery room, intensive care unit, or nursing unit. In some hospitals, the circulating nurse accompanies the patient and anesthesiologist to give a nursing report to the nurse receiving the patient which includes a review of the nursing care plan.

SPONGE, NEEDLE, AND INSTRUMENT COUNTS

The kinds and numbers of sponges, needles, and instruments needed for different operations will vary. Each item must be considered a foreign object that can cause unnecessary harm should it be left inside the patient. Therefore, to ensure adequate patient protection, these items are counted before and after use.

A *counting procedure* is a method of accounting for items put on the sterile table for use during an operation. Sponge and needle counts are taken on every procedure performed in the OR. Instrument counts also are recommended, although in some hospitals policy specifies that instrument counts be taken only when a major body cavity is entered, or the depth and location of the wound is such that an instrument could accidentally be left in the patient. These would include operations within the chest, abdominal and pelvic cavities, extraperitoneal spaces, vagina, hip or shoulder joint, and along the spine. The specific written policy and procedure for all counts must be followed without deviations.

Counting Procedures

Sponges, needles, and instruments are counted at four or more different times.

First Count The person who wraps items for sterilization counts them in standardized multiple units, for example:

1 Sponges, tapes, peanuts, etc., are usually counted in multiples of 5 or 6; i.e., 10 or 12, 20 or 24 per package. If commercially prepackaged, sterile radiopaque sponges are used, this count is done by machine, usually 10 per package.

2 Needles put in racks or a suture book are counted uniformly into sets in multiples of two or three of each type and size the surgeon will need. Disposable eyed needles are precounted by the manufacturer.

3 Instruments are counted as they are assembled in standardized sets. Groups of six of the basic clamps facilitate handling and counting.

Second Count The circulating and scrub nurses count together when packages are opened before the operation begins and as each additional package is opened during the operation.

All Counts

1 As the scrub nurse fingers each item, he or she and the circulating nurse number each one aloud, quietly, until all items are counted.

2 The circulating nurse immediately records the count for each type of item on the count record. Preprinted forms are helpful for this purpose.

3 Count additional packages far away from the counted items already on the table, in case it is necessary to repeat the count or discard the item.

4 Counting should not be interrupted. If uncertain about the count because of interruption, fumbling, or for any other reason, repeat it.

Sponges

1 Only radiopaque sponges with an x-ray detectable element should be used on the sterile field and table. The types of sponges and the number of different sizes should be kept to a minimum.

2 The scrub nurse holds the entire pack of sponges, of whatever type including tapes, in her hand at one time.

3 Shake the pack to separate the sponges.

4 Holding the thumb over the folded edge of the sponges, pick each sponge separately from the

pack and number it while placing it in a pile on the table.

NOTE. If a pack contains an incorrect number of sponges, the scrub nurse should hand the pack to the circulating nurse to take out of the room immediately. The danger of error is great if attempts are made to correct errors or compensate for discrepancies.

Needles

1 All swaged and eyed, reusable or disposable, needles are counted when packets are added to the table.
2 The scrub nurse retains the packet with descriptive information of number and type of needles to help determine if the count is correct for swaged and disposable needles.

Instruments

1 Remove the top rack of instruments from the instrument tray and place it on a rolled towel on the instrument table or over the lip of the tray. Remove knife handles, towel clips, tissue forceps, and other small instruments from the tray and place these on the instrument table. Do not put instruments on the Mayo stand until they are counted or as they are being counted.
2 Be sure all instruments left in the tray are exposed for counting.
3 Detachable parts, such as screws, blades, etc., must be counted.

Third Count Counts are taken in three areas when the surgeon starts the wound closure.

Sponge Count

1 *Floor count.* The circulating nurse counts sponges that have been discarded from the sterile field. This count should be verified by the scrub nurse.
2 *Table count.* The scrub and circulating nurses together count sponges on the instrument table and Mayo stand.
3 *Field count.* The circulating nurse totals the floor and table counts, subtracts this figure from the total number, and tells the surgeon or first assistant the number needed to complete the count. One of them does the operative field count. If it is the desired number, the circulating nurse tells the surgeon that the count is correct.

Needle and Instrument Counts The procedure is essentially the same as for the sponge count. The circulating nurse adds to the field count any needles or instruments recovered from the floor or passed off the table. The count should be reported to the surgeon as correct only after a physical count by number actually has been completed.

NOTE. If a needle or instrument has broken, the scrub and circulating nurses both must make sure all pieces are recovered.

Fourth or Final Count A fourth count is done if a discrepancy is noted in any of the counts or if policy stipulates additional counts before any part of a cavity or a cavity within a cavity is closed. A final count may be taken during subcuticular or skin closure.

After the final counts are completed, the circulating nurse signs the operative record to indicate that the counts are correct. A registered nurse must participate to verify that all counts are correct and to sign for all counts.

NOTE. Omitted counts due to extreme patient emergency must be documented on the operative record and a patient incident report completed by the circulating nurse.

When the operation is completed, the scrub nurse should sign the operative record also. Hospital records can be subpoenaed and admitted as evidence in court. Therefore, when your name appears in a hospital record, to attest to an act you have performed, you should always write it yourself. Include your role in the act, such as "scrub nurse" signing for "sponge, needle, instrument counts," with your signature.

NOTE. If either the scrub or circulating nurse is relieved by another person during the operation, the incoming nurse should verify all counts before the nurse being relieved leaves the room. The persons who take the final counts are held accountable and must sign the records.

Incorrect Count

1 The entire count is repeated immediately.
2 The circulating nurse looks in the trash receptacles, under the furniture, on the floor, in the linen hamper, and throughout the room.
3 The scrub nurse looks over the drapes and under articles on the table.
4 The surgeons recheck the field and the wound.
5 The circulating nurse should call the supervisor, head nurse, or team leader to check the count.

6 If the item is not found, the surgeon may wish an x-ray taken at once, with a portable machine, to determine whether it has been left in the wound. Due to the condition of the patient or a reasonable assurance, based on wound exploration, that the item is not in the patient, the surgeon may wish to complete the closure first. However, hospital policy should make it *mandatory* to take an x-ray *before* the patient leaves the OR whenever a sponge, needle, or instrument count is incorrect.

7 If a count is wrong, the circulating nurse writes up the incident on the appropriate form as a permanent record. She does this even if the item is located by x-ray. This record has legal significance to verify an appropriate attempt was made to find the missing item. If the item is not found by x-ray, the record brings to the attention of personnel the need for more careful counting and control of sponges, needles, and instruments.

Methods of Guarding Sponges

Regardless of the types and numbers of sponges used, all must be accounted for expediently and conveniently. Various methods may be used to help ensure that a sponge is not left in the patient or misplaced.

By the Scrub Nurse

1 Keep sponges, tapes, peanuts, etc., separated on the instrument table and far away from each other and away from linen, especially towels.
2 Keep sponges far away from small items such as needles and clips that might be dragged into the wound by them.
3 Do not give the surgeon or assistant a sponge to wipe powder off gloves. It may end up in the linen hamper or trash.
4 Never mix sponges and tapes in the solution basin at the same time to avoid danger of dragging a small sponge unknowingly into the wound along with a tape.
5 Do not give the pathologist a specimen on a sponge to take from the room; put it on a towel instead.
6 Discard all soiled sponges into the kick bucket, leaving two clean ones and one tape on the field. If the surgeon needs more, you must waive this rule and leave more. Keep a mental count of the number of sponges or tapes on the field at any given time.
7 Do not be wasteful of sponges. Besides the economy factor, the more sponges that are used, the more there are to count and the greater the chance for error.
8 Once the peritoneum is opened or the incision extends deep into a body cavity where a sponge could be lost, three alternative precautions can be taken:
   a Remove all small sponges from the field and use only tapes. The rings hang over the wound edges.
   b Use 4 by 4 in. (10 by 10 cm) sponges on sponge forceps only.
   c Give sponges to the surgeon one at a time on an exchange basis.
9 *Do not add sponges or remove them from the operative field during the sponge count until the count is verified as completed and correct.* Prior to beginning the final count, the scrub nurse should place adequate tapes and sponges on the field for use while the count is taken.

By the Circulating Nurse

1 To prevent the possibility of a sponge being taken into the OR and causing confusion in the count, different types and sizes should be used on trays such as spinal, shave, or prep trays, and be contained before the incision is made. The tray, including the used sponges, may be bagged in plastic and stored temporarily. Sponges from these trays must never be put in the kick bucket or trash receptacle until after the final sponge count is completed.

2 Unfold each discarded sponge and shake tapes to be sure no sponges are on them. To avoid transmission of hepatitis or other pathogenic organisms, soiled sponges are never touched with bare hands. Use sponge forceps or gloves to separate sponges for counting and stacking.

3 Count sponges into the multiple or submultiple of the total number in a package as recorded on the sponge count record; count and stack into separate units for each type of sponge.

> NOTE. The kick bucket is lined with an antistatic plastic bag. Therefore, either hang the sponges over the rim of the bucket or transfer them from the kick bucket to a moisture-proof surface until the count unit is completed. The number of sponges needed to complete a unit may be placed directly into a waterproof plastic or paper bag. Each bag is closed to await the final count. If this method is used, the scrub nurse should verify the count as the sponges are deposited in the bags. Closed bags can be placed on a table or in a kick bucket under a towel placed over it to await final count. The number of sponges in each bag and number of bags are recorded so that when it is time for the final count the circulating nurse has a record of the number bagged.

4 Give scrub nurse dressings after the final sponge count.

5 Trash and linen should never be taken from the room until the final sponge count is completed.

Method of Accounting for Needles

By the Scrub Nurse

1. Give needles to the surgeon on an exchange basis; that is, one is returned before another is passed. Account for each needle as the surgeon finishes with it. Never let one lie loose on the field or Mayo stand. Keep them away from sponges and tapes.
2. Use needles and needleholders as a unit. Some hospitals go by the rule: no needle on the Mayo stand without a needleholder and no needleholder without a needle.
3. Secure used needles until after final count. Many methods for efficient handling are available.
   - **a** Sterile adhesive pads with or without magnets facilitate counting and safe disposal. Separate pads can be used for needles that may be used again and for those that will not be. When a large number of swaged needles will be used, the scrub and circulating nurses may determine the number of needles a pad will hold and work out a unit system. When the maximum number is reached and counted by them, the pad is closed. This method eliminates the hazard of handling loose needles on the Mayo stand or instrument table.
   - **b** Swaged needles can be inserted through or into their original packet. An empty packet indicates an unaccounted-for needle at the time of the final count.
   - **c** Used needles can be returned to the needle rack, or threaded into the top layer of the suture book.
   - **d** Accumulation of used needles in a medicine cup or other container is the least-desirable method because each must be handled individually to count them. This not only potentially contaminates gloves, but may puncture them as well.

By the Circulating Nurse Open only the number of packets of sutures with swaged needles that will be needed. Overstocking the table not only is wasteful, but also complicates the needle count.

Simplifying the Instrument Count

Reducing the number and types of instruments and streamlining standardized sets makes counting easier. Inform the supervisor if unused, unnecessary instruments are routinely included in basic sets. Instruments peculiar to specific operations, wrapped separately can be added to the basic set only when needed.

ROOM CLEANUP PROCEDURES AFTER THE OPERATION IS COMPLETED

Physical facilities influence the flow of supplies and equipment following the operation. However, the basic principles of aseptic technique dictate the procedures to be carried out immediately after the operation is completed to prepare the OR for the next patient. Every patient merits the same degree of safety in the environment and deserves the same care as every other. In addition, personnel working in the operating room suite must be protected. Therefore, every patient should be considered potentially a contaminant in the environment. Some have known pathogenic microorganisms; the danger of transmission of the hepatitis virus or other infectious organisms may be unknown. Cleanup procedures must be rigidly followed to contain and confine organisms, known or unknown, to prevent contamination of the entire suite; this is done by:

1 Destroying organisms as quickly as possible after the operation is completed

2 Protecting operating room personnel from contact with known infectious material such as frank pus, colon bacilli, gas gangrene, tetanus, tuberculosis, or any other infectious diseases

3 Preventing cross contamination of other patients

The routine cleanup procedure can be accomplished expeditiously by the circulating nurse and scrub nurse working cooperatively. While the circulating nurse assists with the outer layer of the dressing and prepares the patient for transport from the OR, the scrub nurse dismantles the sterile field before removing gown and gloves. All instruments, supplies, and equipment must be either terminally sterilized, decontaminated, or contained for disposal before they are handled by other personnel.

By the Scrub Nurse

1. Push the Mayo stand and instrument table away from the operating table as soon as the intermediate layer of the dressing is applied. *Do not contaminate the Mayo stand* until the patient has left the room (refer to "Note" on p. 141).
2. Assist surgeon and assistant in removing gowns and gloves. Gowns are always removed before gloves. Grasp both shoulders of the gown and pull them downward over the arms. Roll the outside of the gown inward and discard in linen or trash hamper; linen goes to laundry, disposable gown goes into trash. Using glove-to-

glove technique, grasp cuff of gloves and pull them inside out over the surgeon's hands. Discard in trash receptacle.

3 Check drapes for towel clips, instruments, and other items. Be sure no equipment is discarded with disposable drapes or sent to the laundry with linen. Roll drapes off the patient to prevent sparking and airborne contamination; do not pull them off. Disposable drapes are placed in plastic bag for disposal. Roll wettest part of linen drapes into the center as far as possible to prevent soaking through the linen bag, even though it is waterproof.

4 Discard soiled sponges and other waste or disposable items in trash receptacle.

5 Discard unopened packets of suture.

NOTE. The amount of suture put on the table for the operation should be kept to a minimum so that there is very little actual waste. However, undamaged suture packets may be decontaminated and returned to the manufacturer for resterilization. If a packet is grossly stained with blood or a solution, discard it. Clean packets may be soaked for a minimum of 10 minutes in an activated glutaraldehyde solution. They are then rinsed, dried, and placed in the suture collection box to be sent to the manufacturer.

6 Dispose of sharp items safely. Special care must be taken in handling all knife blades, surgical needles, and needles used for injection or aspiration. Place them in an appropriate container for either disposal or cleaning to prevent injury and potential risk of contracting hepatitis, syphilis, malaria, or aspergillosis. The primary cause of accidental cuts and punctures to personnel, both within and outside of the OR, is the disposal of surgical sharps at the end of the operation. Those hospitals with standardized systems designed specifically for safe handling and disposal of sharps avoid virtually all accidental cuts, punctures, or lacerations. Remember, protection of yourself and other personnel is an important part of your job.

Blades and needles are never discarded loose in trash receptacles. They must be enclosed and secured so that they cannot perforate the receptacle. A self-closing, adhesive pad designed for this purpose is the safest device to use. Needles can cut through adhesive tape or puncture paper cups, boxes, or suture and blade packets. Sharps in these containers create a hazard. A safe disposal procedure must be implemented, and the cleaning procedures adhered to.

a Remove knife blades from handles. Point the blade toward the table away from you, so if a blade breaks or slips it will not fly across the room. Remove blades with a needleholder; never use fingers. Never put knife handles in the washer-sterilizer or instrument tray with the blades left on them. Other instruments designed for replaceable cutting blades should have the blades removed; thereafter they may be handled with the other instruments.

b Place reusable surgical needles, either on the needle rack or loose, into a perforated stainless steel box to be run through the washer-sterilizer with the instruments. Check the suture book to see that it is not discarded with needles in it.

c Place reusable needles used for injection or aspiration in the perforated stainless steel box with the surgical needles. Include those used by the anesthesiologist.

NOTE. Whether or not disposable needles are run through the washer-sterilizer as a safety measure before discarding depends upon the individual hospital's rules and regulations. Each hospital should have a safe way of rendering them unfit for use again. Many have a needle-destruction unit available for this purpose.

7 Place instruments directly into perforated trays for processing in a *washer-sterilizer.* Instruments must be terminally sterilized before they are handled for definitive cleaning and checked for proper functioning prior to reuse (see Chap. 14).

a Place heavy instruments in bottom of tray.

b Turn instruments with concave surfaces, such as curettes and rongeurs, with bowl side down to facilitate drainage of the concave surface.

c Open box locks and pivots of hinged instruments to expose the maximum surface area.

d Disassemble instruments designed to be disassembled without tools.

e Sharp or pointed instruments should be carefully spaced in the tray to prevent contact with other instruments that could damage their surfaces. Some hospitals prefer to wash and sterilize sharp instruments separately.

If a washer-sterilizer is not available, an alternative procedure is to carefully wash and rinse instruments and then put them into perforated trays and *autoclave* them. Any soil remaining on instruments is more difficult to remove after they have been heat-sterilized because it becomes baked on them. Soil also inhibits the sterilization process.

a Obtain clean water in the solution basin. A mild soap or noncorrosive, low-sudsing, free-rinsing detergent may be added to the water.
b Wash instruments carefully to guard against the accidental spray of contaminated material around the room. Brushing tends to aerosolize organisms. If brushing is necessary to remove gross soilage, keep instruments beneath the level of the solution.
c Load the instrument tray the same way as recommended above for the washer-sterilizer tray. Autoclave with tray unwrapped.

NOTE. After hand-washing, instruments may be placed into a solid basin, covered with a 2% solution of trisodium phosphate, and autoclaved for 45 minutes at 250°F (121°C).

8 Put glass syringes, medicine glasses, and other glassware, including those used by the anesthesiologist, into a separate tray or the tray with the instruments. Syringes must be separated. Check for disposables and discard them in the trash.
9 Place rubber goods and plastic items not to be disposed of into tray with instruments if they can be steam-sterilized. Many items—gloves, catheters, tubings, etc.—are disposable. Check before putting them into washer-sterilizer.

NOTE. Disposable suction tubing is recommended over reusable tubing, which presents formidable cleaning problems. However, if tubing is reused, special care must be given to cleaning the lumen prior to placing tubing with instruments for terminal sterilization. Suction detergent-disinfectant solution through the lumen.

10 Wash, rinse, and dry items that cannot be immersed in water or steam-sterilized. These must be wrapped for sterilization in ethylene oxide gas.
11 Invert small basins and solution cups over the instruments. Basins and trays too large for the washer-sterilizer or standard instrument sterilizer are washed, dried, and put into a double pillowcase to be autoclaved in the bulk sterilizer. The circulating nurse holds the pillowcase open for the scrub nurse to drop in the utensils. The Mayo tray may be included.
12 Dispose of solutions and suction bottle contents. Disposable suction units simplify disposal. Wall suction units should be disconnected by the circulating nurse to avoid contamination of the wall outlet. If disposable units are not used, decontaminate contents with disinfectant prior to hopper disposal. Wash the container. Thoroughly wash plunger and other areas of wall-mounted suction apparatus. Containers are autoclaved along with the basins and trays.
13 Put trays in the washer-sterilizer and/or autoclave for terminal sterilization.

If the washer-sterilizer and autoclave are in an adjacent substerile room, the circulating nurse opens the doors for the scrub nurse. The scrub nurse places the trays in them. The circulating nurse adds detergent to the washer-sterilizer, and then starts operation of equipment.

If the washer-sterilizer and/or autoclave are not in an immediately adjacent room, the scrub nurse removes gown, covers tray with a clean towel, carries it to the utility room, and places it in the washer-sterilizer or autoclave there. Bring the towel back to the room and discard it in the linen hamper, or trash receptacle if it is disposable. Care must be taken to avoid touching front of scrub clothes with either the tray or towel.
14 Discard all used disposable table drapes in plastic bag with used disposable patient drapes. Unused sponges may be put into the pillowcase with basins to be autoclaved before being placed in the stock cupboard. Some hospitals discard these.

Even if not obviously soiled, all linen from open packs should be subjected to laundering to replace moisture lost to the fabric by sterilization. Therefore, put unused linen along with used linen table drapes in the linen hamper to be sent to the laundry.
15 Remove gown before gloves. The circulating nurse unfastens neck and back closures. Protect arms and scrub clothes from contaminated outside of gown. Grasp right shoulder of gown with left hand and, in pulling gown off arm, turn the sleeve of the gown inside out. Turn the outside of the gown away from body with flexed elbow. Then grasp the other shoulder with the other hand and remove the gown entirely, pulling it off inside out. Discard in linen hamper, or trash receptacle if disposable (see Fig. 8-10).

To remove gloves, use glove-to-glove, then skin-to-skin technique to protect clean hands from the contaminated outside of the gloves, which bear cells of the patient. Gloves are turned inside out as they are removed and then discarded into the trash (see Fig. 8-11, p. 157).

Figure 8-10 (A, B, and C) Sequence of scrub nurse removing soiled gown at the end of the operation. Clean arms and scrub dress are protected from contaminated outside of the gown. **A** With gloves kept on, she loosens cuffs of gown and shakes them down over wrists. She then grasps right shoulder of gown (unbuttoned or untied) with left hand and, **B** in pulling the gown off arms, turns the arm of the gown away from body with flexed elbow. **C** She then grasps the other shoulder with other hand and removes the gown entirely, pulling it off inside out. She has thus kept arms clean.

Cart System Cleanup

All reusable instruments, basins, supplies, and equipment, including suction bottles, are put on or inside the cart. The cart is covered or closed and taken to the central decontamination area outside of the OR suite for cleanup. A closed cart, especially if it has been used as the instrument table, is wiped off with a disinfectant solution before it is taken out of the room. A cart with soiled supplies should be removed from the OR suite via the outer corridor if this is the design of the suite. If dumbwaiters are used, a separate one is provided for the soiled cart. Clean and contaminated supplies are always kept separated.

The cart is designed to go through an automatic steam cart washer or a manual power wash for terminal cleaning, after it is emptied, before it is restocked with clean and sterile supplies.

By the Team

As soon as the patient leaves the room, the circulating nurse is free to assist with cleanup of the room. Nursing assistants and/or housekeeping personnel may be available to assist also. Regardless of which member of the team performs them, specific functions must be carried out to complete the room cleanup.

The personnel and areas considered contaminated during and after an operation are:

1 The members of the sterile team, until they have discarded their gowns, gloves, caps, masks, and shoe covers. These remain in the contaminated area. Some hospitals require personnel to change scrub clothes after known septic operations.

2 All furniture, equipment, and floor, within and around the perimeter of the sterile field, unless accidental spillage has occurred in other parts of the room; then these are considered contaminated also.

3 All anesthesia equipment.

4 Stretchers used to transport patients. These should be cleaned after each patient use.

Clean, but not sterile, gloves are worn to complete the room cleanup. The scrub nurse changes gloves after the sterile field is dismantled. The following must be decontaminated:

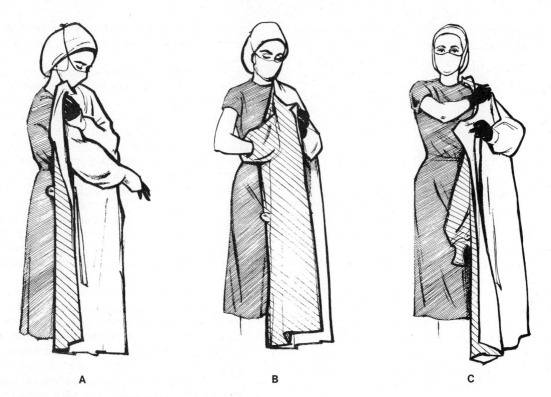

1 *Furniture.* Wash horizontal surfaces of all tables and equipment, including the anesthesia machine, with a disinfectant solution. Apply disinfectant from a pistol-grip sprayer or squeeze-bottle dispenser and wipe with a clean cloth or a disposable wipe that is changed frequently. All surfaces of the mattress, pads, and screw connections of the operating table must be included. Mobile furniture can be pushed through disinfectant solution used for floor care to clean the casters.

2 *Overhead operating light.* Overhead light reflectors should be wiped using a clean cloth wet with disinfectant solution. Lights and overhead tracks become contaminated quickly and present a possible hazard from the fallout of microorganisms onto sterile surfaces or into wounds during each operation. Therefore, it is important to keep them clean.

3 *Anesthesia equipment.* All reusable anesthesia masks and tubing must be *cleaned and sterilized before reusing.* Some of this equipment can be steam-sterilized; if not, it may be sterilized by ethylene oxide gas and aerated prior to reuse. If this method is not available, items should be immersed in activated glutaraldehyde solution for 10 hours.

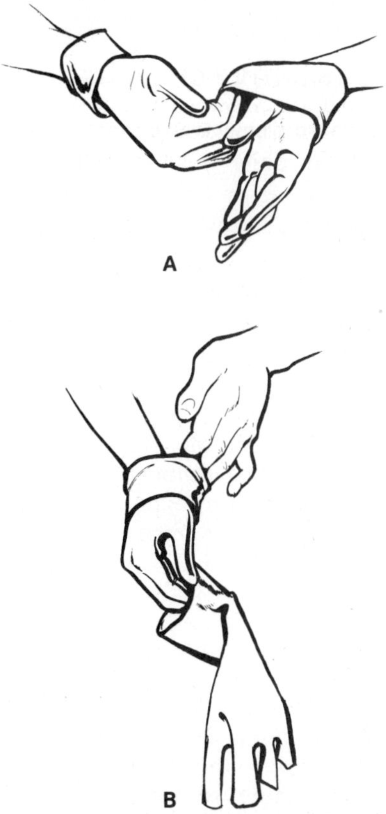

Figure 8-11 (A and B) Sequence of scrub nurse removing soiled gloves at the end of the operation. She uses **A** glove-to-glove, then **B** skin-to-skin technique to protect "clean" hands from the contaminated outside of the gloves, which bear cells of the patient. She turns the gloves inside out when removing them, keeping hands "clean."

4 *Linen.* After all cleaning procedures have been completed, cloths should be discarded or put in the linen bag if they are not disposable. When all linen, used and unused, has been placed inside the linen bag, it is closed securely. After removal from the linen hamper frame, someone outside the room should stand at the door with a clean plastic bag, holding it so that hands are covered by a large cuff in the top of the bag. The sealed linen bag is placed upside down in this clean bag. Take care not to touch the clean bag or the other person with gloved hands. The person holding the clean bag should unroll the cuff and gently expel the air from the bag away from his or her face. A knot is tied in the top of the bag. This entire procedure protects housekeeping and laundry personnel since the outside of the bag is clean and dry for transportation from the OR suite. The hamper frame is cleaned after the linen bag is removed.

5 *Trash.* All trash collected in plastic bags, including disposable drapes, kick bucket and wastebasket liner bags, is combined into one clean plastic bag, if possible, held open by a person outside of the room. It is double-bagged, as described for linen, and discarded per hospital routine.

6 *Floors.* Wet-vacuuming, with a filter-diffuser exhaust cleaner, is the method of choice for floor care in the OR. Machine cleaning is more effective than manual cleaning. If waste, such as suture material and gross soilage, is great, the wet-vacuum equipment may be used dry for first treatment. Then the floor is flooded, half of the room at a time, with detergent-disinfectant solution. This may be dispensed from a pump spray or automatic spraying device attached to the central wet-vacuum equipment system. If portable equipment is used, a spray-type watering can may be used to flood the floor, although this method is slower and may wet it unevenly. Hot water may hasten the cidal action of the disinfectant agent, but may also soften tile adhesive. Room-temperature water requires at least a 5-minute contact time for effectiveness.

Furniture is rolled across the flooded floor area to clean the casters. The wet-vacuum pickup is used to pick up the solution before repositioning furniture. Standing platforms are considered part of the floor and may be flooded with solution to be picked up by wet-vacuum.

The exterior of the equipment and tubing is cleaned following each use, with special attention given to cleaning the rubber blade before the next use. If the hose is equipped with a brush attachment, this is washed and autoclaved between uses.

If wet-vacuum equipment is not available, freshly laundered, clean mops can be used. The floor can be flooded with detergent-disinfectant solution. One mop is used to apply and one to take up the solution. *Mops, treated or nontreated, never should be used dry in the OR.* Following *one-time use,* the mop heads are removed and placed in the linen hamper with other soiled linen. The mop handles may be stored in the housekeeping storage area until needed again.

7 *Walls.* If walls are splashed with blood or organic debris during the operation, those areas should be washed. Otherwise walls are not considered contaminated and need not be washed between operations.

Room Ready for Next Patient

Cleaning procedures, as described, provide terminal sterilization and adequate decontamination following any operation. With appropriate care, special procedures, quarantine of a room, or discrimination of type of operative procedure scheduled to follow in the same room are rarely necessary. With a well-coordinated team, minimal turnover time between operations can be accomplished; in an average time of 15 to 20 minutes the room will be ready for the next patient.

DAILY CLEANING AFTER SCHEDULE IS COMPLETED

In the OR

At the completion of the day's schedule in each OR, more stringent and rigorous cleaning is done in all areas previously discussed:

1 *Furniture* is thoroughly scrubbed, using mechanical friction in addition to chemical disinfection. Disinfectants are only adjuncts to good physical cleaning; "elbow grease" is probably the most important ingredient.

2 *Casters and wheels* should be cleaned and kept free of suture ends and debris. Equipment is available that automatically washes stretchers, tables, and platforms, then steam-cleans and dries them within a matter of minutes.

3 *Equipment,* such as electrosurgical units, should be cleaned with care so as not to saturate surfaces to the degree that disinfectant solution runs into the mechanism causing malfunction and repairs.

4 *Ceiling- and wall-mounted fixtures and tracks* are cleaned on all surfaces.

5 *Kick buckets, linen hamper frames, and other waste receptacles* are cleaned and disinfected; these are even autoclaved when feasible.

6 *Floors* are given a thorough wet-vacuum cleaning with wet-vacuum pickup used dry and then wet.

7 *Walls* should be checked for soil spots and cleaned as necessary.

8 *Cabinets and doors* should be cleaned, especially around handles or push plates where contamination is apt to occur.

Outside OR Itself

1 *Counter tops and sinks* in substerile room should be cleaned.

2 *Scrub sinks and spray heads* on faucets should undergo thorough cleaning daily. A mild abrasive on sinks removes oily film residue left by scrub antiseptics. Spray heads, faucet aerators, or sprinklers should be removed and disassembled, if possible, for thorough cleaning and sterilization of parts. Contaminated faucet aerators and sprinklers can transfer organisms directly to hands or items washed under them. Scrub sinks should not be used for routine cleaning purposes.

3 *Walls around scrub sinks* must receive daily attention. Spray and splash from scrub antiseptics build up around the sink and must be removed.

4 *Transportation and storage carts* need to be cleaned with specific attention to wheels and casters.

WEEKLY OR MONTHLY CLEANING

A weekly or monthly cleaning routine is set up, in addition to the daily cleaning schedule, by the executive housekeeper and OR supervisor. Any routines for housekeeping must, of necessity, be based on physical construction. However, if specific schedules are not established, some areas may never be cleaned. Areas to be considered are:

1 *Walls.* Walls should be cleaned when they become visibly soiled. If they are painted or tiled with wide porous grouting, these factors must be considered in planning cleaning routines. Washing walls in the OR and throughout the suite once a week is reasonable, but less-frequent time intervals for cleaning may be acceptable if spot disinfection is assured on a daily basis. This requires adequate continuous supervision.

2 *Ceilings.* Ceilings may require regular special cleaning techniques because of mounted tracks and lighting fixtures. The types of fixtures are considered in planning cleaning routines.

3 *Floors.* Floors throughout the OR suite should be machine scrubbed periodically to remove accumulated deposits and films. Conductive flooring should never be waxed. Rounded corners and edges facilitate cleaning.

4 *Air-conditioning grilles.* The exterior of air-conditioning grilles should be vacuumed at least weekly. Additional cleaning is necessary when filters are checked and changed.

5 *Storage shelves.* Storage cabinets have been replaced in many OR suites by portable cart storage. Storage areas should be cleaned at least weekly, or more often if necessary, to control accumulation of dust, especially in sterile storage areas.

6 *Sterilizers.* Regular cleaning of all types of sterilizers must be done as recommended by the manufacturer.

7 *Dispensers.* Microbial contamination can be transferred from contaminated dispensers of surgical scrub antiseptics or hand lotions. All contents of dispensers should be drained and discarded on a weekly schedule. The dispensers should be washed, dried, and sterilized before being refilled and returned to use.

Chapter 9

Anesthesia

HISTORICAL INTRODUCTION

The attempts of human beings to relieve suffering from pain are as old as the human race itself. Primitive people considered pain the torture of demons, which they attempted to frighten away by wearing charms and tattooing their bodies. The medicine men continued the use of magic.

A Babylonian clay tablet, circa 2250 B.C., gave a remedy for toothache. During the time of Nero, Greek and Roman surgeons gave their patients a mixture of wine and vinegar. It was also called a "potion of the condemned" and was used to relieve anguish such as that suffered during crucifixion. These surgeons also experimented with a form of local anesthesia by placing a carbonate stone directly over the operative area and pouring vinegar over it; they noted a numbing sensation, due to the formation of carbon dioxide. Sleep-producing inhalations were first used by the Egyptians and Arabians who concocted many potions from plants such as the poppy and the hemlock. Sponges saturated in these solutions were held to the patient's nostrils. However, death often resulted from them and from the root juices used as reviving agents because dosage was unregulated and drug action unknown. The Egyptians and Assyrians produced unconsciousness by pressing on the carotid vessels in the neck, causing cerebral anoxia.

Monks of the Middle Ages emphasized the use of prayer for divine healing. The lack of realistic understanding of human suffering was shown by the fact that a Scotsman was buried alive for trying to alleviate the pain of childbirth. However, early alchemists were then at work in their laboratories and the result was a compound, sweet vitriol, later called *ether.*

Army surgeons have always contributed to medical advancement. Paré dulled the pain of his soldiers by compressing blood vessels and nerves near the operative area. At this time also, half-frozen soldiers were found to have a higher pain threshold. Refrigeration anesthesia was revived in 1941 for use in amputation. However, amputation often without anesthesia was the surgical trademark of the Civil War. In some instances it was performed on a kitchen table, with crude heavy knives and instruments and even table forks as retractors. If the surgeon himself was not the source of morbidity and mortality, infection and/or shock were.

Mesmerism and hypnotism, although advocated by some, were considered ineffective and discredited for pain control.

Progress in anesthesia soon followed the development of chemistry and physics during the Renaissance. The modern concept of anesthesia was based on Joseph Priestley's experiments with oxygen and nitrous oxide. This combination and also ether were first used at parties for entertainment. Traveling chemists administered these agents to induce incoherence and giddy laughter, whence the term *laughing gas.* The anesthetic properties were realized when injuries sustained during inhalation of these agents were unfelt.

Dr. Crawford Long of Georgia administered the first ether anesthesia in 1842 for the painless removal of a tumor of the neck, but did not publish the results of this and subsequent cases until 1849. In 1846, however, two Boston dentists, Morton and Wells, employed nitrous oxide for tooth extraction. In October of that year, Dr. Morton first demonstrated ether for surgical anesthesia before an astounded group of clinicians. With his words, "Doctor, your patient is ready"— the same words so often heard today—a new era in surgery was born. Dr. Oliver Wendell Holmes devised the term *anesthesia* from the Greek words meaning "negative sensation."

Sir James Simpson, a Scottish surgeon, instituted the use of chloroform anesthesia in 1847. It was administered to Queen Victoria during childbirth by England's first anesthetist. However, in the late nineteenth and twentieth centuries, with administration of ether and chloroform for anesthesia, operations within the abdomen, thorax, and cranium evolved. Development of the surgical specialties was concurrent with the refinement of anesthesia methods and instrumentation as science and surgery evolved. The hot, unair-conditioned OR under the skylight where patients were inducted with rapidly vaporizing drop ether (patient and team alike inhaled the vapors) gave way to the well-ventilated ORs of today. The heat, unpleasant odor, and suffocating feeling of earlier years led patients to fight the prolonged unpleasant induction and to long remember the experience. Near the turn of the century one reference warned the anesthetizer to be careful, when the patient vomited—a not infrequent occurrence—that the ejecta did not enter the wound or proximal area.

Purification of drugs like morphine, invention of the hollow needle, and development of gas machines hastened the finding of new anesthetic techniques and agents. Endotracheal anesthesia, first employed by open tracheotomy, was developed by Dr. Friedrich Trendelenburg. Dr. Chevalier Jackson's development of the laryngoscope greatly aided intubation.

The importance of watching the patient's condition under anesthesia was realized ultimately and supportive measures were developed. First experiments with intravenous therapy, using lamb's blood, began in the seventeenth century. The four blood types and the anticoagulants were not discovered until the twentieth century. Plasma was first used during World War I to combat shock, although saline had been used earlier.

The human race is greatly indebted to the many pioneers in anesthesia. Men like Dr. Heidbrink and Dr. Boothby perfected gas machines and face masks. Eminent surgeons such as Dr. George Crile and Dr. Harvey Cushing emphasized the importance of keeping accurate records of the patient's condition during operation. In 1896, Dr. Cushing brought to the United States from Italy one of the first sphygmomanometers invented. In 1950, the first clinical use of the electroencephalogram in estimating the depth of anesthesia was reported.

Special techniques such as hypothermia (see p. 191) and extracorporeal circulation (see p. 391) opened new vistas to thoracic and cardiovascular surgeons, making possible the advanced, complex surgical procedures in these specialties.

Continuing assessment of vital functions under anesthesia, rapid pleasant induction and recovery, replacement of blood loss, and ever-developing new drugs and techniques are salient features of modern anesthesia that infinitely enhance patient recovery and the operating team's efficacy of performance.

VALUE TO LEARNER

The development of successful, controllable anesthesia has made modern surgery possible. The methods used are constantly being improved by research. Since anesthesia is a necessary adjunct to most operative procedures, all persons caring for surgical patients should know the pertinent facts in order to give intelligent patient care. Anesthetization is no small part of the patient's total experience. The nurse's familiarity with various anesthetic agents, their interaction with certain drugs, and their potential hazards is a necessity. The alert, informed nurse can quietly note onset of complications and help to avert an emergency or fatality.

Working with anesthesiologists in the OR gives the learner an unparalleled opportunity to master immediate resuscitative measures and their effectiveness as well as an understanding of the care of unconscious and critically ill patients.

It is mandatory that all persons who work in areas where explosive agents are stored and used know potential explosion hazards and their control.

Finally, the fact that *no* operative procedure is minor must *never* be forgotten. Operation and anesthesia impose upon the patient certain inescapable risks, even under supposedly ideal circumstances.

DEFINITIONS

Understanding of common terms is essential.

Amnesia Loss of memory.

Analgesia Lessening of or insensibility to pain.

Anesthesia Loss of feeling or sensation especially loss of the sensation of pain.

Anesthesiologist A doctor of medicine who specializes in the field of anesthesia.

Anesthetic A drug that produces local or general loss of sensibility.

Anesthetist A person who has been trained to administer an anesthetic.

Anoxemia Low blood oxygen; subnormal blood-oxygen content.

Anoxia Absence of oxygen.

Apnea Suspension or cessation of breathing.

Arrhythmia Lack of rhythm designating alteration or abnormality of normal cardiac rhythm.

Assisted Respiration The maintenance of adequate alveolar ventilation by supplementing the patient's respirations by manual or mechanical means; respiratory rate and rhythm are controlled by the patient, tidal volume by the anesthesiologist.

Biotransformation Metabolism of anesthetic drugs. They are broken down in the hepatic cells where they may accelerate their own rate of metabolism or be influenced by other drugs. Metabolic products may be inert or highly reactive chemically, possibly causing destruction of liver cells. Biotransformation occurs by one or more than one of four mechanisms: oxidation, conjugation, hydrolysis, reduction.

Bradycardia Slowness of heartbeat; less than 60 beats per minute.

Depolarization Neutralization of polarity; reduction of differentials of ion distribution across polarized semipermeable membranes, as in nerve or muscle cells in the conduction of impulses; to make electrically negative.

Fasciculation Incoordinate skeletal-muscle contraction in which groups of muscle fibers innervated by the same neuron contract together.

Hemodynamics The study of how the physical properties of the blood and its circulation through the vessels affect blood flow and pressure.

Hypercapnia Excessive amount of carbon dioxide in the blood.

Hyperkalemia Above-normal elevation of potassium in the blood.

Hypnosis A state of altered consciousness, sleep, or trance induced artificially in the subject by means of verbal suggestion of the hypnotist or by the subject's own concentration.

Hypnotic A drug, or verbal suggestion, that induces sleep.

Hypotension Lowered blood pressure.

Hypothermia A state in which body temperature is lower than the physiological normal.

Hypovolemia Low or decreased blood volume.

Hypoxia, Hypoxemia Oxygen want or deficiency; state in which an inadequate amount of oxygen is available to or utilized by tissue—inadequate tissue oxygenation.

Induction The period from the beginning of administration of the anesthetic until the patient loses consciousness.

Lung Compliance Ability to expand.

Margin of Safety The difference between therapeutic and lethal dosage.

Narcosis A state in which there is diminution of consciousness, sensation, motor activity, and reflex action.

Neutralization Process that counterbalances or cancels the action of an agent, rendering it inert.

P Expression for partial pressure; the pressure exerted by one of the gases present in a mixture of gases. In such a mixture, the partial pressures of the gases are exerted independently of each other.

$PaCO_2$ Arterial carbon dioxide tension (partial pressure of carbon dioxide in arterial blood). Normal: 38 to 42 torr.

Pain Threshold An individual's tolerance for pain. It may be influenced by certain factors such as apprehension.

PaO_2 Arterial oxygen tension (partial pressure of oxygen in the arterial blood)—degree of oxygen transported in the circulating blood. Normal: 80 to 100 torr.

Perfusion Introduction of fluids into tissues by their injection into blood vessels; passage of a fluid through spaces.

pH Expression for hydrogen ion concentration or acidity of blood. (Alkalemia: values above 7.42; acidemia: values below 7.38; normal: 7.4.)

Polarity The state of having poles or regions of intensity with mutually opposite qualities; demonstration of sedation of a nerve sensation at or near the positive electrode and of irritation at or near the negative electrode.

Regional Anesthesia Insensitivity of a part of the body to pain caused by the interruption of the conductivity of the sensory nerves supplying that area.

Respiratory Acidosis The reduction of carbon dioxide excretion through the lungs caused by respiratory depression or obstruction, or pulmonary disease.

Surgical Anesthesia Stage III of general anesthesia as described by Guedel with diethyl ether anesthesia. It implies the loss of reflexes with accompanying muscle relaxation.

Tachycardia Excessive rapidity of heart action, heart beat. Pulse rate is over 100 beats per minute.

Tachypnea Abnormally rapid rate of breathing.

Tension The partial pressure exerted by a component of a mixture of gases; used interchangeably with **P.**

Ventilation The constant supplying of oxygen through the lungs.

PAIN

Pain is a perceptual phenomenon, a disturbed sensation causing suffering or distress. It is often what induces the patient to seek medical assistance. Realization of pain commences with stimulation of the nerve endings of pain fibers, which in turn produces a nerve impulse that travels to the brain. There the impulse is processed and registered by the individual as an unpleasant feeling state. The quality, intensity, location, duration, and memories of pain influence one's depth of perception of it and the emotional response to it. No pain is undoubtedly purely organic or strictly functional; most pain also carries a psychogenic factor. Therefore, patience and discrimination on the part of health care personnel are basic to alleviation of pain.

Methods of surgical intervention used to relieve intractable pain are discussed in Chapter 24.

Any patient with trauma, tissue damage from operative procedure, ischemia (localized tissue anemia), or infarct (localized area of ischemic tissue necrosis) is a candidate for pain.

The main focus of this chapter is a review of the methods of anesthesia, the various anesthetic agents used to avoid pain of operation, and the appropriate measures that provide comfort and safety for the patient intra- and postoperatively. One of these measures is preanesthetic medication.

PREOPERATIVE PREMEDICATION

History

It is interesting to note that morphine sulfate was used for preoperative medication in 1850 in Italy. In 1870, it was observed that when used in conjunction with inhalation anesthesia, morphine reduced the amount of anesthetic required and prolonged the anesthetic state. In the late nineteenth century, surgeons advocated the use of atropine with morphine to dry secretions and speed heart rate due to its parasympatholytic action. Certain problems associated with premedication, however, led Blumfield to state in 1913 that it was "a great help to the patient, but no help either to the surgeon or anesthetist." While narcotic premedication was considered still in its infancy in 1912, considerable progress has been made since then with the addition of other drugs and a better understanding of their pharmacology. Today premedication is a very essential feature of preoperative preparation.

Purpose

Preoperative medication is given to allay preoperative anxiety, produce some amnesia, and dull awareness of the OR environment. These drugs may decrease secretions in the respiratory tract, counteract undesirable side effects of the anesthetic, and raise the pain threshold. The preoperative medication constitutes to a greater or lesser extent a part of the overall anesthetic technique. Certain drugs may prolong the effect of the anesthetic and increase a respiratory-depressant effect.

The administration of anesthetic actually begins with the giving of preanesthetic drugs. Discerning choice can lead to a smooth, effective anesthetic management and an uncomplicated postanesthetic course as opposed to a stormy, unsatisfactory experience for all concerned.

Choice of Drugs

The selection of drugs is made by the anesthesiologist based on an assessment of the patient's physical and emotional status, including age and weight, the surgeon's requirements for minimal or maximal relaxation, and the anesthesiologist's own skills and personal experiences. If the patient is scheduled for local anesthesia (see p. 178), the surgeon may order the preoperative drugs. In choosing premedication, the anesthesiologist aims to disturb respiration and circulation as little as possible. Since more than one pharmacological response is desired, a combination of drugs is used. For example, an analgesic is given to patients who are to be anesthetized with the less potent general anesthetic agents. Most anesthesiologists prefer to have the patient arrive in the OR awake but drowsy, free of apprehension, and fully cooperative. Drowsiness and lack of fear are not synonymous; for many patients relief from anxiety is attained only by dulling the consciousness. The nature and quantity of drugs ordered depend on the anesthesiologist's goals.

Time Given

The time is calculated so that maximum effect is reached before induction. It is usually given 45 to 60 minutes prior to induction. Adequate action is desired for induction and maintenance, but residual postoperative depression is to be avoided.

Drugs Used

These may be classified as sedatives and tranquilizers, narcotics, and anticholinergics. The efficacy depends greatly on the rate and extent of absorption, distribution in the tissues, degree of protein binding, site and rapidity of detoxification and excretion.

Individual patients may experience side effects and special sensitivities or undesirable interactions (effect of one drug upon another) between two or more drugs. Drugs taken simultaneously or in close sequence may act independently; they may interact to reduce or increase the intended effect of either; or they may produce an undesired reaction. For example, a number of antibiotics enhance the effect of anticlotting agents. Conversely, barbiturates and glutethimide decrease the anticlotting effect of anticoagulants. The anesthesiologist inquires about a patient's previous drug intolerance, incidence of adverse reactions, and carefully notes any medication the patient is currently taking.

NOTE. An estimated 1,500,000 adverse drug reactions annually result in hospital admissions.

Sedatives and Tranquilizers

1 *Barbiturates*—secobarbital (Seconal), pentobarbital (Nembutal), phenobarbital—for hypnotic and sedative effect. In normal doses they cause minimal respiratory and circulatory depression. They do not counteract pain and unless a narcotic is also given, painful stimuli may cause restlessness and excitation. They may be given for sleep the night before operation and to allay apprehension. Each barbiturate is metabolized or excreted characteristically. For example, phenobarbital is excreted mainly by the kidney so may be used for patients with reduced liver function. Barbiturates may react with other drugs such as Dilantin, causing variation in the latter's effectiveness. Nausea and vomiting occur less frequently postoperatively with barbiturates than with narcotics.
2 *Nonbarbiturate sedatives and major tranquilizers.* Sometimes it is preferable to give one of these drugs, especially in aged patients and those allergic to barbiturates. In such cases, chloral hydrate, ethinamate (Valmid), or glutethimide (Doriden) may be used.
   a Phenothiazine derivatives—promethazine (Phenergan), hydroxyzine (Vistaril), meprobamate (Equanil), chlorpromazine (Thorazine), triflupromazine (Vesprin). These produce sedation, act as antiemetics and antihistamines, potentiate narcotics and general anesthetics, and block autonomic reflexes. They may produce postural hypotension. Chlorpromazine lowers the body temperature, inhibits shivering, and decreases myocardial irritation. It has a prolonged action and may be used in premedication for hypothermia (see p. 191). These drugs are qualitatively alike but differ quantitatively. They have an additive effect in combination with narcotics and hypnotics so that the dose of the latter may be decreased and their side effects minimized.
   b The tranquilizers—diazepam (Valium), a benzodiazepine derivative, and droperidol (Inapsine) and haloperidol (Haldol)—which are butyrophenone derivatives, are also used. Diazepam, for example, may be given as a premedicant before electric cardioversion of arrhythmias, cardiac catheterization, or endoscopy.

Narcotics This classification includes the natural alkaloids of opium (morphine), mixtures of the alkaloids (omnopon—Pantopon), semisynthetic modifications of these compounds (hydromorphone—Dilaudid), and the synthetic narcotics (meperidine—Demerol). These drugs are analgesics. All decrease alveolar ventilation and are respiratory depressants. Lesser doses are indicated for the elderly and patients in poor physical condition or with circulatory instability because of the increased incidence of side effects related to respiration and circulation. Hepatic failure and pulmonary complications may induce unfavorable reaction.

1 *Narcotics,* such as morphine sulphate which is the most commonly used, produce narcosis, analgesia, and decrease of reflex irritability. They are thought to produce a moderate decrease in the amount of anesthetic needed. They pave the way for a faster, smoother induction; there is less anxiety, pain, and excitement. The drugs may decrease respiratory minute volume and ability of the circulation to react to stress as a result of vasodilating action on the peripheral vascular smooth muscle. There is an increased incidence of hypotension. Their duration of effect may be longer than is generally expected. Narcotics are especially valuable when the patient is in pain preoperatively but are best avoided in the asthmatic patient. Their narcotic effect may extend to the postoperative period if the operation is of short duration and help alleviate pain and restlessness. They constrict and stimulate smooth muscles, sometimes causing pre- and postoperative nausea, vomiting, and constipation. The latter may result because after initial stimulation, peristalsis and intestinal tone are reduced.

2 *Synthetic narcotics*—meperidine (Demerol), alphaprodine (Nisentil), methadone, phenazocine (Prinadol), and fentanyl (Sublimaze). These potent drugs give good analgesia and produce fewer undesirable side effects than morphine. Meperidine is the most commonly used of these drugs. It is an effective anesthetic adjuvant and analgesic. The availability of a liquid preparation of meperidine makes it useful in postoperative pain management in pediatric patients where an oral medication is preferred. The large selection of narcotic drugs are more alike than different. No one has been found that is strikingly superior to another in equivalent doses. Anesthesiologists favor one or another, depending on the situation.

NOTE. Naloxone (Narcan) is a specific narcotic antagonist. It has no depressant action, even in the absence of a narcotic. Pentazocine (Talwin) is a nonnarcotic drug. It is a weak analgesic and narcotic antagonist with a minimal dependence potential. Adverse effects are similar to those of other narcotics. Hallucinatory phenomena may occur.

Anticholinergic Drugs Atropine and scopolamine are given for parasympathetic depressant action, mainly for inhibition of mucous secretion. (The routine use of the less irritating anesthetic agents has diminished this problem.)The patient usually complains of dry mouth after their administration. The drugs are also useful in the prevention or treatment of reflex slowing of the heart, which may occur intraoperatively with stimulation of the carotid sinus, intrathoracic manipulation, traction on the extraocular muscles or intraabdominal viscera. While these drugs are bronchodilators, some anesthesiologists eliminate them in bronchitis patients because resulting thickness of secretions and inability to cough them up may contribute to pulmonary problems. Dosage is reduced or the drug eliminated in febrile dehydrated children, or in the presence of tachycardia.

NOTE. Glycopyrrolate (Robinul) is a synthetic anticholinergic agent preferred by some anesthesiologists. This drug is believed not to cross the blood-brain barrier, but it reduces volume and acidity of secretions.

Premedication for Pediatric Patients See Chapter 26.

Premedication for Ambulatory Surgery Patients In general, minimal, if any, premedication is given, and after the patient has been admitted. Agents associated with prolonged effects such as depression, vomiting, or a return to amnesia or a sedated state after awakening are best avoided.

Special Considerations in Premedication

1 Hypnosis is valuable as a premedicant, especially in children, and for anesthesia in selected cases (see p. 193).

2 The patient's metabolic rate varies with age, body build, and general condition. Heavy smokers, alcoholics, hyperthyroid, toxic, emotional, or high-fever patients all have a higher rate requiring more medication, oxygen, and anesthetic for effect. A lower metabolic rate, as accompanies debilitating diseases, asthenia, and hypothyroidism, requires smaller dosage.

3 Persons with drug addiction (abuse of barbiturates, narcotics, cocaine, or amphetamines) present the anesthesiologist with special problems concerning premedication, anesthesia, and venipuncture. These patients may have contracted infectious hepatitis and, in rare cases, malaria. Usually opium addicts are given their accustomed drug for premedication but they must be closely observed for premonitory withdrawal symptoms, especially during and after prolonged operative procedures. Cessation of drug intake and withdrawal may be life-threatening.

CHOICE OF ANESTHESIA

Anesthesia selection is made by the anesthesiologist and/or surgeon. The primary consideration with any anesthetic is that it should be associated with low morbidity and mortality. Choice of the safest agent and technique must be a personal decision predicated on thorough knowledge, sound judgment, and evaluation of the individual situation. The anesthesiologist aims to use the lowest concentration of anesthetic agents compatible with patient analgesia and relaxation.

Anesthetic drugs are not specific but depress activity of all cells. There is no perfect agent that would suppress only selected cells. Therefore, the ideal anesthetic agent or technique for all patients does not exist but the one selected should include some or all of the following:

1 Provide maximum safety for the patient
2 Provide optimum operating conditions
3 Provide patient comfort
4 Have a low index of toxicity
5 Provide potent, predictable analgesia extending into the postoperative period
6 Produce adequate muscle relaxation
7 Provide amnesia
8 Have rapid onset and easy reversibility
9 Produce minimum side effects

The following factors are of importance:

1 Age of patient
2 Physical and mental status of patient
3 Presence of complicating systemic disease or concurrent drug therapy
4 Previous anesthesia experience
5 Position required for operation
6 Type and expected length of procedure
7 Local or systemic toxicity of the agent
8 Expertise of the anesthesiologist
9 Presence of infection at the site of operation
10 Preference of the patient

THE ANESTHETIC STATE

Over the years attempts have been made to account for the action of anesthetic agents. Important theories have evolved, none of them wholly satisfactory. It is not within the scope of this text to detail these theories, only to touch briefly on them. The learner should review neuroanatomy and physiology to facilitate understanding.

Both the central nervous system and the autonomic nervous system play essential roles in clinical anesthesia.

The central nervous system possesses a powerful control system throughout the body. The effect of anesthetic drugs is one of progressive depression of the central nervous system beginning with the higher centers (cerebral cortex) and ending with the vital centers in the medulla. The sequence of brain depression by anesthetic agents was long used to explain clinical signs of anesthesia but the system is more complex than that. It is realized that the cerebral cortex is not inactive during deep anesthesia but that afferent impulses continue to flow into the cortex along primary pathways and to excite cells in the appropriate sensory areas. Also, the cerebral cortex is integrated with the reticular system. The brain represents approximately 2 percent of body weight but receives about 15 percent of cardiac output. Various factors cause alterations in cerebral blood flow and are of considerable importance in anesthesia. These factors are oxygen, carbon dioxide, temperature, arterial blood pressure, drugs, age of patient, anesthetic techniques, and neurogenic factors.

The autonomic nervous system is equally important because of its role in the physiology of the cardiovascular system, the anesthesiologist's ability to block certain autonomic pathways with local analgesic agents, specific blocking effects of certain drugs, and the sympathomimetic and parasympathomimetic effects of many anesthetic agents.

The anesthetic state involves motor, sensory, mental, and reflex functions. Anesthetic depression is referred to as presurgical anesthesia, surgical anesthesia, or overdosage. The anesthesiologist constantly assesses the patient's response to stimuli.

KNOWLEDGE OF ANESTHETICS

Using discerning observation, astute deduction, and meticulous attention to the minutiae, the anesthesiologist provides skilled induction, careful maintenance of anesthesia, and prophylaxis to avoid postoperative complications. Responsible for the vital functions of the patient, the anesthesiologist must know the varying physical and chemical properties of all gases and liquids used in anesthesia. These properties determine how the agents are supplied, their stability, the systems used for their administration, and their uptake and distribution in the body. Important factors are their diffusion, solubility in body fluids, and the relationships of pressure, volume, and temperature. The most recently synthesized general anesthetic agents are nonflammable in contrast to the older agents.

Also, operating room and recovery room nurses need to be cognizant of the pharmacologic characteristics of the most commonly used anesthetics.

Anesthesia and operative trauma produce multiple systemic effects.

TYPES OF ANESTHESIA

Anesthesia may be produced in a number of ways.

1 *Neuroleptanalgesia; neuroleptanesthesia.* The terms *neurolepsis* and *neuroleptanalgesia* describe the state resulting from the combination of a narcotic (potent analgesic) and a tranquilizer (neuroleptic, psychotropic drug). The analgesia, amnesia, and sedation produced are not true anesthesia. Supplementation is necessary for extensive surgical procedures. When the narcotic-tranquilizer combination is reinforced by use of an anesthetic such as nitrous oxide (inhalation agent), the resulting state is referred to as *neuroleptanesthesia.*

2 *General anesthesia.* Pain is controlled by general insensibility. Basic elements of general anesthesia include loss of consciousness, analgesia, interference with undesirable reflexes, and muscle relaxation.

3 *Balanced anesthesia.* Balanced anesthesia is a technique whereby the properties of anesthesia, i.e., hypnosis, analgesia, and muscle relaxation are produced, in varying degree, by a combination of agents.

4 *Local or regional anesthesia.* Pain is controlled without loss of consciousness. One area or region of the body is anesthetized. This is sometimes called *conduction anesthesia.*

NEUROLEPTANALGESIA NEUROLEPTANESTHESIA

Different combinations of narcotics and tranquilizers are possible. Neuroleptanalgesics are administered intravenously, whether used alone or in combination with inhalation of nitrous oxide. Neuroleptic drugs reduce motor activity and anxiety, produce detached apathetic state, and potentiate the hypnotic, analgesic effects of the narcotic as well as nitrous oxide. The narcotic produces marked analgesia. Dosage can be regulated so that the patient can still cooperate and respond to command (neuroleptanalgesia).

Innovar, a commonly used neuroleptanalgesic, is a combination of droperidol, a potent tranquilizer, and fentanyl, a potent, short-acting synthetic narcotic. Fentanyl may cause profound respiratory depression, hypotension, bradycardia. Therefore, some anesthesiologists prefer to measure these drugs separately. An advantage of this combination is the apparent absence of toxic effects on the kidneys, liver, heart (only slight cardiac depressant effect; alpha-blocking property). Droperidol also exerts an antiemetic effect. Consciousness returns within minutes but the psychotropic drug effects will persist for 4 to 6 hours after administration, causing drowsiness and indifference to discomfort. Respirations must be closely watched and patients encouraged to breathe deeply.

This technique is one of the forms of balanced anesthesia (see p. 177).

GENERAL ANESTHESIA

Anesthesia is produced as the central nervous system is affected. Association pathways are broken in the cerebral cortex to produce more or less complete lack of sensory perception and motor discharge. Unconsciousness is produced when blood circulating to the brain contains an adequate amount of the anesthetic agent. General anesthesia permits procedures involving large operative fields usually without time limitations. It provides an immobile, quiet patient who does not recall the operative procedure.

Most anesthetic agents are potentially lethal substances. The anesthesiologist must constantly observe the body's reflex responses to stimuli and other guides to determine the degree of central nervous system, respiratory, and circulatory depression during induction and operation. No one clinical sign can be used as a reliable indication of anesthesia depth. Continuous watching and appraisal of all clinical signs, in addition to other available objective measurements, are necessary. In this way, the anesthesiologist judges the level of anesthesia, referred to as *light, moderate,* or *deep,* and provides the patient with optimum care (see monitoring, p. 187).

The three methods of administering general anesthesia are *inhalation, intravenous injection,* or *rectal installation.* The latter method is now obsolete because absorption in the colon is unpredictable. Control of each method varies.

Induction of General Anesthesia

Induction of and emergence from general anesthesia are two crucial periods requiring maximum attention from the operating team. The following key points are repeated here because they are critical to the patient's welfare:

1 The circulating nurse should remain at the patient's side to protect him physically, support him emotionally, assist the anesthesiologist, and closely observe the monitors.

2 While this period may be quiet and uneventful for most patients, untoward occurrences are possible. Excitement, cough, retching, vomiting, or laryngospasm in turn lead to hypoxia. Secretions in the air passages, from irritation by the anesthetic, can cause obstruction and arrhythmias. Induction must be gentle and not so rapid as to cause physiologic insult.

3 In order to prevent the above, absolute avoidance of stimulation of the patient is mandatory. (Avoid venting steam from the sterilizer in the adjacent substerile room or clattering instruments. Do not touch the patient until the anesthesiologist says it is safe to do so.)

4 Precautions to be taken during induction are: continuous electrocardiography, use of chest stethoscope, ready availability of resuscitative equipment, including defibrillator.

5 Induction is individualized. For example, a very obese patient may be inducted with the head raised slightly to avoid pressure of the abdominal viscera against the diaphragm. The patient is placed horizontally, however, if the blood pressure begins to drop.

Small children need much reassurance and gentle handling. The circulating nurse can be of considerable help to the anesthesiologist in making the induction period less frightening. Sometimes a drop of artificial flavoring (orange, peppermint) put inside the face mask facilitates the child's acceptance of it.

The speed of induction depends on the relationship among potency of the agent, administration technique, partial pressure administered, and rate at which the anesthetic is taken up by the blood and tissues.

Techniques for Administering General Anesthesia

Inhalation This is the most controllable method in that uptake and elimination of anesthetic agents are accomplished mainly by pulmonary ventilation. The lungs act as the avenue of entrance and escape for the anesthetic although the agents are metabolized in the body in varying degrees. *The anesthetic vapor of a volatile liquid or an anesthetic gas is inhaled and carried into the bloodstream by passing across the alveolar membrane into the general circulation and on to the tissues.* Obviously, ventilation and pulmonary circulation are two critical factors involved in the process. Each can be affected by components of the anesthetic experience such as change in body position, preanesthetic medication, alteration in body temperature, or respiratory gas tensions.

In inhalation anesthesia, the aim is to establish balance between the content of anesthetic vapor or gas inhaled and that of the body tissues, the blood and lungs functioning as the transport system. Anesthesia is produced by the development of an anesthetizing concentration of anesthetic in the brain, the depth of anesthesia being related to the concentration.

One must remember that while the respiratory system is being employed as a distributing agent for the anesthetic, it is also carrying on its normal function of ventilation, i.e., meeting tissue demands for adequate oxygenation and elimination of carbon dioxide, and helping to maintain normal acid-base balance. The amount of anesthetic vapor inspired is influenced by the volume and rate of respirations. Gas or vapor concentration and rate of delivery are also significant. Pulmonary circulation is the vehicle for oxygen and anesthetic transport to the general circulation. The large absorptive surface of the lungs and their extensive microcirculation provide a large gas-exchanging surface. In optimum gas exchange, all alveoli share the inspired gas and cardiac output equally (ventilation-perfusion match). Because respiratory and anesthetic gases interact with the pulmonary circulation, alveolar anesthetic concentrations are rapidly reflected in the circulating blood.

Alveolar concentration results from a balance between two forces: ventilation that delivers anesthetic to the alveoli and uptake that removes anesthetic from alveoli. Certain factors influence uptake of the anesthetic and therefore induction and recovery. *Uptake* has the following two phases:

1 *Transfer of anesthetic from alveoli to blood.* The rate of transfer is determined by solubility of the agent in the blood, rate of pulmonary blood flow (related to cardiac output), and partial pressure of anesthetic in arterial and mixed venous blood.

2 *Transfer of anesthetic from blood to tissues.* The factors influencing uptake by individual tissues are similar to those for uptake by blood. They are solubility of the gas in the tissues, tissue volume relative to blood flow (flow rate), and partial pressure of anesthetic in arterial blood and tissues. Tissues differ; therefore their uptake of anesthetic differs. Highly perfused tissues (heart) equilibrate more rapidly with arterial tension than poorly perfused tissue (fat), which has a slow rise to equilibrium and retains the anesthetic longer. *Elimination* of anesthetic is affected by the same factors that affected uptake. As an anesthetic is eliminated, its partial pressure in arterial blood drops first, followed by that in the tissues.

Clinical Aspects of Inhalation Anesthesia

1 Pulmonary blood-gas exchange is important because defective gas exchange is the commonest cause of hypoxemia and respiratory failure. It also interferes with delivery of anesthetic.

2 Potent inhalation agents, as myocardial depressants, affect oxygenation. Most of them induce a dose-related hypoventilation, e.g., the deeper the anesthesia the more decreased the ventilation. Operative stimulation partly corrects depression and ventilation, but controlled respiration (carbon dioxide kept constant) is advised with these agents to prevent hypoventilation and reduce cardiac depression.

Controlled Respiration. Respirations may be assisted or controlled. Assistance, to improve ventilation, may easily be given by manual pressure on the reservoir bag of the anesthesia machine and implies that the patient's own respiratory effort initiates the cycle. *Controlled respiration* may be defined as the completely controlled rate and volume of respirations. The latter is best accomplished by means of a mechanical device that automatically and rhythmically inflates the lungs with intermittent positive pressure, requiring no effort by the patient. Gas moves in and out of the lungs. The combination of a volume preset ventilator with an assist mechanism maintains integrity of the respiratory center. Controlled ventilation is used in all types of operations, especially in lengthy ones. The anesthesiologist's artificial control of respiration or the patient's respiratory efforts influences the minute-to-minute level of anesthesia.

The advantages of controlled respiration are that it:

1 Provides for optimum ventilation
2 Puts the diaphragm at rest for thoracic procedures
3 Gives access to deep regions of the thorax and upper abdomen
4 Permits deliberate production of apnea to facilitate surgical manipulation below the diaphragm, ligation of a deep vessel, or taking an x-ray

The patient is taken off a respirator gradually near the end of operation and spontaneous respiration is resumed. Or, assisted ventilation may be continued postoperatively, as in the case of an obese patient or after lengthy or open-heart procedures.

An anesthesia machine is used to deliver anesthetic-oxygen mixtures to the patient through a breathing system. Inhalation anesthesia methods available through use of the machine may be classified as open, semiopen, semiclosed, or closed. In the *open method,* valves direct the expired gases into the atmosphere and the patient inhales only the anesthetic mixture delivered by the anesthesia machine. With this method, the composition of inspired mixture can be accurately determined. However, anesthetic gases are not confined to the breathing system. High flows of gases are necessary. Water vapor and heat are lost. For children or long operations the inspired gases should be humidified. Also, the resistance to breathing varies. With the *semiopen system,* there is some rebreathing of the mixture; exhaled gas can pass into the surrounding air with some return to the inspiratory part of the apparatus. The degree of rebreathing is determined by the volume of flow of fresh gas. Expired carbon dioxide is not chemically absorbed by the machine. The *semiclosed system* is characterized by the passing of exhaled gases into the atmosphere, or else they mix with fresh gases and are rebreathed. A chemical absorber for carbon dioxide is placed in the breathing circuit. This reduces carbon dioxide accumulation in the blood. Induction is slower, but there is less loss of heat and water vapor. A *closed system* allows complete rebreathing of expired gases. The expired carbon dioxide is absorbed by a chemical absorber (soda lime) on the machine, and the body's metabolic demand for oxygen is met by adding oxygen to the inspired mixture. This system provides maximal conservation of heat and moisture; increases resistance to breathing; reduces the amount and therefore cost of the gases; confines the gases to the machines, minimizing the problems of odor, environmental contamination, and explosion.

The *techniques of inhalation anesthesia* used are:

Mask Inhalation The vapor of a volatile liquid or anesthetic gas itself is inhaled through the closed system of the anesthesia machine via a face mask. Excess carbon dioxide from the patient's breathing is absorbed by soda lime in a container on the machine.

Endotracheal Administration Anesthetic vapor or gas is inhaled directly into the trachea through a nasal or oral tube inserted between the vocal cords by direct or blind laryngoscopy. Endotracheal tubes are open at both ends. Tracheal intubation is widely used. The tube must be securely fixed in place. *Intubation* (insertion of tube directly into trachea) and *extubation* (removal of tube) are precarious times for the patient who may cough, jerk, or experience spasm of the larynx from massive tracheal stimulation. In light anesthesia cardiac arrhythmias may occur. Hypoxia is a common complication.

Advantages: Assurance of a patent airway and control of respiration. Protection from aspiration of blood, vomitus of gastric contents, or foreign material. No interference with the operative field in procedures such as cleft-palate repair. Airway can be preserved with many operative positions. Positive pressure can be given immediately by pressing the reservoir bag on the machine without danger of dilating the stomach. Less vapor is spilled into the room. Easy removal of secretions from trachea.

Complications: Possible trauma to teeth, pharynx, vocal cords, or trachea. Accidental esophageal or endobronchial intubation, the latter resulting in ventilation of only one side. Sore throat, tracheitis, laryngitis, laryngeal edema (more common in children). Ulceration and granuloma of vocal cords (late effect), ulceration of tracheal mucosa. Laryngospasm can follow extubation (removal of tube) especially in children. Aspiration of gastrointestinal contents can occur in patients with intestinal obstruction who are extubated before protective reflexes return. Tracheal collapse following extubation.

Open Drop Technique Formerly used for children, this method has been supplanted by the use of nonexplosive agents. Ether or another volatile liquid is dropped onto a permeable face mask. Vapor, formed on contact with air, is inhaled. Vaporization rate is influenced by room temperature and humidity. Minimal resistance to respiration accompanies this simple technique.

Inhalation Anesthetic Agents

The advantages and disadvantages of all the various agents discussed are entirely relative. The most important factor influencing the safe administration of any anesthetic is the knowledge and skill of the anesthesiologist. The perfect anesthetic has not yet been found and there is no such thing as an entirely safe anesthetic agent. With the synthesis of potent nonflammable agents, most hospitals discontinued use of flammable anesthetics.

Anesthetic Gases

Nitrous Oxide A very commonly used, inorganic gas of slight potency. It has a pleasant sweet fruitlike odor and supports combustion. When combined with oxygen, the range over which explosion may occur is increased. Many techniques of modern anesthesia are based upon its use.

Administration: Inhalation

Advantages: Comfortable, rapid induction and recovery; nontoxic, nonirritating; few aftereffects except headache, vertigo, and drowsiness; excellent analgesic for minor operations not producing severe pain; when combined with a minimum of 20 percent oxygen, causes minimal physiological change.

Disadvantages: Poor relaxation; possible excitement or laryngospasm; hypoxia a hazard. Lacks sufficient potency for most general surgery but can be used widely when potentiated by intravenous barbiturates, narcotics, and muscle relaxants.

Use: In short procedures not requiring much relaxation. As an adjunct to thiopental sodium, halothane, methoxyflurane (potent agents). The combination of nitrous oxide with a potent agent reduces concentration of the latter needed for surgical anesthesia, thereby lessening circulatory and respiratory depressions of the more potent agents.

Cyclopropane A very potent gas that is very seldom used because it is highly explosive. It is heavier than air so tends to accumulate near the floor.

Administration: Inhalation.

Advantages: Pleasant, rapid induction; wide margin of safety if alveolar ventilation is maintained; produces moderate relaxation; low concentration required for anesthesia. Supports circulation: myocardial contractile force is well maintained.

Disadvantages: Flammable; explosive. Decreases respiration amplitude. Sensitizes the heart to catecholamines and may cause cardiac arrhythmias (increasing with depth of anesthesia).

Volatile Liquids

Halothane (Fluothane) A widely used, synthesized, haloginated compound. It has a pleasant odor.

Administration: Inhalation.

Advantages: Nonflammable, potent, versatile, chemically stable; rapid, smooth induction. High potency makes possible the use of high concentrations of oxygen for adequate ventilation. Nonirritating to respiratory tract; does not stimulate respiratory tract secretions. Depth of anesthesia can be rapidly altered. Little excitement; permits early intubation because of minimal laryngeal irritation. Spontaneous ventricular arrhythmias are rare if anoxia and respiratory acidosis are avoided. Useful for patient with bronchial asthma as it induces bronchodilation.

Disadvantages: Special vaporizer must be used for administration because of its marked potency. Potentially toxic to liver. Progressively depressant to respiration. Especially depressant to the cardiovascular system, causing hypotension, bradycardia, and, in rare cases, cardiac arrest. Limited relaxation of abdominal muscles (necessitating muscle relaxants). Exerts undesirable effects on rubber, some metals, and plastics. Is highly soluble in rubber and is retained in it during prolonged administration. Emergence may be accompanied by muscle rigidity or shivering and pallor, counteracted by methylphenidate. Complete elimination of halothane takes some time.

Use: Wide spectrum—all types of operative procedures except routine obstetrics where uterine relaxation is not desired. It is a profound uterine relaxant. It is valuable as a pediatric induction agent. Because of its possible effect as a hepatotoxin, some anesthesiologists avoid repeated administration within an arbitrary time, for example, a 3-month period in adults. Recent jaundice, known or suspected liver disease (past or present) are usually contraindications to its use.

NOTE. Halothane sensitizes the heart to catecholamines. Injection of epinephrine during halothane anesthesia may cause cardiac arrhythmias of varying severity including ventricular fibrillation. Its use is avoided by some anesthesiologists, permitted in very limited dosage by others.

Enflurane (Ethrane) A widely used, nonflammable, stable, halogenated ether, similar in potency and versatility to halothane.

Administration: Inhalation.

Advantages: Rapid induction and recovery with minimal aftereffects. Pharyngeal and laryngeal reflexes are obtunded easily, salivation is not stimulated, and bronchomotor tone is not affected. Cardiac rate and rhythm remain relatively stable, although caution is advisable when used with epinephrine. Muscle relaxation is produced but small, supplementary doses of muscle relaxants may be required; nondepolarizing relaxants (see p. 175) are potentiated by enflurane.

Disadvantages: Respiration and blood pressure are progressively depressed with deepening anesthesia. Although biotransformation (metabolism) of enflurane is less than occurs with other halogenated agents, small amounts of fluoride ion are released. Severe renal disease is a contraindication to use. At deeper levels, an electroencephalographic pattern resembling seizures may occur. The agent is absorbed by rubber.

Use: Wide spectrum of procedures.

Methoxyflurane (Penthrane) The least volatile and most potent of the synthesized, nonexplosive inhalation anesthetics in use. It is a stable clear liquid, a halogenated ether, with a pleasant fruitlike odor.

Administration: Inhalation.

Advantages: Nonexplosive and nonflammable in the usual clinical ranges employed; depth of anesthesia is readily reversible; excellent muscular relaxation although a certain degree of hypotension may accompany its achievement; relatively wide margin of safety; minimal salivation; ability to stabilize heart from arrhythmias.

Disadvantages: Dose-related nephrotoxicity. Potent respiratory depressant (decreases tidal volume and respiratory rate); depressant to cardiovascular system producing hypotension with deeper levels of anesthesia; prolonged induction and emergence; highly soluble in fatty tissue; strong tracheal irritant. Some nausea and vomiting may accompany recovery. It is soluble in rubber and difficult to vaporize.

Use: In general, limited to low concentrations for short duration, e.g., for analgesia in the first stage of labor, because of potential for nephrotoxicity. Liver and renal disease are contraindications to use. Many hospitals have abandoned this agent.

NOTE. It minimally sensitizes the heart to catecholamines.

Diethyl Ether Very rarely used because of its flammability and other disadvantages. It has been supplanted by newer agents. However, it produces excellent analgesia and anesthesia and has a wide margin of safety. It has a burning taste, penetrating odor, high potency, high volatility. It is a bronchodilator.

Administration: Inhalation.

Advantages: Excellent relaxation; level of anesthesia is easily defined; near-normal ventilatory volume and blood pressure can be maintained.

Disadvantages: Long induction and recovery; flammable and explosive; increases secretions; irritating to mucous membranes, lungs, and kidneys.

NOTE. Ether is irritating. Patient's skin and eyes must be protected.

Intravenous Administration

For general anesthesia, the anesthetic agent is injected directly into the circulation, usually via a peripheral vein in the arm. Upon intravenous injection, the drug is diluted by blood in the heart and lungs, passing in high concentration to the organs of highest blood flow (brain, heart, liver, kidneys). Concentration in the brain is therefore rapid. With recirculation, redistribution in the body occurs and cerebral concentration decreases. Dissipation of effects depends on redistribution and biotransformation. Since prompt removal of the agent from circulation is not possible with this method, the safety of the agents is related to their metabolism. The technique is simple and well received (often requested) by patients. Extravascular or intra-arterial injection are to be avoided and it is advisable to give a small test dose at induction. Intravenous anesthesia, a widely used technique, became popular with the introduction in the 1930s of the rapidly acting barbiturates.

Nonvolatile Liquids The thiobarbituric-acid derivatives are commonly used for anesthesia and offer a rapid, pleasant induction, but do not provide relief from pain, merely marked sedation and amnesia. Because solutions of them are highly alkaline and extravasation can cause thrombophlebitis, nerve injury, or tissue necrosis, they are administered via the tubing of a common intravenous solution infusion. The range of central nervous system depression produced by barbiturates is from mild sedation to coma, or cardiac arrest. They are respiratory depressants and can also produce hypotension. Transition from consciousness to operative anesthesia is very rapid. An anesthesia machine, oxygen, and assorted airways and resuscitation equipment must always be at hand prior to administration, i.e., injection. Also, because excessive secretions in the respiratory passage predispose the patient to cough or laryngospasm, he or she should be requested to clear them as necessary prior to induction.

> NOTE. 1. Intravenous barbiturates are not appropriate for all patients, for example, those with poor superficial veins. Caution is necessary in patients with bronchial asthma, acute or chronic respiratory infections, or porphyria.
> 2. Since intravenous barbiturates do not effectively block motor impulses, relaxant drugs are frequently used in conjunction with them. Sometimes during recovery the patient may have muscular shivering or rigidity, slight cyanosis, or stertorous respiration. This is thought to be due to a temporary disturbance of control of body temperature. These aftereffects are treated by the application of warm blankets and oxygen inhalation if cyanosis occurs.

Thiopental Sodium (Pentothal Sodium) The most frequently used barbiturate. It is short-acting in small dosage used for induction but repeated administration may lead to acute tolerance and/or more prolonged effect. It is potent, has a cumulative effect, and very rapid uptake from the blood.

Administration: Intravenous.

Advantages: Pleasant rapid induction (30 to 60 seconds) and recovery; nonflammable; nausea and vomiting are rare; does not irritate mucous membranes of trachea or bronchi or stimulate salivation; easy administration.

Disadvantages: Administration of large doses can cause rapid, pronounced respiratory and circulatory depression but small, divided doses are well tolerated. However, patients bear close watching as some may seem to awaken rapidly but return to an anesthetized state when undisturbed. Respiratory depression may be marked immediately following injection.

> NOTE. Inadvertent intra-arterial injection is evidenced by sudden excruciating pain that requires immediate treatment to prevent a chemical endarteritis with tissue destruction. Spasm and ischemia must be counteracted to prevent gangrene of the fingers. Treatment: intra-arterial 1% procaine, which dilutes the barbiturate solution; local heparinization via the arterial needle to prevent arterial thrombosis; stellate ganglion block for vasodilatation.

There are wide variances in individual tolerance. Minor laryngeal or pharyngeal stimulation from movement of head or neck, early stimulation of the pharynx and trachea by airway insertion, blood or secretion in the pharynx, or painful peripheral stimulus can precipitate the most common complications—coughing, laryngospasm. (If spasm persists to cyanosis, a muscle relaxant and oxygen are given.) The drug cannot be removed or its effect stopped once it is injected. Must be supplemented with another agent to produce analgesia and relaxation for operation. Possible excitement during recovery. Ease of administration can make it susceptible to abuse. It has been said that thiopental sodium is fatally easy to give!

Use: Excellent induction agent, its most common use, prior to administration of more potent anesthetics such as the inhalants. Short procedures not requiring relaxation, e.g., cervical dilatation, incision and drainage of abscess, closed reduction of fracture. As basal anesthetic. For control of convulsions. As adjunct to spinal or nitrous oxide and/or curarizing drugs. For hypnosis during regional anesthesia. Adapts to many different surgical procedures.

NOTE. Morphine sulfate (and nitrous oxide) have a synergistic action with thiopental sodium, i.e., when they are given together each potentiates the action of the other. They are given together with caution. Because of their combined respiratory-depressant effect, postoperative narcotics should be reduced in dosage until the patient has fully reacted. A lowered metabolic rate from the anesthetic and narcotic may also greatly prolong the usual 4-hour destruction rate of morphine in the body.

Other Intravenous Barbiturates (methohexitol—Brevital), sodium thiamylal (Surital). Rapidity of action, duration, and potency vary. Uses are similar to thiopental sodium. These are circulatory and respiratory depressants. Methohexitol is used most frequently.

Dissociative Agents General anesthesia may be produced also by drugs called *dissociative agents,* the resulting state referred to as *dissociative anesthesia.* The drugs are thought to act by selectively interrupting associative pathways of the brain before producing sensory blockade. They permit operation on patients who appear to be awake (eyes remain open and movement may occur) but are anesthetized. The patient is unaware and amnesic.

Ketamine Hydrochloride A phencyclidine derivative administered intravenously (IV) or intramuscularly (IM) to yield profound analgesia. It produces rapid induction (IV—30 seconds, IM—2 to 4 minutes); it is swiftly metabolized. Respirations are not depressed unless it is administered too rapidly or in too large a dose. It is potentiated by narcotics and barbiturates. Individual response varies depending on dose, route of administration, and age of the patient; there is a dose-response relationship. Its mild stimulant action on the cardiovascular system may elevate blood pressure.

Use: Mainly for children, ages 2 to 10 years, for short procedures not requiring skeletal-muscle relaxation; in plastic and eye procedures when combined with local agents; as induction agent prior to use of other general agents and to supplement low-potency agents (nitrous oxide) when adequate respiratory exchange is maintained. For longer procedures repeated doses are given that may prolong recovery time. If relaxation is needed, muscle relaxants and controlled ventilation are indicated.

Contraindications: Intraperitoneal and obstetrical procedures involving tracheobronchial stimulation since pharyngeal and laryngeal reflexes are usually active. If the drug is used alone, mechanical stimulation of the pharynx should be avoided.

Disadvantages: Emergence reactions with psychologic manifestations may occur in the recovery period. Incidence of disturbances such as emergence delirium, vivid imagery, hallucinatory-like actions, and terrifying dreams can be reduced by preanesthetic diazepam and by allowing the patient to lie quietly, not stimulated or disturbed except for such essential procedures as monitoring vital signs. The reactions are more common in adults.

Maintenance of General Anesthesia

The anesthesiologist attempts to maintain the lightest level of anesthesia compatible with safety and good operating conditions. The anesthesiologist, as well as every other team member, must constantly watch the operative field so as to make pertinent observations. For instance, he or she must note the color of the blood, one indication of the adequacy of oxygenation, and the amount and kind of bleeding. Slow bleeding may denote poor circulation, oozing—a clotting defect, profuse bleeding—the need for transfusion. Muscle relaxation must be constantly assessed in order to provide the varying amounts of anesthesia needed at specific times. Observation of tissue manipulation is important. For example, bradycardia and cardiac arrhythmia may be caused by compression of the eye or traction on the extraocular muscles, whereas traction on abdominal viscera, placing of packs, or rapid decompression of the abdomen such as suction of a large amount of fluid can cause hypotension. Factors such as these affect the quality of anesthesia and patient outcome.

Emergence from General Anesthesia

The anesthesiologist aims to have the patient as nearly awake as possible at the end of the operation so that pharyngeal and laryngeal reflexes are recovered to prevent aspiration and respiratory obstruction. Retching, vomiting, and restlessness may accompany emergence, which is often similar in pattern to the patient's induction. Tracheal tubes are carefully removed by the anesthesiologist when he or she deems the maneuver safe. Undesirable sequelae may be associated with extubation, such as cough and especially laryngospasm. The tube is not removed in the presence of cyanosis or inadequate respiratory exchange or in the absence of a means of respiratory control as when the operation endangers the airway (maxillofacial procedure). Extubation is delayed until spontaneous respiration is assured.

When he or she considers it safe to move the patient, the anesthesiologist assists in transferring the patient to a stretcher or bed, safeguarding the head and neck. Transfer must be carefully and gently made to avoid trauma, strain of ligaments or muscles. The relaxed, unconscious patient must be adequately supported. The anesthesiologist gives the recovery room nurse an adequate report, including specific problems in regard to *that* patient, and the records before transfer of responsibility for the patient.

General Considerations

1 Anesthetic agents vary in potency and therefore in the amount of analgesia they produce.

2 A deficit in pulmonary and/or cardiac function is detrimental because abnormalities of pulmonary ventilation and diffusion influence the course of anesthesia and diminish one's tolerance to stress or to insults from the anesthetic and the procedure. Subnormal cardiac reserve or oxygen-transporting ability, combined with anemia or hypoxia in an arteriosclerotic patient, for example, can be lethal. Some degree of impairment of pulmonary function accompanies general anesthesia in varying degrees.

3 Circulation is affected at many points during anesthesia, with circulatory alterations occurring both centrally and peripherally. Individual agents are associated with characteristic hemodynamic patterns. Generally, the agents are circulatory depressants that reduce myocardial contractility and cardiac output.

4 During anesthesia, respiratory patterns vary from breathholding and apnea to deep breathing or tachypnea. Drug action affecting respiratory stimulation or depression is related to changes in oxygen tension—PaO_2—or arterial carbon dioxide—$PaCO_2$ (see page 162). Hypoxia, anemia, and decreased cardiac output may produce inadequate tissue oxygenation.

5 The liver and kidneys are affected by general agents, for example, the rate of visceral blood flow. Alteration in liver-function tests may follow anesthesia. Halogenated hydrocarbons have been associated with hepatotoxicity. Kidney function is affected by disturbances in the systemic circulation since kidneys normally receive 20 to 25 percent of the cardiac output. Reduced renal plasma flow and glomerular filtration rate are depressions in renal function. They are related to hemodynamics and to water and electrolyte excretion. Oliguria, with reduced sodium and potassium excretion, accompanies induction. Postoperative fluid retention may result from reduction in urine volume from anesthesia and operative trauma, and use of narcotics. In the absence of renal disease, changes in renal function are usually transitory and reversible. Endocrine effects on renal function during anesthesia are important.

6 Biotransformation of agents varies with metabolites excreted by the kidneys. Urinary secretion of intravenous agents may be slow and unpredictable. Studies indicate that nitrous oxide may be exhaled as long as 56 hours after anesthesia and metabolites of halothane have been recovered from patients' urine as long as 20 days after anesthesia.

7 Agents differ in the amount of muscle relaxation produced.

8 General anesthesia is usually more complicated than local or regional anesthesia. The agents may cause nausea, emesis, or systemic complications. General anesthesia is also more expensive.

9 General anesthesia may be contraindicated for elective type procedures in a variety of medical diseases (cardiorespiratory, severe debilitation) and in emergency operations on patients who recently ingested food or fluids. Gastric suction and intubation are indicated. General anesthesia is avoided by some anesthesiologists for elective procedures during the first 5 months of pregnancy because of unknown teratogenic effects of inhalation anesthetics.

10 Endotracheal intubation is common except for the shortest of procedures.

11 Induction is usually by intravenous technique.

12 After recovery from anesthesia, the patient should be attended when he or she gets out of bed until it is safe for the patient to do so alone.

CARE OF THE ANESTHETIZED PATIENT

While safety factors are stressed throughout the text, important factors are reiterated for emphasis:

1 The patient's position must be changed *slowly* and *gently* in order to allow circulation to readjust.

2 Patients' ability to detoxify anesthetic agents and tolerate stress differ greatly but any anesthetized patient has a diminished ability to compensate for physiologic changes caused by motion or operative positions.

3 Anesthetic agents are basically depressants that affect the vasomotor and respiratory centers, predisposing the patient to postoperative respiratory complications. It is imperative that the lungs be adequately ventilated intra- and postoperatively either by voluntary or mechanical means. The patient's chest must be free for adequate respiratory excursions during operation. The airway must be patent and pressure must not be exerted on the chest. Remember that the patient under the drapes is unable to complain!

4 Team members, especially the circulating nurse and anesthesiologist, must be constantly aware of potential trauma to the patient since he or she is unable to produce a normal response to painful or injurious stimuli.

NEUROMUSCULAR BLOCKERS (MUSCLE-RELAXANT DRUGS)

The employment of certain skeletal muscle-relaxant agents in conjunction with anesthetics is common and has had a marked effect on clinical anesthesia. These powerful drugs give surgical relaxation in light anesthesia and are administered as adjuncts to many anesthetic agents. Deep anesthesia with its untoward effects has therefore practically been eliminated.

The drugs are administered intravenously in small amounts at intervals and may cause circulatory disturbance. They produce major alterations in respiration and the chief danger in their use is that they decrease pulmonary ventilation, thereby causing respiratory depression. Special attention to anesthesia depth, ventilation, and electrolyte balance is required. The drugs are excreted through the kidneys.

Use of Neuromuscular Blockers

Neuromuscular blockers may be used:

1 To increase muscular relaxation during operation; to create smoother working conditions; to shorten duration of operation

2 To widen scope of less potent anesthetics such as nitrous oxide; to lessen overall amount of anesthetic needed

3 To facilitate controlled breathing and tracheal intubation by relaxing jaw or larynx

4 To prevent contraction of the diaphragm and to give a quiet field, for example, for cardiotomy in open-heart procedures, prior to circulatory occlusion

5 To control or prevent shivering, which accompanies systemic hypothermia

6 To facilitate diagnostic endoscopy under light general anesthesia

Types

Relaxants are classified as *nondepolarizing agents* or as *depolarizing agents.* Briefly, the differences between them are as follows:

1 Nondepolarizing agents.
- **a** These agents do not cause muscular fasciculation on intravenous injection.
- **b** Their effects are decreased by anticholinesterase drugs, lowering of body temperature, acetylcholine, depolarizing relaxants, and epinephrine.
- **c** Paralysis is increased by nondepolarizing agents, halothane, and ether.
- **d** Tetanic electrical impulses produce a gradual fade in response.

2 Depolarizing agents. These agents have the opposite effect. For example, they cause muscular fasciculation on intravenous injection.

Although theoretically antagonistic, combinations of nondepolarizing and depolarizing blockers are used during anesthesia.

Action

The neuromuscular blockers interfere with the passage of impulses from the motor nerves to the skeletal muscles. They act primarily at the neuromuscular junction causing a paralysis of variable duration. They also can affect transmission of impulses at pre- and postganglionic endings in the autonomic nervous system.

Depolarizing and nondepolarizing drugs behave differently. The duration of their action should be balanced against the duration of the clinically significant effect they produce on the muscles of ventilation. A nerve stimulator is a useful tool for assessing neuromuscular transmission as a guide to dosage, degree and nature of blockade, and evidence of muscle-response recovery during and after use of nondepolarizing agents.

Interaction with Drugs

Interaction between nondepolarizing relaxants and other drugs can result in delayed recovery. For example, antibiotics may act synergistically with nondepolarizing agents to produce prolonged paralysis. Such drug interactions reportedly are more apt to occur if the peritoneal cavity is irrigated with an antibiotic solution or the antibiotic is injected intravenously. Patients with renal failure are especially susceptible since antibiotics are excreted through the kidneys. There is also synergism between inhalation anesthetics and the nondepolarizing agents. The use of relaxants is avoided in patients with myasthenia gravis to avoid delayed recovery due to the disease state.

Neuromuscular Blocking Agents

Nondepolarizing Agents

Curare (Tubocurarine chloride) Derived from a poison obtained from certain South American plants first used centuries ago by the Indians. Their poison arrows caused death by suffocation from respiratory paralysis. The action is predominantly a paralysis of voluntary muscles, resulting from blocking of transmission of nerve impulses to muscle fibers. The muscle relaxation is potentiated by certain anesthetics (halothane, enflurane, diethyl ether, methoxyflurane) and by some antibiotics. It may be prolonged by extreme debility and widespread cancer. Autonomic blockade can cause hypotension. The drug releases histamine.

Pancuronium Bromide (Pavulon) A long-acting, synthetic muscle relaxant similar in action to curare but about five times more potent. It increases arterial pressure and heart rate.

Gallamine Triethiodide (Flaxedil) Similar to curare in mechanism and duration of action. Its advantage over curare is an absence of hypotension and bronchospasm. It may cause tachycardia and increase in arterial pressure.

Depolarizing Agents

Succinylcholine Chloride (Quelicin, Anectine) An ultra-short-acting, synthetic muscle relaxant of rapid onset used mostly in intubation; it may also be used as a dilute solution to provide continuing muscle relaxation. Caution is necessary in intraocular operations or in the presence of glaucoma because it increases intraocular pressure. Its use is contraindicated in recent burns, massive muscle trauma, degenerative neuromuscular disease, or electrolyte imbalance, as hyperkalemia may accompany its use. Presence of low or abnormal plasma cholinesterase (enzyme responsible for metabolism of acetylcholine) may prolong its action. Repeated intravenous administration may effect changes in heart rate and rhythm (bradycardia, ventricular arrhythmia) but this action is blocked by atropine. Return of normal function after injection is dependent on metabolism by enzymes.

Muscle contractions, caused by depolarization of the nerve-muscle end plate, are seen following injection. After this, the end plate is blocked by the drug. Muscle pain may occur after its use unless fasciculation is prevented by a small preliminary dose of a nondepolarizing agent.

Decamethonium (Syncurine) A very potent, synthetic substance of rapid onset and short duration of action. It is not cumulative and has little effect on vital systems. It is used for deep relaxation of short duration such as that needed for endoscopy, treatment of laryngeal spasm, abdominal closure, endotracheal intubation. It is excreted through the kidneys and prolonged blockade may result if given to a patient in renal failure.

Blockade during Operation

The anesthesiologist must constantly verify the degree of paralysis present. He or she does this by noting the amount of relaxation of the abdominal wall or the limpness of extremities, or by using a nerve stimulator connected to the patient through needle electrodes. The use of neuromuscular blockers should demonstrate surgeon-anesthesiologist teamwork and communication at its best. Use of these drugs always presents the hazard of overdosage, a danger alleviated by the anesthesiologist's familiarity with the surgeon's technique and the requirements of the particular operation; thus, the anesthesiologist can regulate dosage of anesthetic and relaxant necessary to produce the conditions required at the appropriate time. For example, a major use of the blockers is in intra-abdominal procedures. At different times during the operation, blockade may be more or less essential. Although tightness of tissues and inadequate exposure may be due to factors other than relaxation, such as too many packs improperly placed, it is helpful to the anesthesiologist to be told before pertinent action, such as closure of the peritoneum, is taken. Inadequate muscle relaxation makes closure difficult. Another example: controlled respiration during upper abdominal manipulation can prevent descent of the diaphragm into the operative field.

At the conclusion of the operation the degree of residual blockade must be determined and treated if necessary for respiratory adequacy before the patient is released from the anesthesiologist's care. Sufficient ventilatory reserve must be demonstrated to overcome soft tissue obstruction and for the patient to be able to cough and breathe deeply. There must be clinical confirmation that all respiratory muscles are active.

Treatment of Residual Blockade

Although the blockers are relatively safe as long as ventilation is supported, serious problems relating to their use (hypoxia, hypotension, respiratory abnormalities) may result after discontinuance, if recovery is delayed beyond expectation. Time is required for their elimination from the body. The need for constant, minute-to-minute postoperative observation of patients cannot be overemphasized.

The primary treatment of residual neuromuscular blockade after anesthesia and operation is maintenance of patent airway and adequate manual or mechanical ventilation until full recovery. The action of nondepolarizing muscle relaxants may be reversed with antagonists such as neostigmine or pyridostigmine bromide. These drugs must be accompanied or preceded by atropine sulfate to minimize side effects such as excessive secretions and bradycardia.

BALANCED ANESTHESIA

Balanced anesthesia is one of the most widely used techniques in modern anesthesia. A combination of agents are used to provide hypnosis, analgesia, muscle relaxation, and obtunding of reflexes with a minimum disturbance of physiological functions. Many variations are possible, depending upon the condition of the patient and the requirements of the operative procedure.

Induction can be accomplished with a thiobarbiturate (Pentothal, Brevital), diazepam (Valium), Innovar, or a dissociative agent (ketamine). Analgesia is provided by nitrous oxide and intravenous use of narcotics (morphine, meperidine, fentanyl). Oxygen is administered in physiologic quantities. Muscle relaxants permit control of ventilation while providing optimum conditions for the surgeon. Residual effects of narcotics or relaxants may require reversal by antagonists at the conclusion of the operation.

OCCUPATIONAL HAZARD AMONG OPERATING ROOM PERSONNEL

It has long been a recognized fact that substantial amounts of anesthetic gases escape into the operating room air during operative procedures, thereby polluting the air. Complacency about this fact is no longer acceptable since anesthesia is thought to involve risk to all persons in the operating room as well as to the patient. Data obtained from studies demonstrate that personnel receiving chronic exposure to waste anesthetic gas face a serious occupational health hazard, although unknown related factors may be involved. *Waste anesthetic gas* refers to anesthetic gases and vapors that escape from the anesthesia machine and equipment and those released through the patient's expirations. These health hazards to OR personnel include significantly increased risk of spontaneous abortion in females working in the OR, congenital abnormalities in their children as well as in the offspring of unexposed wives of exposed male personnel, cancer in females administering anethesia, hepatic and renal disease in both males and females. Volunteers exposed to trace amounts of anesthetic gases corresponding to amounts present in the OR environment during a 4-hour period showed significant behavioral changes including decreased perception, cognition, and motor reaction. A dose-response relationship also was seen between the least and the most exposed persons, with anesthesiologists at the high-exposure level and OR nurses and technicians at the lower level. Studies of retention of anesthetic agents in anesthesiologists following administration of clinical anesthesia have demonstrated traces of gas in expired air for varying lengths of time, from 7 hours following nitrous oxide to 64 hours following halothane administration. Since an estimated 25 million inhalation anesthetics are administered annually, a substantial number of OR staff are occupationally exposed to these gases.

The United States government is concerned with the problem of the environmental effects of waste gas. In 1970, Congress passed the Occupational Safety and Health Act. This act created the National Institute for Occupational Safety and Health (NIOSH), which has public health authority and responsibility in the research area. The responsibilities include:

1 Determination of the effects of exposure to materials, processes, and stresses that carry potential for illness, disease, or loss of functional capacity

2 Development of criteria for recommended standards which, based on research, describe exposure levels safe for various periods of employment

To reduce occupational morbidity, proper and consistently conscientious use of scavenging equipment and procedures is strongly recommended. Scavenging involves removal of waste anesthetic gases, mainly by trapping them at the site of overflow on the breathing circuit followed by disposal to the outside atmosphere and good dilution. The rate of removal of gases by the disposal system depends on the rate at which fresh (pure) air enters the OR and the patterns taken by air currents as they circulate through the room. Exposure to trace concentrations of gas can thus be reduced by 90 to 95 percent.

Personnel exposure should be reduced to the lowest practicable limits by reducing waste gas to the most technically feasible level. A waste-gas control program to ensure the continuing purity of environmental air includes the following measures:

1 Good work practices of anesthesiologists. The major source of waste gas in the OR is the intentional outflow of gases from the anesthesia breathing system. The quantity of gases discharged may vary greatly depending on the type of breathing system, gas-flow rate, and gas concentration.
2 Use of a well-designed, well-maintained scavenging system. Inexpensive, practical, effective exhaust systems are available. The gas evacuation system can be attached to anesthesia machines and ventilators.
3 Use of proper anesthesia technique.
   a Different techniques of administration result in different exposure levels.
   b Components of the breathing system should fit well.
   c Liquid anesthetic agents should not be spilled.
   d Masks, tubing, reservoir bags, endotracheal tubes should be inspected after each cleaning for leaks, holes, abnormalities.
4 Proper maintenance of anesthesia equipment through:
   a Daily routine checking of anesthesia machines for leaks.
   b Periodic preventive maintenance of all machines and fittings.
5 Maintenance of a high flow rate of fresh air into the air-conditioning system through engineering control procedures.
6 Use of an OR atmospheric monitoring program to determine effectiveness of the above measures.

Preemployment medical examination of personnel, periodic examinations for surveillance and early detection of disease, rotation of duty, and keeping employees informed about hazards are advocated until further research is completed.

LOCAL OR REGIONAL ANESTHESIA

Action

Local anesthesia depresses superficial nerves and blocks the conduction of pain impulses from a specific area or region. The sensory nerves are the first affected. The patient remains conscious. Regional anesthesia (for example: spinal) may be employed when general anesthesia is contraindicated or undesired.

Sometimes local anesthesia is used as an adjunct to general anesthesia for decreasing operative stimuli, thereby diminishing the general stress response to trauma. The local anesthetic is used during manipulation of highly sensitive tissues to reduce sensory reflexes to painful stimuli in the operative field. Injected at the site of operation, it temporarily disconnects the operative site from the central nervous system.

Preparation of the Patient

Patients who are to receive a local anesthetic need preparation that may differ somewhat from that of patients about to receive a general anesthetic. These preparations depend on the extent of the procedure to be performed and on the anticipated technique of administration. Although it is anticipated that the patient will remain conscious, it is sometimes desirable or necessary to supplement local anesthesia with narcosis or light general anesthesia in which case preparation for a general anesthetic is followed. Careful preoperative assessment, history taking, preanesthetic medication, and a clear explanation of what to expect, such as paresthesias, are as essential as for general anesthesia. Preoperative orders regarding the time when the patient should cease taking anything by mouth vary with the circumstances; at least 4 hours prior to operation is a frequent cutoff time since the patient may vomit from apprehension or untoward reaction. Often a preoperative barbiturate or diazepam is ordered before the use of a local anesthetic agent. Medication is given as ordered. Patients are transported via stretcher.

Care of the Patient during Operation

The patient must be cooperative and willing to be awake, although drowsy from premedication. Psychological support must be given during the operation. However, supplementary agents should be available for analgesia or anesthesia as necessary. Gentle manipulation of the patient, including concern for the hearing sense, cannot be overemphasized for the patient in a conscious or semiconscious state.

These patients need careful observation throughout the operation, and for a period of time afterward, for symptoms of delayed reaction or complications. The patient may not be attended by an anesthesiologist. The surgeon may inject or topically apply the anesthetic drug. This depends, however, on the type or length of the procedure. For example, in breast biopsy and possible radical mastectomy, an anesthesiologist is present. However, for a simple excision of a skin lesion or drainage of an abscess, an anesthesiologist probably is not present. When an anesthesiologist is present, the operation is scheduled for *attended local.*

The circulating nurse is responsible for *every* patient's safety and nursing care. In the absence of an anesthesiologist, she is totally responsible for monitoring the patient's vital signs and intravenous infusion, and for recording these data as well as the total amount of anesthetic and supplementary drugs administered to the patient.

In addition, resuscitative equipment must be at hand prior to the administration of any anesthetic. If any reaction is observed, the patient is informed of it for his or her protection in future anesthesias.

Advantages of Local Anesthesia

1 Infiltration anesthetic agents are nonexplosive.

2 It needs minimal simple equipment, provides economy.

3 Loss of consciousness does not occur, unless supplemented. Local anesthesia avoids the undesirable effects of general anesthesia.

4 It is suitable for patients who recently ingested food or fluids (as in obstetrics and emergency operation); for ambulatory patients; for minor procedures; for procedures where it is desirable to have the patient awake and cooperative.

5 The surgeon can administer the anesthetic in instances of unavailability of an anesthesiologist.

Disadvantages of Local Anesthesia

1 It is not practical for all types of procedures. For example, too much drug would be needed for some major operations such as radical mastectomy; the duration of anesthesia is insufficient for others.

2 There are individual variations in response to local anesthetic drugs.

3 Too rapid absorption of the drug into the blood, usually from overdosage, can cause severe, potentially fatal reactions.

4 Apprehension may be increased by the patient's consciousness and ability to see and hear. Some patients prefer to be unconscious and unaware.

Contraindications to Local Anesthesia

These factors are variable and exceptions may be found. Local anesthesia is generally contraindicated in patients with:

1 Allergic sensitivity to the local drug.

2 Local infection or malignancy, which may be carried to and spread in adjacent tissues by injection. A bacteriologically safe injection site should be selected.

3 Septicemia. In a proximal nerve block, a needle may open new lymph channels that drain through a region, thereby causing new foci and local abscess formation from the perforation of small vessels and exit of bacteria.

4 Highly nervous, apprehensive, excitable patients or those unable to cooperate because of mental state or age.

Techniques of Administration

Topical Application The anesthetic is applied directly to a mucous membrane, to a serous surface, or into an open wound. It is most often employed for anesthesia of respiratory passages to eliminate laryngeal reflexes and cough, for insertion of airways before induction or during light general anesthesia, or for therapeutic and diagnostic procedures such as laryngoscopy or bronchoscopy. It is also used in cystoscopy. Mucous membranes readily absorb topical agents because of their vascularity. Onset of anesthesia occurs within a minute. Volume of the topical agent in the blood may equal the same level obtained by intravenous injection. Duration of anesthesia is 20 to 30 minutes. Ointments or solutions may be used. If a spray or atomizer is used it should contain a visible reservoir so that the quantity of drug administered is clearly observed because droplets vary in size.

Preanesthetic sedation and atropine are important prior to topical application within the respiratory tract. The atropine is necessary as saliva can dilute the anesthetic and prevent adequate duration of contact with the mucous membrane. Also, a dry throat is necessary to prevent aspiration until the anesthetic effect has disappeared and throat reflexes have returned. Adverse reaction to topical anesthetic agents is not uncommon unless dosage is carefully controlled. Sudden cardiovascular collapse occurs most frequently following topical anesthesia of the respiratory tract, according to statistics.

Simple Local Infiltration The agent is injected intracutaneously and subcutaneously into the tissues at the incisional site to block peripheral nerve stimuli at their origin. It is used in suturing superficial lacerations or in the excision of minor lesions.

Regional Application The agent is injected into or around a specific nerve or group of nerves to depress the entire sensory nervous system of a limited, localized area of the body. The injection is at a distance from the operative site. A wider, deeper area is anesthetized than with simple infiltration. There are several types of regional anesthesia:

Nerve Block Anesthetizing of a selected nerve at a given point. Nerve blocks may be used operatively, to prevent pain of the procedure; diagnostically, to ascertain cause of pain; or therapeutically, to relieve chronic pain. Each type of block carries unique complication potential. Some examples of blocks employed are:

1 Operative blocks: paravertebral (cervical plexus) block, for the area between the jaws and clavicle; intercostal block, for relatively superficial intra-abdominal procedures; arm (brachial plexus) block; block at the elbow or wrist (median, radial, or ulnar nerve); hand and digital block, for fingers. In the latter, epinephrine is not added to the local agent as gangrene can result from inadequate circulation.

2 Diagnostic or therapeutic blocks: utilized to block sympathetic nerve ganglia. Desired vasodilatation is produced by paralysis of the sympathetic nerve supply to the constricting smooth muscle in the artery wall. Stellate ganglion block is used to increase circulation in peripheral vascular disease in the head, neck, arm, or hand. Paravertebral lumbar block increases circulation in the lower extremities.

NOTE. With the proliferation of pain clinics concerned with the management of acute and chronic pain problems, the anesthesiologist plays an essential role as part of the multidisciplinary staff and activities. Because of his or her unusual familiarity with anesthetic drugs, nerve pathways, and nerve block techniques, the anesthesiologist is of great service to both colleagues and patients in assessing and treating pain, especially if amenable to nerve block.

Intravenous Regional Block with Tourniquet Intravenous injection of a local anesthetic in an extremity. It involves draining of blood from the extremity by use of a tourniquet after placement of an intravenous catheter and subsequent injection close to site of operation of a fixed quantity of local drug that is confined to the area by tourniquet (see p. 250). The tourniquet is applied to the leg for foot operation, to the forearm for hand or wrist operation, and to the arm for operation above the wrist. It is used more for upper extremity procedures.

At the conclusion of the operation and release of the tourniquet, entry of a bolus of remaining local anesthetic into the systemic circulation may cause cardiovascular or central nervous system symptoms of toxicity.

Field Block Blocking off of operative site with wall of anesthetic solution by series of injections into proximal and surrounding tissues, as, for example, abdominal wall block for herniorrhaphy.

SPINAL ANESTHESIA

Intrathecal Block

Intrathecal block, commonly referred to as *spinal anesthesia,* is a technique of regional anesthesia. The agent is injected into the subarachnoid space, using a lumbar interspace, causing desensitization of spinal ganglia and motor roots. Absorption into the nerve fibers is rapid. The level of anesthesia attained depends on various factors: position during and immediately after injection; cerebrospinal fluid pressure; site and rate of injection; volume, dosage, and specific gravity (baricity) of the solution; inclusion of a vasoconstrictor (epinephrine); spinal curvature; interspace chosen; coughing or straining, which can inadvertently raise the level. Spread of the anesthetic is controlled mainly by solution baricity and patient position. The period immediately following injection is decisive, when the anesthetic is becoming "fixed," absorbed by the tissues and unable to travel. Further control of the anesthetic level is attained by tilting the operating table at that time. The direction of tilting depends on whether the agent is *hyperbaric* (specific gravity greater than that of the spinal fluid) or *hypobaric* (lighter than spinal fluid). *Isobaric* anesthetics (same weight as spinal fluid) are made hyperbaric by the addition of 5 or 10% dextrose to the anesthetic before injection.

Immediately after injection, the anesthesiologist carefully tests the level of anesthesia by pinprick, tilting the table as necessary to achieve the desired level for the particular operation. After anesthetic fixation, with the anesthesiologist's permission, the patient is placed in operative position. The patient is asked to relax and let the team turn him or her. Incision is never made until it is certain that anesthesia is adequate. Supplementation of spinal anesthesia is necessary if anesthesia or muscular relaxation is insufficient or the patient is unduly apprehensive. Sometimes the patient is kept in a light sleep with an intravenous agent.

Choice of Agent This depends on various factors such as duration, intensity, and level of anesthesia desired, anticipated operative position of the patient, and the operative procedure.

Duration of Agent The variable duration of anesthesia depends on physiologic, physical, and metabolic factors. It is prolonged by addition of a vasoconstrictor. Anesthesia diminishes as the agent is absorbed into the systemic circulation.

Procedure

For injection, the patient is placed in the position desired by the anesthesiologist, depending on solution baricity and anesthesia to be produced.

1 *Lateral Position.* The most common, the patient's back is at the edge of the operating table, parallel to it, the knees flexed onto the abdomen, and the head flexed to the knees. Hips and shoulders are vertical to the table to prevent rotation of the spine.
2 *Sitting Position.* The patient sits on the side of the table with feet resting on a stool. The spine is flexed, with chin lowered to the sternum, the arms crossed and supported on a pillow on an adjustable table or Mayo stand.
3 *Prone Position.* The patient lies face downward on the table.

The circulating nurse or a nursing assistant supports the patient in position, observes and reassures him or her, and assists the anesthesiologist in any way possible. Attention to asepsis is extremely important. The anesthesiologist dons sterile gloves before handling sterile items. A sterile *spinal set,* used only for spinal anesthesia, or a disposable spinal tray is used. (The latter eliminates the need for the essential meticulous cleaning and sterilizing of nondisposable equipment.) The *tray* contains:

1 Drape
2 Ampul file
3 Ampuls of local anesthetic, spinal anesthetic, vasoconstrictor drug, 5 and 10% dextrose
4 Medicine glass
5 Sponges
6 Needles: 25-gauge hypodermic for infiltration of local anesthetic into skin; 22-gauge, 2 in. (5 cm) long, for intramuscular injection; blunt 18-gauge for mixing drugs; 22- and 26-gauge, $3\frac{1}{2}$ in. (9 cm) long, spinal needles with stylets for intrathecal injection
7 Syringes: 5 cc for spinal anesthetic, 10 cc for hypobaric solutions, 2 cc for superficial anesthesia

Forceps and sponges are of a different type than those counted and used during operation. The lumbar puncture site is cleansed with an antiseptic solution and draped with a fenestrated drape. The blood pressure is checked before, during, and after spinal anesthesia as hypotension is common.

Use of Spinal Anesthesia

For abdominal (mainly lower) or pelvic procedures requiring relaxation (for example, intestinal obstruction); inguinal or lower extremity procedures; operative obstetrics (caesarian section—lacks effect on fetus). It is advised for alcoholics, barbiturate addicts, very muscular patients who would need large doses of general anesthetic and muscle relaxant, and for emergency operations in patients who have eaten recently. It is also used in the presence of hepatic, renal, or metabolic disease because of minimal upset of body chemistry.

Advantages Patient is conscious if desired, throat reflexes are maintained; nonirritating to the respiratory system; no difficulty with airway problems; quiet breathing; contracted bowel; reduced bleeding in vascular procedures from relative hypotension; excellent muscle relaxation and anesthesia if properly executed.

Disadvantages Spinal anesthesia produces a circulatory depressant effect and stasis of blood as a result of interference with venous return from motor paralysis and arteriolar dilatation in the lower extremities. Change in body position may be followed by sudden drop in blood pressure. Agent cannot be removed after injection. Nausea and emesis may accompany cerebral ischemia, traction on viscera, or premedication. Possible sensitivity to the agent; danger of trauma or infection. Patient can hear.

Postanesthetic Complications Transient or permanent neurological sequelae from trauma, irritation by the agent, lack of asepsis, loss of spinal fluid with decreased intracranial pressure syndrome. Examples: "spinal headache"; auditory and occular disturbances such as tinnitus, diplopia; arachnoiditis, meningitis; cauda equina syndrome (failure to regain use of legs or control of urinary and bowel function); or temporary paresthesias such as numbness and tingling.

Contraindications to Spinal Anesthesia Spinal cord lesions or tumors; presence of neurologic disease; previous complications following spinal; fear of the technique; severe shock, anemia, dehydration, hypovolemia; young age, or emotional instability; skin sepsis at or near injection site; blood coagulopathies that may result in hematoma and cord depression; abnormalities of the vertebral canal.

NOTE. 1. High levels of anesthesia are necessary for upper intra-abdominal procedures. Extreme caution is essential to prevent respiratory paralysis (diaphragm, intercostal muscles), an emergency situation requiring artificial ventilation until the level of anesthesia has receded.
2. Anesthesia machine, oxygen, and intravenous infusion must be in readiness before injection. Constant vigilance of respiration and circulation is mandatory.
3. Serial injection, "continuous" technique—intermittent injections of anesthetic given via plastic catheter—may be used for long procedures or where better control of anesthesia is desired.

EPIDURAL ANESTHESIA

Injection is made into the space surrounding the dura mater within the spinal canal. Spread of the anesthetic and duration of action are influenced by the concentration and volume of solution injected (total drug mass), and rate of injection. The anesthetic diffuses toward the head and caudad. In contrast to spinal anesthesia, position, baricity, and gravity have little influence on anesthetic distribution. The high incidence of systemic reactions is attributed to absorption of the agent from the highly vascular peridural area and the relatively large mass of anesthetic injected. Epinephrine is usually added to retard absorption. The following two approaches may be used: the lumbar, the more common, and the caudal.

Lumbar Approach

The lumbar approach is a peridural block. Equipment is similar to spinal, with addition of 19-gauge, $3\frac{1}{2}$ in. (9 cm) long, thin-walled spinal needle with stylet with a rigid shaft and short bevel tip to minimize danger of inadvertent dural puncture. Lateral position is used for injection with less flexion of the back than for spinal to avoid dural puncture.

Caudal Approach

The caudal approach is an epidural sacral block. Injection epidurally is through the caudal canal, desensitizing nerves emerging from the dural sac. Position for injection: prone, with hips flexed, sacrum horizontal, and heels turned outward to expose injection site. The sacral area is prepared and draped, care being taken to protect the genitalia from irritating solution. Lateral position is used in pregnant patients. Spinal tray with addition of 20-gauge, $1\frac{1}{2}$ in. (4 cm) long spinal needle with stylet. Skin and ligaments are infiltrated with a local anesthetic agent before inserting spinal needle.

Use of Epidural Anesthesia

Uses include: anorectal, vaginal, perineal procedures; obstetrics; intractable or prolonged pain. "Continuous" technique is sometimes employed, requiring additional equipment in the setup—needles, stopcocks, plastic catheter (referred to as *continuous lumbar epidural block* or *continuous epidural sacral block*). Patient must be constantly attended by trained personnel once the block is initiated as for obstetric analgesia. Continuous electronic monitoring of the fetal heart is recommended because of the patient's insensibility to uterine contractions.

Management and Sequelae Similar to spinal anesthesia.

Disadvantages Less controllable height of anesthesia; more difficult technique; area of potential infection from anaerobic organisms with the caudal approach; unpredictable; time-consuming—longer time for complete anesthesia; larger amount of agent injected; continuous technique may slow the first stage of labor.

LOCAL AND REGIONAL ANESTHETIC AGENTS

Chemically the commonly employed agents are amides or ester compounds. They differ in structure and therefore in action. These drugs are applied to body surfaces or injected around nerves essentially to prevent the pain of surgical procedures but also to treat the pain associated with disease or trauma. They vary in potency, penetration, duration, rapidity of hydrolysis or destruction, and toxicity, detoxification occurring in the liver.

Action

These drugs interfere with the initiation and transmission of nerve impulses by mechanisms based on physical and biochemical changes, interacting with the membrane that ensheaths nerve fibers. The drugs retard and stop the propagation of nerve impulses, eventually blocking conduction. This is accomplished by blocking: a peripheral stimulus at its origin (topical application or local infiltration), transmission of stimuli along afferent nerves from the operative site (regional anesthesia), and conducting pathways in and around the spinal cord (spinal and epidural). Their duration of action depends not only on their pharmacological properties but also on volume and concentration of the solution and whether it is combined with a vasoconstrictor to slow absorption, prolong anesthesia, and decrease bleeding. Epinephrine 1 to 200,000 may be used for these purposes, added to the local agent or commercially supplied in the solutions. If adding it to a solution, it is best to do so with a calibrated syringe rather than with a dropper, an inaccurate method. Pharmacological effects of epinephrine sometimes displayed are palpitation, tachycardia, tremor, pallor, diaphoresis.

Conduction Velocity Nerve fibers vary in their susceptibility to local anesthetic agents. The larger the fiber, the greater the concentration of anesthetic required. In practice, the least amount of the lowest concentration of the anesthetic agent to achieve the desired effect should be administered.

Blocking Quality Depends on potency, latency (time between administration and maximum effect), duration of action, regression time (time between beginning and end of pain perception).

Characteristics of an Acceptable Agent

These include high potency, minimal systemic activity, prompt metabolism, lack of local irritation, reversibility of action, regional as well as topical efficacy, stability during sterilization and storage. Not every agent will possess all attributes; the perfect agent does not yet exist.

Hyaluronidase is a drug that is sometimes added to local anesthetic agents to facilitate spread of a local agent through the tissues and create more certainty of reaching all the desired nerves. This property also causes more rapid absorption of the local anesthetic and may reduce the intensity and duration of its effect. More rapid absorption may also increase the possiblity of a systemic reaction (see p. 185).

Types

A number of different local or regional anesthetic drugs are in use. They may be categorized by potency or duration of action.

Cocaine The first local anesthetic introduced, cocaine is a crystalline powder with a bitter taste in solution. It is the most toxic of local drugs and, in contrast to all but lidocaine hydrochloride, is a vasoconstrictor. It causes temporary paralysis of sensory nerve fibers, produces exhilaration, lessens hunger and fatigue, and stimulates pulse and respiratory rates. Administration is by topical application *only* because of its high toxicity; the solution penetrates mucous membrane. When applied to the throat it abolishes throat reflexes. The patient is awake and can cooperate but disadvantages are its limited use and possible addiction. It is used topically in 4 to 10 percent concentration for anesthesia of the respiratory tract (nose, pharynx, tracheobronchial tree). Untoward reactions may occur rapidly in response to the use of even a very small amount of the drug.

Procaine Hydrochloride (Novocaine) Similar to cocaine but less toxic. Concentrations used: 0.5 to 5.0%. It is injected subcutaneously, intrathecally, intramuscularly. It has low potency; it is of short duration; and it is ineffectual topically. Its advantages include minimal toxicity, easily sterilized solution, low cost, and lack of local irritation. Newer agents are used more frequently.

Lidocaine Hydrochloride (Xylocaine) Probably the most widely used agent, this is a potent anesthetic of twice the duration of procaine. It is also more toxic, being slowly hydrolized in circulating plasma. Its major advantages are rapid onset of anesthesia and lack of local irritant effect. Used extensively for operative procedures and dentistry, it has moderate potency and duration of action. For injection 0.5 to 2% concentration is used. It is a good topical anesthetic (2 to 4%), although not as effective as cocaine. Lidocaine also is used in the management of ventricular arrhythmias during and after cardiac procedures, in resuscitation after cardiac arrest, and in treatment and prevention of irritability in patients who experienced myocardial infarction.

Mepivacaine Hydrochloride (Carbocaine) Similar to lidocaine hydrochloride. It takes effect rapidly but produces 20 percent longer duration of anesthesia. It has moderate potency and duration of action. Epinephrine may *not* be added to it because of its duration. For topical and injection administration, 0.5 to 2% concentrations are used. It is commonly employed for infiltration and nerve block. It produces minimal tissue irritation and few adverse reactions.

Tetracaine Hydrochloride (Pontocaine) A very potent agent. Onset of analgesia is slow but the duration of effect is longer than that of many of the other drugs. It has high potency of long duration. It is also more systemically toxic because of the slow rate of its destruction in the body but low total dosage tends to reduce the chance of reaction. However, the high incidence of reported reaction may be attributed to rapid absorption rate from respiratory tract mucosa. Use: 1 to 2% as topical anesthetic in the eye, pharynx, tracheobronchial tree, 0.5% for corneal anesthesia in ophthalmology. Tetracaine hydrochloride is also a spinal anesthetic made hyperbaric by addition of 10% dextrose. Adverse reactions may have an abrupt onset with no prodromata, and only a brief interval between onset and death.

Bupivacaine Hydrochloride (Marcaine) This drug is more potent and longer-acting than lidocaine hydrochloride or mepivacaine hydrochloride. It has high potency of long duration. Onset of anesthesia is slow but duration is two to three times longer, with toxicity approximate to that of tetracaine hydrochloride. Concentrations used: 0.25 to 0.75% for regional nerve blocks. A 0.75% concentration produces profound motor relaxation for intra-abdominal procedures. The drug affords prolonged pain relief following caudal block for rectal procedures and perineorrhaphy. Cumulation occurs with repeated injection.

Chloroprocaine Hydochloride (Nesacaine) Possibly the safest local anesthetic from the standpoint of systemic toxicity because of its fast metabolism. It has moderate potency of short duration. It is rapidly hydrolyzed in the plasma. Its action is fast but it is not active topically. For injection, 0.5 to 2% is used.

Dibucaine Hydrochloride (Nupercaine, Percaine, Cinchocaine) A very potent anesthetic producing a high rate of systemic toxicity. Lower concentrations are needed to decrease the incidence of adverse reactions. It has long duration of action. It is infrequently used.

Prilocaine Hydrochloride (Citanest) Similar to lidocaine hydrochloride and mepivacaine hydrochloride but somewhat more potent with short onset of action and longer duration. A major disadvantage of this drug is the potential development of methemoglobinemia.

DRUG INTERACTIONS

Anesthesiologists and/or surgeons frequently administer many drugs to patients already under the influence of several different pharmacological agents when they come to the OR. An estimated 18 to 30 percent of all hospitalized patients in the United States experience some form of an adverse drug reaction. All drugs in use must be considered potential "interreactors" with some other drug. A simple shift in pH can cause a significant alteration in action, effectiveness, distribution, and excretion of such common drugs as barbiturates and local anesthetics. Many drugs used in anesthesia are weak acids (barbiturates) and weak bases (local agents and vasopressors). These drugs ionize and are bound to proteins; therefore changes in ionization and protein binding can alter their effectiveness. Advertently or inadvertently the anesthesiologist can modify these physicochemical characteristics and thus alter the effects of such drugs.

In addition, many variables modify the action of anesthetic agents, such as dose, circulatory adaptation, ventilation management, effect of time, disease states, or concomitant operation.

REACTIONS TO ANESTHETICS

Adverse drug reactions occurring during anesthesia and operation are of increasing concern to both physicians and patients. These reactions are relatively frequent, often severe, potentially fatal. Reactions increase in ratio to the number of drugs used.

Systemic reactions manifested by symptoms referable to the central nervous system and the respiratory and cardiovascular systems are caused by absorption into the circulation of toxic amounts of the local or general anesthetic drug. The main factor then in producing these reactions is the circulating blood level of the anesthetic. Toxic amounts of drugs can depress the peripheral vessels as well as the myocardium and medullary centers. Hypotension, apnea, coma, respiratory and circulatory collapse, and cardiac standstill may then result.

In topical anesthesia, extremely rapid systemic absorption from mucous membranes explains the relatively high frequency of toxic reactions. In local or regional anesthesia, inadvertent intravenous injection and use of fairly large quantities in high vascular areas will contribute to local anesthetic toxicity.

Drugs Implicated in Reaction

Many drugs employed in anesthesia release histamine, which in turn is the basis of allergic response.

1 Barbiturates, used as basic hypnotics or operative anesthetics, are a frequent cause of skin rashes.

2 Nonbarbiturates, such as ketamine, may cause cutaneous eruptions.

3 Local anesthetics are associated with numerous reactions such as anaphylaxis, urticaria, dermatitis. Dermatitis is not uncommon among dentists and physicians who develop hypersensitivity because of frequent contact with an agent.

4 Adjuncts to anesthesia, such as tranquilizers and neuroleptics.

5 Neuromuscular blockers. Curare is the strongest histamine releaser.

6 Other agents: nonanesthetic drugs administered during operation such as epinephrine, antibiotics, diuretics; acrylic bone cement.

Predisposing Factors to Reaction

1 Overdosage.
- **a** Inattention to maximal safe quantity.
- **b** Disregard for latent period of onset of anesthesia.
- **c** Too rapid injection.
- **d** Too rapid absorption. Intravenous is the most dangerous route of injection. Injection site is also pertinent. Hazardous sites involve vascular areas: tracheobronchial mucosa, tissues of the head, neck, perivertebral region. The least hazardous areas are subcutaneous tissue of the extremities and trunk.

2 True hypersensitivity (immunological sensitization) produces allergic responses and anaphylaxis. This can occur following very small or minimal dose. However, it is much less frequently encountered than reactions from overdosage.
- **a** Briefly, allergic reactions are classified as four types:
  - **(1)** Classic anaphylactic or immediate reaction (usually mediated by immunoglobulin E antibody) with release of histamine within seconds.
  - **(2)** Cytotoxic reaction resulting in cell destruction.
  - **(3)** Immune complex hypersensitivity, e.g., serum sickness.
  - **(4)** Delayed or cellular type hypersensitivity. (At times there is a delay of 24 hours or more before onset of reaction.)
- **b** Magnitude of allergic response is influenced by a number of factors, such as amount of antigen or antibody present. The antigen is exogenous, the other factors endogenous, which is the reason for extensive variation in individual susceptibility.
- **c** Histamine contracts smooth muscle of bronchioles and large blood vessels, dilates venules, and increases capillary permeability. Establishing the cause and mechanism for reaction is important in future management of the patient.

Symptoms of Systemic Reactions

Symptoms manifested may be those of central nervous system stimulation, central nervous system depression, or stimulation followed by depression and collapse.

1 *Stimulation:* talkativeness, incoherence, excitation, tachycardia, bounding pulse, flushed face, hyperpyrexia, tremors, hyperactive reflexes, muscular twitching, convulsions

2 *Depression:* drowsiness, stupor, syncope, rapid thready pulse or bradycardia, apprehension, hypotension, pale or cyanotic moist skin

3 *Other signs:* nausea, vomiting, dizziness, blurred vision, sudden severe headache, precordial pain, extreme pulse rate or blood pressure change, angioneurotic edema (wheeze, laryngeal edema, bronchospasm), rashes, urticaria, severe local tissue reaction

Treatment of Anesthetic Reactions

Treatment is aimed at preventing simultaneous respiratory and cardiac arrest. Time is of the essence. Administration of the drug is stopped immediately (when possible) at the first indication of reaction. Treatment consists of:

1 Maintaining oxygenation of the vital organs and tissues with ventilation by manual or mechanical assistance. Intubation is done as indicated.
2 Reversing myocardial depression and peripheral vasodilatation before cardiac arrest occurs. Intravenous fluid therapy is begun and a vasoconstrictor drug is given intravenously or intramuscularly for hypotension or a weak pulse, signs of circulatory depression. Drugs used include:
   a Epinephrine (IV)—counteracts hypotension, bronchoconstriction, laryngeal edema. (It also stimulates beta and alpha adrenergic receptors and inhibits further release of mediators.)
   b Ephedrine and other vasoconstrictors such as phenylephrine (Neo-Synephrine)—cause peripheral vasoconstriction, increased myocardial contraction, and bronchodilation.
   c Antihistamines—block histamine release.
   d Steroids—effect is not immediate and their use is directed toward late manifestations of allergic response.
   e Isoproterenol—uses are predominantly in asthma and heart attack.

   When applicable, application of a tourniquet or subcutaneous injection of epinephrine in the area of drug injection may delay absorption of toxic drug.
3 Giving antagonist drug in situations where causative agent is identified.
4 Stopping muscle tremors or convulsions if they are present as they constitute hazard of further hypoxia, possibility of aspiration, body injury. Small doses of a short-acting barbiturate and/or diazepam are given intravenously to inhibit cortical irritation.

NOTE. In patients in whom the adverse response is due to hypersensitivity, the previous measures are applicable. However, aminophylline may be administered to help alleviate bronchospasm, hydrocortisone (IV) to combat shock, and sodium or potassium iodide (IV) to reduce mucosal edema.

The nurse must know resuscitation measures and be able to assist in or initiate them when necessary, as per hospital policy.

Precautions for preventing reactions include:

1 Careful questioning of the patient preoperatively for history of any allergies or hypersensitivities and reactions to previous anesthetics or other drugs.
   a Individuals with multiple allergies are thought to be more prone to adverse reaction.
   b Any drug with known or suspected history of reaction, or any chemically related drug, is not given.
   c If testing for sensitivity to specific drugs is done, it must be executed *very* cautiously under *well-controlled* conditions.
2 Knowledge of patient's general condition.
   a Many surgeons insist on seeing a patient in their office no longer than 1 week prior to operation (general or local anesthesia).
   b Identification must be made of all drugs the patient has recently received or is currently taking.
3 Administration of appropriate premedication drugs and dosages.
4 Careful observing of the patient, including facial expressions, and noting responses to conversation and state of alertness.
5 Limiting the total amount of drug injected or applied to prescribed safe limits and recording this information. Adjust precise amount also to the size of the patient.
6 Immediate cessation of administration at any sign of sensitivity.
7 Slow injection to avoid overdosage.
8 Frequent aspiration or pulling back on syringe plunger while injecting a drug to be sure that the solution is not entering a blood vessel inadvertently.

The anesthesiologist's (or surgeon's) perception of possible occurrence and readiness to treat a reaction is of great help in preventing a fatal one. The circulating nurse also shares this responsibility and that of closely observing the patient.

Care with Drug Ampuls

When you are responsible for placing drug ampuls on the table for use:

1 Be careful to read the label correctly.

2 Discard the ampul if the label is not completely legible or has been disturbed.

3 Observe the solution for clarity and discard any suspicious ampul.

4 Provide a rustproof ampul file for opening.

5 Sterile single-dose ampuls are recommended.

CRYOANESTHESIA

This involves the blocking of local nerve conduction of painful impulses by means of marked surface cooling of a localized area. It is used in topical procedures such as the removal of warts or noninvasive papular surface lesions. Cryotherapy units are commercially available.

MONITORING OF THE PATIENT

During extensive surgery under anesthesia, the body is subjected to much stress. Bleeding, trauma, potent drugs, and operative positions that may not facilitate breathing and circulation all contribute to disturbed physiology.

To continuously measure the patient's responses to these stresses during the intraoperative and postoperative periods, clinical evaluation by listening, observing, and feeling is augmented by the use of electronic or mechanical devices. These devices furnish much valuable information about the patient, reveal trends and subtle changes, give warning of an impending dangerous state, and indicate response to therapy. Much of this equipment is expensive, constitutes an explosion hazard, and takes up much space in the operating room. Some operating room suites have permanently installed apparatus with concealed wiring and conduits in a glass-enclosed room or area adjoining the operating theatre.

Personnel using electronic monitoring equipment must be able to easily determine equipment malfunction. *Instrumentation should augment, not replace, the surgeon's or anesthesiologist's judgment or careful nursing observation.* The use of computers in the operating room improves methods of handling data.

With monitoring, many aspects of respiratory, cardiovascular, and nervous system functions can be constantly observed. This is desirable since anesthetic agents and/or operative manipulation may initiate unwanted circulatory and respiratory reflex responses.

The following parameters may be monitored to show minute-to-minute changes in physiologic variables.

Electrocardiogram (ECG) Shows changes in rhythm, rate, or conduction of the heart (arrhythmias, appearance of premature beats, block of impulses). Electrocardiogram is a recording of electrical forces produced by the heart. It does not provide an index of cardiac output.

There are various types of cardiac monitoring systems but generally they consist of a monitor screen (cathode ray oscilloscope) on which the electrocardiogram is visualized, and a "write-out" system, which transcribes the rhythm strip on paper. The write-out may be controlled or automatic. A heart-rate meter may be set to write out a rhythm strip if the rate should go below a preset figure. Lights and beepers may provide appropriate visual and audible signals of heart rate. Monitor leads or electrodes are attached to the chest or extremities. Chest electrodes are usually attached with self-adhering, disposable disc electrodes; special clamps or small metal plates are used on extremities. Careful placement of leads is important to show the waves and complexes of the ECG rhythm strip.

One tracing is taken before induction as a control. An electrocardiograph is especially valuable during induction and intubation when arrhythmias are prone to occur. Rapid identification of abnormal heart rhythms makes treatment more specific. It permits early recognition of occult irregularities of the heart's action. In cases of cardiac arrest it shows when heart action ceased; it also defines type of arrest, which is of value in treatment. Changes shown may be due to the anesthetic itself, to a change in oxygenation or coronary blood flow, to hypercarbia, or to alteration in electrolyte balance or body temperature. Recording may be affected by use of electrosurgical unit.

Stethoscopy Monitors heart beat. Stethoscope is taped to the precordium and attached to an indwelling plastic earpiece. Pressure-sensitive detecting units may be placed within the esophagus (esophageal stethoscope). Precordial and esophageal stethoscopes can detect both cardiac and pulmonary sounds. A commercially available pulsometer may be connected to pacemaker monitors.

Arterial Blood Pressure (Direct) Assesses respiratory and hemodynamic status. It is obtained through the radial artery via a catheter usually inserted percutaneously. A very slow drip of slightly heparinized saline keeps the catheter open for taking intermittent blood samples and pressure recordings. Continuous monitoring is used in complex operations or those with controlled hypotension. The *indirect method* is by means of the sphygmomanometer, which is used for every operative procedure with very few exceptions. Blood pressure (BP) signifies the pressure forcing blood through the circulation. A machine is available for automatic BP monitoring at 1-minute intervals using ultrasound. Evaluation of BP during anesthesia requires consideration of the blood volume, cardiac output, and state of sympathetic blood volume since tissue perfusion is dependent on these factors. The arm used for the measurement should be protected from contact with the team members standing beside the table.

Arterial Blood Gases and pH This is a diagnostic tool in regard to tissue perfusion. Serial monitoring of these measurements is indispensable in evaluating pulmonary gas exchange and acid-base balance. In planning interventions, the measurements are considered in relation to other parameters such as venous pressure, left atrial pressure, and vital signs.

Respiratory gases in the blood, oxygen and carbon dioxide, exert their own partial pressures (P), the measurements of which are expresed in millimeters of mercury. Identification of the gas being measured is indicated as Pa (arterial) or Pv (venous). For example, the partial pressure of oxygen in arterial blood is expressed as PaO_2 - 95 mm Hg. The pH, measure of blood acidity, usually is determined also when respiratory gases are measured. Newer monitoring techniques permit rapid analysis of pO_2, pCO_2, O_2 saturation, pH, base excess, and actual bicarbonate. Tidal volume, respiratory rate, and concentration of oxygen inhaled can be adjusted to establish adequate oxygenation and carbon dioxide elimination. Differentiation of respiratory or metabolic acidosis or alkalosis is a guide to appropriate treatment.

Hypoventilation, uneven ventilation in relation to blood flow, impairment of diffusion, venous-to-arterial shunting (as in ventricular septal defect) lead to anoxemia unless oxygen in inspired air is increased. Hypoventilation of the whole lung or a major portion leads to retention of carbon dioxide and predisposes the patient to cardiac arrhythmias. Disturbances of acid-base balance have many serious consequences in many organs, and must be corrected to achieve normal physiologic functioning.

Either or both arterial and venous blood-gas determinations and/or pressures may be monitored.

Central Venous Pressure (CVP) Measures the pressure under which blood is returned to the right atrium. This helps to determine the circulatory status and aids in assessing the relationship between circulating blood volume and pumping action of the heart. It may reflect incipient heart failure. It is an indicator of the heart's competence to accept increased fluid volume, and of the adequacy of blood volume being presented to the heart for its pumping action. It is not, however, a measure of blood volume or cardiac output. Serial measurement, portraying a trend, is more valuable than an isolated reading. CVP serves as a guide during fluid or blood administration, and is an important determinant in preventing too great or too rapid replacement, which can cause pulmonary edema. It is especially useful for avoiding circulatory overload in patients having a limited cardiopulmonary reserve. It is used during shock and hypotension to judge the adequacy of blood replacement. CVP may be measured indirectly, but most accurately, by means of a manometer attached to a radiopaque polyethylene catheter passed to the right atrium or adjacent vena cava through a vein such as the subclavian or internal jugular. The catheter is inserted aseptically to avoid infection. Normal CVP reading is 3 to 10 cm of water or 2 to 8 mm of mercury (1 cm H_2O = 1.3 mm Hg). Pressures from 12 to 20 cm are borderline elevations requiring close observation. Pressures above 20 cm indicate possible myocardial incompetence.

Pulmonary Artery (PA) Pressures Provide precise information about cardiac performance that is useful in preventing and treating heart failure. For example, an increase in PA pressure is seen before symptoms of left-sided heart failure or fluid overload are apparent. Hypovolemia is associated with low pressures. In the failing heart, the left ventricle ejects a greatly decreased amount of blood, cardiac output falls, arterial-oxygen tension drops, and respiratory insufficiency follows. PA pressures serve as guidelines for therapy: administration of fluids, diuretics, and cardiotonic drugs to obtain optimal cardiac output. These pressures are measured through a flow-directed pulmonary artery (PA) catheter, e.g., Swan-Ganz,* a sophisticated monitoring tool. The multiple-lumen catheter also permits monitoring of central venous pressure, cardiac output, and/or vascular tone.

Cardiac Output Determines the quantity of blood pumped from the left ventricle. It depends on contractile strength of the heart, peripheral resistance of the vessels, and venous return. The average in an adult is 5 liters per minute. It is measured by a *thermodilution technique.* A bolus of cold physiologic saline is injected into a lumen of an arterial catheter and temperature gradient at a point downstream is measured via a second lumen. A transistorized intravascular thermistor in a thermodilution catheter detects changes in

*Edwards Laboratories, Santa Anna, Calif.

blood temperatures that are then used to compute cardiac output.

Cardiac output measurement provides an index of the amount of blood pumped by the heart during a time of observation. A reduced cardiac output results in decreased perfusion of the capillary circulation.

Total Blood Volume (BV) Is useful in determining the total amount of blood replacement required. Calculation of BV depends upon venous hematocrit value. The dilution principle is utilized in determination. An accurate method of BV measurement involves measuring the plasma and red-cell volumes separately, then adding the results together. To measure red-cell volume, cells are tagged with detectable, nontoxic, radioactive chromium, subsequently injected intravenously, and counted after an appropriate mixing time. Or radioactive iodinated human serum albumen (RIHSA), in standard-dose packages, can be injected, mixed, and counted. Counting may be done rapidly by an electronic device. This technique may be used in place of estimation of operative blood loss.

Estimation of Operative Blood Loss May be made in all operations where a major blood loss and need for replacement is necessary since a deficit of blood volume is the most frequent cause of postoperative hypotension. The gravimetric method of weighing sponges is a simple and common method. Previously dry sponges are weighed after use as they are discarded from the operative field. Dry weight is subtracted from wet weight. Blood in the suction bottle may be measured but allowance must be made for presence of irrigating solution if used. The amount of blood on drapes is visually estimated.

Respiratory Tidal Volume (V_T) Reveals the volume of air moved with each breath. A respirometer may be placed on the expiratory limb of anesthesia machine; mechanical or electronic meters are available.

Body Temperature Measures surface (skin) or deep (core) body temperatures by thermistors and thermocouples. A thermistor is inserted in the patient's esophagus or rectum and connected to a meter. Changes in central body temperature can predict important incidents. Convulsions may follow hyperpyrexia, which increases metabolism and demand for oxygen. A falling temperature, the most common change, may precede increased irritability of the heart and ventricular fibrillation. Hypothermia also delays metabolism of drugs and alters effects of neuromuscular blockers. Changes in body temperature may be marked during anesthesia. Cutaneous temperature changes are a clue to vasoactivity at a given time, helping diagnose vasoconstriction or vasodilatation. They parallel changes in cardiac output.

Hypothermia under anesthesia may result from air-conditioning, massive blood replacement or cool infusion solutions, anesthetic effect (decreased metabolic rate and vasodilatation), prolonged exposure of body cavities to air, high inflow anesthesia circuits with water loss from the respiratory tract. Transfusion reactions under anesthesia may be accompanied by profound hypotension and temperature change. The common undisguised physical reaction and chill are not seen in the anesthetized patient. Retention of heat and *hyperthermia* may be caused by premedication such as atropine, the sterile drapes covering the patient, a warm OR, a closed anesthesia breathing circuit, or sepsis in the patient.

Electroencephalogram Uses scalp electrodes to provide an index of many processes. The patterns reveal the presence of organic brain damage, abnormal physiologic alterations, and the action of drugs. It is also a means of determining cessation of circulation, an index of expected prognosis, and brain vitality.

Hourly Measurement of Urinary Output via Indwelling Catherter Is of diagnostic value in assessing effective blood volume and fluid administration. Volume, electrolytes, osmolarity, pH are important. A urometer is useful in measuring output.

Chest X-ray This is essential for checking position of: pulmonary artery catheter (Swan-Ganz), central venous pressure line, endotracheal tube, chest tube; for observing changes in lung and heart during therapy.

INVASIVE MONITORING

Measurements involving invasive monitoring techniques yield specific information that is usually otherwise not obtainable or as accurate. Although these measurements may be pertinent in guiding patient care, they present additional risk because their obtainment requires invasion of the great vessels and/or heart. The benefits of invasive monitoring must be balanced against the risks.

Complications are cardiac arrhythmias, embolism, thrombosis, and infection.

The *insertion of catheters into vital areas is always performed by a physician.* The nurse must understand the function and significance of the monitors and thus design nursing care on the basis of this knowledge while working closely with the anesthesiologist. *Direct arterial puncture for blood samples is performed only by a physician.* However, when arterial or venous catheters are in place, the circulating nurse may be asked to collect blood samples for analysis or to take measurements, although this is not universal practice. These procedures require skill and knowledge of the equipment and the hazards involved.

Drawing Blood Samples

Samples for arterial gas measurements are sometimes drawn from an indwelling arterial (radial or femoral) catheter line kept open by a continuously running, intra-arterial infusion, the tubing of which incorporates a plastic three-way stopcock, usually close to the catheter insertion site. One lumen of the stopcock goes to the infusion solution, one to the cannulated artery, and one to the outside air. The latter is normally closed, covered with a sterile cap, or a sterile syringe is kept inserted in the lumen to prevent bacteria and air from entering. With a three-way stopcock, two of the three lumens are always open.

In drawing blood samples from an indwelling arterial line, always *use strict sterile technique* in drawing the blood through the stopcock.

1 Place conveniently and open a package of sterile gloves and tray of sterile equipment.

2 After donning gloves, attach a sterile, 5-cc syringe to the stopcock lumen going to the outside air. Turn off (close) the infusion lumen. This automatically opens the line between the patient and the syringe. Aspirate 3 cc of blood and close the lumen to the patient. Discard this syringe and blood because it is diluted with IV solution and would give an inaccurate determination.

3 Quickly attach a second sterile syringe (coated with heparin to obtain unclotted blood) to the lumen to the outside air, and open the lumen to the patient. This closes the lumen to the infusion, permitting aspiration of undiluted blood for analysis.

4 Close the lumen to the patient and flush the line and stopcock by letting infusion solution run through them to prevent clot formation inside the catheter wall or stopcock, which could result in arterial embolization.

5 Close and recap the lumen to the outside air (being careful not to contaminate cap), thereby restarting the infusion to the patient. Regulate the infusion rate with the clamp on the infusion tubing.

6 If any air bubbles are in the syringe, remove them, and see that the samples are *immediately* taken to the laboratory. If more than 10 minutes elapse between blood drawing and analysis, the analysis cannot be considered accurate. In event of delay, the syringe with blood should be immediately immersed in ice and refrigerated at near-freezing temperature.

Assisting with Insertion of a Central Venous Pressure Line

1 Preparation.
- **a** Collect necessary *sterile* supplies. A catheter insertion tray is convenient.
- **b** Set up the line: connect the IV bag to the tubing; insert the manometer into the line, attached by stopcock between IV tubing and the anesthesia extension tubing; run air out of the line and clamp; secure manometer upright to IV pole.

2 Assisting the physician.
- **a** Insertion: the line is usually inserted by cutdown or percutaneously into the subclavian vein or one of its feeding tributaries. Catheter insertion is a sterile procedure.
- **b** As soon as the line is in place. a central venous pressure reading is taken as a baseline measurement and as a presumptive check for proper placement of the cannula tip. Since the expansion of the lungs will increase intrathoracic pressure (deflation decreases it), the column of fluid in the manometer should fluctuate with each breath while a reading is being taken.
- **c** A chest x-ray is taken to assure accurate placement of the catheter. The connections to the three-way stopcock should be taped to prevent their inadvertent disconnection.

3 Taking a CVP reading.
- **a** Shut off the lumen of the stopcock to the patient, thereby running IV fluid into the manometer. At the desired level, shut off the stopcock lumen to the IV infusion.
- **b** Take a reading on the manometer (make certain zero scale is on a level with the patient's right atrium), then close the stopcock lumen to the manometer, thereby opening the infusion to the patient again, to keep the line open.

Assisting with Insertion of a Pulmonary Artery (PA) Catheter

Strict sterile technique is used. A pulmonary artery catheter insertion tray is convenient. Catheter selection, e.g., the number of catheter lumens, depends on what is to be measured. The major lumen of the catheter terminates at the catheter tip. The external end of that lumen is attached to a transducer that converts vessel pressure to an electronic signal. PA pressure waveforms are displayed on an oscilloscope. The pressures can be measured from the monitor. Pressure wave and ECG are recorded simultaneously.

The catheter is inserted through a peripheral vein, such as the antecubital, using a cutdown incision or a percutaneous needle introducer. The catheter is threaded into a thoracic vein where the balloon on its tip is partially inflated. When a right atrial pressure-wave pattern is seen on the oscilloscope, the balloon is fully inflated and the blood flow rapidly carries the catheter through the tricuspid valve into the right ventricle, and then to the main pulmonary artery. The catheter finally stops when it wedges in a pulmonary vessel slightly smaller than the diameter of the inflated balloon. During this time, the pressure-wave patterns on the oscilloscope quickly change from right atrial to right ventricular to pulmonary artery to pulmonary capillary wedge (PCW) patterns.*

The nurse should consult the procedure book. Nurses' responsibilities in this procedure vary according to hospital policy, and may include:

1 Interpreting the procedure to the patient.
2 Gathering equipment; prepping the skin and assisting the physician with cutdown.
  a Attaching plastic three-way stopcocks to both distal and proximal lumen outlets of the catheter.
  b Flushing lumina with heparinized solution to eliminate air bubbles and ensure patency.
  c Testing balloon by injecting air or carbon dioxide. *Never use water,* which interferes with deflation.
  d Checking equipment for damage or electrical current leakage (see p. 000).
3 Calibrating the monitor.
4 Watching the monitor for premature ventricular contractions (PVCs) during insertion. Have lidocaine hydrochloride and defibrillation equipment ready.
5 Taking and recording pressure readings as ordered.

INDUCED HYPOTHERMIA

Hypothermia is the artificial, deliberate lowering of body temperature below the normal limits. Expert skill, knowledge, and vigilance are required, and the patient is carefully monitored.

Systemic hypothermia may be light (37 to 32 °C or 98.6 to 89.6 °F), moderate (32 to 26 °C or 89.6 to 78.8 °F), deep (26 to 20 °C or 78.8 to 68 °F), or profound (20 °C or below, 68 °F or below).

This procedure either alone or in conjunction with extracorporeal circulation (see p. 391) is used to lower body temperature in order to reduce the metabolic rate and oxygen needs of the tissues in conditions causing hypoxia or during a decrease or interruption of circulation. Bleeding is also decreased and less anesthetic is needed. The patient can therefore better tolerate the operative procedure. Hypothermia may be used:

1 For direct-vision intracardiac repair of complex congenital defects in infants and in other cardiac procedures. This is the most common usage.
2 After cardiac resuscitation, to decrease oxygen requirement of vital tissues and limit further damage to the brain following anoxia.
3 In treatment of hyperpyrexia and some other nonsurgical conditions (hypertensive crisis).
4 To increase tolerance in septic shock.
5 In neurosurgery, to decrease cerebral blood flow, brain volume, and venous and intracranial pressures.
6 To aid in transplantation of tissues and organs.

Attaining Hypothermia

To achieve hypothermia, heat must be lost more rapidly than it is produced. The following methods may be used.

1 *Surface-induced hypothermia:* attained by means of thermal blankets or mattresses circulating ice water through their coils, immersion in ice-water baths, ice packing of the body, alcohol sponging. External cooling is used for infants and small children under 20 lb (10 kg) because of their smaller surface area.
2 *Internal cooling:* achieved through decrease or interruption of blood flow by placing ice packs around a specific internal organ or cold fluids within a body cavity (ice-water enema, intragastric, intraperitoneal lavage—but carries risk of infection); drugs may be used to lower metabolism and resistance to shivering.
3 *Systemic hypothermia:* bloodstream is cooled by diverting the blood through heat-exchanging devices of extracorporeal circulation and returning it to the body (continuous flowing circuit), e.g., core cooling by cardiopulmonary bypass; intravenous administration of cold fluids. Systemic hypothermia is used in adults and larger children

*American Journal of Nursing, 76:1766, Nov 1976.

to 26°C (78.8°F). Oxygen consumption and metabolism of different organs vary so uniform hypothermia is impossible.

NOTE. A hypo-hyperthermia machine, an electronic system, is available. The temperature is not deliberately taken below about 29°C (84.5°F) unless arrest of the heart is desired by means of deep hypothermia (below 26°C). This is accompanied by perfusion of the rest of the body with the extracorporeal-circulation method, permitting an open, motionless dry field while the blood flow is interrupted. A noncontracting heart requires very little oxygen.

The patient is progressively rewarmed at the close of the operation until his or her temperature is 35°C (95°F) or until consciousness returns. Sometimes a degree of hypothermia is maintained for a day or two postoperatively to allow the patient to adapt more readily. Oxygen therapy and tracheotomy, if advised, are part of the postoperative care.

Complications in Use

Hypothermia carries many inherent risks. Primarily it affects the myocardium, decreasing its resistance to ventricular fibrillation and predisposing the patient to cardiac arrest. This is more likely to happen with deep hypothermia or during manipulation of the heart itself. Other dangers are heart block, effects on the vascular system, atrial fibrillation, embolism, microcirculation stasis, undesired downward drift of temperature ("overshooting"), tissue damage and metabolic acidosis, numerous effects on other organs and systems.

Time is required for cooling and rewarming. Shivering and vasoconstriction, normal defenses of the body against cooling, can be problems during use of hypothermia. This muscle activity increases the oxygen needs greatly. Shivering can be overcome by the administration of a muscle-relaxant drug or intravenous injection of chlorpromazine or an analgesic such as meperidine. Rewarming carries certain problems such as the possibility of reactive bleeding or circulatory collapse. Rewarming can be accomplished by circulating warmed blood by means of extracorporeal circulation, or by using a mattress with circulating fluid, and warm blankets. If external heat is applied, take care not to burn the patient. "Rewarming shock" may be prevented by slow warming, adequate oxygenation, prevention of vasoconstriction and shivering.

CONTROLLED HYPOTENSION

Controlled hypotension is the deliberate lowering of the blood pressure during anesthesia, as an adjunct to operation. It is done to produce an essentially bloodless field in order to shorten operating time, decrease need for transfusion, improve results in radical procedures, increase operability by improving surgical access, and give the surgeon greater technical freedom and visibility.

Naturally, controlled hypotension is not indicated as a routine procedure. It is used only when the expected gain, for a particular patient requiring a specific operation, outweighs the risk involved. It is employed to diminish the risk of operation, and to improve the chances for its success and for the recovery of the patient.

Adequate oxygenation of the blood and tissue perfusion in vital organs (heart, liver, kidneys, lungs) must be maintained to prevent damage. Capillary flow must be sustained and blood pressure carefully controlled. Absence of vasoconstriction prevents ischemia. The degree and duration of hypotension must be carefully controlled so that the state can be rapidly terminated at any time.

Precautions in Use

1 Careful selection of patient
2 Administration and evaluation by expert anesthesiologists only
3 Choice of appropriate but not arbitrary level of blood pressure
4 Preoperative cardiac, renal, and hepatic evaluation of patient
5 Utilization for only a short time and lowering of blood pressure only enough to obtain desired result
6 Maintenance of blood volume at optimum level and assistance of respirations with adequate oxygenation

Uses of Controlled Hypotension

1 Total hip replacement.
2 Operation where excessive blood loss is expected, such as vascular surgery, to decrease gross hemorrhage or vascular oozing.
3 In neurosurgery, where control of intracranial vessel hemorrhage may be difficult (hemangioma, meningioma, cerebral aneurysm). In the latter case it also decreases leakage and makes the aneurysm less turgid.
4 Operation where blood transfusions should be avoided, as when compatible blood is unavailable or transfusion is against religious belief of patient.

Complications

Potential complications of controlled hypotension are cerebral or coronary thrombosis, reactionary hemorrhage, anuria, delayed awakening.

Hypotension is contraindicated in patients with anemia; arteriosclerosis (indicated by myocardial ischemia, failing cerebral function, cerebral thrombosis, or cerebrovascular accident); history or clinical evidence of cardiovascular, renal, or liver disease; hypotension (increases susceptibility to hypoxia).

HYPNOANESTHESIA

Hypnoanesthesia refers to hypnosis when used as a method of anesthesia. Hypnosis produces a state of altered consciousness characterized by heightened suggestibility, selective wakefulness, reduced awareness, and restricted attentiveness. Although hypnosis has a long history of misuse, modern application by highly trained medical specialists is humane. Hypnoanesthesia has been successfully employed in adult and pediatric patients, especially the latter. Motivation is an important factor. The method may be combined with the use of a small dose of chemical anesthetic or muscle-relaxant drug. *It must not be used indiscriminately in place of standard treatment.*

Hypnosis may be used as a therapeutic aid in *very selected* patients under the following circumstances:

1 When chemical agents are contraindicated. The patient may be kept pain-free, asleep or awake, without toxic side effects.
2 When it may be of value as an adjunct to chemical anesthesia to decrease the amount of anesthesia needed.
3 When it is desirable to free the patient from certain neurophysical effects of an anesthetic.
4 When apprehension and fear of anesthetic are so great as to contribute to serious anesthetic risk.
5 When posthypnotic suggestion may be valuable in the postoperative period.
6 When it is desirable to raise the pain threshold.
7 When it is desirable to have the patient able to respond to questions or commands.

Prehypnotic Preparation

1 Careful psychiatric evaluation of the patient to determine feasibility of hypnosis
2 Establishment of rapport with the patient so that he or she will listen to and obey commands; explanation of procedure
3 Use of trial trances to see if sleep is deep enough

Limitations

1 Hypnoanesthesia requires skill and special training.
2 It is time-consuming.
3 Muscular relaxation induced by hypnosis is limited. Hypnoanesthesia may need to be supplemented.
4 It may release an underlying psychiatric disorder.
5 Hypnoanesthesia is unreliable compared to chemical anesthesia.
6 Contraindications: patient's refusal to be hypnotized; patient's being under psychiatric care.

ACUPUNCTURE

Acupunture has a long history of use in Asia and Europe but it has not been employed extensively in the United States. This ancient medical practice is a complex phenomenon, not well understood, and numerous theories have emerged about it. Research continues in the hope of establishing credibility on a scientific or physiologic basis for its effectiveness for analgesia and anesthesia in a certain percentage of cases.

Acupuncture is a technique of providing local, intense stimulation at specific locations in the body known as acupuncture or meridian points. The stimulation is effected by rotation of or by electric current applied to very fine gauge needles of varying lengths inserted into these points, which generally correspond to the area where the somatic nerve supply is located. The appropriate points can be selected to produce analgesia or anesthesia in the desired region of the body.

Acupuncture has had limited use in operative and dental procedures as well as for postoperative or intractable pain. The patient remains conscious during the procedure. Studies show that the technique may have a place among treatment modalities for patients with chronic pain unrelieved by other methods. Procedures should be limited to use by physicians or under their direct supervision in keeping with acceptable standards of medical practice.

ANESTHESIA FOR AMBULATORY SURGERY PATIENTS

Anesthetic management is rarely difficult for the usual procedures of short duration (15 to 90 minutes) if careful selection of patients, preoperative evaluation, and instruction are adhered to.

Local anesthesia is preferable if appropriate. Spinal anesthesia is not frequently used because of the danger of postoperative postural hypotension. Intravenous agents associated with prolonged recovery (ketamine, Innovar) are avoided unless there is specific indication for their use. Doses of intravenous agents such as narcotics and barbiturates may be reduced to avoid delayed recovery. General anesthesia patients are operated on early in the day to allow maximum recovery time.

Prime considerations in selecting patients for ambulatory (outpatient) surgery are the anticipated period of recovery from anesthesia, of whatever type is deemed appropriate, and possible postoperative complications. Preoperative written forms explicitly state instructions for the patient such as "nothing by mouth after midnight" before admission and "notify the surgeon of a change in physical condition such as fever or a cold." Patients receive recovery room care as required. For example, elective endotracheal intubation is frequently used in children. Cautious recovery room observation is made. If croup develops, most patients are hospitalized for treatment.

Patients are discharged on written order of the surgeon and/or anesthesiologist, in the company of a responsible adult. Discharge is contingent on patient safety in all respects.

ANESTHESIA IN AGE-EXTREME PATIENTS

Age-extreme patients, both the geriatric and pediatric age groups, present a special challenge to the anesthesiologist. It has been estimated that by the year 2006 about one in three Americans will be 65 years of age or older. The implication of this statistic is obvious to the OR team. The mortality rate associated with operative procedures is higher among the aged than the general population, especially if the operation is an emergency one not allowing sufficient time for thorough preoperative evaluation and preparation. Operative morbidity can be reduced, however, by skillful management of anesthesia. This is also true for the other age extreme—the pediatric patient.

Pediatric surgery involves many complex procedures that present an equal challenge for anesthesia management. Small deviations in administration of anesthetic agents can rapidly change an optimal situation into a life-threatening emergency. The uniqueness of infants and children is discussed in Chapter 26.

ANESTHESIA AND INFECTION

Anesthesiologist

Like everyone else in contact with the patient, the anesthesiologist is a potential vector in the spread of infection. He or she has a personal responsibility for practicing the highest standards of both personal cleanliness and asepsis in the OR. As the scope of duties takes the anesthesiologist to areas outside the OR suite, he or she must change contaminated attire on return from those areas. The anesthesiologist must also change masks between patients, and meticulously and repeatedly wash his or her hands with antiseptic soap. It is the duty of the anesthesiologist to see that the equipment used is properly cleaned and sterilized to protect the patient.

Hazards of Equipment

Anesthesia techniques encompass the use of drugs for parenteral administration, as well as of gases and liquids for inhalation administration by means of anesthesia machines. These machines and their component parts (reservoir bags, canisters, connecting pieces, ventilators, etc.) accumulate large numbers of microorganisms during use. Consequently, the parts that come in contact with the patient's skin or respiratory tract are sources of cross contamination. Inhalation, exhalation, and the forcible expulsion of secretions create moist conditions favorable to the survival and growth of a multitude of organisms (streptococci, staphylococci, coliforms, fungi, yeasts, etc.). Therefore, the anesthesia circuit can become a veritable reservoir for microorganisms and a pathway for transmission of disease. There is additional risk when the apparatus is used on a patient with known respiratory disease such as tuberculosis. All used accessories must be cleaned and sterilized before reuse, as clinical cross infection has been traced to contaminated apparatus. It has been shown that the valves of the anesthesia circuit become contaminated from essentially healthy patients at an average rate of 35 organisms per minute. *Pseudomonas aeruginosa* has been cultured from anesthesia absorbers. Many microorganisms accumulate in the valves and air passages, including the soda lime. While the alkalinity of soda lime inhibits many organisms, it is not a dependable germicide or effective mechanical filter, nor meant to be one. Respiratory therapy equipment, mechanical ventilators, resuscitators, suction machines and bottles present the same problems. Resistant strains of organisms, as well as opportunists, have caused nosocomial infections to become a national health problem. The danger of patient-to-patient infection must be eliminated. Included in the requirements for correction is the fundamental recognition that:

1 The patient's respiratory tract is a portal of entry for pathogenic organisms as well as a source of delivering pathogens into the environment.

2 The respiratory tract loses some of its inherent defense mechanisms during operation under anesthesia.

3 Aseptic precautions are necessary to prevent needless exposure of air passages to foreign, potentially pathogenic organisms from the equipment and the hands of anesthesia personnel.

4 Anesthesia machines and equipment, unless properly treated, harbor microorganisms capable of causing postoperative wound infections.

> NOTE. In the presence of tuberculosis or virulent respiratory infection, the anesthesiologist may wear gown and gloves. The patient should wear a mask during transportation and until induction of anesthesia.

Every patient is entitled to have sterile all items that can be sterilized. Manufacturers strive to make the machines that cannot be sterilized more amenable to adequate cleaning and freedom from microorganisms.

Disposable Equipment

The increasing availability of disposable equipment warrants its use for reasons of safety, efficiency, and convenience. Presterilized, disposable airways, endotracheal tubes, tracheostomy tubes, breathing circuits and canisters (with soda lime sealed in the plastic) reduce the hazard of infection. They are especially indicated for the compromised host and for the bacteriologically contaminated patient.

Care of Reusable Equipment

All parts of the patient-exposed, reusable equipment must be thoroughly cleaned after *every* use to prevent pulmonary complications. Thorough cleaning to remove debris and drying must precede any sterilization process.

1 The anesthesia machine should be disinfected immediately whenever soiled by blood and secretions.

2 Surfaces of anesthesia machines, carts, or cabinets should be disinfected after *each* patient use, including the specific work area used for airways, endotracheal tubes, etc. The top of a cart or tray should be draped with a disposable impervious material that is *changed between operations. All* equipment for maintenance of airway should be set up on and returned to this drape. Disposable items should be discarded in suitable containers after use. Nondisposable equipment must be set aside after use for terminal cleaning and testing, thereby diminishing the risk of contaminating clean equipment needed for subsequent patients.

3 All equipment that comes in contact with the patient and the inside of the breathing circuit must be terminally cleaned and maintained in a sterile state.

- **a** Endotracheal tubes, airways, laryngoscope blades, face masks, suction equipment must be sterile for each patient. They are packaged and sterilized individually or in sets.
- **b** After sterilization, the interior of breathing circuits remain sterile if they stand unused in their normal position on the machine but contamination rapidly occurs when used on patients. The parts of the circuit nearest the patient are the most heavily contaminated parts. Therefore, corrugated hoses, breathing tubes, reservoir bags are sterilized between each patient use.
- **c** Items located farther away, such as circle systems and ventilators, are cleaned and sterilized according to a regular schedule, at least once or twice a month.

4 For cleaning, an automated process is available for decontamination. Machines wash equipment in mild detergent and hot water, rinse and dry it. Some machines incorporate a chemical-disinfection cycle. If automatic equipment is not used, anesthesia and respiratory therapy equipment must be disconnected and manually cleaned prior to sterilization. Prompt immersion in detergent-disinfectant solution prevents crusting of secretions. Tubing takes a long time to dry. Commercial dryers are available.

5 Sterilization methods (see Chap. 5).

- **a** Autoclaving is the preferred method for all heat-stable materials including some drugs in ampuls.

> NOTE. Local anesthetic drugs do not tolerate repeated heat sterilization. They should not be resterilized.

- **b** Ethylene oxide is used for materials deteriorated by heat, such as rubber, plastics, mechanical ventilators, electronic equipment. Thorough aeration, according to the manufacturer's recommendations, is necessary before use to remove all residual gas from the material sterilized. Otherwise, facial burns, laryngotracheal inflammation and obstruction or bilateral vocal cord paralysis may be caused by use of the equipment.
- **c** Two percent buffered glutaraldehyde solution does not impair conductivity of antistatic rubber. While the least convenient method, it is the preferred method if ethylene oxide is not available for heat-sensitive items. If glutaraldehyde is used, the items must be thoroughly rinsed with *sterile* water since tap water contains microorganisms.

6 Sterile packaged equipment should be stored in a closed clean dry area. Anesthesia and respiratory therapy equipment should be kept sterile until used.

Checking Anesthesia Equipment

Inhalation systems are tested biologically at regular intervals.

COMPLICATIONS OF OPERATION UNDER ANESTHESIA

The anesthesiologist must be constantly aware of the surgeon's actions, and do everything possible to ensure the safety of the patient and reduce the stress of operation. Continuous appraisal of the patient's overall condition helps avoid complications. Some complications may occur as a direct result of anesthesia; others may have additional contributing factors. Some of the conditions that may occur during the procedure are discussed in the following paragraphs. These same complications, as well as others (see Chap. 29), may appear in the postoperative period. Tragically, catastrophic emergencies may sometimes arise when least expected, and a matter of minutes can make the difference in life or death for the patient. Anticipation and preparedness may spell that difference.

Aspiration

Pulmonary aspiration of gastric contents is highly dangerous and may occur during abolition of throat reflexes when the patient is unconscious or when he or she is conscious with the throat anesthetized, as for bronchoscopy. Aspiration results in residual effects on lung function and blood-gas exchange. A chemical pneumonitis results from aspiration of highly acidic gastric juices. Aspiration of solids or particulate matter results in respiratory obstruction. Bronchospasm and atelectasis may be followed by pneumonitis or bronchopneumonia. Most aspiration is irritative, but it can be infectious if nasopharyngeal flora are aspirated. Pneumonia or lung abscess may result. Every patient who has food in the stomach is a poor risk for anesthesia; for example, a patient with traumatic injuries on whom operation is attempted without adequate preparation of the patient. Increased intragastric pressure is an aspiration hazard and may result from conditions such as pylorospasm, gastrointestinal bleeding, intestinal obstruction, or gas forced into the stomach by application of positive-pressure ventilation without use of a cuffed endotracheal tube.

Symptoms Cyanosis, dyspnea, tachycardia, followed by cardiac embarrassment, lung collapse and consolidation.

Treatment Lower head of table for postural drainage. Suction oropharynx and tracheobronchial tree. If the patient has aspirated particulate matter that causes obstruction of airways, bronchoscopy must be performed to remove it. Suctioning must be interrupted every 10 to 15 seconds to give oxygen. Aspiration of acid gastric content injures the alveolar capillary interface resulting in intrapulmonary shunting and pulmonary edema. Intensive pulmonary care is aimed at improving ventilation-perfusion ratios and decreasing the abnormal gas exchange. This may require tracheal intubation for mechanical ventilation with continuous positive pressure. Careful cardiovascular monitoring and frequent blood-gas and acid-base determinations guide therapeutic measures. Prophylactic antibiotics may be given to prevent infection, and a bronchodilator (aminophylline) to treat spasm.

Prevention Adequate preoperative preparation and careful administration of anesthetic agents. Use of nasogastric tube pre- and intraoperatively where indicated. Anesthetic is decreased near the end of the operation, hastening the return of throat reflexes. Obstetric patients who receive light general anesthesia, near vomiting-reflex level, bear close watching; regurgitation is possible from hand pressure on the abdomen during delivery; gastric evacuation is delayed by labor and medications.

Laryngospasm and Bronchospasm

The latter often follows the former.

Etiology Certain anesthetics and/or drugs; allergic conditions such as asthma; vagal reflex; stimulation of pharynx and larynx under light anesthesia; foreign material in tracheobronchial tree; movement of head or neck; painful peripheral stimuli. Degree of spasm varies from mild to severe.

Symptoms Wheezing respirations or stridor, cyanosis, respiratory obstruction.

Treatment Depends on precipitating factor. Methods generally used: positive-pressure oxygen; tracheal intubation as indicated; neuromuscular blockers for relaxation; bronchodilator drugs such as atropine, epinephrine, aminophylline, and isoproterenol (with great caution as they act as cardiac stimulators and, in the presence of hypoxia, they may contribute to cardiac arrhythmia and cardiac arrest). If etiology is allergic, steroids and antihistamines may be given. Vagal reflexes are inhibited by atropine. If reflex is the cause, anesthesia is deepened; if irritation of anesthetic vapor is the cause, concentration of the agent is reduced. Drying agents are given for excessive secretions. Immediate effective treatment is mandatory to counteract hypoxia and prevent cardiac arrest.

Prevention Patent airway, appropriate premedication such as atropine; avoidance of factors stimulating vagal reflex.

Respiratory Obstruction

Etiology Blocking of the airway by a foreign body, soft tissue, excessive secretions; poor position; laryngospasm or bronchospasm resulting in hypoxia and carbon dioxide retention.

Symptoms Increased respiratory effort with inadequate respiratory exchange; respiratory motion of chest and abdomen without audible air movement at the airway. Pallor and cyanosis rapidly follow hypoxia. The latter develops more slowly if the patient has been breathing high concentration of oxygen. Respirations may or may not be noisy.

Treatment Eliminate the cause; administer oxygen by positive pressure.

Prevention Patent airway; chin held up and forward if endotracheal tube is not used; adequate oxygen intake; prevention of foreign bodies in the airway; proper positioning on operating table; avoidance of pressure on the chest.

Hypoxia and Hypercarbia

The ability to oxygenate depends on hemoglobin concentration, cardiac output, and oxygen saturation, therefore, any deficits in any of these factors affects oxygenation. The body compensates for mild hypoxia with increased heart and respiratory rates, bringing more oxygen to the blood and tissues. If hypoxia progresses, this compensation is inadequate. If hypoxia is prolonged, cardiac arrhythmia or irreversible brain, liver, kidney, and heart damage results.

Etiology Inadequate pulmonary ventilation from depression of the respiratory center by narcotics and/or anesthetic, reduced cardiac output, severe blood loss, or obstruction to respiratory passages, ventilation-perfusion ratio abnormality.

Symptoms Pallor or cyanosis; decreased volume of respirations; dark blood in the operative field.

Treatment Immediate adequate oxygen intake to stimulate the medullary centers and prevent respiratory-system failure.

Prevention Patent airway, adequate oxygenation, proper positioning, intraoperative measurement of arterial pH, pCO_2, and pO_2 to enable the anesthesiologist to evaluate oxygenation and carbon dioxide removal. Patients may be given oxygen and assisted ventilation during transportation to the recovery area to prevent hypoxia from hypoventilation.

Intercostal Muscle Spasm ("Rigid Chest")

This may occur after large doses of intravenous Innovar or on emergence from general anesthesia. It may reverse itself, or neuromuscular blockers may be needed.

Convulsions

Convulsions occur most often in patients with hyperactive metabolic rate, especially in hyperpyretic or dehydrated children. It is important to maintain as normal a body temperature as possible in all patients. Anoxia and death can result.

Etiology Severe hypoxia and carbon dioxide retention; hyperthermia; overdose of regional anesthetic drugs; air embolism; epilepsy.

Symptoms Muscular twitching, dilated pupils, rapid snorting respirations, rapid pulse, grimacing, cyanosis.

Treatment Administer oxygen to maintain respiration; rapid-acting intravenous barbiturate or neuromuscular blocker to stop convulsions; artificial ventilation for apnea; support circulation.

Injuries

Injuries are many and varied. Some of the more common ones are injury to nerves and bones from faulty positioning and careless handling of anesthetized patients, which can result in paralysis, fractures, and postoperative pain (see Chap. 8 for instructions for lifting an unconscious patient). Eyes can be injured from irritating anesthetics, face masks, or from drying of the cornea if the eyelids are not closed, as occurs most often in patients with protruding eyes, patients whose faces are covered with drapes, or those in prone positions. Extravasation, thrombophlebitis, or air emboli associated with intravenous infusions are preventable. Keep intravenous needles visible and not entirely hidden beneath drapes; check infusions frequently; fill tubing with solution before connecting to needle or catheter.

Malignant Hyperpyrexia (Hyperthermia)

This is an often fatal complication (over 60 percent mortality when it occurs), characterized by progressive elevation of body temperature monitored as high as 42.8°C (109°F) or 44°C (111°F). Most potent anesthetic agents, depolarizing skeletal muscle relaxants, and also some local anesthetics have been associated with this catastrophe, although it most often occurs during general anesthesia. A favorable prognosis decreases when excessive heat is noted from the patient through the surgeon's gloves or in the reservoir bag or soda lime canister as fever may be a late sign of the syndrome.

Etiology Many agents may trigger this abnormal muscular and metabolic response in susceptible individuals. Suspected patients include those with any type of myopathy (muscle disease), history of muscle cramps or localized areas of muscle weakness, or greater than normal muscle size (large tissue mass with high metabolic potential). A familial genetic (autosomal dominant) transmission exists affecting 50 percent of offspring although many cases are nonfamilial. Unexplained fever during operation under anesthesia has many causes, some obscure. The exact cause of this syndrome is unknown.

Symptoms Tachycardia associated with tachypnea, cyanosis or dark blood in the operative field, skin mottling, fever, hot skin or tissues, diaphoresis. Symptoms usually include rigidity. Spasm of the jaw muscle with rigidity of masseter muscles or severe fasciculations following succinylcholine should suggest development of malignant hyperpyrexia. A sudden, generalized hypermetabolic state is produced. The temperature rises as more heat is produced than the body can eliminate. The body tries to adjust by vasodilatation and increased cardiac output. If rapidly increasing tissue demands are not met, severe acidosis and hypoxia occur, progressing to cardiovascular collapse.

Treatment Success is contingent on complete preparedness (preplanned action), early diagnosis, and vigorous therapy. The surgeon must terminate the procedure as fast as possible. Meanwhile, the anesthesiologist institutes treatment. The inhalation anesthetic is immediately discontinued and the tubing is changed because of rubber/gas solubility of inhalation agents. The patient is hyperventilated with 100 percent oxygen while aggressive measures are taken to reduce the temperature with internal and external cooling: iced intravenous solution such as Ringer's lactate, immersion in ice or placement on a cooling mattress, lavage of body cavities and operative wound with cold solution, partial cardiopulmonary bypass, if readily available, to cool viscera. Cooling efforts should cease when reduced to 38.3°C (101°F). Body temperature must be carefully monitored to avoid accidental cooling to arrhythmic levels. Attempt is made to correct acidosis and electrolyte imbalance. An intravenous alkali such as sodium bicarbonate is infused. Other drugs used include diuretics (mannitol, furosemide) to dislodge myoglobin from renal tubules and sustain high urinary flow; procainamide to relax muscle rigidity, treat ventricular tachycardia, and reverse cytoplasmic calcium elevation; hydrocortisone or dexamethasone to restore integrity of cell membranes; insulin to shift potassium back into cells and improve glucose uptake for utilization; dantrolene sodium (dissolved) to relax skeletal muscles. Chlorpromazine or promethazine may be given to limit or prevent shivering, normally a heat-retaining mechanism to be avoided. Shivering also increases oxygen consumption. Parameters to be monitored include electrocardiogram, temperature, urinary output, arterial blood gases and electrolytes, central venous pressure.

Prevention Mortality would be lowered greatly if the problem could be foreseen. Preoperative history should routinely include questions about the patient's previous anesthesia experiences, unexplained incidents or deaths of family members who underwent anesthesia, and known muscular abnormalities of relatives. The hereditary predisposition has been detected in three generations. Also, the temperature and ECG should be monitored intraoperatively on all general anesthesia patients.

Incidence Occurrence may be in the first anesthetic experience or a later one; one-third of the cases appear in a second or subsequent anesthesia. There is a prevalence in males perhaps due to increased muscularity and in children, adolescents, and young adults.

Late Complications Acute renal failure, inadvertent hypothermia from too vigorous cooling, skeletal muscle swelling or necrosis (from hypoxia and acidosis), coagulopathy, hyperkalemia, pulmonary edema, neurologic sequelae (paraplegia, decerebration), and coma.

Hypovolemia

Hypovolemia is low or decreased blood volume due to a deficit of extracellular fluid volume. Decreased blood volume, if present prior to operation, increases operative risk and morbidity.

Etiology Reduced fluid intake, hemorrhage, extensive burns (plasma loss), loss of gastrointestinal fluids, wound drainage, fever, diaphoresis, diuresis. Impaired renal function and metabolic acidosis are predisposing factors.

Symptoms Dry skin and mucous membranes, depressed blood pressure, elevated pulse, oliguria, decreasing central venous pressure and blood volume determinations, deep rapid respirations.

Treatment Infusion of Ringer's lactate or 5% dextrose in water with added electrolytes as necessary. Increase blood volume. Oxygen may be administered.

Hypervolemia

Hypervolemia is an excess of extracellular fluid in the blood, commonly referred to as *edema.*

Predisposing Factors Intravenous infusions given too rapidly or in excessive amounts, especially isotonic saline solution, or prolonged administration of adrenocorticosteroids. Edema may progress to pulmonary edema.

Symptoms Dyspnea, moist rales, elevated pulse and respiration, diminished urine output. Increasing central venous pressure may indicate fluid overload with venous distention.

Treatment Diuretics, restricted fluids, and prevention or treatment of pulmonary edema.

Arterial Hypotension

Reduced blood pressure, with resultant inadequate circulation, may accompany depression of the myocardium, depression of the vasomotor center in the brain, decline in cardiac output, or dilatation of peripheral vessels. Hypotension may occur also when positive pressure is applied to the airway. Progressive deepening of general anesthesia usually produces peripheral vasodilatation and diminished myocardial contractility. Adequate blood flow to the brain and heart, the two most vulnerable vascular beds due to their high metabolic demand, must be maintained. If arterial hypotension is uncontrolled, it may cause cerebral vascular accident, myocardial infarction, or death.

Etiology Overdosage of general anesthetic or rapid vascular absorption of local agents. Overdosage may be due to an actual excess of the agent for a normal patient under ordinary circumstances, or to an excessive amount at a specific time for a particular patient, exceeding the patient's tolerance. Tendency to overdosage occurs during prolonged anesthesia (large amounts of drugs absorbed), in age-extreme patients, or with unrecognized hypothermia during lengthy abdominal or thoracic procedures. Circulatory effects of spinal or epidural anesthesia, such as diminished cardiac output or reduced peripheral resistance, also produce hypotension. Other causes are: hemorrhage, loss of whole blood, or loss of plasma into tissues during extensive operation; circulatory abnormalities such as cardiac tamponade, heart failure, hypovolemia, cerebral or pulmonary embolism (fat embolism from fracture sites, amniotic fluid emboli during delivery, or air emboli from introduction of air into circulation during infusion or procedure), myocardial ischemia or infarction; changes in position, especially if executed rapidly or roughly (some operative positions are poorly tolerated, see Chap. 10); excessive preanesthetic medication (postural hypotension may follow narcotic administration); potent therapeutic drugs (tranquilizers, adrenal steroids, antihypertensives) given prior to anesthetic; hypoxia. Surgical manipulation may induce hypotension mechanically by obstructing venous return to the heart with packs, retractors, or body rests. Or, hypotension may result from vagal-induced reflex precipitated by intraperitoneal traction, manipulation in the chest or neck areas, or stimulation of periosteum. Other causes are transfusion reaction, suggested by accompanying cyanosis and oozing at operative site; septic shock; severe hyperthermia; anaphylactic reaction.

Symptoms Pallor or cyanosis, damp clammy skin, dilated pupils, decreased urinary output because renal circulation is affected, decreased bleeding in operative field or pallor of organs caused by compensatory vasoconstriction, nausea, vomiting, sighing respirations, or air hunger in conscious patients.

Diagnosis Determination of arterial blood pressure and pulse rate, and an estimation of pulse volume. Arbitrary figures of measured blood pressure are not as important as individual circulatory status. A specific measurement in a healthy adult may be relatively insignificant while the same figure in an aged patient could be hazardous. In critically ill patients, central venous pressure and urine output are monitored.

Treatment Must be prompt to avoid circulatory collapse. The aim is to increase perfusion of vital organs and to treat any specific cause while giving general supportive therapy. Supportive measures include elevation of the legs to increase blood pressure by draining pooled blood, especially after sympathetic blockade; rapid intravenous fluid therapy to increase blood volume. Various solutions are applicable in an emergency since the volume of fluid is more vital than its composition, in early treatment. If whole blood is not available, 5% dextrose in water, physiologic saline, plasma or serum albumin, or 6% dextran (plasma expander) may be given. Vasoactive drugs are given as necessary. Vasopressor drugs exert a vasoconstrictor action through stimulation of alpha receptors of the sympathetic nervous system or increase myocardial contractile force and heart rate by activation of beta receptors. Drug selection must often be empirical. Drugs that may be used are: ephedrine, epinephrine, mephentermine (Wyamine), methamphetamine (Methedrine), phenylephrine (Neo-Synephrine), methoxamine (Vasoxyl), metaraminol (Aramine), isoproterenol (Isuprel), dopamine hydrochloride (Intropin), levarterenol (Levophed). These various drugs have various actions; they increase ventricular contractile force, alter sinoatrial nodal activity, constrict vascular smooth muscles, dilate blood vessels in splanchnic bed, or may produce ventricular arrhythmia. The incidence and severity of the latter action is intensified by hypoxia or hypercarbia. Drug effectiveness is reduced in the presence of respiratory or metabolic acidosis. Oxygen is administered.

Prevention Obviously the reverse of the causes, therefore: minute-to-minute observation of *all* patients receiving *any* type of anesthetic; in suspect individuals, testing cardiovascular response to proposed operative position before induction; avoiding overdosage in premedications and anesthetic drugs; gentle tissue manipulation and position change; administration of minimal amount of anesthetic needed for adequacy; adequate time taken to induce and deepen anesthesia so as not to raise the blood level of anesthetic too rapidly; prudent application of positive pressure to airway; prompt replacement of fluid and blood loss. If major blood loss is anticipated, a large intravenous catheter (14- to 16-gauge) is inserted so blood can be rapidly infused, under pressure if necessary.

Circulatory Shock

Shock is a complex phenomenon, a life-threatening condition in which circulation fails for one or several reasons, resulting in insufficient flow of blood for adequate perfusion or oxygenation. If prolonged, inadequate organ blood flow with deficient microcirculation profoundly depresses vital processes. Since the objective of circulation is achieved in the capillaries, defective cellular metabolism derived from shock interferes further with the body's inherent defenses and metabolic acidosis occurs. The body's normal defense mechanisms are reflex vasoconstriction and increased pulse rate, which tend to redistribute the flow of blood to the heart and brain at the expense of the other vital organs. If shock is promptly recognized, treated, and reversed, permanent damage is avoided. If it progresses to irreversibility, death ensues from cellular dysfunction and organ hypoperfusion.

There are multiple kinds and causes of shock presenting problems in the relationships among the heart, circulatory system, and blood volume. Circulatory inadequacy may originate from a marked decrease in cardiac output, venous return to the heart, or peripheral vascular resistance.

Etiology Loss of circulating volume, loss of pumping power of the heart, or loss of peripheral resistance. Because of the complexity of shock, discussion is brief and addressed to the hypovolemic type.

Hypovolemic Shock Decrease in circulating blood volume from loss of blood, plasma, or extracellular fluid. Excessive fluid loss is greater than compensatory absorption of interstitial fluid into the circulation. Causes: hemorrhage; burns; severe dehydration from vomiting, diarrhea, intestinal obstruction, excessive heat, withholding fluids; metabolic acidosis. Shock resulting from hemorrhage or underestimated blood loss is the type most often seen in the operating room and is usually reversed by prompt restoration of circulating blood volume.

Treatment

1 Fluid-volume replacement. Whole blood, or other intravenous fluid or plasma expander as indicated. In case of hemorrhage, if not previously done, type and cross match blood for transfusion. Hypervolemia must be avoided in replacement.

2 Position. Elevation of the legs may aid venous return and cardiac output except in case of severe oligemia.

3 Temperature. Keep as nearly normal as possible. Keep the patient warm but not overheated as perspiration increases fluid loss.

4 Oxygen. Given when circulation is not delivering enough to the tissues (low pO_2).

5 Drugs. Administered according to the needs of the patient to maintain blood pressure, correct acidosis, protect kidneys from failure.

Venospasm

If caused by cold IV fluid infusion, venospasm may be manifested by very slow flow. It may result from pressure infusion or extravasation. Intravenous procaine relieves spasm. Thrombophlebitis may follow venospasm.

Coronary Thrombosis

This can occur from severe hypoxia and lack of oxygen to coronary vessels. Sometimes its occurrence is the reason for a patient's never regaining consciousness following an operation.

Cardiac Arrhythmias

An alteration of normal cardiac rhythm may decrease cardiac output, exhaust the myocardium, and lead to ventricular fibrillation or cardiac arrest. *Bradycardia* is the slowing of the heart or pulse rate. *Tachycardia* is an excessive rapidity of the heart's action.

Etiology Hypoxia, hypercarbia, acidosis, coronary disease, vagal reflexes, anesthetic agents, toxic doses of epinephrine or other drugs, laryngospasm and coughing initiated by the presence of secretions in the airway following induction. Other causes may be hypotension, hemorrhage, hypovolemia, pneumothorax, mechanical injuries. The most dreaded arrhythmias are:

1 *Ventricular tachycardia.* Rapid heart rate (150 to 200 beats per minute) resulting from ventricular ischemia or irritability, anoxia, or digitalis intoxication. The heart rate does not give time for ventricular filling and the resultant reduced cardiac output predisposes the patient to ventricular fibrillation or cardiac failure. It is treated by prompt intravenous administration of lidocaine or procainamide or intramuscular quinidine. *Synchronized cardioversion* may be used. This is the application of high-intensity, short-duration electrical shock to the chest wall over the heart to produce total cardiac depolarization, i.e., countershock timed to interrupt an abnormal rhythm in the cardiac cycle, thereby permitting resumption of a normal one. Cardioversion is usually applied in instances of nonarrest but nevertheless dangerous arrhythmia. It may be an elective or emergency treatment.

2 *Ventricular fibrillation.* The most serious of all arrhythmias, characterized by total disorganization of ventricular activity. There are rapid and irregular, uncoordinated, random contractions of the small myocardial groups without effective ventricular contraction and cardiac output so that circulation ceases. It is rapidly fatal, since respiratory and cardiac arrest quickly follow, unless successful defibrillation is effected. The patient in fibrillation is unconscious and possibly convulsing from cerebral hypoxia.

Treatment

1 A fast sharp single blow (precordial thump) to the midportion of the sternum (use nipple line as a landmark), delivered with the bottom fleshy part of a closed fist struck from 8 to 12 in. (20 to 30 cm) above the chest. The blow generates a small electrical stimulus in a heart that is reactive, and may be effective in restoring a beat in cases of asystole or recent onset of arrhythmia.

2 Prompt defibrillation by short-duration electrical shock to the heart. This produces simultaneous depolarization of all muscle fiber bundles after which spontaneous beating (conversion to spontaneous normal sinus rhythm) may resume if the myocardium is oxygenated and not acidotic. Defibrillation of an anoxic myocardium is difficult. *The time fibrillation started should be noted.* The electrical shock is coordinated with controlled ventilation and cardiac compression. Cardiopulmonary resuscitation (see CPR, p. 204) begins as soon as the presence of fibrillation is identified.

Defibrillation: Equipment and Technique Necessary equipment for defibrillation includes: defibrillator machine, paddle electrodes, and standard electrode paste or saline-soaked 4 by 4 gauze pads to reduce resistance to passage of electric current offered by the skin. If paste is used on the paddles, it should not extend beyond the electrodes or on any part of the electrode handles. Rapid sponge application provides the advantage that external cardiac compression may be resumed after defibrillation without the hand slipping on the chest. External defibrillation of the heart is used unless the chest is already open, as for intrathoracic operations. For internal defibrillation, sterile electrodes are placed on the myocardium, one over the right atrium, the other over the left ventricle. If these electrodes are gauze-covered, they are dipped in saline before use. Team members must understand the functioning of the defibrillator for the patient's safety and their own.

External paddle positions. (1) Standard position: one electrode is placed just to the right of the upper sternum below the clavicle and the other electrode just to the left of the cardiac apex or left nipple, thus delivering current through the long axis of the heart. The large diameter of the paddles increases the area of skin contact, thus reducing the possibility of skin burns by spreading of the current. Paddles must always be scrupulously clean as foreign material reduces uniformity of shock. (2) Anterior-posterior position: one electrode is placed anteriorly over the precordium, the other posteriorly behind the heart immediately below the left scapula, avoiding the spinal column. This allows for more energy passage through the heart but placement is more difficult.

With the electrodes pressed firmly against the chest wall for good contact, the electrical charge is delivered by the person holding the electrode paddles by pressing a switch on the handle, or a foot switch. The safest method is by switches on both paddles that must be pressed simultaneously for discharge of electric energy. The operator should have dry hands. Some machines require two persons, one to place and hold the paddles, and another to press the switch. A switch that requires another person to discharge the shock is potentially dangerous because the actions of the two persons may not be synchronized. When using a defibrillator, *neither the person holding the electrodes nor anyone else should touch the metal operating table or the patient as the current is applied in order to avoid possible self-electrocution. No part of the operator's body should touch the paste or uninsulated electrodes as well. Warning is given before discharge.* Shock may be repeated at intervals if fibrillation persists.

Myocardial damage resulting from defibrillatory efforts is in direct proportion to the energy used, therefore maximal settings, when not required, may increasingly impair an already damaged myocardium. The energy level delivered through a specific ohm load should be indicated on the front panel of the defibrillator. Delivery output ranges vary with machines. Amount of shock is registered in joules or watt seconds. If the patient's chest muscles do not contract, no current reached the patient. Check the defibrillator's connection to the electrical source and "off" button to the synchronizer. If the machine is battery operated, the battery must be charged enough to energize the capacitor. Be familiar with and follow the directions for the defibrillator that you use.

Adjunct drug therapy is used as necessary: vasopressor-cardiotonic and myocardial stimulant drugs to maintain a useful heartbeat, antiarrhythmic drugs to prevent recurrence, sodium bicarbonate to combat acidosis (see p. 208). Continuous monitoring of the heart and laboratory analysis, such as arterial blood gases, are essential.

Prevention Appropriate preoperative sedation and skillfully administered anesthesia help to avoid hazardous cardiovascular reflexes. As premature ventricular contractions are precursors to fibrillation, in itself a precursor to cardiac arrest, any cardiopulmonary emergency in a prearrest phase requires:

1 *Monitoring of heart rhythm and rate.* Ability to recognize rhythms that precede arrest permits intervention that may prevent arrest. If cardiac status is not under constant monitoring, hypoxia and acidosis may be present and require correction prior to effective use of other therapeutic modalities.

2 *Establishment of an intravenous lifeline.* Venous cannulation provides access to peripheral and central venous circulation for the following purposes: administering drugs and fluids, obtaining venous-blood specimens for laboratory analysis, and inserting catheters into the right heart and pulmonary arteries for physiological monitoring and electrical pacing. Peripheral venipuncture sites: external jugular vein, vein in dorsum of hand or antecubital space, long saphenous vein in leg. Central venipuncture sites: femoral vein, subclavian vein, internal jugular vein. If cardiac arrest appears imminent, or has occurred, cannulation of a peripheral or femoral vein should be attempted first so as not to interrupt cardiopulmonary resuscitation (see p. 204). If the patient is awake, an 18-gauge needle or catheter may be used initially; if unconscious, a 14- or 16-gauge (adult) catheter may be inserted by cutdown and 5% dextrose in water infusion started. If solution is in a plastic bag, squeeze the bag before use to detect a puncture that could permit contamination. No drug should be added to the solution that might be absorbed by the plastic. To keep the infusion open, the rate should be kept low. The usual complications to all intravenous techniques should be guarded against, e.g., hematoma formation, catheter fragment or air embolism, inadvertent entry to an artery, sepsis.

Cardiac Arrest

In cardiac arrest, there is cessation of cardiocirculatory action; the pumping mechanism of the heart ceases. Cardiac standstill represents total absence of electrical cardiac activity, reflected as a straight line on an ECG rhythm strip. It may occur as primary cardiac failure or secondary to failure of pulmonary ventilation. The three types of circulatory arrest are profound vascular collapse, ventricular fibrillation, and ventricular asystole. This may precede or follow failure of the respiratory system since the systems are interrelated.

Etiology A single or combination of factors may precipitate arrest but the general cause is inadequate coronary arterial blood flow. Defective respiratory function produces systemic hypoxemia, causing myocardial hypoxia and depression. It also increases myocardial irritability and the heart's susceptibility to vagal reflexes. Some of the specific precipitating factors are arrhythmias, emboli, extreme hypotension or hypovolemia, respiratory obstruction, aspiration, effects of drugs, anesthetic overdosage, excessively rapid, unsmooth induction, pharyngeal stimulation, metabolic abnormalities (acidosis, toxemia, electrolyte imbalance), poor cardiac filling due to positioning, manipulation of the heart, central nervous system trauma, anaphylaxis, electrical shock.

Symptoms Loss of heart beat and blood pressure; fixed dilated pupils; cyanosis; cold clammy skin; absence of reflexes; unconsciouness in previously conscious patient.

Diagnosis Arrest is readily detected during anesthesia by the absence of blood pressure and precordial heart sounds, and lack of a palpable carotid pulse. Onset of pupillary dilatation is within 45 seconds after cerebral anoxia; full dilatation is reached about 90 to 110 seconds after cessation of cerebral circulation.

Prevention Use of intraoperative electrocardiogram monitoring; use of intravenous lines prior to operation; maintenance of intact airway, adequate oxygenation, and adequate arterial blood pressure; proper timing and judicious use of medications; proper patient positioning; gentle handling of tissues with minimal traction and manipulation, especially in the region of the heart and great vessels; skillful anesthetic administration and testing for sensitivities; optimal preoperative preparation. Hypoxemia of respiratory origin, for which there is no commonly used monitor, is especially hazardous and may be diagnosed too late to permit brain survival.

Incidence Estimated occurrence is 1 in 3400 operations. It may occur during induction, intraoperatively, or postoperatively. Occurrence during cardiac operations or following massive hemorrhage is not uncommon. Patients more prone to arrest include those at age extremes, those with previously diagnosed paroxysmal arrhythmias as well as those with primary cardiovascular abnormalities, or digitalis toxicity. Unexpected arrest is one that happens in a patient of general good health who is undergoing a low-risk or relatively routine procedure. These arrests are associated with major morbidity and mortality.

CARDIOPULMONARY RESUSCITATION

Cardiopulmonary resuscitation (CPR) is aimed at reversing the processes that lead to death. CPR is an emergency procedure requiring special training to recognize arrest and perform artificial ventilation and artificial circulation. Resuscitative measures must be instituted immediately (within 3 to 5 minutes after arrest) to prevent irreversible brain damage. *No time must be lost!* The combination of anoxia and acidosis can make restoration of normal function impossible. Resuscitation is not a one-man job. *The team must be completely familiar with the preplanned routine before the necessity for its use arises.* Success depends on prompt diagnosis and immediate effective treatment. Outcome is directly related to the rapidity with which a functional, spontaneous heart rhythm can be restored. Patients who experience arrest in an operating room may be on monitors with an intravenous line already in place, and resuscitation equipment on hand. These arrests are referred to as *witnessed arrests. Note time of onset of arrest and start the time-elapsed clock.* Basic Life Support is instituted at once with the aim of reestablishing the oxygen system and restoring the heartbeat.

Basic Life Support

The ABCs of resuscitation are:

A Airway: patent, free of secretions or foreign body, for effective pulmonary ventilation
B Breathing: prompt restoration and maintenance of oxygenation through artificial ventilation
C Circulation: provision of oxygen to vital tissues by means of cardiac massage

These methods must be in effect until the patient can resume normal, spontaneous respiration and circulation or until cardiac or central nervous system biological death warrant their discontinuation.

The following discussion presumes the arrested patient to be in the operating room with anesthesiologists and other team members present. In a witnessed arrest, the head is tilted to open the airway and simultaneously the carotid pulse is palpated. If the pulse is absent, a precordial thump on the chest is given. If the patient has respiratory arrest, four quick, full lung inflations are given. If pulse and breathing are not immediately restored, CPR is begun. If the patient is being monitored at the time of arrest, a fast precordial thump is given and the monitor checked for cardiac rhythm while the carotid pulse is checked. If ventricular fibrillation or tachycardia without a pulse is evident, countershock is given as soon as possible. Meanwhile CPR is started. In infants and small children, a hand is placed over the precordium to feel the apical beat in lieu of checking a carotid pulse.

Pulmonary Resuscitation Begun to combat respiratory failure. Immediate opening of the airway is mandatory. If respiratory obstruction is present, it must be cleared. During operation under general anesthesia, either an oro- or nasopharyngeal airway or endotracheal tube is in place to maintain a patent air passage. One hundred percent oxygen can be delivered at once under positive pressure by manual ventilation. If not, ventilation by other means, such as an esophageal obturator airway or expired-air technique, should be initiated to sustain oxygenation, followed by tracheal intubation as soon as possible. A cuffed endotracheal tube permits continual delivery of high-oxygen concentration without hazard of stomach distention or aspiration. It facilitates adequate ventilation since, with its use, interposed breaths are not necessary, thereby permitting a faster, uninterrupted cardiac compression rate of 80 per minute. When a tube or airway is lacking, the most rapid means of reestablishing oxygenation is by an *expired-air technique or mouth-to-mouth or mouth-to-nose artificial ventilation.* When combined with cardiac compression, tissues receive oxygen.

Procedure With the patient on his or her back and airway patent, extend the head backward as far as possible so that the chin is pointed upward. Keep the head in this position to extend the neck and lift the tongue away from the back of the throat.

For *mouth-to-mouth technique,* the mandible may be thrust forward also by placing the fingers of one hand behind the angle of the jaw and pushing it forward. Hold the mouth open with the thumb of this hand by retracting the lower lip. With your other hand, pinch the nostrils together with thumb and index finger while exerting pressure on the forehead to maintain backward tilt (see Fig. 9-1). Pressure of your cheek against the patient's nose to prevent air leakage is an alternative method. Deliver four quick, full lung inflations in rapid succession, tightly sealing your lips over the patient's open mouth for each breath. Take a deep breath, seal your lips over the patient's mouth, and blow forcefully into it, watching for the chest to rise (see Fig. 9-2). Remove your mouth, allowing the patient to exhale passively, while watching for the chest to fall. Repeat this procedure every 5 seconds as necessary. If the chest does not rise, improve the jaw support and head tilt. Also blow more forcefully.

For *mouth-to-nose technique,* lift the patient's lower jaw with one hand, thus sealing the lips, and tilt the patient's head back with the other hand on his or her forehead. Take a deep breath, seal your lips around the nose, and blow into it until you feel the lungs expand. Remove your mouth, allowing passive exhalation. It may be necessary to separate the patient's lips during exhalation for air to escape as the soft palate may cause nasopharyngeal obstruction. Repeat the maneuver every 5 seconds. For infants and children: cover both mouth and nose with your mouth and use smaller breaths (less volume) to inflate the lungs every 3 seconds. Also, do not tilt the head as much since an infant's neck is pliable and air passages may become obstructed.

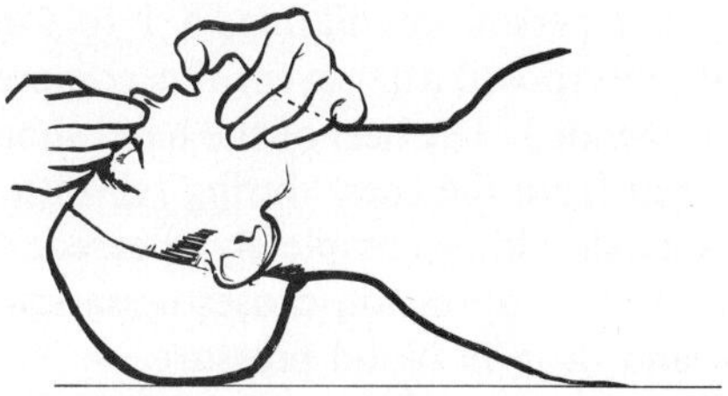

Figure 9-1 Positioning for mouth-to-mouth resuscitation. Patient is supine with neck hyperextended to straighten the airway. Resuscitator pinches nostrils with one hand and elevates the mandible with the other, holding the mouth open with thumb.

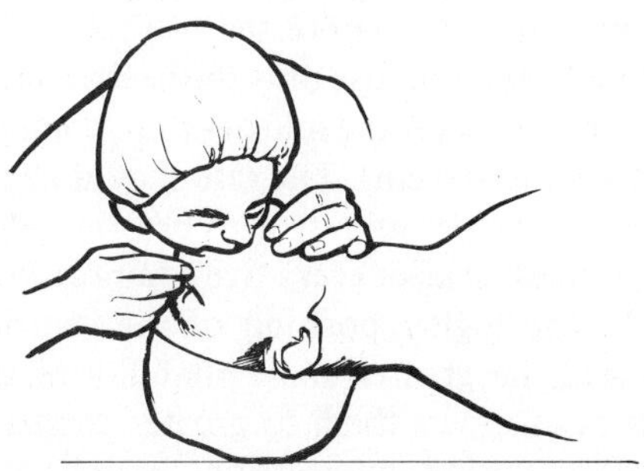

Figure 9-2 Mouth-to-mouth resuscitation. Resuscitator takes a deep breath and, tightly sealing lips over the patient's open mouth, blows forcefully into it, watching for the patient's chest to rise.

Mouth-to-stoma direct ventilation is possible for patients who have a tracheostomy or laryngectomy tube. Delete head tilt or jaw thrust. Seal the mouth and nose with your hand or a tightly fitting face mask to prevent air leakage when you blow into the tube. This problem is prevented if the tube has an inflatable cuff.

Mouth-to-airway technique may be used through either an endotracheal tube or oral airway.

These techniques, except when practiced through an endotracheal tube, carry a risk of inflating the patient's stomach with air, possibly followed by regurgitation of gastric contents. There is also danger of passing infection from patient to resuscitator. The advantages of the method are simplicity and immediate availability.

NOTE. 1. If attempts to ventilate are unsuccessful despite proper opening of airway, further attempts to remove obstruction should be made. Laryngoscopy, cricothyrotomy, or tracheotomy may be indicated.
2. Tracheal suctioning should last no longer than 5 seconds at a time without ventilation.
3. If there is a possibility of a fractured neck due to traumatic injury, extention of the neck is avoided and a modified technique employed.
4. Ventilation is assured by seeing the chest rise and fall, by feeling in your own airway resistance and compliance of the patient's lungs as they expand, by hearing and feeling air escape during the patient's exhalation.
5. In the operating room the anesthesiologist handles artificial ventilation.

Cardiovascular Resuscitation Must accompany ventilation in a pulseless patient to maintain adequate blood pressure and circulation, thereby keeping tissues viable, preserving cardiac tone and reflexes, and preventing intravascular clotting. This may be accomplished by *external* (closed-chest) *cardiac compression,* the rhythmic application of pressure over the lower one-half of the sternum, *except for the xiphoid process.* Since the heart occupies most of the space between the sternum and the thoracic spine, depression of the sternum compresses the ventricles against the spinal column (see Fig. 9-3). In this way, a pulsatile circulation is produced by sending blood into the pulmonary artery and aorta. During relaxation of pressure, the negative, intrathoracic pressure causes venous blood to flow back into the heart from the pulmonary and systemic circulatory systems (see Fig. 9-4). Blood moves in the arterial direction through the heart valves. Carotid artery blood flow from this technique usually is only one-quarter to one-third of normal although systolic blood pressure is raised. Artificial ventilation is *always* required when external cardiac compression is employed as ventilation volumes from compression are inadequate for oxygenation of the blood. The brain and myocardium must be perfused effectively for survival. External cardiac compression must be instituted immediately on cessation of circulation. It must be performed with knowledge and care. Prior manikin practice is recommended.

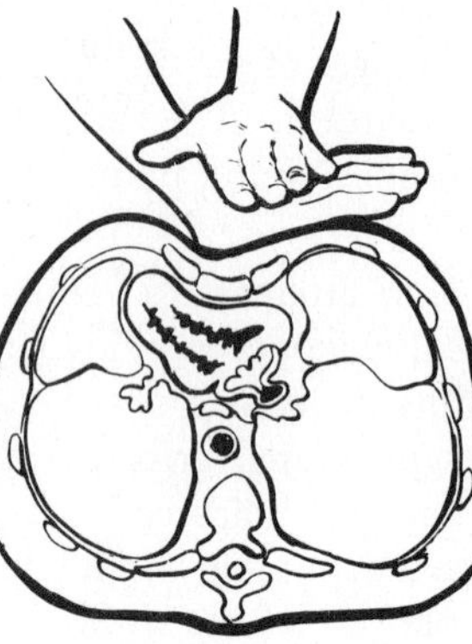

Figure 9-3 Manual depression of the sternum compresses the cardiac ventricles against the spinal column, sending blood into the pulmonary artery and aorta.

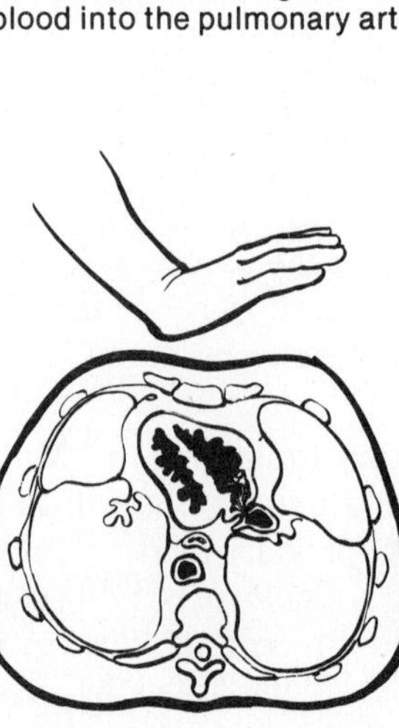

Figure 9-4 Releasing the pressure on the sternum allows the heart to fill with venous blood.

Procedure The patient should lie on a hard flat surface such as the operating table. A bedboard may be needed in other locations. The resuscitator stands or kneels close beside the patient. Place the long axis of the heel of one hand parallel to and over the long axis of the lower half of the sternum about 1 to $1\frac{1}{2}$ in. (2.5 to 4 cm) above the xiphoid process. Place your other hand on top of the first one, parallel to it. The fingers may be interlocked for greater stability, or they should be arched so that the force will not extend to the ribs (see Figs. 9-5 and 9-6). Bring your shoulders directly over the patient's sternum, keeping your arms straight. Using the weight of your shoulders, exert pressure vertically downward to depress the sternum at least $1\frac{1}{2}$ to 2 in. (4 to 5 cm), then release the pressure, allowing the heart to fill with venous blood. Compressions must be smooth, regular, and uninterrupted, not sudden or jerking. Fast jabs can cause injury and do not enhance stroke volume. Compression and relaxation should be of equal duration. Sixty intermittent compressions per minute are recommended in a two-person resuscitation team. With the other person ventilating, a 1 to 5 ratio, one breath interposed after every five compressions, is recommended. The heel of the hand should not be removed from the chest during relaxation but the pressure should be completely released. Any interruption in compression causes cessation of blood flow and drop in blood pressure.

For infants and small children, proceed as follows: For infants, use only the tips of the index and middle fingers to exert pressure over the midsternum, compressing it $\frac{1}{2}$ to $\frac{3}{4}$ in. (1 to 2 cm). Or, an infant's chest can be encircled with the hands and the midsternum compressed with both thumbs. For small children, use only the heel of one hand to exert pressure over the midsternum, compressing it $\frac{3}{4}$ to $1\frac{1}{2}$ in. (2 to 4 cm). The rate should be 80 to 100 compressions per minute with breaths delivered as fast as possible after every five compressions (1 to 5 ratio). The higher position of the ventricles and liver and the greater chest pliability of these patients predisposes them to greater danger of liver laceration during compression. Since backward tilt of their heads also lifts their backs, a firm back support can be provided by the resuscitator's putting one hand beneath a child's back while compressing the chest with the other hand. A folded blanket beneath the shoulders provides support.

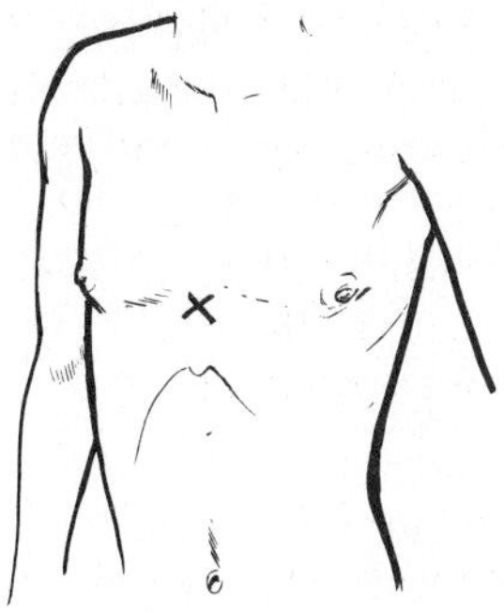

Figure 9-5 The cross indicates the correct spot to place the hands for performing closed-chest cardiac massage—over the lower third of the sternum, but above the xiphoid process.

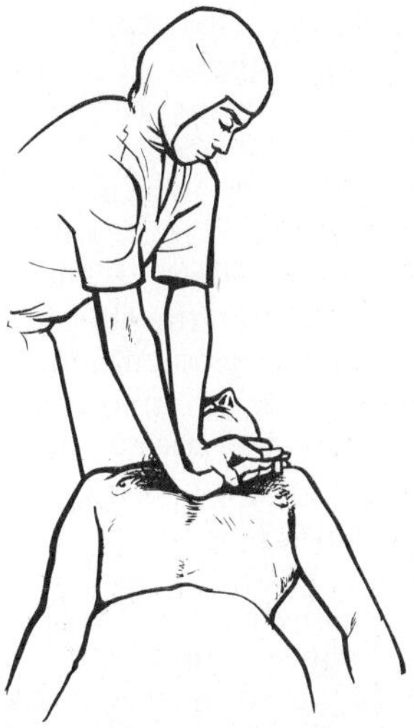

Figure 9-6 Closed chest cardiac massage. Patient is supine on a hard flat surface. Resuscitator places the heel of one hand over the lower third of the sternum, the heel of the other hand on top of it. The fingers are arched upward so as not to exert any force on the ribs.

Basic life support should not be interrupted for more than 5 seconds at a time. If intubation is difficult, the patient must be ventilated between short attempts.

Elevation of the legs to a 60° angle with the trunk aids venous return. Cardiac compression is successful only if the heart fills with blood between compressions and the resuscitator can move an adequate volume of oxygenated blood. The carotid pulse is checked every few minutes to indicate compression effectiveness or return of spontaneous effective heartbeat.

Manual cardiac pumping causes fatigue leading to variation in cardiac output; therefore it is preferable to have alternate resuscitators. Commercially available, manually operated mechanical chest compressors or automatic compressor-ventilators that provide simultaneous compression and ventilation eliminate this problem. When such devices are used, *compression must always be started with the manual method first.* Compressor-ventilators should be used only with a cuffed endotracheal tube or mask, and only by experienced operators.

Complications of external compression are minimized by careful attention to detail. Compression must be performed with extreme caution to prevent injuries such as: rib or sternal fracture; costochondral separation; fat embolism; intercostal muscle hemorrhage; rupture, laceration, or hematoma of liver or spleen; lung contusion; pneumothorax, hemothorax, hemopericardium; rupture of vena cava. *Never compress the xiphoid process at the tip of the sternum or exert pressure on the ribs to prevent fractures.*

Internal Cardiac Compression Instituted if the patient's chest is already open as during a cardiothoracic procedure. Thoracotomy may be performed and internal compression administered in some rare instances where external compression may be ineffective, e.g., internal thoracic injuries such as penetrating wounds of the heart, flail chest, pericardial tamponade due to hemorrhage, chest or spinal deformities. Internal compression may be used if the patient is salvable. The advantage of internal compression is a constantly high blood outflow. Disadvantages are delay in compression, potential contusion of the heart, lack of sterility to save time.

Procedure If the chest is not already open, incision is made through the left fifth intercostal space and the pericardial sac is opened to permit direct manual cardiac compression. A rib spreader is placed to avoid strangulation of the operator's hands. By cradling the heart in the hands, the ventricles are compressed between the thumb and fingers of one hand or the fingers of both hands 60 to 80 times a minute. The heart should not be bruised to avoid impairment of myocardial function. Adequate venous filling is necessary for adequate ventricular stroke volume. The same definitive therapy applies as for external cardiac compression.

Checking Effectiveness of CPR Signs suggestive of effective compression are constricted reactive pupils; palpable peripheral pulse; audible heart beat; improvement in color of mucous membranes, skin, blood. Additional signs indicative of potential recovery are prompt return of spontaneous respiration and consciousness. Continuous compression is stopped when arterial blood pressure remains above 70 to 90 mm of mercury and a strong spontaneous pulse is resumed. It may be performed intermittently as necessary to assist the restored heart.

Persistent dilatation of pupils and lack of reaction to light are ominous signs usually indicative of brain damage. Cell destruction is also manifested by convulsions, hyperpyrexia, and persistent coma. Survival in relation to these symptoms is usually accompanied by tragic consequences such as decerebration or paralysis. Serial electroencephalograms are valuable in determination of degree of damage or improvement.

If oxygenation and sternal compression (basic life support) do not promptly produce spontaneous cardiac action, additional supportive therapy is also used (advanced life support).

Advanced Life Support

This consists of definitive therapy: supplemental oxygen administration, intravenous fluid or intravenous drug therapy, and defibrillation. Continual electrocardiogram and supplemental monitoring are essential.

Compression is usually accompanied or followed by the judicious use of *intravenous drugs* to manipulate cardiovascular variables to benefit the patient's cardiorespiratory status. The various drugs correct hypoxia, correct metabolic acidosis, increase perfusion pressure during cardiac compression, stimulate spontaneous or more forceful myocardial contraction, accelerate cardiac rate, suppress abnormal ventricular activity, treat pulmonary edema. Controversy continues concerning the use of potent vasoconstrictors in treatment of hypotension because of the possibility of ischemic damage to organs associated with their use. Patients who do not respond to one catecholamine often respond to another. The important factor in optimal therapy is the prompt recognition of the causes of hypotension, shock, and cardiac arrest and the prompt correction of reversible precipitants. A number of agents are discussed below.

1 *Oxygen:* administered immediately by inhalation. In arrest, numerous factors contribute to severe hypoxemia. Oxygen raises arterial-oxygen tension, increases arterial-oxygen content, and improves tissue oxygenation. Efficient ventilation combats respiratory acidosis. Supplemental oxygen is needed because mouth-to-mouth ventilation delivers only 16 to 17 percent oxygen and external cardiac compression provides a cardiac output only 30 percent of predicted normal.

2 *Sodium bicarbonate:* an antacid to counteract metabolic acidosis generated during anaerobic metabolism. The extent of metabolic acidosis is dependent on the time interval between arrest, initiation of CPR and supplemental oxygen, and resumption of cardiac function. As a result of acidosis in arrest, myocardial contractility is impaired, reducing response to countershock; myocardial irritability is enhanced so fibrillation threshold is lowered; myocardium will not respond to catecholamines. Blood gas and pH determinations should be obtained to guide antacid therapy. Catecholamines should not be injected with the bicarbonate because the high pH inactivates the catecholamine.

3 *Epinephrine (Adrenalin):* an endogenous catecholamine with both alpha- and beta-receptor stimulating actions. By vasoconstriction, in the face of acidosis, it helps maintain cerebral and myocardial blood supply. It elevates perfusion pressure produced during cardiac compression, improves myocardial contractility, stimulates spontaneous contractions during ventricular standstill, and increases myocardial tone so that defibrillation is more effective. Intracardiac injection may be given but the intravenous route is preferred to prevent the potential complications of heart injection such as myocardial laceration. Epinephrine may be useful in treatment of asystole, allowing electric energy to be converted to mechanical energy.

4 *Atropine:* reduces vagal tone, enhances atrioventricular conduction, increases cardiac output, and accelerates cardiac rate in cases of sinus bradycardia. It is used to treat severe bradycardia particularly in the presence of hypotension (potentially lethal because of grossly impaired cardiac output).

5 *Lidocaine (Xylocaine):* commonly used for management of cardiac arrhythmias, especially those of ventricular origin. It is valuable in instances where successful defibrillation reverts back repeatedly to ventricular fibrillation.

6 *Morphine:* an analgesic used in myocardial infarction, it also is employed for treatment of acute pulmonary edema. Morphine pools blood peripherally and decreases venous return to assist in relieving pulmonary congestion and in decreasing myocardial oxygen requirement.

7 *Calcium chloride:* useful in profound cardiovascular collapse, it increases myocardial contractility, enhances ventricular excitability, and prolongs systole. Calcium gluconate or other calcium salt may be used. Calcium cannot be given together with sodium bicarbonate as a precipitate forms from the mixture.

8 *Norepinephrine or levarterenol (Levophed):* a naturally occurring catecholamine with some actions similar to epinephrine. It is a potent peripheral vasoconstrictor so is useful in peripheral vascular collapse, such as hypotension or cardiogenic shock. It elevates blood pressure.

9 *Metaraminol (Aramine):* a sympathomimetic amine that increases cardiac output, systolic and diastolic blood pressure. It produces marked vasoconstriction and is used to treat hypotension, but not during arrest.

10 *Isoproterenol hydrochloride (Isuprel):* increases cardiac output and heart rate and is useful for profound bradycardia resulting from complete heart block. A potent cardiac stimulant, it is contraindicated when tachycardia is present.

11 *Propranolol hydrochloride (Inderal):* useful in instances of repetitive ventricular fibrillation or tachycardia where rhythmic heart beat was not achieved with lidocaine or other agents. It is hazardous when cardiac function is depressed.

12 *Corticosteroids (synthetics):* may be used for prompt treatment of cardiogenic shock or shock lung as complication of arrest, or cerebral edema following arrest.

13 *Dopamine hydrochloride (Intropin):* a chemical precursor of epinephrine that occurs naturally. It dilates renal and mesenteric blood vessels in doses that may not increase heart rate or blood pressure. Its actions differ with dosage and it has both alpha- and beta-receptor stimulating actions. Cardiogenic shock is an indication for use. It may cause tachycardia. It is inactivated in alkaline solution so must not be added to sodium bicarbonate. It will maintain urinary output by increasing renal blood flow, and increase blood pressure due to peripheral vasoconstriction.

14 *Procainamide hydrochloride (Pronestyl):* useful in suppressing premature ventricular contractions and recurrent ventricular tachycardia not controlled by lidocaine. Electrocardiogram and blood pressure must be carefully monitored as marked hypotension may ensue.

15 *Furosemide (Lasik) and ethacrynic acid (Edecrin):* potent diuretics useful in treating postarrest cerebral or acute pulmonary edema. Dehydration and blood volume depletion leading to circulatory collapse must be guarded against.

In summary, the first seven agents listed are the ones most commonly used during CPR. The following eight may be employed for definitive therapy, primarily after resuscitation. Vasoconstrictors improve tissue perfusion by maintaining perfusion pressure, prevent or diminish blood loss, decrease tissue vascularity, and improve coronary blood flow. Among indications for use are anesthetic overdose, hypotension associated with blood loss, adrenergic insufficiency. Vasodilators improve tissue perfusion, prevent or diminish blood loss, and decrease myocardial oxygen demand. Indications for use are regional perfusion for hypo- or hyperthermia, controlled hypotension during operation, hypertensive crises such as renal failure, impaired cardiac performance such as ischemic heart disease.

Nurses' Responsibilities

During cardiopulmonary resuscitation, the nurses on the team must remain calm and give fast alert assistance.

1 *Circulating nurse.* Start time-elapsed clock and record time of arrest. Provide and prepare necessary equipment, including ECG and defibrillator. Keep the room quiet and free from confusion. One person, usually the anesthesiologist, commands resuscitation efforts with support from surgeons and other available professional personnel. Resuscitation teams are multidisciplinary.
   - **a** An *emergency cart* should be available at all times, including defibrillator, paste, electrodes, ECG monitor and recording sheets, endotracheal equipment, intravenous solutions and tubings, stopcocks, cutdown tray, angiocatheters, tourniquet, alcohol swabs, armboard, drapes, sutures, sterile sponges, sterile gloves, airways, Ambu bag, face mask, pharyngeal suction, flashlight, hemostat, cardiac pacemaker, syringes and needles, medications. Many frequently used emergency drugs such as diluted epinephrine, lidocaine, and sodium bicarbonate are in commercially prepared, sterile, prefilled syringes to avoid delay in preparation. Drugs other than those listed on page 208 are potassium, digitalis preparations, amobarbital, aminophylline, Benadryl, Narcan, diazepam. Specific drugs and equipment will vary from hospital to hospital depending on how well equipped the anesthesiologist is for emergencies.
   - **b** Help with and observe intravenous and monitoring lines.
   - **c** Keep a record of all medications given: time and amount.

2 *Scrub nurse.* Give attention to the field and surgeon's needs. Keep syringes of medications filled and ready for use. Keep track of sponges. If arrest occurs during operation, when the chest is not open, the wound is packed and the patient repositioned as necessary for CPR. If the wound can be rapidly closed during resuscitation, this may be done.

CPR Duration Cardiopulmonary resuscitation may be done as long as necessary to restore cardiocirculatory function if adequate ventilation and good peripheral pulse have been restored. It is not uncommon for arrest to reoccur following successful resuscitation. The time frame for survival is shortened drastically if the arrest is unwitnessed. When the patient's condition is adequately stabilized, and the wound closed, he or she is transferred to the intensive care unit.

Postresuscitation Care Postarrest supportive therapy depends on the etiology and duration of arrest. Care centers on maintenance of circulation and ventilation, and minimizing of sequelae, such as cerebral edema. The patient must be carefully monitored and closely observed for 48 to 72 hours postarrest. In select patients, hypothermia may be used to reduce oxygen needs. Vital signs, acid-base and electrolyte balances, and urinary output are closely watched. The patient is observed for signs of embolism, pulmonary edema, fractured ribs, or hemopericardium. A chest x-ray is taken as soon as feasible after arrest. An intravenous fluid lifeline must be left in place. If there is evident cerebral damage, the prognosis is guarded.

ANESTHESIA OF THE FUTURE

Any new anesthetic should:

1 Be nonexplosive
2 Be nonirritating to the respiratory tract
3 Have a low incidence of nausea and vomiting
4 Be nondamaging to any organ system
5 Not produce cardiac arrhythmias

Today's research is tomorrow's practice. The search for new anesthetic drugs tailored to suppress only selected cells continues.

Research is also addressed to the development and refinement of processes for continuing automatic assessment of many vital functions. Patient and personnel safety in the operating room remains a vital concern.

Chapter 10

Positions

PRELIMINARY CONSIDERATIONS

Proper positioning of the patient for operation is a facet of patient care that is as important as adequate preoperative preparation and safe anesthesia in regard to patient outcome. It requires knowledge of anatomy and application of physiologic principles as well as familiarity with the necessary equipment.

Position for operation is determined by the procedure to be performed, with consideration of the surgeon's choice of surgical approach, and of anesthetic administration technique. Factors such as age, height, and weight also influence position. See Chapter 26 for positioning and restraining of pediatric patients.

Responsibility

The choice of position for operation is made by the surgeon in consultation with the anesthesiologist and adjustments made as necessary for anesthesia. The responsibility for placing the patient in the operative position is that of the circulating nurse, with guidance, approval, and sometimes assistance of the anesthesiologist and the surgeon or assistant. In essence, it is a shared responsibility among these team members. In cases of complex positioning or obese, heavy patients, the nurse will need help in lifting and/or positioning the patient.

Time

The patient is usually supine, on his or her back face up, after transfer from the stretcher to the operating table. The patient may be anesthetized in this position and then positioned for operation, or may be positioned and then anesthetized. Factors influencing the time at which the patient is positioned are: site of operation, age and size of patient, anesthetic administration technique, pain upon moving if the patient is conscious.

Safety Measures

The safety measures included in Chapter 8 also apply while positioning patients. These include:

1 The patient must be properly identified when transferred to the operating table and the operative site affirmed.

2 The table must be securely locked in position with the brake applied, when the patient is on it and during transfer to and from the table.

3 The anesthesiologist guards the patient's head at all times and supports it during movement.

4 A physician assumes responsibility for protecting an unsplinted fracture during any movement.

5 If an armboard is in use, it must be guarded. Do not hyperextend the arm or dislodge infusion needle.

6 Anesthetized patients and the aged must be moved slowly and gently to allow the circulatory system to adjust.

7 If a patient is on his or her back, the ankles and legs must not be crossed, which would create pressure on blood vessels and nerves.

8 If a patient is on his or her side, a pillow must be placed lengthwise between the legs to prevent pressure on blood vessels.

9 If a patient is prone, the thorax must be relieved of pressure to facilitate respiration.

10 Adequate assistance in lifting patients and constant vigilance are necessary to prevent falls.

11 The position should not obstruct tubings (catheter, intravenous, etc.).

12 The patient is not moved without permission of the anesthesiologist.

Preparations for Positioning

Before the patient is brought into the operating room the circulating nurse should:

1 Review the proposed position by referring to the procedure book and surgeon's preference card

2 Ask for assistance if unsure of how to position patient

3 Consult the surgeon as soon as he or she arrives if the nurse is not sure which position is to be used

4 Assemble the necessary equipment so as to expedite the procedure

CRITERIA FOR POSITIONING

The ability to tolerate the stresses of operation depends greatly on the normality of functioning of vital systems. Criteria that must be met for proper positioning are:

Maximum Safety and Comfort

This is the most important criterion and the sum total of all others. The physical condition of the patient must be considered. Proper body alignment is important.

No Interference with Respiration

Unhindered diaphragmatic movement and a patent airway are essential to maintain respiratory function, to prevent hypoxia, and to facilitate induction by inhalation. There should be no constriction about the neck or chest. Patients' arms should be at their sides, on armboards, or otherwise supported, not crossed on the chest.

No Interference with Circulation

Adequate circulation is necessary to maintain blood pressure, to facilitate venous return, to prevent thrombus formation, and to prevent circulatory disturbances. There must be no pressure on blood vessels. Body support and restraining straps must not be fastened too tightly.

No Pressure on Any Nerves

Prolonged pressure to or stretching of peripheral nerves can result in serious injury or paralysis. Extremities as well as the body must be well supported at all times. Appliances, restraints, and equipment in contact with skin must be well-padded. Most frequent sites of injury are divisions of the brachial plexus and the ulnar, radial, peroneal, and facial nerves. Extremes of position of the head and arm easily cause injury to the brachial plexus. The ulnar, radial, and peroneal nerves may be compressed against bone, stirrups, or operating table if the patient is improperly positioned. Femoral nerve injury may be caused by retractors during pelvic procedures. Facial nerve injury may result from too vigorous a manual effort to elevate the mandible to maintain airway, or from too tight a head strap.

Accessibility of Operative Site

The operative procedure determines the position in which the patient is placed. The surgeon must have adequate exposure to minimize trauma and operating time.

Accessibility for Anesthetic Administration

The anesthesiologist must be able to attach monitoring electrodes, administer anesthesia, observe its effects, and maintain an intravenous lifeline.

No Undue Postoperative Discomfort

Strain on muscles results in injury and/or needless postoperative discomfort. An anesthetized patient lacks protective muscle tone. If a patient's head is extended for a prolonged time he or she may suffer more pain from a resulting stiff neck than from the operative wound.

Individual Requirements Met

If a patient is extremely obese, for example, with torso occupying the table width, his or her arms may be placed on armboards. Patients with arthritis deformans need special individualized care. An obstetric patient at term or a cardiac patient may experience dyspnea when lying flat.

EQUIPMENT FOR POSITIONING

Operating Table

Many different tables with suitable attachments are in use. Practice is necessary to master adjustments. The tables are versatile and adaptable to a number of diversified positions for all surgical specialties. However, orthopaedic and urinary tables are utilized frequently for specialized procedures. Most tables consist of a rectangular metal top that rests on an electric or hydraulic lift base. Some models have interchangeable tops for the various specialties. The table top is divided into three or more hinged sections. Basically, these are the head, body, and leg sections. Each can be manipulated. These individual sections can be flexed or extended so that the desired position can be attained. This procedure is often called *breaking the table,* and the joints of the table referred to as *breaks.* Some tables have a metal crossbar or body elevator between the two upper sections that may be used as a gallbladder or kidney elevator when raised. Tables may be tilted laterally from side to side, raised or lowered in their entirety. The head section is removable, permitting insertion of special headrests for cranial procedures. An extension may be inserted at the foot of the table to accommodate an exceptionally tall patient. Some tables are electrically controlled; movement of others is manual. All have a brake for stabilization. A tiltometer indicates the degree of tilt between horizontal and vertical, of use when spinal anesthesia is used. An x-ray penetrable tunnel top extending the length of the table permits the insertion of an x-ray cassette holder at any area. A self-adhering, conductive rubber mattress covers the table top.

Special Equipment and Table Attachments

Equipment used in positioning is designed to stabilize the patient in the desired position, thus permitting optimal exposure of the operative area. All attachments that come into contact with skin must be well-padded to prevent trauma or abrasion.

Safety Belt (sometimes called *knee strap*) A sturdy, wide strap of conductive material, such as nylon webbing or conductive rubber, is placed over the legs, around the table top, and fastened to restrain leg movement. Some straps are attached at each side of the table and fastened together at the center. This strap or belt must be secure but not so tight as to impair circulation. It is used during all inductions and during operation except for certain positions, e.g., lithotomy. Placement depends on body position, e.g., above the knees for supine (also known as dorsal), and below the knees for prone.

Anesthesia Screen A metal bar that holds the drapes from the patient's face and separates the nonsterile area from the sterile area. It is adjustable, allowing rotation or angling in any plane. It is placed after induction and positioning of patient.

Wrist or Arm Strap Narrow conductive strap placed around the wrist to secure the hand and arm to an armboard or to the table at the patient's side for protection. Hands must never be placed under body areas as compression results.

Arm Band (also known as *lift sheet*) Two large, separate layers of broad, heavy linen, stitched vertically through the middle. It is placed horizontally across the table on top of the clean sheet before the patient is transferred. The arms are enclosed in the lower flaps and the upper flaps brought down over the arms and tucked under the mattress. In this way the full length of the arm is supported at the patient's side, protected from injury, and restrained. It should be applied just before induction. The patient can be told it is to keep his arms comfortable on the table when he is asleep and relaxed. The word "restraint" is avoided.

Armboard Used to support an arm not resting at the patient's side. It is used when: giving intravenous infusions; the arm or hand is site of operation; the arm at the side would interfere with access to the operative area; there is not adequate room on the table for the arm; the arm on the unaffected side requires support (lateral position).

NOTE. For operation on an arm or hand, an adjustable *extremity table* may be used in lieu of an armboard. It is slipped under the mattress at one end. The other end of the table is supported by a metal leg (similar to a Mayo stand). By removing the top panel, a solution drain pan may be fit into the table top. After the skin prep or irrigation, the pan is removed and the top panel reinserted. A conductive foam-rubber pad is placed and covered to receive the arm, which is then draped. The table provides a large, firm surface for operation.

Double Armboard Supports both arms, one directly above the other (lateral position).

Elbow Pads or Protectors Padded linen may be used to protect the elbows from pressure. A hard plastic shell with soft liner is commercially available.

Shoulder Bridge (*thyroid elevator*) A metal bar, which can be raised or lowered, is slipped onto the table under the mattress between the head and body sections by temporarily removing the head section. It is used to hyperextend the shoulder or thyroid area for operative accessibility.

Shoulder Braces or Supports Adjustable, concave metal pieces well-padded with foam rubber or conductive rubber are used to prevent the patient from slipping toward the head of the table when in Trendelenburg position. Braces should be placed equidistant from the head of the table with a $\frac{1}{2}$ in. (13 mm) space between the shoulders and the braces to eliminate pressure against the shoulders. A shoulder brace is not used when an arm is extended on an armboard to avoid nerve compression.

Shoulder Roll A solid roll of cloth placed under each side of the patient's chest to raise it off the table to facilitate respiration. This type of equipment may be referred to as a *bolster*.

Elevating Pads Pads used to elevate a specific part of the body (hyperextend spine for laminectomy).

NOTE. Commercially available bolsters and elevating pads are commonly used. They are covered with conductive materials.

Body Rests or Braces Metal brace with a foam-rubber pad covered with conductive rubber is placed in metal clamps on the side of the table and slipped in from the table edge against the body at various points to stabilize it (lateral position).

Kidney Rests Concave metal pieces with grooved notches at the base. They are placed under the mattress on the body elevator (part of the table) and slipped in from the table edge snugly against the body to stabilize it in kidney position. Be careful that the upper edge of the rest does not press too tightly against the body, even though padded.

Body-Restraint Strap A belt, the center portion of which is a pad to protect the skin, is placed over the patient and secured by hooks to the sides of the table. This strap helps to hold the patient securely in position.

Hemorrhoid Strap Made of a piece of 3-in. (7.5 cm) adhesive 6 in. (15 cm) in length with a buckle and canvas strap on one end. A hemorrhoid strap is placed on each buttock, 4 in. (10 cm) lateral to the operative site, to separate the buttocks. Each strap is fastened to the table frame at the side (Kraske position).

Adjustable Arch Bar Consists of two padded rolls mounted on a frame. The rolls extend from the shoulders to the knees. The patient is placed on the abdomen on this arch. The degree of flexion desired for thoracic or lumbar vertebral operations is achieved by adjusting the height of the arch by means of a lever.

Stirrups Metal stirrup posts are placed in holders, one on each side of the table to support the legs and feet in lithotomy position. The feet are supported by canvas loops, thus suspending the legs at a right angle to the feet. During extensive surgery, special leg holders supporting the lower legs may be used.

NOTE. Metal knee-crutch stirrups are available. Even if well-padded, they create some pressure on the back of the knees and lower extremity, jeopardizing popliteal vessel and nerve. This is avoided with the canvas-sling stirrups.

Metal Footboard It can be left flat as a horizontal extension of the table or raised perpendicular to the table to support the feet, the soles resting securely against it. It must be padded for reverse Trendelenburg position.

Special Padded Headrests and Attachments Available for neurosurgical procedures, headrests attach to the table, supporting and exposing the occiput and cervical vertebrae. They are used with supine, prone, sitting, or unilateral position.

Pillows (Soft or Hard) and Sandbags Various sizes and shapes to fit anatomic structures are used to support or immobilize parts. A doughnut-shaped sandbag may be used for procedures on the head and face. It is about 10 in. (25 cm) in diameter with a 3-in. (7.5 cm) hole in the center, in which the occiput rests. It keeps the operative area in a horizontal plane. The sandbags (positioning weights) and pillows are covered with washable, conductive rubber.

Surgical Positioning System* A convenient, efficient, comfortable means of patient positioning that eliminates sandbags, bolsters, and adhesive tape. Soft pads filled with tiny plastic beads are put under or around the body part to be supported and the patient is placed in operative position. Suction is attached to the pad and, as air is withdrawn, the pad becomes firm. During air evacuation, the circulating nurse and her assistant mold the pad to the body area with their hands. The suction is disconnected. With vacuum inside the pad, the surrounding atmospheric pressure presses the beads together and friction between them prevents their moving, creating a solid mass that keeps its molded shape. Various sizes and shapes of pads provide firm, yet pressure-point relieving support for many procedures. Slip-on conductive pad covers are used. To change a patient's position during operation, the valve on the pad is squeezed until the pad is slightly soft. The patient is repositioned, and suction to the pad is reapplied as the latter is remolded.

OPERATIVE POSITIONS

Many positions for operation are used. Only the most commonly employed ones are included. If IV fluids will be infused in the arm during the operation, an arm will be on an armboard. This fact is assumed in the following discussion because IV fluids are usually given.

Supine Position (Also Known as Dorsal Position)

See Figure 10-1. This is the most natural position for the body at rest. Patient lies flat on the back with arms secured at the sides, palms down. The legs are straight and parallel, in line with the head and spine. The hips are parallel with the spine. The safety belt is placed above the knees. Small pillows may be placed under the head and the lumbar curvature. Heels must be protected from pressure on the table by a pillow, ankle roll, or doughnut. The feet must not be in prolonged plantar flexion. The soles may be supported by a pillow or padded footboard to prevent footdrop. The position is used for procedures on the anterior surface of the body such as abdominal, abdominothoracic, or some lower extremity procedures.

Modifications of supine position are used:

Position 1 For procedures on the *face* or *neck*. The neck may be slightly hyperextended by lowering the head section of the table or by placing a narrow pad between the scapulae. With the patient in supine position, the head may be supported in a headrest or doughnut and/or turned toward the unaffected side. The eyes must be protected from injury or irritating solutions. They should be kept closed, and eye pads taped in place during skin preparation and operation. They should be inspected at the end of the operative procedure.

Position 2 For *shoulder* or *anterolateral* procedures. The patient is in supine position with the affected side elevated. A small sandbag, roll, or pad is placed under the shoulder to elevate it off the table for exposure. The length of the body must be stabilized to prevent rolling or twisting of the spine. Hips and shoulders should be kept in a plane.

Position 3: Dorsal Recumbent Used for vaginal examination. The patient is in supine position except that the knees are flexed and thighs externally rotated. Soles of feet rest on the table. Pillows may be placed under knees if needed for support.

Position 4: Modified Recumbent See Figure 10-2. Used for saphenous ligation or operation in the region of the groin. The patient is in supine position except that the knees are *slightly* flexed with a pillow beneath each. Thighs are externally rotated.

Position 5: Arm-Extension Used for radical mastectomy, axillary dissection, upper extremity or hand operation. The patient is in supine position with the arm on the affected side on an armboard that locks into position at a right angle to the body. The affected side of the body must be close to the table edge for access to operative area. If the axilla is involved, the arm is even with the lower edge of the armboard for accessibility.

*Vac-Pac, Olympic Medical Corporation, Seattle, Wash.

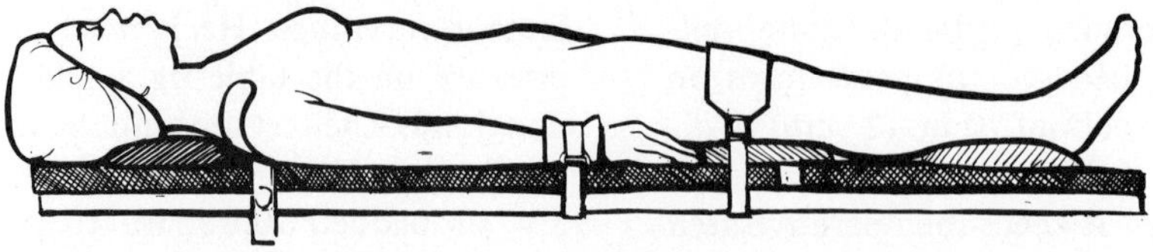

Figure 10-1 Supine position. The patient lies in a straight position on back, face upward, with arms at sides, the legs extended parallel and uncrossed, the feet slightly separated. Strap is placed above the knees. The head is in line with the spine. Note small pillow supporting feet to prevent foot drop.

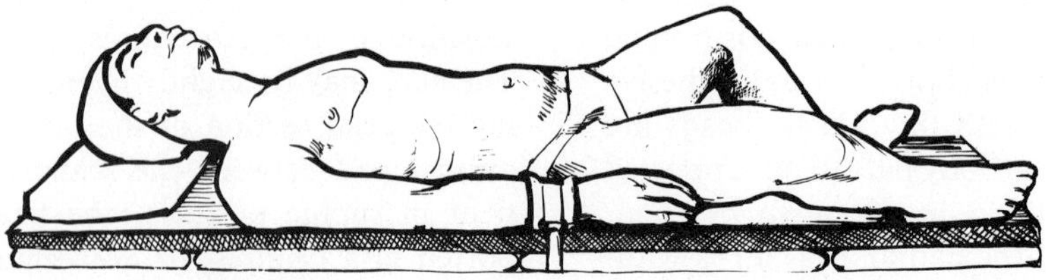

Figure 10-2 Modified recumbent position. The patient lies on back with arms at sides. The knees are slightly flexed, with a small pillow under each. Thighs are externally rotated.

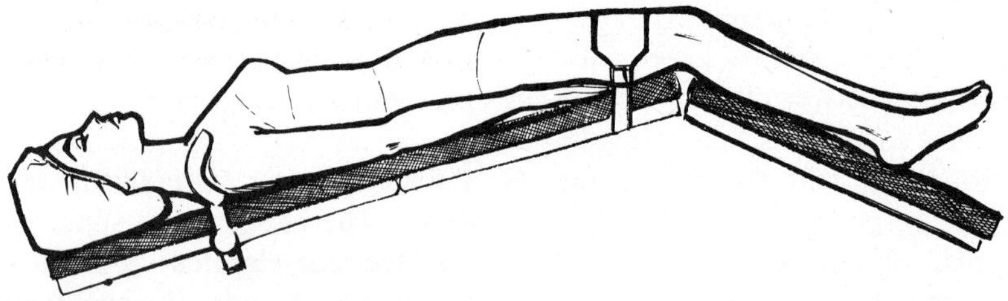

Figure 10-3 Trendelenburg position. Note that the knees are over the lower break in the table, knee strap is above the knees, and shoulder braces are in place.

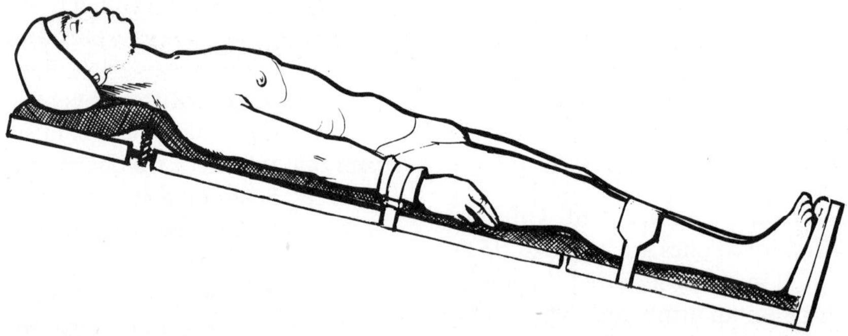

Figure 10-4 Reverse Trendelenburg position. The patient lies on the back. The footboard is padded and raised. The entire table is tilted so the head is higher than the feet. The strap is above the knees. Note operative area is over the raised thyroid elevator on the table.

Hyperextension of the arm must be avoided to prevent neural or vascular injury such as brachial plexus injury or occlusion of the axillary artery. The armboard must be well-padded.

Trendelenburg Position

See Figure 10-3. The patient lies on the back with knees over the lower break of the table. The knees must bend with the table break to prevent pressure on the peroneal nerves and veins in the legs. Shoulder braces are applied. The entire table is tilted downward about 45° at the head, depending upon the surgeon's wish. The foot of the table is lowered the desired amount. It is used for procedures in the lower abdomen or pelvis in which it is desirable to tilt the abdominal viscera away from the pelvic area for better exposure. The patient is left in this position for as short a time as possible. While increasing operative accessibility, lung volume is decreased by pressure of the organs against the diaphragm. In returning to horizontal position, *the leg section should be raised first and slowly* while reversing venous status in the legs. Then the entire table is leveled. A modification of the position is used for patients in hypovolemic shock. Many anesthesiologists prefer to keep the trunk level and elevate the legs by raising the lower part of the table at the break under the hips. Others prefer to tilt the entire table downward. Either position reduces venous stasis in the lower extremities.

Reverse Trendelenburg Position

See Figure 10-4. The patient lies on his or her back. The mattress is adjusted so the operative area is over the elevator bridge on the table. The entire table is tilted so that the head is higher than the feet. A padded footboard may be used, depending on the degree of tilt. The position is used for thyroidectomy to facilitate breathing and to decrease the blood supply to the operative area (blood will pool caudally). It is used also for gallbladder or biliary-tract procedures to allow abdominal viscera to fall away from the epigastrium, giving access to the upper abdomen. Small pillows may be placed under the knee and lumbar curvature. A small pillow or doughnut may stabilize the head. If an elevator bridge is not used, the operative area may be hyperextended by a pad.

Fowler's Position

The patient lies on his or her back with knees over the lower break in the table. The footboard is raised and padded. The foot of the table is lowered slightly, flexing the knees. The body section of the table is raised 45°, thereby becoming the backrest. Arms rest on a large, soft pillow on the lap. The safety belt is above the knees. The entire table is tilted slightly head downward to prevent the patient's slipping caudad. Used for cranial procedures with the head supported in a headrest.

Sitting (Upright) Position

The patient is positioned as for Fowler's except that the torso is in an upright position. The shoulders and torso should be supported with body straps but not so tight as to impede respiration and circulation. Pressure points must be well-padded. Flexed arms rest on a large pillow on the lap or on a pillow on an adjustable table in front of the patient. The head is in a cranial headrest for neurosurgical procedures. An antigravity suit is used to counteract postural hypotension. This position is used for some otorhinology procedures.

Lithotomy Position

See Figure 10-5. Cotton boots are put on the patient's legs prior to transfer to the operating table. The patient's buttocks rest along the break between the body and leg sections of the table. Stirrups are secured in the holders on each side of the table. They must be adjusted at equal height on both sides of the table and at an appropriate height for the length of the patient's legs to maintain symmetry when the patient is positioned. After the patient is anesthetized, the legs are raised simultaneously by two persons. Each grasps the sole of a foot in one hand and supports the knee area with the other. The feet are then placed in the canvas slings of the stirrups. One loop of canvas encircles the sole and the other loop goes around the ankle. Simultaneous movement is essential as the knees are flexed to avoid straining the lower back. If legs are properly placed, undue abduction and external rotation are avoided. There must be no pressure of the lower leg or ankle against the stirrup. Padding is placed if necessary.

The lower section of the mattress is removed and the leg section of the table lowered. The mattress is pulled down on the table, as necessary, until the *buttocks are even with the table edge.* They must not extend beyond the edge, causing strain to the lumbosacral muscles and ligaments, as the body weight rests on the sacrum.

The arms may be placed on armboards or loosely cradled over the lower abdomen and secured by

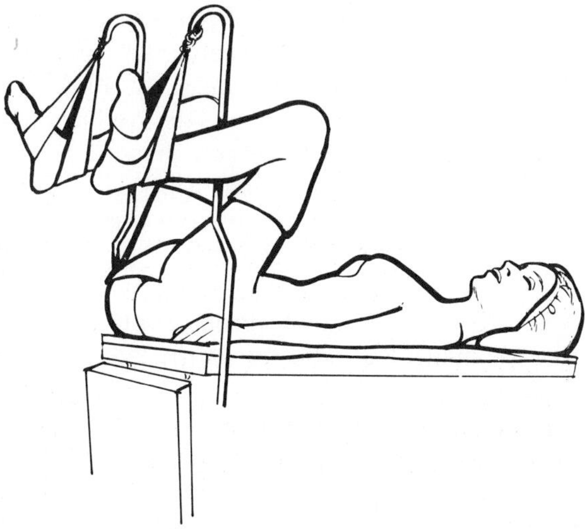

Figure 10-5 Lithotomy position. Patient is on back with the foot section of the table lowered to a right angle with the body on the table. The knees are flexed and the legs are on the outside of the metal posts with the feet supported by canvas straps. Note that the buttocks are even with the table edge.

the lower end of the blanket. Arms must not rest on the chest and impede respiration. Lung compliance is decreased by pressure of the thighs on the abdomen, which hinders descent of the diaphragm. Hands should *not* extend along the table where they could be injured in the table break during manipulation of the table or movement of the patient. Hands have been crushed in the break as the leg section of the table was raised at conclusion of the operation.

For prolonged procedures the legs may be wrapped in elastic bandages prior to operation. During operation, blood pools in the lumbar region of the torso. Legs must be lowered *slowly* when removed simultaneously from stirrups to prevent hypotension as blood reenters the legs and leaves the torso. The position change places an added burden on the heart and circulation. Raise the leg section of the table and replace the lower section of the mattress. As they are lifted from the stirrups, the legs are fully extended to avoid wide abduction of the thighs.

Used for perineal and rectal procedures.

Prone Position

See Figure 10-6. The patient is usually anesthetized and the endotracheal tube inserted in supine position. When the anesthesiologist gives permission, the patient is slowly and cautiously turned to the abdomen by rotation. Shoulder rolls or bolsters under the axillae and along the sides of the chest raise the weight of the body from the abdomen and thorax, facilitating respiration, although the position reduces vital capacity. The arms may be placed on armboards, lie supported along the sides of the body, or raised above the head. The head is turned to the side. A pillow under the ankles and feet prevents pressure to the toes. The safety belt is placed below the knees. Used for procedures on the posterior chest, trunk, legs, and sometimes the rectal area.

Modified Prone Position Prone position except that the mattress is adjusted on the table so that the hips are over the break between body and leg sections of the table. A large, soft pillow is placed under the abdomen, the upper break of the table is flexed, and the table is tilted so the operative area is horizontal. Used for operation on the spine.

Prone Position on an Adjustable Arch Prone position except that the patient is lifted and an adjustable arch is placed under him or her with the affected part of the spine at the highest point of the arch. This point can be lowered or raised as desired by means of a lever. The arms are on armboards with the elbows slightly flexed to prevent overextension. The head is placed in a padded headrest or supported by a roll of a cotton blanket. If the electrosurgical unit ground plate is placed beneath a thigh, the scrotum may require padding for protection. A pillow protects the feet and toes; bolsters protect the chest and abdomen. Entire table is tilted so that operative area is horizontal. Safety belt is below the knees. Some surgeons prefer a special assembly for the orthopaedic table for laminectomy rather than the adjustable arch.

Prone Position with Headrest Patient is in prone position except that the head rests in a cranial headrest exposing the occiput and cervical vertebrae. Safety belt is below the knees. Used for neurosurgical procedures.

> NOTE. When the patient's head is in prone position or face down on a cerebellar headrest, the head should be raised from time to time to prevent pressure necrosis of the cheeks and forehead. Eyes must be protected also.

Kraske (Jackknife) Position

See Figure 10-7. Patient is usually supine until anesthetized, then turned onto the abdomen by rotation with hips over center break of table between body and leg sections. Shoulder rolls or bolsters are placed to raise the chest. Feet and toes are protected by a pillow. The head is to the side, with arms resting on armboards. The safety belt is placed below the knees. The leg section of the table is lowered the desired amount, usually about 90°, and the entire table tilted head downward so that the hips are elevated above the rest of the body. The patient must be well balanced on the table. Used for procedures in the rectal area such as pilonidal sinus or hemorrhoidectomy. Buttocks are retracted with hemorrhoid straps. Because of the dependent position, venous pooling occurs cephalad (toward the head) and caudad (toward the feet). It is very important to return the patient slowly to horizontal from this unnatural position.

Knee-Chest Position

An extension is attached to the foot section. The table is flexed at the center break. The lower section is broken until it is at a right angle to the table. The patient kneels on the lower section and the entire table is tilted cephalad to elevate the

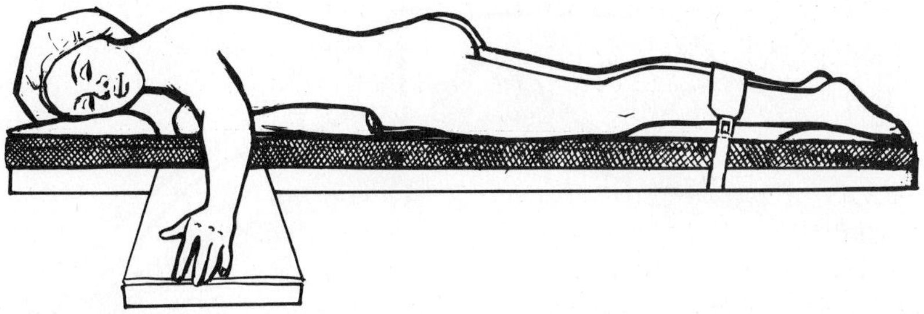

Figure 10-6 Prone position. The patient lies on abdomen. Note shoulder rolls under axillae and sides of chest to raise body weight from the chest to facilitate respiration. The patient is anesthetized and the endotracheal tube inserted in supine position before turning into prone position.

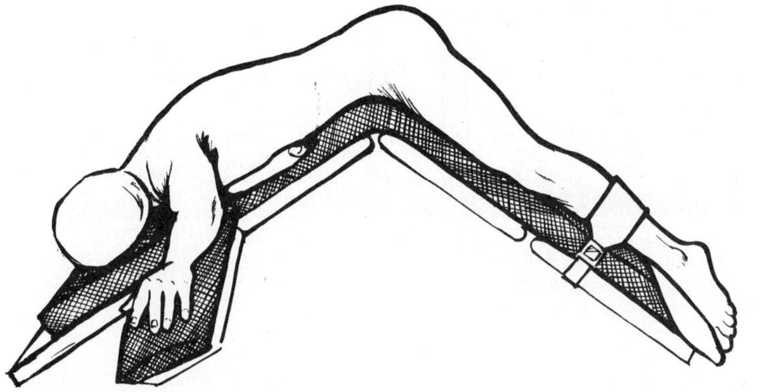

Figure 10-7 Kraske position. The hips are over the central break in the table and the knee strap is below the knees. Note shoulder rolls in place and pillow under the feet.

pelvis. The knees are thus flexed at a right angle to the body. The upper portion of the table may be raised slightly to support the head, which is turned to the side. Arms are placed around the head with elbows flexed, with a large soft pillow beneath. The chest rests on the table. Safety belt is above the knees. The table is titled head downward so the hips are at the highest point—modified jackknife. Used for sigmoidoscopy or culdoscopy.

Kidney Position (Lateral)

See Figure 10-8. The patient is usually anesthetized in supine position, then turned to the unaffected side with back near the table edge. Kidney area is over the elevator. Arms may be placed on a padded double armboard. The knee on the unaffected side is flexed to aid in stabilization; the upper leg is straight. A large soft pillow is placed lengthwise between the legs to prevent undue pressure and circulatory complications. A short kidney rest is attached to the table at the patient's back. A long kidney rest is placed at the front of the patient. Both must be well-padded. In an obese patient, folds of abdominal tissue may extend over the end of the rest and be bruised if caution is not taken. Head may be supported on a small pillow. The table is flexed so the kidney elevator can be raised the desired amount to increase the space between lower ribs and iliac crest. A kidney (body) strap is placed over the hip to stabilize the patient. The safety belt is placed over the legs. The entire table is tilted slightly downward toward the head so that the operative area is horizontal. Upper shoulder, hip, and ankle should be in a straight line. Ankles and feet should be supported from pressure and footdrop. A pillow may be used to support the chest and protect the breasts. Before closure, the table is straightened for better approximation of tissues. Used for procedures on the kidney and ureter. The position contributes to physiologic alterations and is not well tolerated. Blood tends to pool in the lower arm and leg. The circulation is further compromised because of increased pressure on abdominal vessels when the kidney elevator is raised. Respiration is affected as well since gas exchange ratios in the lungs differ. Because of gravity, the lower lung receives more blood from the right heart, is better perfused, has less residual air because of body weight, and is therefore more effective than the higher lung. Controlled respiration is helpful.

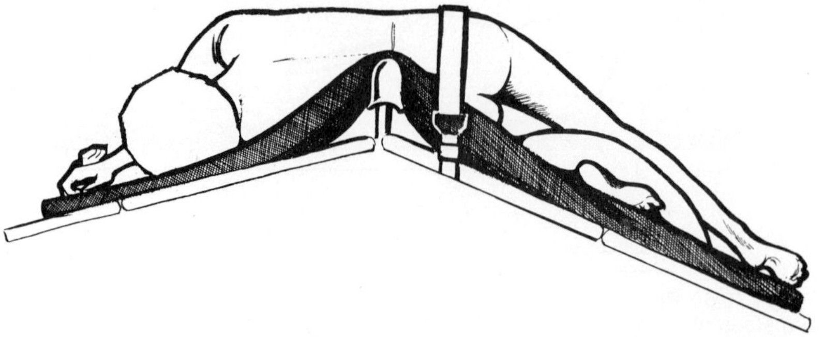

Figure 10-8 Right kidney position. The patient is in a lateral position with the kidney region over the table break. Note the kidney strap across the hip for stabilizing the body, raised kidney elevator for hyperextending operative area, and pillow between legs. Patient's side is horizontal from shoulder to hip.

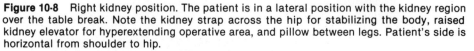

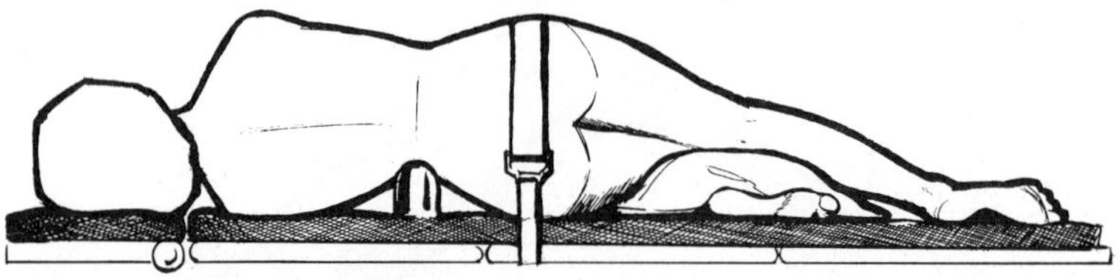

Figure 10-9 Right lateral position. Note the strap across the hip and body rest for stabilizing the body. Pillow between legs relieves pressure.

Lateral Chest Position

See Figure 10-9. Modifications of lateral position also are used. Position for unilateral transthoracic procedures with lateral approach. The patient is anesthetized supine, then turned onto the unaffected side with the back drawn to the table edge. The lower leg is flexed, the upper leg straight, with a large soft pillow between them. Additional stability is provided by placing a strap over the hip. A second strap may be placed over the shoulder unless it interferes with skin preparation. The safety belt is placed over the legs. The arms are extended on a padded, double armboard with the upper arm slightly flexed, thus stabilizing the shoulders; or an armboard is used for the lower arm while the upper arm is brought forward and down over a pad to draw the scapula from the operative area. Position depends on the site and length of the chest incision. The head may be on a small pillow. A small firm pillow or pad under the operative area relieves pressure on the arm of the unaffected side, permitting free flow of intravenous fluids. It also assists in spreading the intercostal space for better exposure. One body rest is placed at the lumbar area, another at the chest at axillary level. The latter must be well-padded so as not to bruise the breasts. Sandbags or towel rolls may be used instead of body rests. A pad at the lumbar area facilitates respiratory movements and adds support. The shoulders and hips should be level. Lowering the head of the table slightly assists postural drainage during operation. This position also is restricting to the cardiorespiratory systems, especially if prolonged.

Anterior Chest Position

Used for thoracoabdominal procedures, with anterior approach. It is more supine than the lateral chest position. After the patient is anesthetized, a small firm pillow is placed under the shoulder and another under the buttocks on the affected side. The knee on the affected side is flexed slightly, with a large soft pillow beneath it to relieve undue strain on abdominal muscles. The safety belt is above the knees. The arm on the unaffected side is supported at the side. The arm on the affected side is padded well and bandaged loosely to the anesthesia screen. It must not be hyperextended to avoid injury to the brachial plexus. The head of the table is lowered slightly for postural drainage.

PATIENT AS AN INDIVIDUAL

The patient's individual needs must be met in positioning as in everything else. Anomalies and physical defects are accommodated. The avoidance of unnecessary exposure, whether the patient is unconscious or conscious, is an essential consideration for all patients. The nurse should objectively observe the patient's position once again, to see if it adheres to physiological principles, before skin preparation and draping.

Chapter 11

Preparation of the Operative Site and Draping

PHYSICAL PREPARATION OF THE PATIENT PRIOR TO OPERATION

The type of operation to be performed, the age and condition of the patient, and the preferences of the surgeon will determine the specific procedures to be carried out before the incision is made. Consideration must be given to control of urinary drainage, to skin antisepsis, and to establishment of a sterile field around the operative site.

URINARY TRACT CATHETERIZATION

The patient should void to empty the urinary bladder just before transfer to the OR suite, unless an indwelling retention catheter is in place. If the patient's bladder is not empty or the surgeon wishes to prevent bladder distention during a long procedure or following operation, catheterization may be necessary after the patient is anesthetized. A retention catheter may be inserted. This maintains bladder decompression to avoid trauma during a lower abdominal or pelvic operation, to permit accurate measurement of output during or following operation, or to facilitate output and healing after operation on genitourinary tract structures. Catheterization is performed before the patient is positioned, except for a patient who will remain in lithotomy position.

Urinary tract infection can occur following catheterization from contamination or traumatism of structures. Sterile technique must be maintained during catheterization. A sterile, disposable catheterization tray is used, unless the patient is being prepared for an operation in the perineal or genital area. For these latter procedures, the sterile catheter and lubricant may be added to the skin preparation setup. For other operations, the perineal area should be scrubbed (wearing clean gloves) with an antiseptic agent to reduce normal microbial flora and remove gross contaminants prior to the catheterization procedure.

Urinary catheterization is a minor operative procedure requiring aseptic technique. Sterile gloves are worn to handle the sterile catheter. The catheter size should be small enough to minimize trauma of the urethra and prevent necrosis of the meatus; usually a 14 French is inserted in an adult female, 16 to 18 French in an adult male.

If a Foley retention catheter is to be inserted, check the integrity of the balloon by inflating it with the correct amount of sterile water or air prior to insertion. Balloon size may be 5 or 30 cc (5 cc is used most frequently); 10 ml of sterile water are needed to properly inflate a 5-cc balloon to compensate for the volume required by the inflation channel. Most Foley catheters have a rubber valve over the lumen to the inflation channel that can be penetrated by a plain Luer slip tip syringe. Some require a needle on the syringe to penetrate the rubber cover over the lumen. Solution or air must be evacuated prior to insertion of the catheter into the urethra.

The hand used to spread the labia or stabilize the penis is considered contaminated and should not be used to handle the catheter. Sponges used to cleanse the labia minora or glans penis should be handled to avoid contaminating the gloved hand that is used to insert the catheter. To facilitate insertion and minimize trauma, lubricate the tip of the catheter with a sterile antimicrobial lubricant. Urine will start to flow when the catheter has passed into the bladder. Drain the bladder. Inflate the balloon of a Foley catheter.

Attach catheter to a sterile closed-drainage system. Secure tubing to patient's leg with enough slack in it to prevent tension or pull on the penis or urethra. The drainage tubing should be positioned to enhance downward flow, but must not fall below the level of the collection container. Attention to the catheter and tubing must be paid during positioning of the patient for the operation to prevent compression or kinking of the tubing. If the container must be raised above the level of the bladder during positioning, clamp or kink the tubing until the container can be lowered and secured under the operating table to avoid contamination of retrograde, backward flow of urine.

SKIN PREPARATION OF THE PATIENT

Purpose of the Patient's Skin Preparation

The purpose of skin preparation (usually called *prep*) is to render the operative site as free as possible from transient and resident microorganisms, dirt, and skin oil so the incision can be made through the skin with a minimal danger of infection from this source.

Preliminary Preparation of the Patient's Skin

Mechanical Cleansing Bathing removes many microorganisms from the skin. This action can be enhanced to progressively reduce the microbial population with daily use of a bar or liquid soap containing 3% hexachlorophene. The bacteriostatic action is due to the cumulative deposit of hexachlorophene that dissolves in the fatty acids of the skin. Many surgeons advise their patients to use such a product at home for several days prior to hospital admission for an elective operation.

Patients whose operations will be on the face, eye, ear, or neck are advised to shampoo their hair prior to hospital admission as this may not be permitted for a few weeks postoperatively.

All patients should shower or be bathed after hospital admission as close to the time of departure from the unit to the OR suite as possible. The operative site and surrounding area should be thoroughly cleansed with a rapid-acting, skin-degerming, antiseptic agent. *History of allergies must be obtained before applying any chemical agent to a patient's skin.*

Hair Removal Hair removal from the skin surrounding the operative site may be necessary. Usually the surgeon is responsible for designating in the patient's preoperative orders the limits of the skin area and how it is to be prepared. Also, the procedure book specifies the anatomical areas that must be mechanically cleansed and hair removed for each type of operation (see Figs. 11-1 through 11-6). The procedure is carried out by personnel, per hospital policy, either on the unit or in the OR suite prior to operation. This can be done in a preoperative holding area only if privacy is assured. Hair may be removed by shaving with a razor or application of a depilatory cream.

> NOTE. Skin preparation may be an embarrassing procedure for the patient. Drape the patient to expose the area to be prepared, but avoid unnecessary exposure. Hair removal after the patient is anesthetized avoids this emotional trauma for the patient.

Shave Prep Breaks in the skin surface afford opportunity for entry of microorganisms and are a potential source of infection. Therefore:

1 Use a sharp, clean straight or safety razor blade. Blades are either discarded after each patient use or terminally sterilized. If disposable razors are not used, razors should be terminally sterilized also between uses.

2 Have good lighting. Because lighting at the patient's bedside may be inadequate, shaving may be more satisfactorily accomplished in the OR under the operating lights or in an isolated well-lighted preoperative holding area in the OR suite. In the latter areas, hair must be contained to prevent a potential source of contamination.

3 Wear gloves to prevent cross contamination even though this is a surgically clean procedure.

4 Wash skin from the incision site to the periphery to raise a generous lather. Loose hair rarely strays from a lather. If dry shaving is preferred, the sticky side of adhesive tape can be used to pick up loose hair.

5 Hold the skin taut and shave by stroking in the direction of hair growth.

6 Avoid making nicks and cuts in the patient's skin. Nicks made in the OR immediately prior to operation are considered clean wounds. However, nicks made the evening before may present themselves as infected wounds at the time of operation.

7 Observe the general skin condition. An abnormal skin irritation, infection, or abrasion on or near the operative site might be a contraindication to operation and must be reported to the surgeon.

Depilatory Cream Hair removal by depilation offers the primary advantage of intact skin free from cuts. If patient is not sensitive to depilatories, a depilatory should be used; it is a safer method of hair removal than shaving. After the cream has remained on the skin for the required number of minutes, wipe it off. Hair is removed simultaneously. Rinse the skin thoroughly.

PATIENT'S SKIN PREP ON THE OPERATING TABLE

Area

After the patient has been anesthetized and positioned on the operating table, the skin of the operative site and an extensive area surrounding it is mechanically cleansed again with an antiseptic agent immediately prior to draping (see Figs. 11-1 through 11-6).

Setup

A sterile skin prep tray is opened on a small table. Some disposable trays include containers of a premeasured amount of antiseptic solution. Solution of choice must be added to others. If prepackaged trays are not used, the table must be prepared with a sterile cover and the following sterile items added:

1 Two towels to define the upper and lower limits of the area to be prepared.

2 Small basins for solutions—usually at least two.

3 Sponges—may be 4 by 8 in. (10 by 20 cm) for large areas: 4 by 4 (10 by 10) or 3 by 3 (7.5 by 7.5) for small areas. *These must not be confused with counted sponges on the instrument table.* Textured foam sponges may be preferred.

4 Cotton applicators as necessary.

Antiseptic Solutions

The infection control committee usually determines the chemical agent(s) to be used in the OR for skin antisepsis. The maximum concentration of a germicidal chemical that can be used on skin and mucous membranes is limited by its toxicity for these tissues. The agent should have the following qualities:

1 It rapidly decreases microbial count.

2 It can be quickly applied and remains effective against microorganisms.

3 It can be safely used without skin irritation or sensitization.

4 It effectively remains active in the presence of alcohol, organic matter, soap, or detergent.

Iodine and Iodophors A solution of 1 or 2% iodine in water or in 70% alcohol is an excellent broad-spectrum, rapid-acting, cidal antiseptic. However, the potential hazard of skin irritations and burns have led to a decline in its use. After application, iodine should be allowed to dry and then rinsed off with 70% alcohol to reduce potential of burns.

Iodophors, an iodine complex combined with detergents, are excellent cleansing agents to remove debris from skin surfaces while slowly releasing 1% iodine to act effectively as a cidal antiseptic. These agents are relatively nontoxic and virtually nonirritating to skin or mucous membranes. The brown film left on the skin clearly defines the area of application. This should not be wiped off after application because the cidal activity is sustained by the release of free iodine as the agent dries and color fades from the skin.

> NOTE. To hasten drying of skin, alcohol may be painted on the area without friction before a self-adhering drape is applied (refer to p. 229).

Alcohols Isopropyl and ethyl alcohol are useful as antiseptic agents if the surgeon prefers a colorless solution that permits observation of true skin color. Since alcohol coagulates protein, it is not applied to mucous membranes or used on an open wound. Isopropyl alcohol is a more effective fat solvent than ethyl alcohol. Seventy percent concentration is satisfactory for skin antisepsis.

Hexachlorophene Since this agent slowly develops a cumulative suppressive action only over a period of frequent routine use, 3% hexachlorophene should only be used as the final skin prep solution on patients who have washed for several days exclusively with soap products containing this agent. Hexachlorophene is neutralized by alcohol. It is relatively ineffective against gram-negative organisms and fungi.

Chlorhexidine Gluconate Chlorhexidine gluconate significantly reduces and maintains a reduction of microbial flora for at least 4 hours after mechanical cleansing with this agent.

Basic Prep Procedure for Clean Areas

1 Expose the skin area to be prepared by folding back the cotton blanket and gown as necessary. Double-check the operative site.

> NOTE. If the operation is unilateral, be sure which is the affected side and expose the proper one. Consult the chart and x-rays. Before an amputation of an extremity, expose the opposite one also for comparison. Check with the surgeon.

2 Don sterile gloves.
3 Place sterile towels above and below the area to be cleansed to mark the limit of the area and also to protect gloved hands from touching the nonsterile blanket or gown.
4 Wet sponge with antiseptic agent, but squeeze out excess solution.

> NOTE. Solution should not run off the skin area onto the operating table to pool under the patient. A patient lying in solution may develop skin irritation, even though the solution itself is nonirritating.

5 Scrub the skin, starting at the site of incision, with a circular motion in ever-widening circles to the periphery. Use enough pressure and friction to remove dirt and microorganisms from the skin and pores. Effective skin antisepsis is achieved through a combination of mechanical and chemical action (see Fig. 11-1 for abdominal prep).

> NOTE. Some surgeons prefer to have the antiseptic agent applied over cancerous areas by painting rather than scrubbing. During vigorous scrubbing, cancer cells may be freed, picked up by the blood and lymph streams, and carried to other parts of the body. To paint, secure a folded sponge in a sponge forceps, dip in solution, squeeze out excess solution, and apply to the skin in circular motions from the incision site to the periphery.

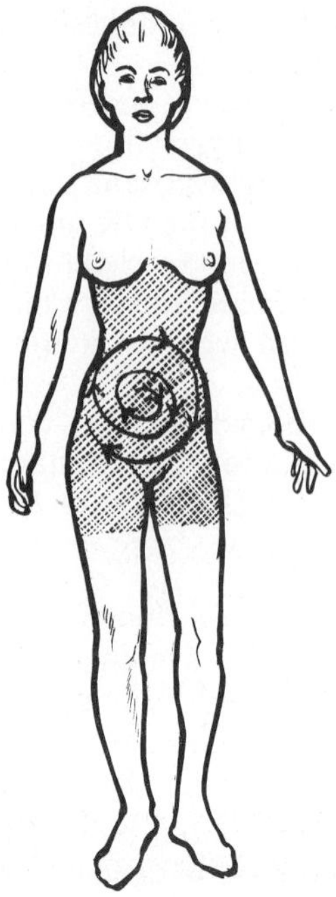

Figure 11-1 Abdominal preparation. The area includes breast line to upper third of thighs, from table line to table line, with patient in supine position. Shaded area shows anatomic area of hair removal. Arrows within area show direction of motion for skin preparation on operating table.

6 Discard the sponge after reaching the periphery. *Never* bring a soiled sponge back toward the center of the area.
7 Repeat the scrub with a separate sponge for each round. Scrub for a minimum of 5 minutes and apply the antiseptic agent according to the manufacturer's recommendations.

Contaminated Areas within the Operative Field

Umbilicus The abdomen contains an area, the umbilicus, which is considered a contaminated area in relation to the surface surrounding it, because it may harbor microorganisms in the detritus that often accumulates there. Solution from the first scrub sponge may be squeezed into the umbilicus to soften the detritus while the remainder of the abdomen is scrubbed. Come back to the umbilicus and scrub it before discarding the sponge. Or discard each sponge after reaching the periphery and use a separate sponge, each round, on the umbilicus only. Also cleanse it thoroughly with cotton applicators.

Stoma The external stoma (orifice) of a colostomy, ileostomy, etc., may be sealed off from the operative site with a self-adhering towel drape. If this is not possible, follow the same rule in the use of sponges as for the umbilicus; come back to that area last, or use a separate sponge each round for the contaminated area only. The opening of the stoma may be packed with a sponge while the surrounding area is scrubbed.

Other Contaminated Areas Draining sinuses, skin ulcers, vagina, anus, etc., are considered contaminated areas also. In all these, follow the general rule of scrubbing the most contaminated area last or with separate sponges.

Foreign Substances Adhesive, grease, tar, and similar foreign materials must be removed from the skin before the area is mechanically cleansed with the antiseptic agent. A nonirritating solvent, such as Freon, will cleanse the skin. The solvent must be nonflammable and nontoxic. However, do not allow solution to collect underneath the patient.

Traumatic Wounds When preparing an area in which the skin is not intact due to traumatic injury, wound irrigation may be part of the skin preparation procedure. The wound may be packed or covered with sterile gauze while the area around it is thoroughly scrubbed and shaved if necessary.

After changing gloves, the wound itself is cleansed and irrigated. The extent and type of injury will determine the appropriate procedure. Solutions irritating to a denuded area must not be used. Small areas may be irrigated with warm sterile solution, usually normal saline, in a bulb syringe. When a bulb syringe is used, care must be taken not to force debris and microorganisms deeper into the wound. The wound is irrigated gently to dislodge debris and flush it out.

Copious amounts of warm sterile solutions may be needed to flush out a large wound. A bottle of warm sterile saline or Ringer's solution attached to intravenous tubing can be hung on a standard near the area to be copiously irrigated. If the area is on an extremity, a sterile irrigating pan with a heavy wire screen fitted over the top is placed under the extremity. During irrigation, the solution runs from the wound into the pan. A piece of tubing connected to an outlet on the pan carries the irrigating solution into a kick bucket on the floor at the edge of the table.

It may be necessary to place dry towels or sheets under the patient if the area has not been protected during irrigation. A moistureproof pad placed under the wound before irrigation will help channel solutions into a drainage pan.

Debridement of the wound (excision of all devitalized tissue) usually follows irrigation. The surgeon may wish to have sterile tissue forceps and scissors on the preparation table for removal of nonviable tissue along with the irrigation.

Areas Prepared for Grafts

1 Separate setups are necessary for skin preparation of recipient and donor sites prior to skin, bone, or vascular grafting procedures.

2 The donor site usually is scrubbed first. The recipient site for skin grafts usually is more or less contaminated, e.g., following a burn or other traumatic injury. Items used in preparation of the recipient site must not be permitted to contaminate the donor site. Also, microorganisms on the skin of the donor site must not be transferred to a denuded recipient site.

3 The donor site for a skin graft should be scrubbed with a colorless antiseptic agent so the surgeon can properly evaluate the vascularity of the graft postoperatively.

Special Considerations in Specific Anatomic Areas

Eye

1 Eyebrows are never shaved or removed unless the surgeon deems this essential. Eyebrows do not grow back completely.

2 Eyelashes are trimmed, if ordered by the surgeon, with fine scissors coated with sterile petrolatum to catch the lashes.

3 Eyelids and periorbital areas are cleansed with a nonstaining antiseptic agent.

4 Conjunctival sac is flushed with a nontoxic agent, such as benzalkonium chloride.

Ears, Face, or Nose

1 Usually it is not possible to define the area with towels.

2 Protect the eyes with a piece of sterile plastic sheeting. If the patient is awake, ask that eyes be kept closed during the prep.

3 As much of the surrounding area is included as is feasible and consistent with aseptic technique. Skin surfaces should be cleansed at least to the hair line.

4 Cotton applicators are used for cleansing the nostrils and external ear canals.

Neck

1 One sterile towel is folded under the edge of the blanket and gown, which are turned down almost to the nipple line.

2 The area includes the neck laterally to the table line and up to the mandible, tops of the shoulders, and chest almost to the nipple line.

3 For combined head and neck operations, include the face to the eyes, shaved areas of the head, the ears, the posterior neck, and the area over the shoulders.

Lateral Thoracoabdominal

1 The gown is removed. The blanket is turned down well below the lower limit of the area to be prepared. A towel is folded under the edge of the blanket.

2 The arm is held up during the preparation.

3 Beginning at the site of incision, the area may include the axilla, chest, and abdomen from the neck to crest of the ilium. For operations in the region of the kidney, it extends up to the axilla and down to the pubis. The area also extends beyond the midlines, anteriorly and posteriorly (see Fig. 11-2).

Chest and Radical Breast

1 The anesthesiologist turns the patient's face toward the unaffected side.

2 One towel is folded under the blanket edge, just above the pubis. The other is placed on the table under the shoulder and side.

3 The arm on the affected side is held up for the prep, by grasping the hand and raising the shoulder and axilla slightly from the table.

4 The area includes the shoulder, upper arm down to the elbow, axilla, and chest wall to the table line and beyond the sternum to the opposite shoulder (see Fig. 11-3).

Shoulder

1 The anesthesiologist turns the patient's face toward the opposite side.

2 One towel is placed under the shoulder and axilla.

3 The arm is held up by grasping the hand and elevating the shoulder slightly from the table.

4 The area includes the circumference of the upper arm to below the elbow, from the base of the neck over the shoulder, scapula, and chest to midline.

Upper Arm

1 One towel is placed under the shoulder and axilla.

2 The arm is held up by grasping the hand and elevating the shoulder slightly from the table.

3 The area includes the entire circumference of the arm to the wrist, the axilla, and over the shoulder and scapula.

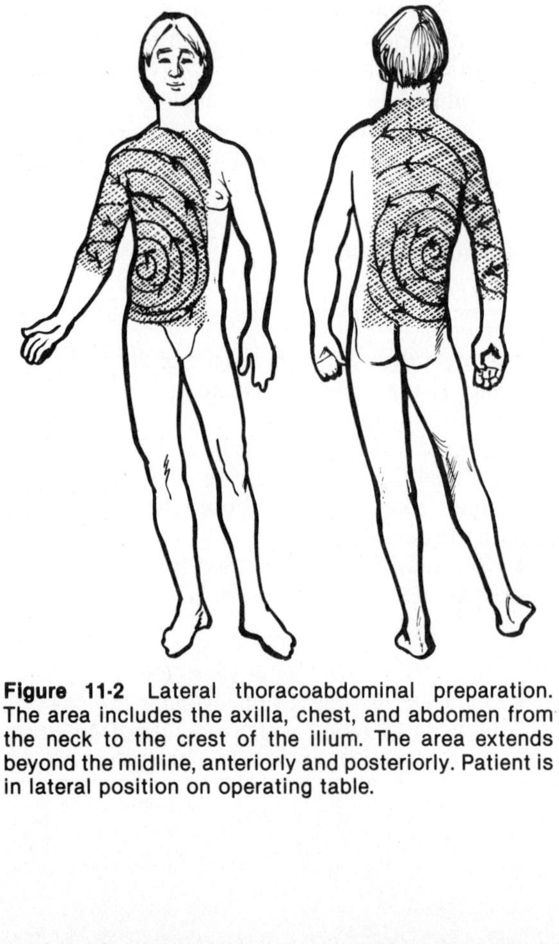

Figure 11-2 Lateral thoracoabdominal preparation. The area includes the axilla, chest, and abdomen from the neck to the crest of the ilium. The area extends beyond the midline, anteriorly and posteriorly. Patient is in lateral position on operating table.

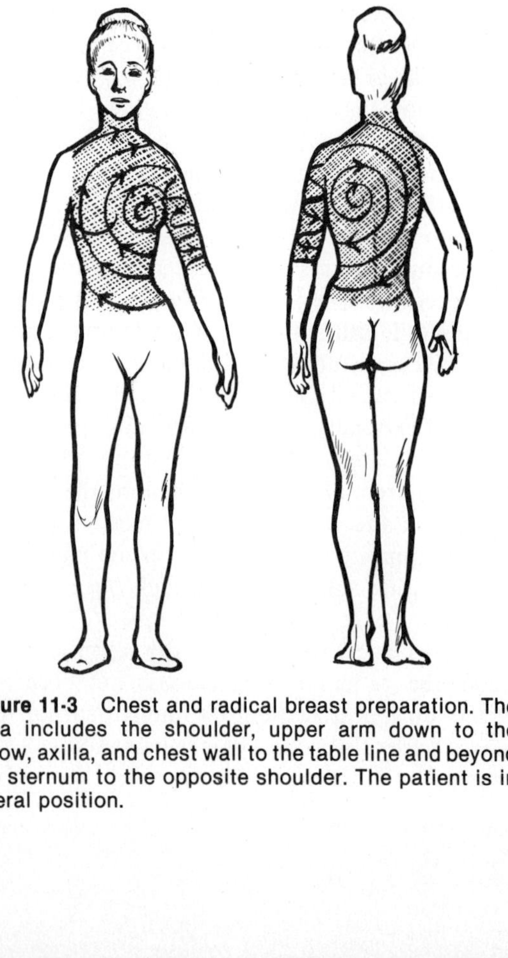

Figure 11-3 Chest and radical breast preparation. The area includes the shoulder, upper arm down to the elbow, axilla, and chest wall to the table line and beyond the sternum to the opposite shoulder. The patient is in lateral position.

Elbow and Forearm

1 One towel is placed under the shoulder and axilla.
2 The arm is held up by grasping the hand.
3 The area includes the entire arm from the shoulder and axilla to and including the hand.

Hand

1 The towels use to define the area on a flat surface are omitted. The anatomy of the part furnishes sufficient landmarks to define the area, and towels are apt to slip over the scrubbed area.
2 The arm must be held up by supporting it above the elbow so the entire circumference can be scrubbed.
3 The area includes the hand and arm to 3 in. (7.5 cm) above the elbow.

Rectoperineal

1 One towel is folded under the edge of the blanket above the pubis. The other towel is placed under the buttocks.
2 The area includes the pubis, external genitalia, perineum and anus, and inner aspect of the thighs (see Fig. 11-4).
3 Begin scrub over the pubic area, scrubbing downward over the genitalia and perineum. Discard sponge after going over the anus.
4 The inner aspect of the upper third of both thighs are scrubbed with separate sponges.
5 The rectoperineal area is prepped first, with the patient in lithotomy position, followed by the abdominal prep, with the patient in supine position, for a combined abdominoperineal operation. Two separate prep trays are used.

Vagina

1 A sponge forceps must be included on the preparation table for a vaginal prep because a portion of the prep is done internally.
2 A moistureproof pad is placed under the buttocks and extends to a kick bucket that receives solutions and discarded sponges.
3 One towel is folded under the edge of the blanket above the pubis.
4 The area includes the pubis, vulva, labia, perineum, anus, and adjacent area, including the inner aspect of the upper third of the thighs. *The vagina is prepped last* (see Fig. 11-4).
5 Begin over the pubic area, scrubbing downward over the vulva and perineum. Discard sponge after going over the anus.
6 The inner aspects of the thighs are scrubbed with separate sponges from the labia majora outward.

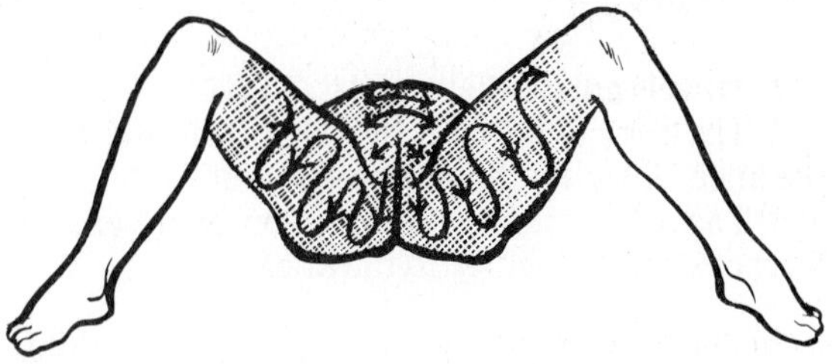

Figure 11-4 Rectoperineal and vaginal preparation. The area includes the pubis, vulva, labia, perineum, anus, and adjacent areas, including the inner aspect of the upper third of the thighs.

7 The vagina is cleansed with sponges on sponge forceps after the external surrounding areas are scrubbed. The cleansing agent should be applied generously in the vagina because the vaginal mucosa has many folds and crevices that are not easily cleansed.
8 After cleansing the vagina, wipe it out with a dry sponge to prevent the possibility of fluid entering the peritoneal cavity during operation on the pelvic organs.
9 Catheterize, if indicated.

Hip

1 One towel is placed under the thigh on the table. The other towel is placed on the abdomen and folded under the edge of the gown, just above the umbilicus.
2 The leg on the affected side is held up by supporting it just below the knee.
3 The area includes the abdomen on the affected side, thigh to the knee, buttocks to table line, groin, and pubis (see Fig. 11-5).

Thigh

1 One towel is placed under the thigh on the table. The other towel is placed on the abdomen and folded under the edge of the gown, just below the umbilicus.
2 The leg is held up by supporting the foot and ankle.
3 The area includes the entire circumference of the thigh and leg to the ankle, over the hip and buttocks to the table line, the groin and pubis.

Knee and Lower Leg

1 One towel is placed over the groin.
2 The leg is held up by supporting it at the foot.
3 The area includes the entire circumference of the leg and extends from the foot to the upper part of the thigh (see Fig. 11-6).

Ankle and Foot

1 Towels are omitted.
2 The foot is held up by supporting the leg at the knee. A leg-holder device is useful.
3 The area includes the foot and entire circumference of the lower leg to the knee.

NOTE. 1. A moistureproof pad should be placed on the operating table under a lower extremity to retain drops of solution. This is removed after the prep so that the table will be dry.
2. An extremity remains supported and elevated until sterile drapes are applied under and around the prepped area.
3. A full extremity prep may be done in two stages to provide adequate support to the joints and to assure that all areas are scrubbed. It may include the foot for hip, thigh, knee, and lower leg operations.
4. Caution must be taken to prevent solution from pooling under a tourniquet. If a tourniquet is used (refer to Chap. 12), it is positioned prior to prep. A towel tucked under the tourniquet cuff absorbs excess solution. This is removed before the tourniquet is inflated.

Skin Marking

Some surgeons use a staining solution to mark the incision lines on the skin. This may be done before the patient is prepped. If so, the stain must withstand scrubbing without washing off. If the skin is marked after the prep, a sterile dye solution and applicator or sterile marking pen must be used. Methylene blue or alcoholic gentian violet are used for this purpose.

DRAPING

Draping is the procedure of covering the patient and surrounding areas with a sterile barrier to create and maintain an adequate sterile field during the operation. An effective barrier eliminates the passage of microorganisms between nonsterile and sterile areas. Criteria to be met in establishing an effective barrier are:

1 Blood and aqueous fluid-resistant to keep drapes dry and prevent migration of microorganisms.
2 Abrasion-resistant to prevent abrasive damage that causes fiber breakdown and thus permits microbial penetration.
3 Lint-free to reduce airborne contaminants or shed into the operative site. Cellulose and cotton fibers can cause granulomatous peritonitis or embolize arteries.
4 Antistatic to eliminate risk of a spark from static electricity. Material must meet the requirements of the National Fire Protection Association.

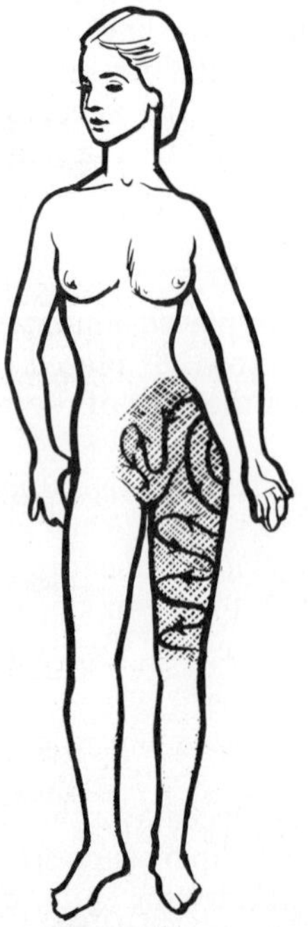

Figure 11-5 Hip preparation. The area includes the abdomen on the affected side, thigh to the knee, buttocks to table line, groin and pubis.

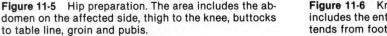

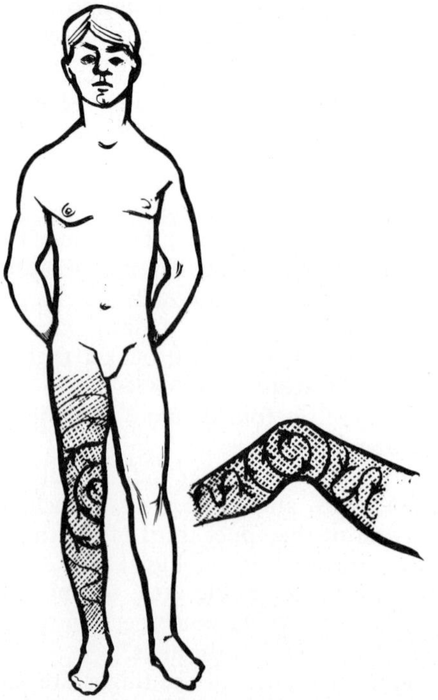

Figure 11-6 Knee and lower leg preparation. The area includes the entire circumference of affected leg and extends from foot to upper part of thigh.

5 Sufficiently porous to eliminate heat build-up.

6 Drapable to fit around contours of the patient, furniture, and equipment.

Draping Materials

Self-Adhering Plastic Sheeting Sterile, waterproof, antistatic, plastic sheeting may be applied to dry skin. It is available in various sizes as:

An Incise Drape The entire drape has an adhesive backing that is applied to the skin. This may be applied separately or the sheeting may be incorporated into the drape sheet. The skin incision is made through the plastic.

A Towel Drape The plastic sheeting has a band of adhesive material along the edge. This can be used as a draping towel and will remain fixed on the skin without towel clips. This is advantageous when clips might obscure the view of a part to be exposed to x-rays during operation. It also is used to wall off a contaminated area, such as a stoma, from the clean skin area to prevent spilling contents and causing infection or chemical irritation.

An Aperture Drape Adhesive surrounds a fenestration (opening) in the plastic sheeting. This secures the drape to the skin around the operative site, such as an eye or ear.

NOTE. Caution must be used in applying this type of drape around face of patient who is awake. Be sure patient has breathing space. Some patients experience claustrophobia. Drape towels, which do not feel as confining, are used for them.

Advantages of a self-adhering plastic drape:

1 Resident microbial flora from skin pores, sebaceous glands, and hair follicles cannot migrate laterally to the incision.

2 Microorganisms do not penetrate through impermeable material.

3 Landmarks and skin tones are visible through the transparent plastic.

4 Inert adhesive holds drapes securely, eliminating need for towel clips and possible puncture of the patient's skin.

A nonporous material, such as plastic sheeting, should not cover more than 10 percent of the body surface as it may interfere with the patient's thermal regulatory mechanism of perspiration evaporation. The heat-retaining property of plastic causes the patient to expire excessively, but its nonporous nature prevents evaporation. The material is used in the following manner:

1 The usual skin preparation is done.

2 The scrubbed area must be dried. It may dry by evaporation, or excess solution may be blotted or wiped off with a sterile sponge or towel.

NOTE. Alcohol may be applied after an iodophor scrub to hasten drying by evaporation. Alcohol will neutralize hexachlorophene, however, ether, a highly flammable agent, is not recommended for skin preparation. A combination of alcohol and Freon can produce chemical irritation on the skin.

3 The transparent plastic material is firmly applied to the skin with the initial contact along the proposed line of incision. Smooth the drape away from the incision area.

4 Regular fabric drapes are applied over the plastic sheeting, unless the plastic is incorporated into the fenestrated area of the drape.

Nonwoven Fabric Drapes Often referred to as *paper* drapes, nonwoven disposable materials are compressed layers of synthetic fibers, i.e., rayon, nylon, or polyester, combined with cellulose and held together chemically or mechanically without knitting, tufting, or weaving. Material may be either nonabsorbent or absorbent. Those fabrics that comply with the criteria for establishing an effective barrier have the following advantages as disposable drapes:

1 Moisture repellancy retards blood and aqueous fluid moisture strike-through to prevent contamination.

NOTE. Not all nonwoven fabrics have this characteristic: only nonabsorbent materials or those laminated with plastic are impermeable to moisture.

2 Lightweight, yet strong enough to resist tears.

3 Lint-free.

4 Contaminants are disposed of along with drapes.

5 Antistatic and flame-retardant for use in the OR.

6 Prepackaged and sterilized by the manufacturer. This eliminates the washing, mending, folding, and sterilizing processes.

Some drapes have a reinforced area, roughly 2 ft (61 cm) wide, surrounding the fenestration that contains a layer impermeable to strike-through.

Other drapes are completely laminated with a plastic layer. Although lamination of nonwoven materials with a plastic layer provides a complete microbial barrier, some laminated materials can only be used for instrument table covers, but not over the entire body of the patient because of their heat-retention property.

Woven Textile Fabrics The weight and thread count of woven natural fibers determine integrity and porosity of the fabric. Double-thickness, 140-thread-count muslin, as used for wrappers, is permeable to steam under pressure for sterilization. However, if used for drapes, once wet by blood or aqueous fluids even four thicknesses of muslin are ineffective as a barrier to the migration of microorganisms because of the wicking action of absorbent fibers.

Tightly woven, reusable textile fabrics are less absorbent so may inhibit migration of microorganisms. Cotton fibers swell when they become wet. This swelling action closes the pores or interstices so that liquid cannot diffuse through the tightly woven fibers. Tightly woven cotton cloth can be treated to repel fluids and be impermeable to moisture strike-through. However, these fabrics have essentially the same heat-retaining qualities as plastic lamination and cannot be used for complete patient draping.

Points concerning textile drapes:

1 When packaged for sterilization, drapes must be properly folded and arranged in sequence of use. Drapes may be fanfolded or rolled.

2 All material must be steam-permeable.

3 Material must be free from holes and tears. It is the responsibility of the person who folds the drape to see that it is free from holes. Those detected may be covered with heat-seal patches. Occasionally holes may not be detected until the drape is laid down. The hole must be covered with another piece of linen or the entire drape discarded.

4 Drapes should be sufficiently thick to prevent moisture from soaking through them, or a plastic waterproof drape should first be placed over the operative area and the drapes placed over it.

Style (Type) of Drapes

Towels May be used to outline the operative site. The folded edge of each towel is placed toward the line of incision. When packaging reusable linen, four towels for this purpose can be placed together with the folded edges graduated. Nonabsorbent disposable towels are used for this technique. Towels are secured with towel clips.

Laparotomy Sheet Often called a *lap* sheet. At least 108 by 72 in. (274 by 183 cm), it has a longitudinal fenestration that is placed over the operative site on the abdomen, the back, or a comparable area. The opening, about 40 in. (102 cm) from the top in the center of the sheet, is 9 by 4 in. (23 by 10 cm), which is large enough to give adequate exposure in the usual laparotomy. A 24-in. (60-cm) reinforcement around the opening provides an extra thickness. The sheet is long enough to cover the anesthesia screen at the head and extend down over the foot of the table. It is wide enough to cover one or two armboards. The sheet is unfolded toward the feet first.

NOTE. Fenestrated sheets are usually marked to indicate the direction in which they should be unfolded. This may be an arrow or label designating *Top* or *Head, Bottom* or *Foot.*

Thyroid Sheet The same size as a laparotomy sheet. The fenestration is transverse and closer to the top of the sheet.

Breast Sheet The same as a laparotomy sheet except the fenestration is 11 by 11 in. (28 by 28 cm), which provides for a larger exposure. Besides its use for radical mastectomy, it is used for operations within the chest cavity.

Kidney Sheet The same size as a laparotomy sheet. The fenestration is transverse to accommodate the transverse kidney incision.

Hip Sheet The same as a laparotomy sheet except that it is somewhat longer to completely cover the orthopaedic fracture table.

Split Sheet The same size as a laparotomy sheet. Rather than fenestrated, one end is cut longitudinally up the middle at least one-third the length of the sheet to form two free ends (tails). The upper end of this split may be U-shaped. Bands may be sewn on each tail approximately 8 in. (20 cm) from the end of the split to snug the sheet around an extremity or head.

Perineal Sheet A sheet of a size to create an adequate sterile field with the patient in lithotomy position. It has large boots incorporated into it to cover the legs in stirrups. It contains an opening $6\frac{1}{2}$ to 7 in. (17 cm) in diameter with a 10-in. (25-cm) reinforcement around it.

Combined Sheet A combination laparotomy and perineal sheet, used for combined abdominoperineal resection of the rectum when the entire procedure is done with the patient in lithotomy position. The rectum is removed before the abdomen is closed.

While many hospitals use them for most operations, fenestrated sheets are not always feasible. The openings may be much too large for small incisions, such as taking specimens for biopsies, operations on hands or feet, etc. Smaller, separate sheets may be used for these purposes, leaving exposed only the small operative area, or to provide underdrapes on the operative field.

Minor Sheet This sheet is 36 by 45 in. (91 by 114 cm). It has many uses. Wrapped around an extremity, it permits the extremity to remain on the sterile field for manipulation during operation. It is used under an arm to cover an armboard for shoulder, axillary, arm, or hand operations.

Medium Sheet About 36 by 72 in. (91 by 183 cm). It is used to drape under legs, as an added protection above or below the operative area, or for draping areas in which a fenestrated sheet cannot be used.

Single Sheet This sheet is 108 by 72 in. (274 by 183 cm). Folded lengthwise, it is placed above the operative field to shield off the anesthesiologist and anesthesia machine or other equipment near the patient's head or operating table.

Stockinet May be used to cover an extremity. This seamless tubing of stretchable material contours snugly to the skin. An opening is cut through it over the line of incision. The material may be secured with a plastic incise drape before the incision is made, or it may be clipped to the wound edges after incision.

Techniques to Remember in Draping

Since draping is a very important step in the preparation of the patient for operation, it must be done correctly. The entire team should be familiar with the draping procedure. The scrub nurse must know it perfectly and be ready to assist with it. Check beforehand to see that the necessary articles are arranged in proper sequence on the instrument table.

The person responsible for draping the patient may vary, as do the materials and styles of drapes used to create a sterile field. The surgeon or assistant usually places the self-adhering drape and/or the towels and towel clips to outline the site of incision. The scrub nurse assists with placing the remainder of the drapes.

During any draping procedure, the circulating nurse should stand by to direct the scrub nurse as necessary and to watch carefully for breaks in technique. A contaminated drape or exposure of a nonsterile area might well be the source of an infection for the patient.

1 Place the drapes on a dry area. The area around or under the patient may become damp from the solutions used for skin preparation. The circulating nurse must remove damp items or cover the area to provide a dry field on which to lay the sterile drapes.

2 Allow sufficient time to permit careful application.

3 Allow sufficient space to observe sterile technique.

4 Handle the drapes as little as possible.

5 Never reach across the operating table to drape the opposite side; go around the table.

6 Take the towels and towel clips, if used, to the side of the table from which the surgeon is going to apply them before handing them to him or her.

7 Carry the *folded drapes* to the operating table. Watch the front of the sterile gown; it may bulge and touch the nonsterile table or blanket on the patient. Stand well back from the nonsterile table.

8 Hold the drapes high enough to avoid touching nonsterile areas, but avoid touching the overhead operating light.

9 Hold the drape high until it is directly over the proper area, then lay it down where it is to remain. Once a sheet is placed, do not adjust it. Be careful not to slide the sheet out of place when opening the folds. If a drape is incorrectly placed, discard it. The circulating nurse peels it from the table without contaminating other drapes or the operative site.

10 Protect the gloved hands by cuffing the end of the sheet over them. Do not let your gloved hands touch the skin of the patient.

11 In unfolding a sheet from the operative site toward the foot or the head of the table, protect the gloved hand by enclosing it in the turned-back cuff of the sheet provided for this purpose. Keep the hands at table level.

12 If a drape becomes contaminated, do not handle it further. Discard it without contaminating gloves or other items.

13 If the end of a sheet falls below waist level, do not handle it further. Drop it and use another one.

14 If in doubt as to its sterility, consider a drape contaminated.

15 A towel clip that has been fastened through a drape has its points contaminated. Remove it only if absolutely necessary, then discard it from the sterile setup without touching the points. Cover the area from which it was removed with another piece of sterile draping material.

16 If a hole is found in a drape after it is laid down, the hole must be covered with another piece of draping material or the entire drape discarded.

17 A hair found on a drape must be removed and the area covered immediately. Although hair can be sterilized, the source of a hair is usually unknown when found on a sterile drape. It would cause foreign-body tissue reaction in the patient if it got into the wound. Remove the hair with a hemostat and hand the instrument off the sterile field; cover the area with a towel or another piece of draping material.

Procedures for Draping Patient

Draping procedures may vary from one hospital to another. However, standardized methods of application should be practiced using adequate draping materials for each operation. The most common procedures are discussed here merely to elaborate the principles. The following details procedures using only *absorbent* draping materials because it is more complex to establish a microbial barrier with them. The draping procedure is simplified when single-thickness, impermeable materials are used. Consult procedure book for specific draping procedures.

Laparotomy The term *laparotomy* refers to an incision through the abdominal wall into the abdominal cavity. All flat, smooth areas are draped as follows in the same manner as the abdomen. These areas include the neck, chest, flank, and back.

1 Hand up four towels and the towel clips. With practice these can be held in the hands at the same time and separated one by one as the surgeon takes them. Go to the side of the table on which the surgeon is draping to avoid reaching over the nonsterile table. The surgeon places these towels far within the scrubbed area, leaving only enough skin exposed for the incision.

2 Hand one end of the fanfolded medium sheet across the table to the assistant, supporting the folds, keeping it high, and holding it taut until it is opened; then lay it down. Place this medium sheet below the site of incision and the edge of it at the skin edge, covering the draping towel. This sheet provides an extra thickness of material under the area from the Mayo stand to the incision, where instruments and sponges are placed, and closes some of the opening in the laparotomy sheet if necessary. This sheet may be eliminated if a self-adhering incise drape is used, or impermeable drapes are used.

3 Place the laparotomy sheet with the opening directly over the skin area outlined by the towels in the direction indicated for the foot or head of the table. Drop the folds over the sides of the table. However, if an armboard is in place, hold the folds of the sheet at table level until the sheet is opened all the way. Open it downward over the patient's feet and upward over the anesthesia screen (see Figs. 11-7 and 11-8).

NOTE. Sheets with appropriate fenestrations are used to expose the operative site.
1. For neck, use a thyroid sheet.
2. For chest, with patient in either supine or lateral position, use a breast sheet.
3. For flank, with patient in kidney position for transverse incision, use a kidney sheet.
4. For back, use a laparotomy sheet the same as for the abdomen.

4 Place the large, single sheet crosswise of the table above the operating area. This sheet provides

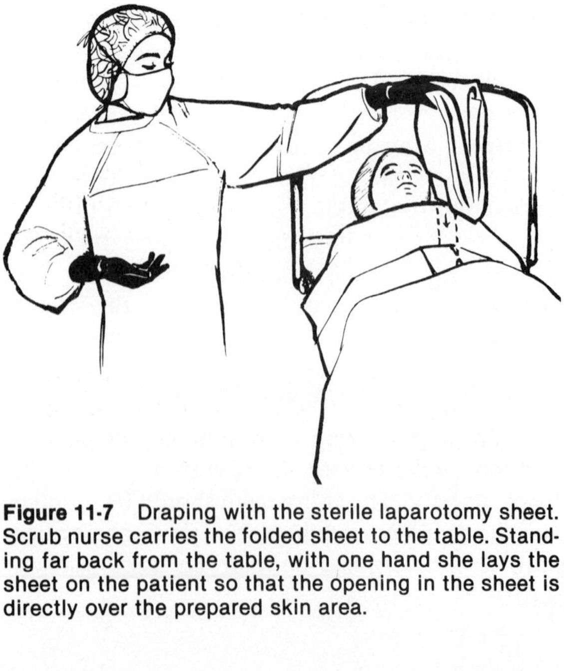

Figure 11-7 Draping with the sterile laparotomy sheet. Scrub nurse carries the folded sheet to the table. Standing far back from the table, with one hand she lays the sheet on the patient so that the opening in the sheet is directly over the prepared skin area.

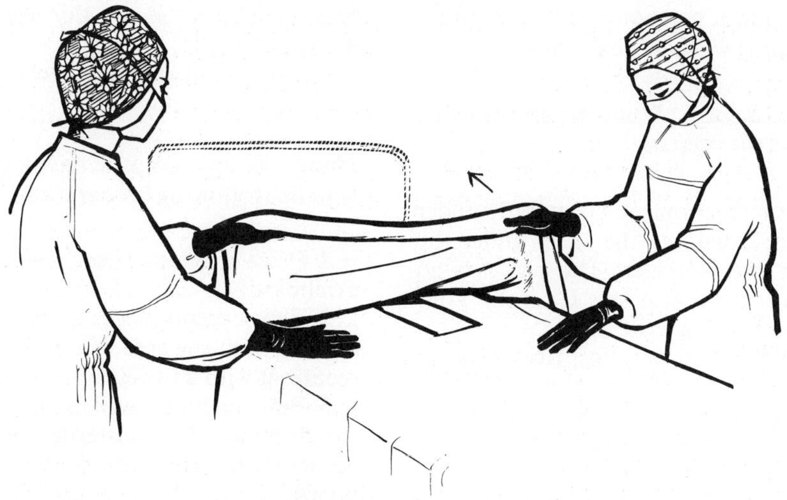

Figure 11-8 Unfolding the upper end of the laparotomy sheet over the anesthesia screen. Note that the hands approaching the unsterile area are protected in a cuff of the drape and the sheet is stabilized with the other hands.

extra thickness above the area and closes some of the opening in the laparotomy sheet if necessary. It also covers the armboard if one is in use. A single sheet may be needed for this latter purpose even if an impermeable lap sheet is used.

Head An overhead instrument table may be positioned over the patient. The table drape is extended down over the patient's shoulders to create a continuous sterile field between the instrument table and the operative site.

1 The surgeon places four towels around the head and secures them with towel clips or sews them in place. Towel clips are not used if x-rays will be taken during operation.
2 Hand one end of a fanfolded medium sheet to the assistant. Holding it taut, unfold, and secure it over the head end of the operating table below the operative area at the skin edge of the draping towel.
3 Place a fenestrated sheet with the opening over the exposed skin area of the head. Unfold the sheet across the front edge of the overhead table and secure it before allowing the remainder of the drape to drop over the head of the operating table toward the floor.

NOTE. If a split sheet is used, the tails are placed toward the head end of the operating table, draped around the patient's head, and secured with towel clips.

Face Even if the operation is unilateral, the surgeon may want the entire face exposed for comparison of skin lines.

1 The surgeon places a drape under the head while the circulating nurse holds up the head. This drape consists of a towel placed on a medium sheet. The center of the towel edge is 2 in. (5 cm) in from the center of the sheet edge. The towel is drawn up on each side of the face, over the forehead or at the hairline, and fastened with a clip. This leaves the desired amount of the face exposed.
2 Hand up three towels and four towel clips. These four towels surround the operative site.
3 Place a medium sheet just below the site. This sheet must overlap the one under the head.
4 A fenestrated drape may be placed to complete the draping.
5 Cover the remainder of the foot of the table, as necessary, with a single sheet.

NOTE. 1. If the patient is receiving inhalation anesthesia, use a minor sheet instead of a towel on the medium sheet for the first drape under the head. The minor sheet is large enough to draw up on each side of the face and to enclose the tubes from the anesthesia machine for a considerable distance, thus keeping them from contaminating the sterile field.
2. If the operation on the face is unilateral, the anesthesiologist may sit at the unaffected side, near the patient's head with an anesthesia screen placed on this side of the table.

Eye and Ear The basic procedure is the same as draping the patient for a facial operation, except that only the eye or ear is exposed.

NOTE. If local anesthesia will be administered, drapes must be raised off the patient's nose and mouth to permit free breathing. A

Mayo stand or screen positioned over the lower face before draping will elevate the drapes.

Chest and Radical Breast While the arm is being held up, following the preparation:

1 Place a minor sheet on the armboard, under the patient's arm, extending the sheet under the side of the chest and shoulder. The person who has been holding up the arm lays it on the armboard and fastens it with a wrist strap.
2 Hand up towels and towel clips; five or six are required.
3 Apply breast sheet so that the axilla is exposed for anticipated axillary dissection.

Shoulder While the arm is still being held up, following the preparation:

1 Place a medium sheet over the chest and under the arm.
2 Place a minor sheet under the shoulder and the side of the chest.
3 The surgeon outlines the site of operation with towels and secures them with clips.
4 Place a minor sheet over the patient's chest, covering the patient's neck. Keep this sheet even with the edge of the towel that limits the operative site laterally.
5 Wrap the arm in a minor sheet and secure it with a sterile gauze bandage. At this point, a sterile member of the team relieves the person who has been holding up the arm.
6 Place a medium sheet above the area and secure these sheets together with towel clips.
7 A laparotomy or a breast sheet may be used. Pull the arm through the opening. Or a single sheet may be placed above the area and the foot of the table covered with a medium sheet.

Elbow While the arm is still being held up, following the preparation:

1 Place a medium sheet across the chest and under the arm, up to the axilla.
2 The surgeon limits the operative area on the upper arm by placing a towel around the arm and securing it with a clip.
3 Wrap the hand and lower arm in a minor sheet or a double thickness of towels and secure with a sterile bandage. At this point, a sterile member of the team relieves the person who has been holding up the arm.
4 Draw stockinet over the exposed operative area.
5 Place a medium sheet across the chest, on top of the arm, even with the towel on the upper arm and covering it. Secure this sheet around the arm with a towel clip.
6 Lay the laparotomy sheet over the hand and pull the arm through it.

Hand While the arm and hand are still being held up, following preparation:

1 Place a minor sheet, folded in half, on the armboard.
2 The surgeon places a towel around the lower arm, to limit the area of the site of operation, and secures it with a towel clip.
3 Pull stockinet over the hand. At this stage in the draping, the nonsterile person is relieved of holding the arm. The arm is laid on the armboard.
4 Place a minor sheet across the armboard just above the operative site.
5 Place the laparotomy sheet on the hand with the foot end toward the patient. Do not drop the folds *below* the level of the armboard. Open the lap sheet.
6 Place a medium sheet below the laparotomy sheet to finish covering the patient.
7 Place a single sheet over the anesthesia screen.

Perineal With patient in lithotomy position:

1 The scrub nurse hangs a towel, folded in half, over a strip of 1-in. (2.5 cm) adhesive tape held by the circulating nurse, if a sterile plastic towel drape is not used. The circulating nurse places this towel over the anus and fastens the adhesive around the patient's buttocks, if the operation is vaginal or genital.
2 Hand up three towels and four towel clips.
3 Apply the perineal sheet by handing one end of it to the assistant, opening out the folds, and drawing the boots onto the feet and legs. Keep the hands on the outside of the sheet to avoid contaminating gloves and gown.

Hip If the leg will be manipulated during operation, while the leg is still being held up, following preparation:

1 Place a medium sheet on the table under the leg, up to the buttock.
2 Place another medium sheet on the table, overlapping the first one, to cover unaffected leg.
3 The surgeon wraps a towel around the thigh, just below the operative area, and clips it or sews it in place if x-rays will be taken.
4 Hand up enough additional towels to surround the operative area, with towel clips to secure them.

5 The surgeon wraps the foot and leg, including the towel around the thigh, in a minor sheet and bandages it on. The leg has been held up to this point.

6 Place a minor sheet lengthwise of the table on each side of the operative site, even with the skin. The sheets under the leg and above the site do not overlap.

NOTE. Some surgeons prefer to omit step 6 and draw the leg through the opening of a hip sheet or place a split sheet under the leg with the tails crossed over it toward the patient's head.

7 Place a medium sheet above the operative area. Secure these last three sheets with towel clips.

8 Place a single sheet above the operative area and over the anesthesia screen.

If manipulation of the leg is not necessary during operation, drape the same as for a laparotomy, using a hip sheet instead of a laparotomy sheet.

Knee While the leg is still being held up, following the preparation:

1 Place a medium sheet lengthwise on the table, under the leg, up to the buttock.

2 Place another medium sheet on the table overlapping the first sheet to cover the unaffected leg.

3 The surgeon limits the sterile field above the knee by placing a towel around the leg and securing it with a towel clip.

4 Lay a minor sheet on the sterile sheets under the leg. The person who has been holding up the leg lays it on this minor sheet. The surgeon wraps the leg in the minor sheet and secures it with a sterile bandage. Stockinet may be preferred for this step.

5 Place a medium sheet above the operative area, at the skin edge, over the draping towel, and fasten it with a towel clip.

6 Place the laparotomy sheet, with the opening on the foot and the longer part of the sheet toward the table head. Open it and draw the leg through the opening. A split sheet may be used.

Lower Leg and Ankle While the leg is still being held up, following the preparation:

1 Place a medium sheet under the leg and over the unaffected leg to above the knees.

2 The surgeon limits the sterile field by placing a towel around the leg above the area of intended incision and securing it with a towel clip.

3 Put stockinet over the foot and draw it up over the leg to above the skin edge of the towel. The person who has been holding the leg is relieved and the leg is held by a sterile team member.

4 Place a medium sheet above the operative area and secure around the leg with a towel clip.

5 Place the laparotomy sheet or split sheet with the leg drawn through the opening.

6 Cover the remainder of the table over the anesthesia screen with a single sheet as necessary.

Foot The general method of draping a foot is the same as that for the hand. While the foot is being held up, following the preparation:

1 Place a medium sheet on the table, under the foot.

2 The surgeon limits the operative area on the foot by placing a towel around the ankle and securing it with a towel clip.

3 Enclose the foot in stockinet. A sterile member of the team relieves the person who has been holding up the leg.

4 Place a medium sheet above the operative area, and secure it around the ankle with a towel clip.

5 Place the laparotomy sheet with the opening over the foot and the longer part of the sheet toward the head of the table.

Draping of Equipment

Equipment that is brought into the sterile field but cannot be sterilized must be draped before it is handled by sterile team members.

1 Tailored disposable drapes are available to cover the operating microscope so it can be manipulated in the sterile field by the surgeon.

2 If x-ray films are to be taken during operation, the cassette holder may be placed on the operating table, under the patient, before the patient is positioned, prepped, and draped. The circulating nurse raises the drape for the radiology technician to place and remove the cassette. The holder and/or cassette may be covered with a sterile Mayo stand cover or specially designed disposable cover and placed on the sterile drapes when a lateral view is needed.

3 Cords, attachments, or tubings that are not sterile must be inserted into sterile coverings before they are placed on the sterile field.

Nonsterile equipment that must stand near the sterile field must be excluded from the sterile area by a drape shield. IV poles frequently are used to attach drapes to shield off power-generating sources of mechanical and electrical equipment, such as electrosurgical and cryosurgical units, fiberoptic lighting units, air-powered or electrical instruments, etc. The drape over the patient or a separate single sheet is extended from the operating table upward in front of or over the nonsterile equipment. The circulating nurse fastens the drape to IV poles on each side of equipment that stands above the level of the sterile field or near it.

NOTE. Heat-generating equipment must have adequate ventilation to dissipate the heat. Impermeable, heat-retaining materials cannot completely encase these units.

Some nonsterile equipment, of necessity, will be moved over the sterile field. The sterile field must be protected.

1 Sterile disposable drapes are available to cover x-ray equipment, image intensifiers, etc.
2 When ready to move the x-ray tube or image intensifier over the sterile field, cover the field with a minor sheet. Discard this sheet after use.
3 Photography and television cameras should be draped as much as feasible when used over the operative area.

PLASTIC ISOLATOR

A plastic isolator (shield around the patient's bed or the operating table) may be used to exclude microorganisms from the environment immediately surrounding the patient. It may isolate a patient who is highly susceptible to infection, such as a burned or immunosuppressed patient, or may isolate a patient with a gross infection as a protection for others. In the OR, plastic isolators are used to isolate the operative field from both the room air and OR team and thus exclude microorganisms that are normally in the operating room environment.

The isolator is suspended from a steel frame to form a bubble over the patient. Its floor provides a sterile drape that adheres to the prepared skin around the incision site. Built into the sides are cuffs for gloves, helmets, and jackets. Provision is made for air-conditioning, communication, and the passing of sterile supplies by the circulating nurse.

Chapter 12

Wound Healing and Methods of Hemostasis

HISTORY OF WOUND MANAGEMENT

From ancient times, warfare made necessary some means of controlling hemorrhage and closing wounds. It is probable that the first operation performed was surgery of trauma although the date is not known. Egyptian writings, dating back to 3000 B.C., tell of treatment of various injuries including all kinds of fractures. Tourniquets were used to control bleeding. Mummies have been exhumed that revealed wounds sewed together with sutures.

Early Hindu surgeons surpassed those of Egypt in their skill in treating fractures and other injuries and in performing plastic surgery. The Hindu military surgeons were responsible for the food and sanitary conditions of the army as well as for treating the wounded.

Arabian surgeons used harp strings for sutures. They were made from sheep's intestines, twisted, and sun-dried. Religious laws of the Mohammedans required caravan leaders to carry sutures and needles to take care of injuries. Sometimes camel hair was used for sutures.

Greek surgery is first mentioned by Homer in 1000 B.C. Wounds of battle were cleansed, hemorrhage was checked with crushed roots and leaves, and then covered with compresses that were bandaged on.

Hemostasis, as practiced by early surgeons, combined styptics with pressure, bandages, and elevation of the part. Surgeons used materials at hand to cover the wound as a framework for the blood clot. Hare's fur, shredded bark of trees, egg yolk, dust, or cobwebs were bandaged on the bleeding part. Cold and heat were used. The early lithotomists controlled bleeding by assigning an assistant to compress the ends of the vessels between his fingers until bleeding stopped. The practice of pouring boiling oil into the wound or searing it with hot irons to stop bleeding and infection was torture in the extreme, and the patients usually were crippled if they survived.

Hippocrates (460 to 377 B.C.) noted the analgesic action of cold as a therapeutic entity and used ice and snow to check hemorrhage. Although the effects of cold and the ligature were known to him, Hippocrates recommended hot irons to stop hemorrhage and his custom persisted for over 2000 years. He also wrote of insertion of a "hollow tin tube" with flushings of wine and tepid oil to treat empyema. This was the first wound-drainage system. In his writings, he also stated that the best dressing for one side of a wound was the healthy tissue on the other side of the wound. This was a profound observation.

It was well known in early times that loss of blood meant loss of life. However, the circulation of blood was not understood. Through the writings of Aristotle (384 to 322 B.C.), blood vessels as conceived by Diogenes were described. Veins were thought to contain all, or almost all, the blood. Arteries were thought to contain air, with only a very small amount of blood.

Celsus, a Roman of the first century A.D., described the treatment of abdominal wounds. He mentioned the use of sutures as well known and ancient. Writings that are 4000 years old tell of the use of ligatures and sutures. However, Celsus used clumsy, grasping forceps to stop bleeding and covered the wound with cotton lint wet with vinegar.

The doctrine of air in the arteries continued until the physiologist Galen demonstrated in the second century that arteries, like veins, contain blood. Galen wrote on the treatment of war wounds and emphasized the importance of knowing about arteries, muscles, and nerves so as not to injure them further during treatment. To stop the flow of blood from a vein, he suggested grasping it with a hook and twisting moderately. If bleeding was from an artery, a ligature of linen should be applied. He also mentioned the use of gut for sutures, although he recommended silk when it could be obtained. He used gut sutures for primary closure of wounds in Roman gladiators. Knowledge of the ligature seems to have been lost until Galen spoke of using it after trying all other known methods to stop bleeding.

Sutures fell into disuse during the Middle Ages, accompanying a general regression in surgical technique. Their use appears to have been forgotten until Ambroise Paré, a French surgeon, revived it in the sixteenth century. He was an army surgeon at 19 years of age. In his time, it was thought that gangrene was the natural result of wounds. The accepted treatment for bleeding and infection was still the use of boiling oil or hot irons. One day in treating many wounded, Paré's supply of oil was inadequate, and he was forced to use a hastily concocted poultice of egg yolk, oil of roses, and turpentine. The next day he found these men much better than the ones treated with boiling oil. The difference impressed him so much that he never used the old method again. Paré rediscovered the use of the ligature and is best known for his use of it following amputation to control bleeding. He was the first person known to have used it for this purpose. In 1552, he explained to surgeons the advantages of the ligature. He also was the first to grasp vessels with a pinching instrument. His bullet-grasping forceps is the predecessor of the hemostat in use today.

So slow was the progress of surgery that, 200 years later, surgeons were still using the inhuman, destructive irons. The use of gunpowder in warfare opened up a new field of surgery. It was thought that gunpowder poisoned the wounds, so they were cauterized and cleansed with hot oil. Mention is made of ligatures and sutures again in writings of the early eighteenth century and at various times throughout that century, as is use of pressure on bleeding points to control bleeding.

Research in wound healing did not exist before the eighteenth century, when John Hunter observed and recorded for the first time some of the various patterns of healing. He differentiated primary from secondary healing by calling the first "adhesive inflammation" and the second "suppurative inflammation." He also distinguished between epithelization and granulation. The process of coagulation was recognized also during this century, but it was believed to be the result rather than the cause of hemostasis.

Early in the nineteenth century, Dr. Philip Syng Physick found, while performing animal experiments, that the body absorbs sutures made from animal tissue. It is thought he was the first surgeon to realize this. He wrote a paper on the use of sutures made from animal tissue.

During this period, pus and infection were everpresent in wounds. They were thought to be due to the suture itself. The long ends of silk or flax, left hanging from wounds, sloughed out. Secondary hemorrhage from abscess formation and ulceration of ligatures through the vessels was common. Many types of devices were used to drain the wounds.

William Stewart Halsted, a teaching surgeon at Johns Hopkins Hospital in Baltimore from 1893 to 1922, is acknowledged to have been one of the greatest surgeons of all times. Halsted perfected and brought into use the fine-pointed hemostat for occluding vessels, the Penrose drain, and rubber gloves. However, he is best known for his principles of tissue handling. In addition to his operative techniques of the highest order, he had the ability to inspire his assistants with his high ideals—as near perfection as possible in all operations. The silk-suture technique that he initiated in 1883, or a modification of it, is in use today. Its features are as follows:

1 Interrupted sutures are used for greater strength. Each stitch is taken and tied separately. If one knot slips, all the others hold. Halsted also believed that interrupted sutures were a barrier to infection, for he thought that if one area of a wound became infected, the microorganisms traveled along a continuous suture to infect the entire wound. A continuous suture is a running stitch tied only at the ends of the incision.

2 Sutures are as fine as is consistent with security. A suture stronger than the tissue it holds is not necessary.

3 Sutures are cut close to the knots. Long ends cause irritation.

4 A separate needle is used for each skin stitch.

5 Dead space in the wound is eliminated. *Dead space* is that space caused by separation of wound edges that have not been closely approximated by sutures. Serum or blood clots may collect in a dead space and prevent healing by keeping the cut edges of tissue separated.

6 Two fine sutures are used in situations usually requiring one large one.

7 Silk is not used in the presence of infection (see Chap. 13 for discussion of all types of suture materials).

8 Tension is not placed on tissue. Halsted warned against bringing tissue together under tension and thus endangering blood supply.

The two world wars of the twentieth century called for great numbers of surgeons to be educated in the care of the injured. Study of the total patient, not just of physical injury, and investigation into the cause of shock were carried on during World War I. Further study of shock was done during World War II, and much was learned concerning the effects of wounds on the functions of body organs. Great emphasis was placed upon assisting the patient's own defenses against injury by maintaining fluid and electrolyte balance. The treatment of the total individual is of prime importance in all surgical intervention. The high degree of skill of surgeons in all specialties, the instruments and equipment available to them, the refinements in anesthesia, added to the concept of total patient care, have increased the rate of survival and the return of patients to usefulness following surgical intervention.

Within reasonable limits, in the absence of hemorrhage and sepsis, wound healing is predictable. Yet abuse of the time-honored Halsted principles of operative technique can lead to such complications as hematoma, infection, wound disruption, scarring, stricture, and contracture.

Violation of the integrity of tissue, either by intent to explore or remove pathology or to repair traumatic injury, demands understanding of the mechanism and various factors that influence wound healing. Wound healing is nature's way of restoring continuity and strength to injured or incised tissue.

MECHANISM OF WOUND HEALING

When tissue is cut, the body's inherent defense mechanisms respond immediately to begin repair. Three types of wound healing are recognized: first intention, second intention, third intention. Each has practical applications in the making and closing of incisions or traumatic wounds.

First Intention

Healing by first intention is desired following primary union of an incised, aseptic, accurately approximated wound. It shows:

1 No postoperative swelling
2 No serous discharge or local infection
3 No separation of wound edges
4 Minimal scar formation

The rate and pattern of wound healing differ in different tissues. In general, first-intention wound healing consists of three distinct phases:

1 *Lag phase.* Tissue fluids containing plasma, blood cells, and fibrin exude from the tissues into the wound depositing fibrin, which weakly holds the wound edges together for the first 4 to 6 days. Fibrin and serum protein dry out, forming a scab that seals the wound from further fluid loss. At the same time, fibroblasts, fibrous-tissue germ cells, and epithelial cells migrate from the general circulation. Subsequent adhesion of these cells, a process known as *fibroplasia,* holds the wound edges together. Leukocytes and other cells produce proteolytic enzymes to dissolve and remove damaged tissue debris.

2 *Healing phase.* After the sixth postoperative day, fibroblasts multiply rapidly, bridging wound edges and restoring continuity of body structures. *Collagen,* a protein substance that is the chief constituent of connective tissue, is secreted from the fibroblasts and formed into fibers. This results in the rapid gain in tensile strength and pliability of the healing wound. *Tensile strength* is the ability of the tissues to resist rupture. Healing phase begins rapidly, diminishes progressively, and terminates on about the fourteenth day.

3 *Maturation phase.* During the fourteenth through twenty-first postoperative days, scar formation occurs by deposition of fibrous connective tissue. The collagen content remains constant, but the fiber pattern reforms and cross-links to increase the tensile strength. Wound contraction occurs over a period of weeks up to 6 months. As collagen density increases, vascularity decreases, and the scar grows pale.

Second Intention

The mechanism of second-intention healing is by wound contraction rather than primary union. Granulation tissue containing fibroblasts forms in the defect and closes it by contraction with secondary growth of epithelium. In this type:

1 Infection, excessive trauma, loss of tissue, or poorly approximated tissue is present.
2 The wound may be left open and allowed to heal from the bottom toward the outer surface.
3 Healing is delayed.
4 Scar formation is excessive.
5 Healing may produce a weak union, which may be conducive to incisional herniation (rupture) later.

Third Intention

Suturing is delayed or secondary for the purpose of walling off an area of gross infection where much tissue was removed, as in a debridement. In healing by third intention:

1 Two surfaces of granulation tissue are brought together.
2 A deeper and wider scar usually results.

FACTORS INFLUENCING WOUND HEALING

Physical Condition of the Patient

Age Skin and muscle lose tone and elasticity as natural characteristics of the aging process. The rate is variable in the population, however.

Weight In obese patients, the increase in bulk and weight of excess fat causes difficulty in confining it and securing good closure. Of all tissues, fat is the most vulnerable to trauma and infection.

Nutritional Status Wound healing is impaired by deficiencies in vitamins A, B, and C, zinc, proteins, and carbohydrates. Protein provides essential amino acids for new tissue construction. Vitamin C permits collagen formation. Carbohydrates are necessary for healing. Vitamin B is necessary for carbohydrate metabolism. Although known to be important in collagen synthesis, the mechanism of vitamin A and zinc in wound healing is unknown.

Fluid and Electrolyte Balance As a result of illness or injury, the patient may not be able to maintain normal fluid and electrolyte balance. Changes in this balance can affect kidney function, cellular metabolism, oxygen concentration in the circulation, or hormonal function.

General Health Associated diseases such as diabetes, uremia, anemia, cirrhosis, leukemia, etc., can delay the wound-healing processes. Malignancies, debilitating injuries, and systemic or localized infections can also adversely affect wound healing.

Immune Responses The body normally responds at once to repair the inflammatory reaction of the tissues to injury or foreign substances. The cells liberate a tissue extract that starts an immune response for repair of the tissue. This is known as *tissue reaction.* Some foreign materials normally cause more tissue reaction than others. Abnormalities in function of these immune responses, such as an allergic reaction, can contribute to delayed wound healing.

Drug Therapy Wound healing is basically collagen synthesis. Any agents that interfere with cellular metabolism have a potentially deleterious effect on the healing process. Prolonged high dosage of steroids preoperatively, such as cortisone, inhibit fibroplasia and formation of collagen.

RadiationTherapy Healing is delayed if the patient has had radiation in large doses preoperatively. The blood supply in irradiated tissue is decreased. However, little change from the normal healing pattern occurs if radiation has been given in low doses (see Chap. 27).

Postoperative Complications Edema, vomiting, or coughing can place stress on the healing wound before fibroplasia takes place. Complications in other parts of the body, far from the site of operation, such as pneumonia, thrombus, or embolus, can inhibit oxygen supply to the wound site. Collagen synthesis is partly a function of oxygenation of tissues.

Physical Activity Early ambulation postoperatively is one of the most important factors in the recovery of the surgical patient. Ambulation may be started immediately after recovery from anesthesia if the patient's condition does not contraindicate it. Some surgeons exempt only those whose blood pressure is not stable, those with a cardiac problem, and those whose general condition is poor. If the patient's physical condition does not safely permit ambulation, the surgeon orders otherwise.

Ambulation is started gradually by the patient first turning on his or her side. The patient then sits up with feet over the side of the bed. He or she then stands on the floor for a minute before returning to bed. After repeating this several times, the patient takes a few steps and finally increases the distance walked. Sitting in a chair for prolonged periods is discouraged, as it contributes to stasis of blood. A patient is fearful at first and needs a nurse at his or her side to provide confidence and safety. The nurse and patient must understand the value of early ambulation.

1 It speeds up circulation, which aids in the healing process and eliminates stasis of blood that may result in thrombus and embolus formation.

2 The patient is better able to cooperate in deep-breathing exercises to raise bronchial secretions; thus pulmonary complications are reduced.

3 Early ambulation decreases gas pains, distention, and the tendency toward nausea and vomiting.

4 Increased exercise aids digestion. Thus the patient's oral intake progreses sooner after operation so less supplementary intravenous fluid is necessary for hydration and nutrition.

5 Bodily functions return to normal more readily. In studies of early and late ambulatory groups, the latter group required twice as many catheterizations.

6 Early ambulation eliminates the general muscle weakness that follows bed rest.

7 Fewer pain-relieving drugs are necessary.

8 It boosts patients' morale to know they will be out of bed early after the operation, able to care for themselves, and soon ready to go home. This helps the mental outlook and through it the physical recovery.

9 It shortens hospitalization—an economic factor for the patient. From the point of view of the hospital, space is utilized more efficiently through more rapid turnover of beds.

Type of Wound

Surgical Incision The surgeon cuts through *intact* tissue. A sterile sharp scalpel (knife), scissors, or other cutting instrument may be used to separate skin and underlying tissue. The location, length, and depth of the incision is individually designed to achieve the best results for the patient following the operation the surgeon has planned. A safe operative procedure requires exposure through an adequate incision.

The surgeon spreads the skin taut between thumb and index finger in preparation for making the skin incision. With one stroke of evenly applied pressure on the scalpel, a clean incision is made through the skin. A number of factors influence the ease with which the skin incision is made:

1 Sharpness of knife blade
2 Resistance of self-adhering plastic drapes
3 Toughness of skin
4 Thickness of subcutaneous tissue

A clean stroke of a sterile surgical scalpel, followed by attention to all the principles of sterile technique and tissue handling, are the best insurances of primary healing by first intention. However, the direction of the incision may be a factor in wound healing. Wounds heal side-to-side, not end-to-end.

Traumatic Injuries Following traumatic injury, preservation of life is the first critical concern for the patient. No specific pattern of treatment suits all patients. The patient's general condition is of prime consideration. Injuries are evaluated and the one or ones that pose the greatest hazards to life or to the return to normal function are cared for first. The primary objective, following life support, in the traumatic wound is closure with minimal deformity and functional loss. Minor injuries are cared for in the emergency department. Patients with major injuries receive treatment in the emergency department prior to going to the operating room as quickly as the condition warrants.

Traumatic wounds can be classified as simple or complicated, clean or contaminated. Type of wound closure is predicated upon the classification of the wound.

Simple Wounds Continuity of skin is interrupted but without loss or destruction of tissue or implantation of a foreign body. These lacerations are usually due to a sharp-edged object cutting or penetrating at low velocity.

Complicated Wounds Tissue is lost or destroyed by crush or burn, or a foreign body is implanted by high-velocity penetration. If a penetrating wound was made by an object, such as a knife or bullet, this is not removed until the surgeon explores the wound in the operating room. Movement of a foreign object may cause further trauma. The depth of a penetrating wound is irrigated and may be excised. Skin grafting may be required following destruction of dermis (see Chap. 25).

Clean Wounds These will heal by first intention after closure of all tissue layers and wound edges. The cosmetic care of lacerated areas is important, as well as treatment to provide normal function of a part.

Contaminated Wounds Infection will result if treated by primary closure. Dirty objects have penetrated the skin. Microorganisms multiply rapidly, and within 6 hours contamination can become infection. Debridement is done to thoroughly wash and irrigate the wound. Devitalized tissue is removed because it acts as a culture medium. In excision of each area of contaminated tissue, clean instruments are used and discarded. Irrigation is continued during this excision of tissue. After initial debridement to remove foreign bodies, including dirt and dead or devitalized tissue, the wound heals by second or third intention. Delayed primary closure may be performed several days later.

> NOTE. Following traumatic injury that has resulted in broken skin, the patient is immunized against the tetanus bacillus. The individual is checked for sensitivity. If tetanus toxoid has been given previously, a booster dose of adsorbed tetanus toxoid may be given.

Operative Technique

Good operative technique is more important for good wound healing than any patient factor. Dr. John Deaver (1855 to 1931) of Philadelphia had a good adage: "If the surgeon cuts well and sews well, the patient gets well." Careful wound management involves the following:

Aseptic Technique Healthy tissues are able to combat a certain amount of contamination. Microorganisms are normally present in the skin and the air. Devitalized tissues have little power of resistance. Infection may occur from any one of a variety of causes resulting in a breakdown of the wound postoperatively. The surgeon gives meticulous attention to sterile technique throughout the operation to minimize contamination of the operative site. The entire OR team carefully carries out the rules for aseptic and sterile technique. In addition, many precautions are taken by all OR personnel. Strict adherence to housekeeping techniques, air engineering, sterilization procedures, and all the principles of aseptic technique is necessary. Infection may be due to a break in the chain of asepsis.

Hemostasis Complete hemostasis must be achieved to prevent loss of the patient's blood, to provide as bloodless a field as possible for accurate dissection, and to prevent hematoma (blood clot) formation.

Blood loss is caused by tissue trauma. The extent of dissection and injury done during operation can affect healing if the delivery of oxygen to the tissues is affected. Healing tissues consume oxygen avidly. Hence any condition that lowers circulatory flow and delivery of oxygen to the tissues impairs healing (hypoxia and hypovolemia were discussed in Chap. 9).

Because they are so critical, the mechanisms and methods of hemostasis are discussed in detail later in this chapter.

Tissue Handling All tissues should be handled very gently and as little as possible throughout the operation. The surgeon plans an incision just long enough to afford sufficient operating space. Careful consideration is given to underlying blood vessels and nerves to preserve as many as possible. Retractors are placed to provide exposure, but without causing undue pressure on tissues and organs or tension on muscles. Trauma to tissue in dissecting, handling with instruments, ligating, or suturing may cause edema and necrosis, death of tissue cells, with resultant slow healing. The body must rid itself of necrotic cells before the healing phase takes place.

Tissue Approximation Tissue edges are brought together with precision, avoiding strangulation and eliminating dead space, to promote wound healing. Too tight a closure or closure under tension causes *ischemia,* a decrease of blood supply to the tissues.

Dead space is caused by separation of wound edges that have not been closely approximated or by air trapped between layers of tissue. Serum or blood may collect in a dead space and prevent healing by keeping the cut edges of tissue separated. Wound edges not in close contact cannot heal readily. A drain may be inserted to aid in removal of fluid or air from the operative site postoperatively, or a pressure dressing may be applied over the closed wound to help obliterate dead space.

The choice of wound closure materials and the techniques of the surgeon are prime factors in the restoration of tensile strength to the wound during the healing process. Materials used to approximate tissues are discussed in Chapter 13.

Wound Security The quality of the approximated tissue and the type of the closure material are two factors that will determine the strength of the wound. Tensile strength of the tissues themselves will vary; some are more friable than others. Drains or catheters may be placed in the wound to evacuate serum or fluid from accumulating in dead space postoperatively. Drainage tubes may cause a weak spot in the incision, and underlying tissue may protrude. Also, drains may provide an inlet for microorganisms as well as an outlet for drainage. When possible, drains are placed through a stab wound in the skin rather than through the operative incision.

When sutures are used, the suture material provides all the strength of the wound immediately after closure. Closely spaced sutures give a stronger suture line. The strength of a suture should not be greater than the strength of the tissue on which it is used. To minimize tissue reaction to sutures, the least amount and the smallest size suture consistent with the holding power of the tissues is used.

Immediately after closure, an incision is at about 40 percent of its original strength. It reaches its greatest strength in 7 to 15 days. The wound is about one-third healed on the sixth postoperative day and two-thirds healed on the eighth day. The condition of the patient, type of operation, and many other factors may cause variance from the norm. As the tensile strength of the wound increases, the reliance on other support for wound security gradually lessens.

MECHANISM OF HEMOSTASIS

Hemostasis is essential to successful wound management. Literally, *hemostasis* is the arrest of a flow of blood or hemorrhage. The mechanism is *coagulation,* formation of a blood clot. The clotting of blood takes place by enzyme reaction, in several stages.

When severed by incision or traumatic injury, a blood vessel constricts and the ends contract somewhat. Platelets rapidly clump and adhere to the connective tissue at the cut end of the constricted vessel. Interaction with the collagen fibers causes the platelets to liberate adenosine diphosphate (ADP), epinephrine, and serotonin from their secretory granules. In turn, ADP causes other platelets to clump to the initial layer and to each other, forming a platelet plug. This may be sufficient in small vessels to provide primary hemostasis.

The reaction of plasma to connective tissue activates the clotting factors and causes a series of other reactions. *Prothrombin,* normally present in blood, reacts with *thromboplastin,* which is released when tissues are injured. Prothrombin and thromboplastin, along with calcium ions in the blood, form *thrombin.* This requires several minutes. Thrombin unites with *fibrinogen,* a blood protein, to form *fibrin,* which is the basic structural material of blood clots. This last reaction is very rapid.

The fibrin strands reinforce the platelet plug to form a resilient hemostatic plug capable of withstanding arterial pressure when the constricted vessel relaxes. Massive thrombosis within the vessels would occur, once coagulation is initiated, if it continued. However, fibrin is digested during the process. The products of this digestion, as well as the antithrombins normally present in the blood, act as anticoagulants. The coagulation mechanism rapidly and efficiently inhibits excessive blood loss so that excessive coagulation does not occur.

Hemorrhagic Disorders

Hemostasis can be effectively provided for patients with hemorrhagic disorders by giving concentrated human coagulation factors. These patients then can undergo operation without undue risk of bleeding, and without additional risk of overloading the vascular system.

Anticoagulants In operations on the blood vessels or heart and in patients who have a history of thromboembolic disease, anticoagulants are used. The dosage is adjusted to minimize the tendency of the blood to clot in the vessels, yet not to lead to excessive bleeding during or following the operation. The following drugs are commonly used:

Heparin Acts to inhibit the reaction wherein prothrombin is converted to thrombin.

Coumarin Derivatives Depress the blood prothrombin and decrease the tendency of blood platelets to cling together, thus decreasing the normal tendency of the blood to clot.

Warfarin Sodium Interferes with the action of vitamin K to prevent synthesis of prothrombin and fibrinogen.

Low Molecular Weight Dextran Reduces platelet adhesiveness and aggregation to prevent sludge from forming in the bloodstream. It coats the blood platelets to keep them from massing together.

Aspirin Diminishes the clumping of platelets by inhibiting the release reaction of the platelet factors.

Vitamin K Vitamin K enables the liver to produce clotting factors in the blood. To reduce the possibility of hemorrhage during operation, it is given preoperatively to:

1 Patients who have been on anticoagulant therapy.

2 Patients having faulty metabolism or improper utilization of bile with consequent low vitamin K absorption.

3 Elderly or debilitated patients requiring eye surgery to minimize the possibility of intraocular hemorrhage.

4 Newborns who require operative procedures.

5 Mothers just before delivery to help prevent postdelivery hemorrhage. It also assures the baby of an adequate prothrombin level until a sufficient amount is produced by the liver.

METHODS OF HEMOSTASIS

Basically, two different types of bleeding may occur during operative procedures: diffuse oozing from large denuded surfaces and gross bleeding from transected or penetrated vessels. Many of the present methods of hemostasis make use of the principles applied by the ancient surgeons. However, today bleeding is controlled and wounds are closed or covered to minimize trauma to tissue and to enhance healing without complication. Numerous agents, devices, and sophisticated pieces of equipment are used to achieve hemostasis and wound closure. These various methods can be classified as chemical, mechanical, and thermal.

Chemical Methods

Biological Dressings A biological dressing temporarily covers an open surface defect of the skin and underlying tissue in complicated, contaminated wounds. It is used to arrest the loss of fluid, reduce or eliminate microbial growth, and promote the production of granulation tissue and epithelialization prior to healing by second or third intention. A fibrin-elastin biologic bonding system adheres the dressing to the exposed surfaces. Biological dressings are skin grafts (refer to Chap. 25). These may be:

Autografts Skin grafted from one part of the patient's body to another part.

Homografts Skin taken from one genetically dissimilar person to another. A cadaver may be the source of skin for a homograft biological dressing. Controlled freezing preserves skin for use when needed.

Heterografts (Xenografts) Skin taken from a dissimilar species placed on human tissue (refer to porcine heterografts in Chap. 13).

Controlled Hypotension In selected situations when excessive blood loss is anticipated or encountered, blood pressure may be deliberately lowered to produce an essentially bloodless field for the surgeon. When induced, hypotension is carefully controlled by the anesthesiologist (refer to Chap. 9).

Gelatin Sponge Available in either powder or compressed-pad form, gelatin sponge is an absorbable hemostatic agent made from purified gelatin solution that has been beaten to a foamy consistency, dried, and sterilized by dry heat. As a pad, it is available in an assortment of sizes that can be cut as desired without crumbling. When it is placed on an area of capillary bleeding, fibrin is deposited in the interstices and the sponge swells, forming a substantial clot. The sponge is not soluble; it absorbs 45 times it own weight in blood. It is denatured to retard absorption, which takes place in 20 to 40 days. It is frequently soaked in thrombin or epinephrine solution, although it may be used alone. Before handing a gelatin sponge to the surgeon, dip it into warm saline, if used without thrombin or epinephrine, and press it between your fingers or against the sides of the basin to remove the air from it. Use the same procedure with thrombin or epinephrine solution, but then drop the sponge back into solution and allow it to absorb solution back to its original size.

Hyperbaric Oxygenation (OHP) *Hyperbaric oxygen therapy* is the administration of oxygen under several times greater than normal atmospheric pressure. The therapeutic aim is twofold: to raise the tissue-oxygen tension to normal levels or to raise it to above-normal levels. The physiological effects of oxygen at increased atmospheric pressure are: intense vasoconstriction, bone formation and resorption, bone marrow suppression, vascular proliferation, and a bacteriostatic or bactericidal agent. These effects may be used selectively.

The therapy is administered in specially designed chambers that vary in size from one that contains a fully equipped operating room to a single-patient unit. In the larger, the patient and the OR team enter a chamber filled with compressed air. The patient is given 100 percent oxygen to breathe by mask. Some surgical conditions for which the chamber is used include cardiac and peripheral vascular disease, chronic pulmonary disease, crush injuries and suturing of severed extremities, thermal burns, and gas gangrene.

In a single chamber, the patient is compressed with and breathes pure oxygen. This chamber is used for primary treatment of gas or air embolism, decompression illness, carbon monoxide poisoning, and exceptional blood-loss anemia. It also may be used for adjunctive therapy in the treatment of anaerobic infections, chronic and refractory osteomyelitis, preservation of compromised skin grafts, acute cerebral edema, acute traumatic peripheral ischemia, acute peripheral arterial insufficiency and thermal burns.

These chambers are not in common use, due mainly to high cost. Hospitals that have a hyperbaric chamber accept patients from other hospitals when it is thought the treatment will benefit the patient.

Microcrystalline Collagen Microcrystalline bovine collagen is an off-white, fluffy, flour-like material used as a topical hemostatic agent. It is produced from highly purified bovine corium (dermis) via shredding, hydrochloric acid treatment, and microfragmentation into threads or fibrils less than 1 micron in diameter. When placed in contact with a bleeding surface, hemostasis is achieved by adhesion of platelets and prompt fibrin deposition within the interstices of the collagen. Tissue cohesion is an inherent property of the collagen itself. It functions as a hemostatic agent only when it is applied directly to the source of bleeding from raw, oozing surfaces including bone and friable tissues or from around vascular anastomoses.

Supplied sterile in glass jars, small dry quantities are picked up with dry smooth tissue forceps and applied directly to active bleeding from irregular contours, crevices, and around suture lines. Firm pressure is then quickly applied over a dry gauze sponge, held either by the fingers in accessible areas or a sponge forceps in less accessible areas. It is important that the material be firmly compressed against the bleeding surface before excessive wetting with blood can occur. Effective application is evidenced by a firm adherent coagulum with no break-through bleeding from either surface or edges. If desired, excess collagen can be removed from around the site without recreating bleeding. The remaining coagulum absorbs during wound healing.

Oxidized Cellulose Absorbable oxidation products of cellulose are available in the form of a pad of oxidized cellulose similar to absorbent cotton, or a knitted fabric strip of oxidized regenerated cellulose. Either of these products is laid dry on an oozing surface or held firmly against a bleeding site until hemostasis is obtained. When oxidized cellulose comes into contact with whole blood, a clot forms rapidly. As it reacts with blood, it increases in size to form a gel and stops bleeding in areas difficult to control by other means of hemostasis. Except in situations where packing is required as a life-saving measure, only the minimal amount required to control capillary or venous bleeding or small arterial hemorrhage is used. If left on oozing surfaces, it will absorb with minimal tissue reaction. It is not recommended for use on bone unless it is removed after hemostasis as it may interfere with bone regeneration.

Oxidized cellulose is supplied in sterile vials. It cannot be steam-sterilized because high temperature causes physical breakdown of the product and loss of tensile strength. It may be stored at room temperature. It is used dry; do not moisten in either hemostatic or antibiotic solutions. Oxidized regenerated cellulose has some inherent antibacterial properties.

Oxytocin Oxytocin is a hormone produced by the pituitary gland. It is prepared synthetically for therapeutic injection. This is sometimes used to induce labor and also given to cause contraction of the uterus after delivery of the placenta. It is a systemic agent used to control hemorrhage, rather than a hemostatic agent per se.

Phenol and Alcohol Some surgeons use 95% phenol to cauterize tissue when cutting across the lumen of the appendix or gastrointestinal tract. Phenol coagulates proteins and in high concentration is so extremely caustic that it can cause severe burns. Therefore it must be neutralized with 95% alcohol as soon as the surgeon has used it; the burning action continues until the phenol is neutralized with alcohol (see Chap. 17, for use in general surgery).

Styptics A styptic is an agent that checks hemorrhage by causing *vasoconstriction,* contraction of the blood vessels. While styptics, especially epinephrine, are used to some extent, they have the disadvantage of being rapidly carried away by the bloodstream.

Epinephrine A hormone of the adrenal gland, epinephrine (Adrenalin) is prepared synthetically for use as a vasoconstrictor to prolong the action of local anesthetic agents or to decrease bleeding. Used in local anesthetic agents to constrict the vessels locally, epinephrine keeps the anesthetic concentrated within the area injected and reduces the amount of bleeding when the incision is made. However, it is rapidly dispersed, leaving little local effect. Within the incision, gelatin sponges soaked in 1:1000 epinephrine may be applied to bleeding surfaces. These are especially useful in ear and microsurgical procedures where localized hemostasis is critical.

Tannic Acid A powder made from an astringent plant, tannic acid is used occasionally on mucous membranes of the nose and throat to help stop capillary bleeding.

Thrombin An enzyme extracted from beef blood is used therapeutically as a topical hemostatic agent. Thrombin accelerates coagulation of blood and controls capillary bleeding. It unites rapidly with fibrinogen to form a clot. Topically, it may be used as a dry powder to sprinkle on an oozing surface or as a solution, alone or to saturate a gelatin sponge. Topical thrombin is used on areas of capillary bleeding that do not lend themselves to other means of hemostasis, such as sealing a skin graft onto a denuded area.

Thrombin is used for local application only. *It is never injected.* When a solution of it is on the instrument table, it must be kept separated from any other solutions. Use a careful, sure means of identification. It is recommended that thrombin be mixed just before use, as it loses potency after several hours. Refer to instructions of the manufacturer for mixing the solution.

Mechanical Methods

Bone Wax Composed mainly of beeswax, bone wax is used to control bleeding from bone in some orthopaedic and neurosurgical procedures. The surgeon rubs a small amount of this soft material over cut bone surfaces to stop oozing. The scrub nurse places several pieces, each rolled into a ball, around the rim of a medicine cup. When needed, hold the cup at the sterile field so the surgeon can pick a ball of wax off the rim.

Drains Drains may be used prophylactically or therapeutically during the operation and/or postoperatively. Used prophylactically to evacuate intestinal fluids, urine, or fluids from any source, drains can stimulate a walling-off process about an operative site in which subsequent drainage may accumulate. Therapeutically, drains aid in removal of fluid or air from the operative site to obliterate dead spaces and to enhance apposition of tissues. Although technically not a method of hemostasis in the context of arresting the flow of blood, drainage of body cavities helps prevent tissue trauma and restore organs to normal function.

Drainage during Operation

1 *Gastrointestinal decompression* with a plastic or rubber nasogastric tube inserted through the nostril down into the stomach or small intestine removes flatus, fluids, or other contents. The tube has holes in several locations near the tip to permit withdrawal of contents. Several types of nasogastric tubes are used; most common are the Levin tube into the stomach and Miller-Abbott tube into the small intestine.

The surgeon may ask the anesthesiologist to insert a tube to decompress the gastrointestinal tract during the operation when distention due to obstruction obscures the operative site, to measure blood loss due to gastric hemorrhage, or to evacuate gastric secretions during bowel anastomosis. The anesthesiologist may insert a nasogastric tube preoperatively to empty the stomach before an emergency operation to prevent aspiration of stomach contents.

The nasogastric tube may remain in place postoperatively to prevent vomiting and distention caused by decreased peristalisis following anesthesia, manipulation of the viscera during operation, or obstruction from edema of tissues at the operative site. For this purpose, the tube is connected to a suction apparatus. It also may be used for nasogastric feeding during the healing process after operations on the upper alimentary canal.

2 *Urinary drainage* via urethral or ureteral catheters inserted preoperatively provides constant drainage from the bladder or kidneys during operation. The purpose may be to keep the bladder decompressed or to prevent extravasation of urine into the tissues around the operative site during and after genitourinary operations. Postoperatively, the inflated balloon of a Foley retention catheter maintains an even pressure on the bladder neck, which may help control bleeding following prostatectomy, for example. An indwelling urethral catheter may be connected to a bladder-irrigation or tidal-drainage system until the bladder resumes normal function postoperatively.

Postoperative Drainage

1 *Chest drainage* ensures complete expansion of the lungs postoperatively. Air and fluid must be evacuated from the pleural space following operations within the chest cavity. A chest tube is inserted during closure, clamped shut, and the end covered with a sterile sponge until it can be connected to a sterile closed water-seal drainage system. The drainage system must prevent outside air from being drawn into the pleural space during expiration. Water in the collection unit seals off outside air to maintain a negative pressure within the pleural cavity.

Two tubes vent the leakproof top of the collection unit. A short air-outlet tube extends 1 in. (2.5 cm) or more above the stopper to about 3 in. (7.5 cm) below it into the collection unit. The long inlet tube extends from above the stopper, through it, to about 1 in. (2.5 cm) from the bottom of the collection unit. Sterile water is poured into the collection unit to a level 1 to 2 in. (2.5 to 5 cm) above the end of the long inlet tube. The circulating nurse marks the water level on the outside of the collection unit. Clear sterile tubing connects the inlet tube to the tube placed into the pleural space. Upon the patient's initial expiration, water rises a short distance up into the inlet tube. With each subsequent inspiration-expiration the water level in the tube fluctuates. If the water level in the tube remains stationary, the chest tube or connecting tubing may be clogged or kinked. *The collection unit must be kept well below chest level to prevent water entering the chest.*

Fluid drains by gravity from the chest into the water. The collection unit should be calibrated so that drainage can be measured. Air bubbles through the water and escapes through the outlet tube.

If gravity drainage is not adequate for reexpansion of the lungs, suction may be applied. This requires the addition of one or two collection units to the system, to act as a pressure regulator, and a suction machine to maintain negative pressure. Disposable chest-drainage units are available commercially, as a single unit or in a series of two or three. Some units are modifications based on the principle described for a closed water-seal system. Follow the manufacturer's direction for use. *The chest tube must be clamped tightly,* as a safety measure with some units, *during transportation.* Be sure to check carefully if clamping is needed in the type of unit you use. Be sure it is properly connected before the patient leaves the OR.

2 *Closed-wound suction systems* are used when it is necessary to apply suction to a large, closed-wound site postoperatively. A constant, gentle, negative pressure vacuum evacuates tissue fluid and blood to promote healing by reducing edema and media for microbial growth. It also eliminates dead space by holding skin flaps against underlying tissue.

Sterile plastic tubing connected to a stainless steel needle is placed in the operative area, usually through a small stab wound in the skin. This tubing has several perforations along the length placed in the tissues. It also has radiopaque markings to aid in checking location of tubing on x-ray if desired. The tubing is connected to a sterile, self-contained portable container. This can be attached immediately after placement of the tubing and the vacuum activated. Several different units are available with containers of different capacities as well as sizes of tubings. Directions printed on each unit must be followed to activate the vacuum. An anti-reflux valve guards against backflow of fluids. Calibrations on the side of the container measure the drainage and a line designates when it should be emptied. These units are made entirely or partially of clear plastic so the surgeon can inspect the drainage.

3 *Constant gravity drainage,* without negative pressure vacuum, is often used following operations on the gallbladder, bladder, kidney, or caecum. Each hospital has a supply of tubes, catheters, and various kinds of tubings and adaptors that are kept sterile. Many of the tubes and catheters are radiopaque. They are ready for the circulating nurse to open if needed.

A closed or semiclosed system of drainage may be used. The scrub nurse keeps the end of the tube or catheter sterile until it is connected to the sterile end of the constant-drainage tubing. When necessary to disconnect, protect the end of each with a sterile sponge held with a rubber band. If either end becomes contaminated inadvertently, wipe the tube or catheter off with an alcohol sponge. Obtain another sterile drainage tubing.

Plastic, disposable, constant-drainage bags and tubing are used and changed every 8 hours. They are marked in gradations from 500 to 2000 cc.

Use tubes and catheters or any other drainage tubing for one patient only—never reuse on another. Aside from the aesthetic reasons, the wall absorbs a certain amount of irritating chemicals from the patient's tissues that causes an irritation in the next patient, even though it is thoroughly cleaned and sterilized.

4 *Penrose drain,* made of *gutta-percha,* the coagulated latex of various trees, was described by Dr. Penrose in 1897. Sometimes referred to as a *cigarette drain,* it is still used to maintain a vent for the escape of fluid or air or to wall off an area of exudate in the wound.

A Penrose drain is a thin walled cylinder of radiopaque latex. The diameter may be $\frac{1}{4}$ to 1 in. (6 mm to 2.5 cm), depending upon the surgeon's preference. It is usually supplied to the sterile field in a 6- to 12-in. (15- to 30-cm) length for the surgeon to cut as desired. Penrose drains are commercially available prepackaged and sterilized. However, if they are prepared for steam sterilization in the hospital, a gauze wick must be inserted to permit steam penetration of the lumen.

Although Penrose drains are usually used without a wick, the surgeon may prefer the wick of gauze packing left in the lumen of the tubing. Moisten the drain in saline before handing it to the surgeon. After it is placed into the operative area and brought out through a stab wound in the skin, the drain is secured with a skin suture, or a safety pin is attached on the outside close to the skin, to keep the drain from retracting into the wound.

Penrose drains may be used to gently retract vessels and other small structures.

5 *Sump drain,* a plastic or rubber catheter, may be used for irrigation, aspiration with suction, or to introduce medication to an area. A sump drain has a double or triple lumen for these purposes. Clogging is reduced to a minimum by the large lateral openings. It is connected to a constant-drainage system, with or without suction.

Dressings Dressings give some support to the incision and surrounding skin and absorb drainage (refer to Chap. 8 for types of dressings). Dry gauze is not used on a denuded area because it adheres and acts as a foreign body. Granulation tissue will grow into it. Bleeding can be reactivated when it is removed (refer to Chap. 25 for alternatives).

Hemostatic Clamps Clamps for occluding vessels have two opposing serrated jaws, stabilized by a box lock, and controlled by ringed handles. They are used to grasp or hold a small amount of tissue or to compress blood vessels. The hemostat is the most frequently used surgical instrument and the most commonly used method of hemostasis. This instrument has either straight or curved jaws that narrow to a fine point. Often the pressure of clamping the instrument is sufficient to constrict and seal a vessel with minimal trauma or adjacent tissue necrosis. A wide variety of other hemostatic clamps are used for vessel occlusion, including noncrushing vascular clamps that do not damage large vessels.

Ligating Clips Metallic clips are small pieces of thin, serrated wire, bent in the center to an oblique angle. When placed on a vessel and pinched shut, they occlude the lumen and stop the bleeding. A specific forceps is required for the application of each type available. Clips may be mounted in a sterile plastic cartridge that can be secured in a heavy stainless steel base to facilitate loading the applier forceps.

Ligating clips were devised in 1911 by Dr. Harvey Cushing for use in brain surgery. Cushing clips are made of silver. Stainless steel and tantalum clips are more common today. The serrations across the wire prevent their slipping off the vessels. Many surgeons use them for ligating vessels, nerves, and other small structures.

These metallic clips also may be used to mark a biopsy site or other areas to permit x-ray visualization in order to detect postoperative complications. For example, migration of a marker clip could indicate the presence of a hematoma in the wound.

Ligature A ligature, commonly called a *tie,* is a strand of material that is tied around a blood vessel to occlude the lumen and prevent bleeding from it. Frequently the ligature is tied around a hemostat and slipped off the point onto the vessel and pulled taut to effect permanent hemostasis. Vessels are ligated with the smallest-size strand possible and include the smallest amount of surrounding tissue possible. Ends are cut as near the knot as possible.

Large and pulsating vessels may require a *transfixion suture.* A ligature on a needle is placed through a "bite" of tissue and brought around the end of the vessel. This eliminates any possibility of its slipping off the end of the vessel. All bleeding points should be ligated before the next layer of tissue is incised.

Pressure Pressure is exerted on the bleeding point manually or by mechanical devices. Whether pressure promotes hemostasis or merely constricts the blood vessels is questionable. However, the general belief is that it delays hemorrhage until the normal forces of the blood have time to form a clot.

Digital Compression When digital pressure is applied to an artery proximal to an area of bleeding, such as in traumatic injury, hemorrhage is controlled. The main disadvantage of digital pressure is that it cannot be applied permanently. Firm pressure is applied on the skin on both sides as the skin incision is made to help control subcutaneous bleeding until the vessels can be clamped, ligated, or cauterized. Pressure is applied while sponging the operative area to locate a bleeding vessel.

Mechanical Pressure Devices

1 *Antigravity suit,* commonly known as the *G-suit,* is a method of circumferential pneumatic compression to control hemorrhage, counteract postural hypotension, and maintain venous pressure. An inflatable vinyl plastic envelope, the G-suit is wrapped and laced about the patient from the ankles to the xyphoid process, thereby increasing pressure on the wall of a bleeding vessel. It is most effective in control of intraabdominal bleeding during transport following trauma. It is also used to prevent air embolism during some head and neck operations performed with the patient in a sitting position. The uniform circumferential pneumatic compression reduces the volume of the vascular bed below the diaphragm, thus diverting blood to vital structures above. The increased venous filling the G-suit produces decreases the possibility of air embolus.

   Inflate the section over the lower extremities first to prevent venous stasis in the legs. The entire suit can be inflated or specific sections of it as desired by the surgeon.

2 *Packs* are used to sustain pressure on the wound. The application of sponges or laparotomy tapes effectively controls capillary ooze by occluding the capillaries. The surgeon usually wants these moistened, sometimes with hot saline solution.

   Compressed rayon or cotton radiopaque patties are used for hemostasis when placed on the surface of delicate tissues such as the brain, spinal cord, or nerves. These patties have no loose fibers. They are available in an assortment of sizes. Before use, moisten with saline and press out excess, keeping them flat.

3 *Pressure dressings* are used to eliminate dead space and to prevent capillary bleeding from a wound, serum accumulation or hematoma when closed-wound suction drainage is contraindicated. They may be used as an adjunct to wound drainage to distribute pressure evenly over the wound to minimize edema. (Refer to Chap. 8 for description of materials used.)

4 *Rubber dam,* a piece of thin latex rubber sheeting, placed over an arteriotomy site, can help hold the wound edges together until the bleeding is controlled. This rubber dam can be removed after 4 or 5 minutes of compression.

5 *Suction* is the application of pressure less than atmospheric either continuously or intermittently. It is used during operations for the removal of blood and tissue fluids from the operating field. An appropriate style tip is attached to the sterile conductive suction tubing; many tips are disposable. The kinds of suction tips include:

   a *Poole abdominal,* used on laparotomies or operations within any cavity in which fluid or pus may be encountered. It has an outer filter shield.

   b *Ferguson-Frazier,* used when there is little or no fluid except capillary bleeding and irrigating fluid, such as in brain, spine, plastic, or orthopaedic procedures. It keeps the field dry without the usual sponging. One model has a connection for an electrosurgical unit, and the tip can be used for a fulgurating tip.

   c *Yankauer tonsil suction,* used on mouth or throat procedures. Rather than a straight tube, like an abdominal suction tip, it is angled.

   d *Plain rubber catheter,* used in the nasopharynx, especially in infants.

   e *Aspirating tube,* used through an endoscope.

6 *Tourniquet* may be used when operating on an extremity to keep the operative field free from blood and thus reduce the operating time. Not generally considered a method of hemostasis, bleeding is controlled by other methods prior to wound closure. A firm dressing applied to a closed wound before removing the tourniquet helps to prevent collection of serum in the wound. This is especially true in operations on the knee.

   Regulations for and precautions with tourniquet application and usage must be observed by all persons attending the patient. A tourniquet should never be used when the circulation in the distal part of an extremity is impaired. A tourniquet can cause tissue injury and shut off the entire blood supply to the part below it, causing gangrene and loss of the extremity. Metabolic changes may be irreversible after $1\frac{1}{2}$ hours of tourniquet ischemia. *A tourniquet is dangerous to apply, to leave on, and to remove.* A tourniquet may be applied by the surgeon, one of the assistants, or by the circulating nurse on surgeon's orders. To apply:

   a Protect the patient's skin by placing a folded towel around the extremity under the tourniquet.

   b Elevate the arm or leg to encourage venous drainage before tightening a tourniquet.

   c Record the time the tourniquet is applied and removed. Inform the surgeon when it has been on for 45 minutes and every 15 minutes thereafter. The anesthesiologist may note the time with the surgeon and record it on the anesthesia sheet, thus providing a permanent record of tourniquet time. In some hospitals the circulating nurse posts tourniquet time on the tally board in view of the surgeon.

Kinds of tourniquets include:

a *Blood-pressure cuff.* The surgeon determines the amount of pressure to be sustained.

b *Esmarch bandage.* Friedrich von Esmarch, a great military surgeon of Germany, introduced an elastic bandage for the control of hemorrhage on the battlefield in 1869. As known today, this is a 3 in. (7.5 cm) latex rubber roller bandage used to compress the superficial vessels to force the blood out of an extremity. An Esmarch bandage is not used, however, to empty vessels of blood preoperatively in the patient following traumatic injury or if the patient has been in a cast. Danger exists that thrombi might be in the vessels because of injury or stasis of blood, and these could become dislodged and result in emboli.

Starting at the distal end of an extremity, an Esmarch bandage is wrapped tightly, overlapping spirally, to the level of the blood-pressure cuff or a pneumatic tourniquet. The tourniquet is then tightened and the rubber bandage removed. Or, starting at the distal end of the extremity, the rubber bandage can be partially removed, leaving the last three rounds, which constitute a tourniquet.

To ensure sterilization of all surfaces, a layer of roller gauze bandage is placed between the layers of the rubber bandage. This must be removed and the rubber bandage rerolled before use.

c *Pneumatic tourniquet.* Similar to a blood-pressure cuff, although heavier and more secure, the cuff consists of a rubber bladder shielded by a plastic insert inside a fabric cover. The appropriate size cuff must be used; various cuff sizes are available. Cuffs are inflated automatically with a compressed gas (air, oxygen, or Freon) by means of tubing interconnected between the cuff and a pressure cartridge or piped-in system. The desired pressure is uniformly maintained by a pressure valve and registered on a pressure gauge. Care must be taken to ensure that the gauge registers accurately. Paralysis of the extremity may result from excessive pressure.

d *Rubber band.* This may be used as a tourniquet for a finger or toe.

e *Rubber tubing.* When starting an intravenous infusion, a small piece of rubber tubing is applied around the extremity, usually an arm, momentarily while the needle is being inserted. This stops venous return and makes the vein more obvious.

Thermal Methods

Hemostasis may be achieved or enhanced by application of either cold or heat to body tissues.

Cryosurgery Cryosurgery is performed with the aid of special instruments for local freezing of diseased tissue without harm to normal adjacent structures. Extreme cold causes intracapillary thrombosis and tissue necrosis in the frozen area. The frozen tissue may be removed without significant bleeding during or after operation. Cryosurgery is also used to alter cell function without removing tissue. It tends to be hemostatic and lymphostatic, particularly in highly vascular areas.

Extreme cold, at controlled temperatures ranging from +20 to −196 °C (+68 to −140 °F) is delivered to extract heat from a small volume of tissue in a rapid manner. Liquid nitrogen is the most commonly used refrigerant, however Freon or carbon dioxide gas may be used. The liquid or gas is in a vacuum container and comes through an insulated vacuum tube to a probe. All but the tip of the probe is insulated. The freezing of tissue at this tip is due to the liquid nitrogen becoming gaseous and in the process heat is removed from the tissue. A ball of frozen tissue gradually forms around the uninsulated tip. The extent of tissue destruction is controllable by raising or lowering the temperature of the cells surrounding the lesion.

The machines vary in range of temperatures obtained according to their design and type of refrigerant used. Some are nonelectric with foot-switch operated probes. Special miniature, presterilized, disposable models for single-patient use are particularly suitable for ophthalmic applications (refer to Chap. 22).

Because the process is rapid, involves less trauma to destroy or remove tissue, controls bleeding, and minimizes local pain, cryosurgery is used to alter the function of nerve cells and to destroy otherwise unapproachable brain tumors. Other techniques involve the removal of superficial tumors in the nasopharynx and the skin, destruction of the prostate gland, removal of highly vascular tumors, removal of lesions from the cervix and anus, cataract extraction, retinal detachment, etc. The amount of tissue destroyed is influenced by the size of the tip of the probe and temperature used, duration of use, kind of tissue and its vascularity, and special skill of the surgeon.

Hypothermia Cooling of body tissues to a temperature as low as 26 °C (78.8 °F) in adults and large children and 20 °C (68 °F) in infants and small children, well below normal limits, decreases cellular metabolism and thereby decreases the need for oxygen by the tissues. The decreased requirement for oxygen decreases bleeding. It lowers blood pressure to slow the circulation and increases the viscosity of blood. This process results in hemoconcentration, which contributes to capillary sludging and microcirculatory stasis to provide an essentially dry field for the surgeon. Hypothermia may be localized or generalized (systemic). Refer to Chapter 9 for a detailed description of methods of local and systemic hypothermia by both internal and external body cooling. Hypothermia is used as an adjunct to anesthesia particularly during operations of the heart, brain, or liver.

Diathermy An oscillating, high-frequency electric current generates enough heat to coagulate and destroy body tissues. Heat is generated by the resistance of tissues to the passage of alternating electric current. A short-wave diathermy machine produces a very high frequency of 10 to 100 million cycles per second. The machine should not be activated until the surgeon is ready to deliver this current. Diathermy is useful in stopping bleeding from small blood vessels. It is used primarily to repair detached retina (see Chap. 22) and to cauterize small warts, polyps, and other small superficial lesions.

Electrocautery A small loop heated by a steady, direct electric current to red heat will coagulate or destroy tissue on contact. Heat is transferred to the tissue from the preheated wire. The hemostatic effect is a result of searing or sealing the tissues. Cautery must be of 6-volt hot-wire type, with switch and control at least 3 ft (1 m) from the anesthesia machine and face mask. Hot point of cautery must be at least 24 in. (60 cm) from machine and mask, with a protecting screen between the tip and patient's head. Cautery must *never* be used in the mouth, around the head, or in the pleural cavity when flammable anesthetics are used. *High-frequency cautery must not be used when any flammable agent is present.* Only *moist* sponges should be permitted on the field while cautery is in use, to prevent fire.

Electrosurgery High-frequency electric current provided from an electrosurgical unit frequently is used to cut tissue and to coagulate bleeding points. The concentration and flow of current generates heat as it meets resistance in passage through tissue. Dr. W. T. Bovie, a physicist, developed the first spark-gap tube generator in the 1920s. This was the universal basis of electrosurgical units prior to the 1970s when solid-state units became available. These use transistors, diodes, and rectifiers to generate the current. The current passes through the patient's tissues between two electrodes.

Function of Electrodes

1 *Active electrode.* The active electrode is placed on the tissue by the surgeon. The style of the electrode tip, i.e., blade, loop, ball, needle, etc., will be determined by the type of operation and the current to be used. The electrode tip may be fixed into or detachable from a pencil-shaped handle, or it may be incorporated into a tissue forceps or suction tube. This is attached to a conductor cord, which is connected to the electrosurgical unit. The electrode and cord may be disposable. The electrode may be activated by a hand control or a foot switch to transfer the electric current to the tissue.
2 *Inactive electrode.* Electric current will flow to ground or a neutral potential. Therefore, a proper channel must be provided to disperse the current and heat generated in the tissue. The inactive electrode disperses the current released through the active electrode and provides the return from the tissues back to the electrosurgical unit. Electrosurgical units have either one or both of the following mechanisms to direct the flow of electric current:
   a *Monopolar units.* The inactive electrode is in the form of a patient grounding pad or plate. This electrode is placed in direct contact with the skin. The National Fire Protection Association recommends that grounding area equal 1 $cm^2/1\frac{1}{2}$ watts (W) of applied power output.* A flexible, disposable inactive electrode may be used. Some mold to any body surface. Some are prelubricated. If a stainless steel plate is placed under the patient, a conductive electrode lubricant must be spread evenly over the entire plate to

*Quoted from NFPA 76C, *Safe Use of High-Frequency Electricity in Health Care Facilities,* p. 7, 1975, The National Fire Protection Association, Boston, Mass.

thoroughly wet the skin and thus reduce its electrical resistance to a minimum. Current flows from the active electrode through the body to the inactive electrode. The current then returns to the electrosurgical unit via the conductor cord between the inactive electrode and the unit. *The grounding pad or plate must be properly placed to avoid electrical burn.*

b *Bipolar units.* The inactive electrode is incorporated into the forceps used by the surgeon. One side of the forceps is the active electrode through which current passes to the tissues. The other side is inactive. The current flows only between the tips of the forceps and does not disperse itself throughout the patient as in monopolar units. This provides extremely precise control of the coagulated area and is a safety factor in the use of electrosurgery.

Types of Current

1 *Coagulation.* In coagulation, as the current approaches the active electrode, the density of the current increases to produce an intense heat at the end of the tip. This sears the ends of small or moderate-sized vessels to control bleeding on contact. When the coagulating electrode is held near the tissue, but not in contact with it, a superficial searing called *desiccation* occurs.

2 *Cutting.* The cutting current forms an arc between the tissues and the active electrode intense enough to destroy tissue under it as it moves along the line of incision (reference is not to skin incision). At the same time that it cuts through or across tissue, cutting current accomplishes some coagulation of cells on the surface of the incision and prevents capillary bleeding.

NOTE. Both cutting and coagulation currents are used in many open and closed operative procedures. Some surgeons prefer electrosurgery to other methods of cutting and ligating vessels. Coagulated tissue produces foreign-body reaction, however, and it must be absorbed by the body during healing. If a large amount of coagulated tissue is present, sloughing may result so the wound may not heal by first intention.

The type and amount of current are regulated by controls on the electrosurgical unit. Most units provide up to 400 watts of power. It is seldom necessary to use full-power settings. In the solid-state units, the power output is isolated to prevent overheating and is equipped with a warning buzzer and/or light to warn of a break in the circuit or too high a setting.

Safety Factors Electrical burn through the patient's skin is the greatest hazard in the use of electrosurgery. These burns are usually deeper than flame burns, causing widespread tissue necrosis and deep thrombosis to the extent that debridement may be required. Nursing personnel must be aware, however, of the hazards and safeguard against injury to the patient.

1 A safe general rule for the circulating nurse is to start with the lowest setting of current that accomplishes the desired degree of coagulation or cutting. Increase the current at the surgeon's request. Investigate a repeated request for more current as the inactive electrode or cord may be at fault. Shock to those touching the patient may result. The patient may be burned.

2 Flammable agents, such as alcohol, must not be used in skin preparation if electrosurgery will be used. Fumes may collect in drapes and ignite when an electrosurgical, cautery, or diathermy unit is used. Use aqueous antiseptic solutions.

3 The inactive electrode must be free from bent edges. A metal connection between the plate or pad must not touch the patient. Special care must be taken to ensure that the cord of the inactive electrode does not become dislodged. The safest connectors are threaded and also insulated. The inactive electrode and cord should be carefully checked before use.

4 The connection between the inactive electrode and the electrosurgical unit must be made properly and securely. If the return circuit is faulty, the ground circuit may be completed through inadvertent contact with the metal operating table or its attachments. If the grounded area is small, the current passing through the exposed area of skin contact will be relatively intense. For example, one such contact point may be the thigh touching the leg stirrup in lithotomy position. Older units use a single conductor cord that should be checked each time it is used by grasping the connecting plug and pulling firmly on the cord. If the cord stretches, the wires inside are broken and must be repaired.

5 The inactive electrode must be clean. Some conductive lubricants will dry out and leave a high-resistance film that will prevent proper contact with the patient's skin.

6 The inactive electrode must cover as large an area of the patient's skin as possible in an area free of hair or scar tissue, which tend to act as insulation. Avoid areas where bony protuberances might result in pressure points, which in turn can cause current concentration. The inactive electrode should be as close to the site where the active electrode will be used as possible, to minimize current through the body.

7 Always alert the anesthesiologist to the anticipated use of electrosurgery. Electrosurgery must never be used in the mouth, around the head, or the pleural cavity when flammable anesthetics are used. Follow safety regulations of the hospital for use with all inhalation anesthetic agents.

8 Only moist sponges should be permitted on the sterile field while the electrosurgical unit is in use, to prevent fire.

9 Clean the active electrode tip between uses to remove coagulated tissue.

10 When the electrosurgical unit is not in actual use, although connected, keep the active electrode tip in a container to avoid possibility of a burn from one of the team inadvertently stepping on the foot switch or activating the hand control.

11 If another piece of electrical equipment is being used in direct contact with the patient at the same time as the electrosurgical unit, connect it to a different source of current, such as a battery, if possible. The cutting current of the electrosurgical unit will not work if another piece of electrical equipment is on the same circuit.

12 Electrocardiogram electrodes should be placed as far away from the operative site as possible when electrosurgery will be used. Needle electrodes should be avoided as they could transmit leakage currents into the body.

13 For the safety of the patient and personnel, follow the instructions for use and care in the manual prepared by the manufacturer that accompanies each electrosurgical unit.

Laser Laser is an acronym for Light Amplification by the Stimulated Emission of Radiation. The laser furnishes an intense and concentrated light beam of a single wavelength from a monochromatic source of radiation. Lasers employ ruby, argon, carbon dioxide, or neodymium as their active media. Some lasers emit their energy in brief, repeating emissions that have a duration of only an extremely small fraction of a second. These are called *pulsed laser systems.* Others are capable of producing continuous light beams; these are called *continuous wave lasers.*

The therapeutic use of laser radiation is limited by the inaccessibility of many organs to the laser beam. In organs that can be exposed, lasers are successfully used for the control of bleeding or for the ablation and excision of tissues. For example, the argon laser is used through an endoscope coupled with a flexible fiberoptic bundle (see Chap. 15) to fulgerate or excise lesions in the gastrointestinal tract.

Different lasers have selective uses. For example, the blood vessels (red) do not absorb the red light of the ruby laser. Vessels absorb the blue-green argon light of a different wavelength. (Refer to Chapter 22 for uses of ruby and argon lasers in ophthalmology.) Laser light colors vary from ultraviolet to the invisible near and far infrared.

The carbon dioxide laser possesses two properties of value to the surgeon in treating soft tissue lesions. Its hemostatic action is based on the intense heat of the beam resulting in coagulation of vessels. The laser wound is characterized by minimal bleeding and no visible postoperative edema. The second property is its ability to vaporize tissue not accessible to the surgeon by other means. *Vaporization* is the conversion of solid tissue to smoke and gas. The vapor is removed from the operative field with suction. Large or small masses of tissue can be removed rapidly and efficiently. The amount of tissue destruction is very predictable by adjusting the width and focus of the beam. The carbon dioxide laser is used primarily in laryngology, gynecology, and plastic surgery.

For precautions with the use of all laser equipment follow hospital policy. Nurses and technicians assisting in laser surgery should have special training in its use.

Packs Hot packs are frequently impacted into extensive wounds to control capillary bleeding. The addition of heat accelerates the natural chemical reaction of the blood to hasten clotting.

Photocoagulation The photocoagulator utilizes an intense source of multiwavelength light furnished by a xenon tube to coagulate tissue. Since its use is limited to ophthalmology, refer to Chapter 22.

Plasma Scalpel The plasma scalpel vaporizes tissues and stops bleeding as it simultaneously cuts and coagulates tissue. Within the instrument, which looks like a large ballpoint pen, argon or helium gas passes through an electric arc that ionizes it into a high thermal state of 3000°C (6160°F) or more. These gases are inert and noncombustible. As the instrument moves back and forth over tissue, the gas that flows from the tip is visible so the surgeon can see the depth and extent of the incision. Tissue damage, with resultant inflammatory response during wound healing, is greater than that caused by a steel knife blade but less than that caused by other electrosurgical instruments and lasers. Because it will coagulate vessels up to 3 mm in diameter, the plasma scalpel is useful in highly vascular areas.

Chapter 13

Wound Closure Materials

One of the bases upon which surgery is founded as a distinct discipline of medicine is the control of bleeding and the closure of wounds. The story of sutures, in some measure, is the story of surgery itself. Many kinds of suture materials to close wounds have been known for thousands of years, but only since Lister's discoveries has their use been safe. Only since that time have suturing techniques and other methods of bringing tissue edges together been brought to an advanced state of development.

SUTURES

Common Terms

Suture is an all-inclusive term for any strand of material used for ligating or approximating tissue.

Ties If the material is tied around a blood vessel to occlude the lumen, it is called a *ligature* or *tie*. A *free tie* is a single strand of material handed to the surgeon or assistant to ligate a vessel. A strand attached to a needle before use is referred to as a *stick tie* or *suture/ligature*. The needle is used to anchor the strand in tissue before occluding a deep or large vessel.

Suture The verb *to suture* denotes the act of sewing by bringing tissues together and holding them until healing has taken place. A *suture*, the noun, is the strand of material used for this purpose.

Specifications for Suture Material

1 It must be sterile when placed in tissue. The principles of sterile technique must be rigidly followed in handling suture material. If the end of a strand drops over the side of any sterile surface, discard the strand.

2 It must be predictably uniform in tensile strength by size and material. *Tensile strength* is the measured pounds of tension or pull that a strand will withstand before it breaks when knotted. Minimum knot-pull strengths are specified for each basic raw material and for each size of that material by the United States Pharmacopeia (USP). Tensile strength decreases as the diameter of the strand decreases.

3 It must be as small in diameter as is safe to use on each type of tissue. The strength of the suture usually need be no greater than the strength of the tissue on which it is used. Smaller sizes are less traumatic during placement in tissue and leave less suture mass to cause tissue reaction. The surgeon ties small-diameter sutures more gently, and thus is less apt to strangulate tissue. A small-diameter suture is flexible, easy to manipulate, and leaves minimal scar on skin.

Sizes range from heavy 7 to very fine 11-0; ranges vary with materials. Taking size 1 as a starting point, sizes increase with each number above 1 and decrease with each 0 added. Thus size 7 is the largest and 11-0 is the smallest. The more 0's in the number, the smaller the size of the strand. As the number of 0's increases, the size of the strand decreases. In addition to this system of size designation, the manufacturer's labels on boxes and packets also may include metric measures for suture diameters. These metric equivalents vary slightly by types of materials.

4 It must have knot security, remain tied, and give support to tissue during the healing process. However, sutures in the skin are always removed 3 to 10 days postoperatively, depending on the site of the incision and the cosmetic result desired. Because they are exposed to the external environment, skin sutures can be a source of microbial contamination of the wound that inhibits healing by first intention.

5 It must cause as little foreign-body tissue reaction as possible. All suture materials are foreign bodies, but some are more inert, less reactive, than others.

Choice of Suture Material

Surgical sutures as defined by the USP* are divided into two classifications: absorbable and nonabsorbable.

1 *Absorbable sutures* are sterile strands prepared from collagen derived from healthy mammals or from a synthetic polymer. They are capable of being absorbed by living mammalian tissue, but may be treated to modify resistance to absorption. They may be modified with respect to body or texture. They may be impregnated or coated with a suitable antimicrobial agent. They may be colored by a color additive approved by the federal Food and Drug Administration (FDA).

2 *Nonabsorbable sutures* are strands of material that effectively resist enzymatic digestion or absorption in living tissue. During the healing process the suture mass becomes encapsulated and may remain for years in tissues without producing any ill effects. The strands may be impregnated or coated with a suitable antimicrobial agent. They may be modified with respect to body or texture, or to reduce capillarity. They may be colored by a color additive approved by the FDA.

Capillarity refers to the characteristics of nonabsorbable sutures that allow the passage of tissue fluids along the strand permitting infection, if present, to be drawn into the wound. These suture materials are described as capillary or noncapillary.

a If untreated for reduction of capillarity, the material is designated by USP as Type A, untreated and capillary.

b If treated to reduce capillarity, it is designated Type B, treated and noncapillary. *Noncapillary* is the characteristic of nonabsorbable sutures in which the nature of the raw material or specific processing meets USP tests that establish them as resistant to "wicking" transfer of body fluids.

*United States Pharmacopeia, Nineteenth Revision, Official from July 1, 1975, United States Pharmacopeial Convention, Rockville, Md., 1975.

The two classifications of suture materials are subdivided into monofilament and multifilament strands.

1 *Monofilament* suture is a strand consisting of a single threadlike structure that is noncapillary.

2 *Multifilament* suture is a strand made of more than one threadlike structure held together by spinning, braiding, or twisting. This strand is capillary unless treated to resist capillarity or is absorbable.

The surgeon selects the type of suture material best suited to promote healing. Factors that influence choice include:

1 Biologic characteristics of the material in tissue, i.e., absorbable versus nonabsorbable, capillary versus noncapillary, inertness, etc.

2 Healing characteristics of tissue. Tissues that normally heal slowly such as skin, fascia, and tendons usually are closed with nonabsorbable sutures. Absorbable suture placed through the skin may cause a stitch abscess to develop as it is inclined to act as a culture medium for microorganisms in the pores of the skin. Tissues that heal rapidly such as stomach, colon, and bladder may be closed with absorbable sutures.

3 Location and length of the incision. Cosmetic results desired may be an important influencing factor.

4 Presence or absence of infection, contamination, and/or drainage. If infection is present, sutures may be the origin of granuloma formation with subsequent discharge of suture and sinus formation. Foreign bodies in potentially contaminated tissues may convert contamination to infection. Foreign bodies in the presence of some body fluids may cause stone formation, as in the urinary or biliary tract.

5 Patient problems such as obesity, debility, age, diseases, etc., that influence rate of healing and time desired for wound support.

6 Physical characteristics of the material such as ease of passage through tissue, knot tying, and other subjective preferences of the surgeon.

Absorbable Sutures

Surgical Gut The early surgeons used gut strings discarded by the musicians. The strings on fiddles were called *kitstrings* because the fiddle itself was known as a *kit*. Since these strings were made of sheep intestines, they were called *kitgut*. However, a young cat is a kit, so eventually the word *catgut* replaced kitgut. The more accurate term *surgical gut* has replaced the term catgut.

Surgical gut is collagen derived from the submucosa of sheep intestine or the serosa of beef intestine. The intestines from these freshly slaughtered animals are sent to the processing plants. There they undergo many elaborate mechanical and chemical cleaning processes before ribbons are spun into strands of various sizes, ranging from the heaviest size 3 to the finest size 7-0. Although the larger sizes are made from two or more intestinal ribbons, the behavior of surgical gut is that of a monofilament suture.

Surgical gut is digested by body enzymes and absorbed by tissue; thus no permanent foreign body remains. The rate of absorption is influenced by:

1 *Type of tissue.* Surgical gut is absorbed much more rapidly in serous or mucous membrane. It is absorbed slowly in subcutaneous fat.

2 *Condition of the tissue.* It can be used in the presence of infection, and even the knots are absorbed. However, absorption takes place much more rapidly in the presence of infection.

3 *General health status of the patient.* Surgical gut may be absorbed more rapidly in undernourished or diseased tissue, but in old or debilitated patients it may remain for a long time.

4 *Type of surgical gut.* Plain gut is untreated, but chromic gut is treated to provide greater resistance to absorption.

Plain Surgical Gut Plain (Type A) surgical gut is digested relatively quickly, usually in 5 to 10 days, because the collagen strands are untreated to resist absorption. Plain surgical gut is used to ligate small vessels and to suture subcutaneous fat. It is not used to suture any layers of tissue likely to be subjected to tension during healing. It is available in sizes 3 through 6-0. Usually used in its natural yellowish-tan color, it may be dyed blue or black.

Chromic Surgical Gut Chromic (Type C) surgical gut is treated in a chromium salt solution to resist absorption by the tissues for varying lengths of time depending on the strength of the solution and the duration and method of the process. The chromicizing process either bathes each ribbon of collagen before spinning into strands or applies the solution to the finished strand. This treatment changes the color from the yellowish-tan shade of plain surgical gut to a dark shade of brown. Chromic surgical gut is used for ligation of larger vessels and for suture of tissues in which nonabsorbable materials are not usually recommended because they may act as a nidus for stone formation, as in the urinary or biliary tracts. In closure of muscle or fascia it has the disadvantage of rapidly declining tensile strength. If the absorption rate is normal, chromic surgical gut will support the wound for about 14 days and absorb completely within 120 days. Sizes range from 3 through 7-0. It may be dyed blue or black.

Collagen Sutures Collagen sutures are extruded from a homogeneous dispersion of pure collagen fibrils from the flexor tendons of beef. Both plain and chromic types are similar in appearance to surgical gut and may be dyed blue. Sizes range from 4-0 through 8-0. They are used primarily in ophthalmic surgery.

Handling characteristics of surgical gut and collagen:

1 Surgical gut and collagen sutures are sealed in packets that contain fluid to keep the material pliable. This fluid is chiefly alcohol and water, *but may be irritating to ophthalmic tissues.* Hold packet over a basin and open carefully to avoid spilling fluid on the sterile field or splashing it into your own eyes. Rinsing is necessary *only* for surgical gut or collagen sutures to be implanted into the eye.

2 Surgical gut and collagen sutures should be used immediately after removal from their packets. When the material is removed and not used at once, the alcohol evaporates and the strand loses pliability. Many surgeons prefer that the scrub nurse quickly dip the strand into water or saline to soften it slightly. *Do not soak.* Excessive exposure to water will reduce the tensile strength. Before unwinding the strand, it can be dipped momentarily in water or saline at room temperature, not hot; heat will coagulate the protein.

3 Unwind the strand carefully. Handle it as little as possible. Never jerk or stretch surgical gut; that weakens it. Do not straighten suture by run-

ning fingers down its length; excessive handling with rubber gloves can cause fraying. Take the ends and tug gently to straighten.

Synthetic Absorbable Polymers Polymers, either dyed or undyed, are extruded and braided to form multifilament absorbable sutures. These synthetic sutures are absorbed by a slow hydrolysis process in the presence of tissue fluids. They are used for ligating or suturing except in tissues where extended approximation of tissues under stress is required. They are inert, nonantigenic, nonpyrogenic, and produce only a mild tissue reaction during absorption.

Polyglactin 910 Polyglactin 910 is a copolymer of glycolide and lactide. The precisely controlled combination of these two substances results in a molecular structure that maintains tensile strength longer than surgical gut and then absorbs rapidly within 90 days. Multifilament braided strands are available dyed violet in sizes 2 through 9-0 and undyed in sizes 1 through 7-0. Monofilament strands, dyed violet, are available in 9-0 and 10-0 sizes for ophthalmic procedures.

Polyglycolic Acid Polyglycolic acid suture is a homopolymer of glycolic acid. It is smaller in diameter than surgical gut of equivalent tensile strength. However, polyglycolic acid suture loses tensile strength more rapidly and absorbs significantly more slowly than polyglactin 910 suture. It is available dyed green or undyed natural beige in sizes 2 through 7-0.

Handling characteristics of synthetic absorbable polymers:

1 Synthetic absorbable sutures have an expiration date on the package. Therefore, rotate stock. First in, first out is a good rule to follow.

2 Sutures are packaged and used dry. Do not soak or dip in water or saline. The material hydrolizes in water so that excessive exposure to moisture will reduce the tensile strength. It is smooth, soft, and will retain its pliability.

Nonabsorbable Sutures

Surgical Silk Surgical silk is an animal product made from the fiber spun by the silkworm larvae in making their cocoons. From the raw state, each fiber is processed to remove the natural waxes and gums. Fibers are braided or twisted together to form a multifilament suture strand. The braided type is used more frequently because surgeons prefer its high tensile strength and better handling qualities. Surgical silk is treated to render it noncapillary. It also is dyed, most commonly black, but also is available white. Sizes range from 5 through 9-0.

Silk is not a true nonabsorbable material. It loses much of its tensile strength after about 1 year and usually disappears after 2 or more years. It gives good support to wounds during early ambulation and generally promotes healing a little more rapidly than surgical gut. It causes less tissue reaction than surgical gut, but is not as inert as most of the other nonabsorbable materials. It is used frequently in serosa of the gastrointestinal tract and to close fascia in the absence of infection. It may be used in anastomosing major vessels, especially in young children.

Virgin Silk Virgin silk suture consists of several natural silk filaments drawn together and twisted to form 8-0 and 9-0 strands for tissue approximation of delicate structures, primarily in ophthalmic surgery. It is white or dyed black.

Dermal Silk Dermal suture is a strand of twisted silk fibers encased in a nonabsorbing coating of tanned gelatin or other protein substance. This coating prevents the ingrowth of tissue cells and facilitates removal after use as a skin suture. It is used for suturing the skin particularly in areas of tension because of its unusual strength. It is black in sizes 0 through 5-0.

Handling characteristics of silk sutures:

1 Silk sutures are dry. They lose tensile strength if wet. Therefore, do not moisten before use.

2 If it is necessary to autoclave silk suture, do so at 250°F (121°C) for 15 minutes. Silk shrinks during sterilization and must never be sterilized on a spool, if suppled nonsterile. Some tensile strength is lost during sterilization.

Surgical Cotton Surgical cotton suture is made from individual, long-staple cotton fibers that are combed, aligned, and twisted into a smooth multifilament strand. Sizes range from 1 through 5-0. Usually white, it may be dyed blue or pink.

Cotton is one of the weakest of the nonabsorbable materials; however, it gains tensile strength when wet. Moisten before handing to the surgeon. Tensile strength is increased by 10 percent by moisture. Also, moisture prevents clinging to the surgeon's gloves. Like silk, cotton suture may be used in most body tissues for ligating and suturing, but it offers no advantages over silk.

Linen Surgical linen is spun from long-staple flax fibers, then twisted into tight strands and treated for smooth passage through tissue. Tensile strength is inferior to all other nonabsorbable materials. Linen suture is used almost exclusively in gastrointestinal surgery. It is available in sizes 0 and 2-0.

Surgical Stainless Steel Stainless steel sutures are drawn from 316L-SS (L for low carbon) iron alloy wire. This is the same metal formula used in the manufacture of surgical stainless steel implants and prostheses.

> NOTE. *Two different kinds of metal must not be embedded in the tissues simultaneously.* Such a combination creates an unfavorable electrolytic reaction. Some implants and prostheses are made of vitallium, titanium, or tantalum. Suture material in the wound must be compatible with these metals.

Prior to the availability of surgical stainless steel from suture manufacturers, commercial steel was purchased by weight, using the Brown & Sharpe (B&S) scale for diameter variations. Many surgeons still refer to surgical stainless steel size by the B&S gauge with 18, the largest diameter, ranging to 40, the smallest. One suture manufacturer labels surgical stainless steel with both the B&S gauge and equivalent USP diameter classifications from 7 through 6-0. Both monofilament and twisted multifilament stainless steel strands are available.

Surgical stainless steel is inert in tissue and has high tensile strength. It gives the greatest strength of any suture material to a wound before healing begins and supports a wound indefinitely. Some surgeons use stainless steel for closure following operations on the gastrointestinal tract and thus reduce the danger of wound disruption in the presence of contributing factors. It may be used in the presence of infection or in patients in which slow healing is expected. It is used for secondary repair or resuture. Following evisceration (see Chap. 29), it may be used in place of surgical gut that has been too rapidly absorbed.

Unlike most other suture materials, steel lacks elasticity. A suture tied too tightly may act as a knife and cut through tissue. Stainless steel sutures are harder to handle than any other suture material. A painstaking knot-tying technique is required. This disadvantage more than outweighs the advantages for routine use for most surgeons. However, in selected situations it fills an important need. It is widely used in the respiratory tract, in tendon repair, in orthopaedics and neurosurgery, and for general wound closure.

Handling characteristics of stainless steel:

1 Surgical stainless steel strands are malleable and kink rather easily. Kinks in the strand can make it practically useless. Therefore, care must be taken in handling to keep the strand straight.

2 Use wire scissors for cutting stainless steel sutures. Barbs on the end of the strand can tear gloves, thus breaking aseptic technique, or traumatize tissue.

3 If surgical stainless steel must be threaded to a needle, some surgeons prefer one or two twists of the end around the strand just below the eye of the needle to prevent unthreading during suturing.

Synthetic Nonabsorbable Polymers Although silk is the most frequently used nonabsorbable suture material, synthetic nonabsorbable materials are used because they offer unique advantages in many situations. They have higher tensile strength and elicit less tissue reaction than silk. They retain their strength in tissue. Knot tying with most of these materials is more difficult than with silk. Additional throws are required to secure the knot. The surgeon may sacrifice some handling characteristics and ease of knot tying for strength, durability, and nonreactivity of the synthetics. These advantages may outweigh the disadvantages.

Surgical Nylon Nylon is a polyamide polymer derived by chemical synthesis. It may be used as a monofilament or multifilament strand.

Monofilament nylon is a smooth single strand of noncapillary material, clear or dyed black, blue, or green. The smaller the diameter becomes, the stronger the strand becomes proportionately. Sizes range from 2 through 11-0; the latter is the smallest of all sutures manufactured for use in microsurgery. Monofilament nylon also is used frequently in ophthalmic surgery because it has a desirable degree of elasticity. Larger sizes are used for skin closure, particularly by plastic surgeons where cosmetic results are important. It produces minimal tissue reaction.

Multifilament nylon is very tightly braided and treated to prevent capillary action. Usually used dyed black, but also available white, nylon looks, feels, and handles like silk, but is stronger and elicits less tissue reaction than silk. Sizes range from 1 through 7-0. It may be used in all tissues where a multifilament, nonabsorbable suture is acceptable.

Polyester Fiber A polymer of terephthalic acid and polyethylene, Dacron polyester fiber is braided into a multifilament suture strand. It is available in two forms: uncoated fibers and coated fibers.

1 *Uncoated polyester fiber suture* is closely braided to provide a flexible, pliable strand that is relatively easy to handle. However, uncoated braided polyester fiber suture has a tendency to "drag" and exert a sawing or tearing effect when passed through tissue. It may be used in all tissues where a multifilament nonabsorbable suture is indicated. It is especially useful in the respiratory tract and for some cardiovascular procedures. Available white or dyed green or blue, sizes range from 2 through 10-0.
2 *Coated polyester fiber suture* has a lubricated surface for smooth passage through tissue. It is widely used in cardiovascular surgery for vessel anastomosis and placement of prosthetic materials because it retains its strength indefinitely in tissues. Sutures are available with different coating materials:
   a *Polybutilate* is the only coating developed specifically as a surgical lubricant. This polyester material adheres strongly to the braided polyester fiber. Polyester fiber coated with polybutilate provides a suture that is superior to any other braided material, coated or uncoated, in decreasing drag through tissue. Colored green or white, sizes range from 5 through 7-0.
   b *Silicone* is a commercial lubricant that provides a slippery coating but does not bond well to polyester fiber. It can become dislodged in the tissues as the strand is tied. Sutures with this coating are available white or dyed blue in sizes 5 through 7-0.
   c *Polytetrafluoroethylene,* a commercial product known by the DuPont trade name Teflon, is used as a coating bonded to the surface or impregnated into the spaces in the braid of the polyester fiber strand. Minute particles of this coating can flake off the strand. Since they are insoluble and resistant to enzymes, foreign-body granulomas may be produced. Sutures with this material on them are white or dyed green and available in sizes 5 through 10-0.

Polyethylene Polyethylene is a long-chain plastic polymer extruded into a blue-dyed monofilament suture strand. It is available in sizes 0 through 6-0 for use in some situations in which a monofilament material may be desired.

Polypropylene Polypropylene is a polymerized propylene extruded into a monofilament suture strand. It may be clear or pigmented with blue dye. It is the most inert of the synthetic materials and almost wholly as inert as surgical stainless steel. Polypropylene is an acceptable substitute for stainless steel in situations where strength and nonreactivity are required and the suture must be left in place for prolonged healing. It can be used in the presence of infection. It has become the material of choice for many plastic surgery and cardiovascular procedures because of its smooth passage through tissue as well as its strength and inertness. Polypropylene sutures are available from sizes 2 through 10-0.

SURGICAL NEEDLES

Except for simple ligating with free ties, surgical needles are needed to safely carry the suture material through tissue with the least amount of trauma. The best surgical needles are made of high-quality tempered steel that:

1 Is strong enough so it does not break easily
2 Is rigid enough to prevent excessive bending, yet flexible enough to prevent breaking after bending
3 Is sharp enough to penetrate tissue with minimal resistance, yet not stronger than the tissue it penetrates
4 Is approximately the same diameter as the suture material it carries to minimize trauma in passage through tissue
5 Is appropriate in shape and size for the type, condition, and accessibility of the tissue to be sutured
6 Is free from corrosion and burrs to prevent infection and tissue trauma

Many shapes and sizes of surgical needles are available. The names vary from one manufacturer to another; general classification only, not nomenclature, is standardized. They may be straight (like a sewing needle) or curved. All surgical needles have three basic components: the point, the body or shaft, and the eye. They are classified according to these three components.

Points of Needles

Points of surgical needles are honed to configuration and sharpness desired for specific types of tissue. The basic shapes are cutting, tapered, or blunt (see Fig. 13-1).

Cutting Point A razor-sharp honed cutting point may be preferred when tissue is difficult to pene-

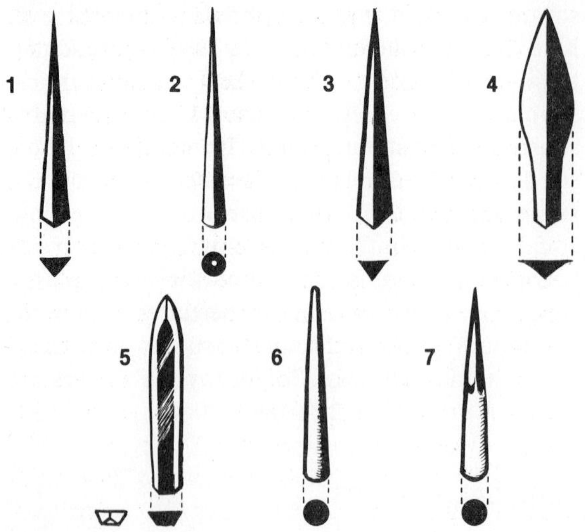

Figure 13-1 Configurations of needle points: (1) precision point cutting, (2) taper, (3) reverse cutting, (4) trocar, (5) side cutting, (6) blunt, (7) cutting edge at end of tapered point.

trate, such as skin, tendon, and tough tissues in the eye. These make a slight cut in tissue as they penetrate. Location and degree of sharpness of cutting edges vary.

Conventional Cutting Needles These have two opposing cutting edges with a third edge forming a triangular configuration on the body of the needle. The cutting edges are on the inside curvature of a curved needle. The cutting edges may be honed to precision sharpness to assure smooth passage through tissue and a minute needle path that heals quickly.

Reverse Cutting Needles These needles have a triangular configuration that extends along the body of the needle. The edges near the point are sharpened or honed to precision points. The two opposing cutting edges are on the outer curvature of a curved needle.

Side Cutting Needles Relatively flat on top and bottom, these needles have angulated cutting edges on the sides. Used primarily in ophthalmic surgery, they will not penetrate underlying tissues. They split through the layer of tissue.

Trocar Points Sharp cutting tips are at the points of tapered needles. All three edges of the tip are sharpened to provide cutting action with the smallest possible hole in tissue as it penetrates.

Taper Point These needles are used in soft tissues, such as intestine and peritoneum, which offer a small amount of resistance to the needle as it passes through. They tend to push the tissue aside as they go through rather than cut it. The body tapers to a sharp point at the tip.

Blunt Point These tapered needles are designed with a rounded blunt point at the tip. They are used for suturing friable tissue, such as liver and kidney. Because the blunt point will not cut through tissue, it is less apt to puncture a vessel in these organs than a sharp-pointed needle.

Body of Needle

The body, or shaft, varies in wire gauge, length, shape, and finish. The nature and location of the tissue to be sutured influence selection of needles with these variable features.

1 Tough or fibrosed tissue requires the use of heavier gauge needles than the fine gauge wire needed in microsurgery.

2 The depth of the "bite" (placement) through the tissue determines appropriate length.

3 The body may be round, oval, flat, or triangular. The point determines the shape: round or oval bodies have trocar, taper, or blunt points; flat or triangular bodies have cutting edges. The shape also may be straight or curved (see Fig. 13-2).

- **a** Straight needles are used in readily accessible tissue. They have cutting points for use in skin, the most frequent use, or tapered points for use in intestinal tissue.
- **b** Curved needles are used to approximate most tissues because quick needle turnout is an advantage. The curvature may be $\frac{1}{4}$, $\frac{3}{8}$, $\frac{1}{2}$, $\frac{5}{8}$ circle or half-curved with only the tip curved. *Curved needles always are armed in a needleholder before being handed to the surgeon.*

4 Curved needles that have longitudinal ribbed depressions or grooves along the body on the inside and outside curvature create a cross-locking action of the needle in the needleholder. This feature virtually eliminates twisting, turning, or rocking of the needle in any position in the needleholder.

5 The body of all needles must have a smooth finish. Many needles have a surface coating of micro-thin plastic or silicone to enhance smooth passage through tissue.

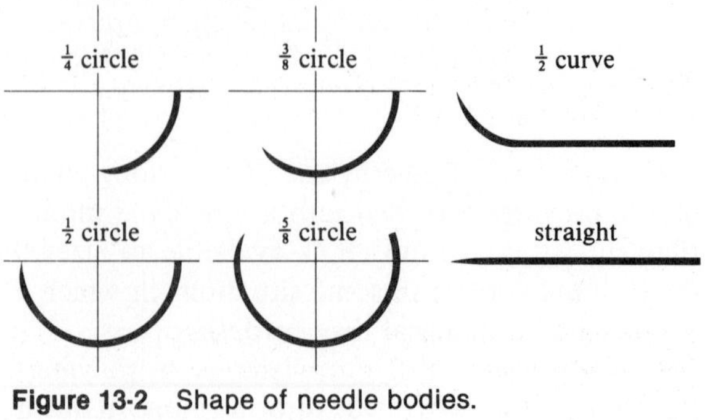

Figure 13-2 Shape of needle bodies.

Eye of Needle

The eye is the segment of the needle where the suture strand is attached. Surgical needles are classified as eyed, French eye, or eyeless (see Fig. 13-3).

Eyed Needle The closed eye of an eyed surgical needle is like that of any household sewing needle. The shape of the enclosed eye may be round, oblong, or square. The end of the suture strand is pulled 2 to 4 in. (5 to 10 cm) through the eye, so that the short end is about one-sixth the length of the long one.

French Eye Needle Sometimes referred to as *spring eye* or *split eye,* a French eye needle has a slit from the inside of the eye to the end of the needle through which the suture strand is drawn. To thread a French eye after arming needle in a needleholder, secure 2 to 3 in. (5 to 7.5 cm) of the strand between fingers holding the needleholder. Pull strand taut across center of V-shaped area above the eye and draw down through the slit into the eye (see Fig. 13-4). French eye needles as a general rule are used with pliable braided materials, primarily silk and cotton, of medium or fine size. These needles are not practical for surgical gut, as the strand may fray or the eye may break because the diameter is usually too large for the slit.

NOTE. Eyed and French eye needles have disadvantages for the scrub nurse, surgeon, and patient.

1. Each needle must be carefully inspected by the scrub nurse for dull or burred points, corrosion, and defects in the eye before and after use.
2. Care must be taken to avoid puncturing gloves with needle point when threading.
3. The scrub nurse may have to choose an appropriate needle to thread. The needle should be the same approximate diameter as the suture size requested by the surgeon.
4. Needles can unthread prematurely. This is both an annoyance to the surgeon and an uneconomical use of time for the patient. To avoid this, the surgeon may prefer the suture strand threaded double with both ends of the suture pulled the same length through the eye; the ends may be tied together in a knot, if desired. Or the scrub nurse may lock the suture strand by threading the short end through the eye twice in the same direction.
5. Two strands of suture material are pulled through the tissue when threaded needles are used. The bulk of the double strand through the eye creates a larger hole than the size of the needle or suture material with additional trauma to tissue.

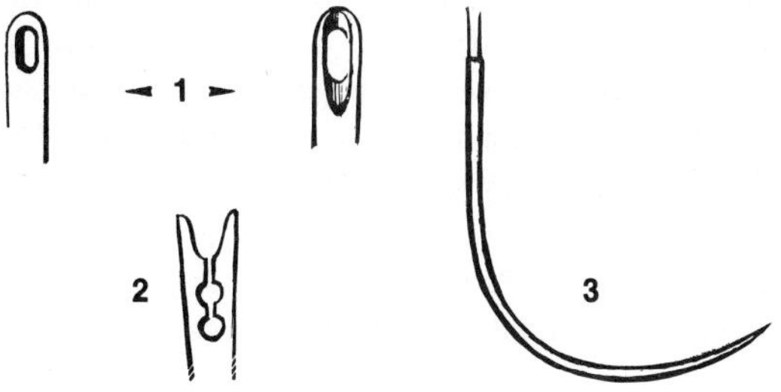

Figure 13-3 Eyes of needles: (1) oblong eyes, (2) French eye, (3) eyeless (swaged).

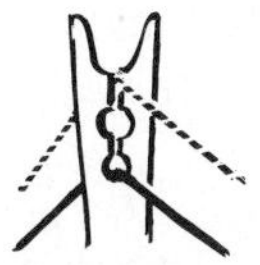

Figure 13-4 To thread French eye needle, pull strand taut across center of V-shaped area and draw down through the split into the eye.

Eyeless Needle An eyeless needle is a continuous unit with the suture strand. The needle is swaged onto the end of the strand in the manufacturing process. This eliminates threading at the operating table and minimizes tissue trauma by drawing a single strand of material through tissue. The diameter of the needle matches the size of the strand as closely as possible. The surgeon uses a new sharp needle with every suture strand. Usually referred to as *swaged needles,* four types of eyeless needle-suture attachments are available.

Single-armed Attachment Has one needle swaged to the suture strand.

Double-armed Attachment Has a needle swaged to each end of the suture strand. The two needles are not necessarily the same size and shape. These are used when the surgeon wishes to place a suture and then continue to approximate surrounding tissue on both sides from a midpoint in the strand.

Permanently Swaged Needle Attachment Is secure so that the needle will not separate from the suture strand under normal use. The needle is separated by cutting it from the strand.

Controlled Release Needle Attachment Is secure so that the suture strand does not separate from the needle inadvertently but does release rapidly when pulled off intentionally. The surgeon grasps the suture strand just below the needle, pulling the strand taut, and releases the needle with a straight tug of the needleholder or the needle. This facilitates fast separation of needle from suture when desired.

Placement of Needle in Needleholder

Needleholders have specially designed jaws to securely grasp surgical needles without damage if used correctly. The scrub nurse should observe the following principles in handling needles and needleholders:

1 Select a needleholder with appropriate size jaws for the size needle to be used. An extremely small needle requires a needleholder with very fine tipped jaws. As the wire gauge of the needle increases, the jaws of the needleholder selected should be proportionately wider and heavier.

2 Select an appropriate-length needleholder for the area of the tissue to be sutured. When the surgeon works deep inside the abdomen, chest, or pelvic cavity, a longer needleholder will be needed than in superficial areas.

3 Clamp the body of the needle in an area about one-fourth or one-half of the distance from the eye to the point. *Never clamp the needleholder over the swaged area.* This is the weakest area of an eyeless needle because it is hollow before the suture strand is attached. Pressure on or near the needle-suture juncture may break it (see Fig. 13-5).

4 Place needle securely in the tip of the needleholder jaws and close it in the first or second ratchet. If the needle is held too tightly in the jaws or the needleholder is defective, the needle may be damaged or notched in such a manner that it will have a tendency to bend or break on successive passes through tissue.

5 Hand the needleholder to the surgeon so the suture strand is free and not entangled with the needleholder. Hold the free end of the suture in one hand while passing the needleholder with the other hand. Protect the end of the suture material from dragging across the sterile field. The assistant may take hold of the free end to keep the strand straight for the surgeon and to keep it from falling over the side of the sterile field.

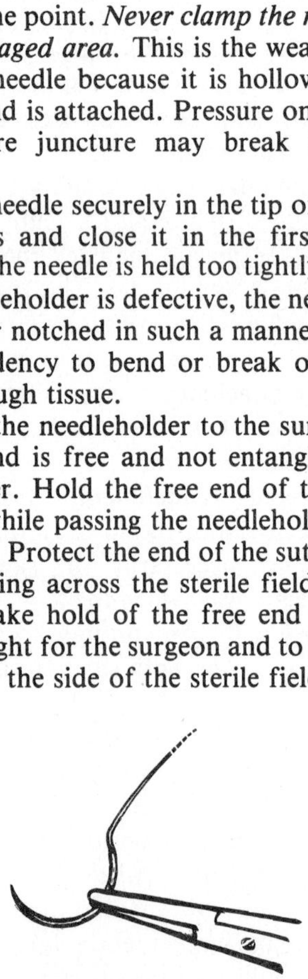

Figure 13-5 Correct position of a curved needle in a needleholder, about one-third down from the swage or eye.

6 Pass the needleholder so the needle point is directed downward toward the surgeon's thumb ready for use without readjustment.

7 Hand a needleholder to the assistant to pull the needle out through the tissue. The needle should be grasped as far back as possible to avoid damage to taper points or cutting edges.

NOTE. Do not use a hemostat or other tissue forceps for this purpose as the instrument may be damaged or it may damage the needle. Refer to Chapter 8 for additional tips in handling needles.

COMMON SUTURING TECHNIQUES

Primary Suture Line

The *primary suture line* refers to those sutures that hold wound edges in approximation during healing by first intention. This line may have one continuous strand of suture material or a series of suture strands. A variety of techniques are used to place sutures in tissues. The most common terms for these techniques are described.

Continuous Suture A series of stitches are taken with one strand of material tied only at the ends of the suture line. This may be referred to as a *running stitch.* Closure is rapid and less suture mass remains in the tissue. A continuous suture is used to close peritoneum because it also provides a temporary water seal. Configuration of the stitches varies with the tissue and desired cosmetic result.

Interrupted Suture Each stitch is taken and tied separately. This is the technique recommended by Dr. Halsted for two reasons: if an interrupted suture breaks or loosens, the remaining sutures may still hold the wound together; in the presence of infection, microorganisms are less likely to follow the primary suture line.

Buried Suture A suture placed under the skin, buried, may be either continuous or interrupted.

Purse-string Suture A continuous suture is placed around a lumen and tightened, drawstring fashion, to close the lumen. This is used when inverting the stump of the appendix, for example.

Subcuticular Suture A continuous suture is placed beneath the epithelial layer of the skin in short lateral stitches. The suture comes through the upper layer of the skin at each end of the incision only. A perforated lead shot may be crushed tightly on each suture end. The suture is drawn tight enough to hold the skin edges in approximation. It is easily removed by cutting off the shot at one end, grasping the other shot, and pulling the entire strand through the length of the incision. It was first used by Dr. Halsted. It leaves a minimal scar.

Secondary Suture Line

The *secondary suture line* refers to those sutures that reinforce and support the primary suture line, obliterate dead space, and prevent fluid accumulation in the wound during healing by first intention. They exert tension lateral to the primary suture line, which contributes to the tensile strength of the wound. Sutures used for this purpose are referred to as retention, stay, or tension sutures.

Retention Sutures Interrupted nonabsorbable sutures are placed through tissue on each side of the primary suture line and a short distance from it to relieve tension on it. Heavy strands of material are used in sizes ranging from 0 through 5. The tissue through which retention sutures are passed includes the skin, subcutaneous tissue, fascia, and may include the rectus muscle and peritoneum of an abdominal incision. Following abdominal operations, retention sutures are used frequently in patients in which slow healing is expected: due to malnutrition, obesity, carcinoma, or infection; in the elderly; for a patient on cortisone; or a patient with respiratory problems. Retention sutures may be used as a precautionary measure to prevent wound disruption when postoperative stress on the primary suture line from distention, vomiting, or coughing is anticipated. They should be removed as soon as the danger of sudden increases in intra-abdominal pressure is over, usually on the fourth or fifth postoperative day. Retention sutures are also used to support wounds for healing by second intention and for secondary closure following wound disruption for healing by third intention.

Retention Bridges, Bolsters, and Bumpers To prevent the heavy suture from cutting into the skin, several different kinds of bridges, bolsters, or bumpers are used with retention sutures.

1 A *bridge* is a plastic device placed on the skin to span over the incision. The retention suture is brought through the skin on both sides of the incision, through holes at each end of the bridge, and fastened over the bridge. One type allows adjustment of tension on the suture during the postoperative healing period.

2 *Bolsters* and *bumpers*—the names are used interchangeably—are segments of plastic or rubber tubing. One end of the suture is threaded through the tubing before the suture is tied. It covers all the suture strand that is on the skin surface (refer to Fig. 17-3, p. 321). Buttons and lead shot are also used as bolsters and bumpers with some other types of suturing techniques, especially in plastic and orthopaedic surgery.

Traction Suture

A *traction suture* may be used to retract a structure to the side of the operative field, out of the way, as the tongue in an operation in the mouth. Usually a nonabsorbable suture is placed through the part. Other materials may be used to retract or ligate vessels.

1 *Umbilical tape.* Aside from its use in tying the umbilical cord on the newborn, this tape has other uses in surgery. In certain cardiovascular operations, it is used as a heavy tie, or as a traction suture. It may be put around a great vessel to retract it. It is available on spools from which the desired lengths are cut or as sterile strands in tubes.

2 *Aneurysm needle.* An aneurysm needle is an instrument with a blunt needle on the end. The eye is on the distal end of the needle. The needle forms a right or oblique angle to the handle, which is one continuous unit with the needle. The needles are made in symmetrical pairs—right and left. The surgeon uses them when he wishes to take a ligature around a deep, large vessel, as in a thyroidectomy or in thoracic surgery.

SURGEON'S CHOICE

The surgeon chooses from the available types and sizes of sutures and needles the ones that best suit each purpose. In general, fine sizes are used for plastic, pediatric, vascular surgery; medium sizes for all kinds of surgery except the above; heavy sizes are used for retention sutures and occasionally for anchoring bone. In general, cutting needles are used in tough tissue such as skin, fascia, tendon, and mucous membranes including the cervix, tonsil, palate, tongue, and nose. Medium tissue calls for round taper point or cutting needles. Round taper point needles usually are used for nerve, peritoneum, muscle, and other soft tissue such as lung and intestine, subcutaneous tissue, and dura.

It is almost impossible to learn the needle-tissue-suture-surgeon combinations by memory alone because of the unlimited number of combinations. Learning the general classification of needles, sutures, and tissues is the first step; practical experience is necessary to fix in mind the combinations. Do not feel discouraged when you cannot anticipate the surgeon's wishes and do not hesitate to ask when you are uncertain of the proper combination at the proper time.

The preference card usually lists the surgeon's usual suture and needle routine by tissue layer. Some hospitals list swaged sutures by code number. Others list sutures by size and materials and needles by size and shape. Remember, suture and needle sizes are as variable as patient sizes. Therefore, the surgeon may unexpectedly request a smaller or larger size out of routine for a particular patient situation.

SUTURES AND NEEDLES: PACKAGING AND PREPARING

Most suture material is individually packaged and supplied sterile by the manufacturer. It is sterilized by cobalt 60 irradiation or ethylene oxide gas. Some materials may be steam-sterilized, but others cannot. The absorbable materials are labeled "not autoclavable" or "nonboilable"; protein in absorbable materials derived from animals will coagulate; synthetic absorbables are affected by moisture and heat. Only stainless steel can be repeatedly steam-sterilized. Nylon, polyester fiber, and polypropylene can be steam-sterilized a maximum of three times without loss of tensile strength. Follow the manufacturer's recommendations for sterilization of nonsterile suture materials.

Many hospitals use only swaged-on needles. As these come in the sterile packets with the suture material, they eliminate the labor and expense of cleaning, packaging, and sterilizing needles. Disposable eyed and French eye needles are packaged and sterilized by the manufacturer.

Preparation of Reusable Needles

Standard sets of reusable eyed and French eye needles may be prepared for each operation or type of operation. This necessitates preparing many more needles in a set than any one surgeon uses if all surgeons' preferences are to be accommodated. An alternative may be to choose needles for each operation on the operating schedule according to each surgeon's preferences listed on a needle card. The basic set for the operation and the names of the surgeons who vary from this and their variations are listed. A needle card is maintained in a file for each operation and kept with the stock needle supply.

Metal racks with a spring to hold the needles are used commonly (see Fig. 13-6). The rack loaded with the eyed needles selected for the operation can be steam-sterilized with the instruments for that operation or it may be wrapped, labeled, and sterilized separately.

Packaging of Suture Materials

A strand of sterile suture material is supplied with as many as four coverings.

Box Each box contains one or three dozen packets of sterile suture material. The label on the box may be color-coded by suture material, i.e., light blue for silk, yellow for plain surgical gut, etc. Most of the boxes fit into a suture cabinet rack.

Overwrap Each packet has a hermetically sealed outer overwrap. This usually has laminated foil on one side and clear plastic film on the other. The overwrap is peeled back to expose the inner primary packet for sterile transfer to the sterile table. The circulating nurse must not contaminate the sterile inner primary packet as she peels back the overwrap.

Primary Packet Suture material, with or without swaged needles, is hermetically sealed in a primary packet that is opened by the scrub nurse. The primary packet may be made of foil, paper, plastic, or combinations of these. The labels may be color-coded by material, the same as the box. A silhouette of the needle is included on the label, if a swaged needle is enclosed, along with the size and type of suture material. A single strand of material or multiple strands may be in the primary packet. The packet may be designed for dispensing individual strands from a multiple suture packet, such as the labyrinth primary packet.

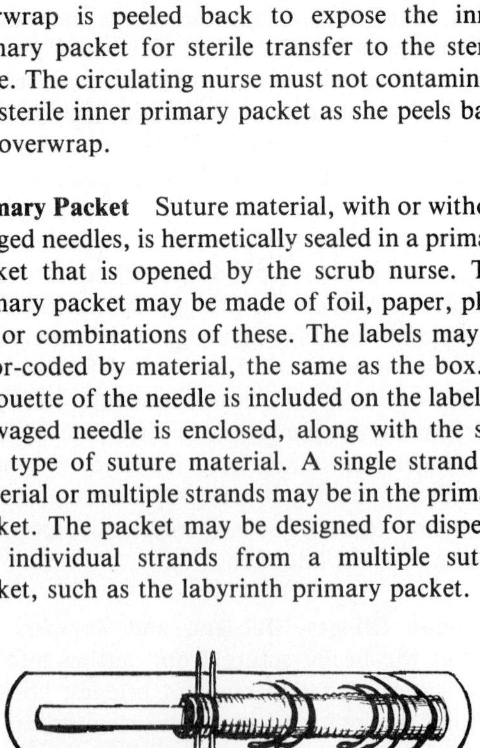

Figure 13-6 Metal needle rack with spring to hold eyed needles. Round and cutting needles are separated.

NOTE. Suture packets, both the overwrap and primary, should be opened only as needed. However, occasionally primary packets are removed from the overwrap, put onto the instrument table, and then not needed. If hermetically sealed primary packets are not opened, they must be decontaminated and may be returned to the manufacturer to be rewrapped and sterilized. The suture material is not resterilized, only the primary packet is; the suture remains sterile. Unopened primary packets must be decontaminated before placing in collection box or other storage container (see Chap. 8). Avoid opening overwrap unless material is needed.

Inner Dispenser Suture material is contained within the primary packet in a manner to facilitate removing or dispensing. This may be a folder, reel, or tube that may or may not be removed with the suture strands.

Preparation of Suture Material

Length of each strand of suture material within the primary packet varies; the shortest is 5 in. (approximately 13 cm) and the longest is 60 in. (150 cm). The most commonly used lengths range from 18 to 30 in. (45 to 75 cm). The length the surgeon prefers should be noted on the preference card. The scrub nurse may have to cut the strands to the desired length, depending upon the lengths available.

Standard Length This term refers to a 60-in. (150 cm) strand of silk or nylon or a 54-in. (135 cm) strand of absorbable material without a swaged needle. It is never handed to the surgeon in this length. The scrub nurse may cut it into a half-length, third-length, or fourth-length for use as a free tie or thread it for a stick tie or suture as shown in Figures 13-7 and 13-8.

Ligating Reels Twelve feet (approximately 4 m) of silk or cotton or 54 in. (135 cm) of absorbable suture are wound in disc-like plastic reels. These reels are color-coded by material and have size identification. The surgeon keeps the reel in the palm of his or her hand for a series of free ties. If these are not stocked, or preferred, the surgeon may ask the scrub nurse to wind a standard length onto a rod or other device for this purpose.

Precut Lengths Most suture materials are supplied in lengths ready for use as free ties or for

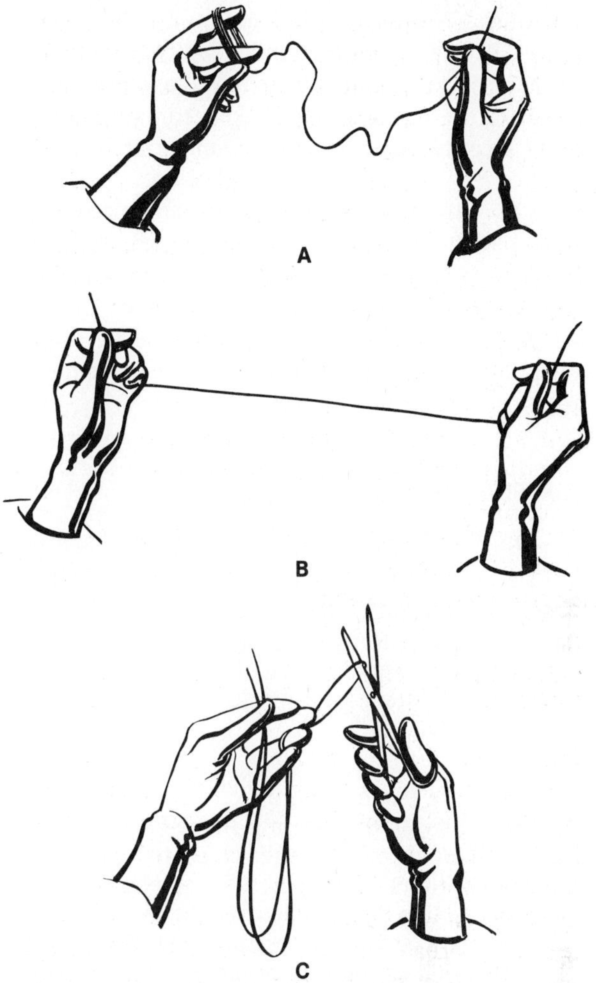

Figure 13-7 (A, B, and C) Sequence of scrub nurse preparing half-lengths of surgical gut suture. **A** The suture loops are separated by the fingers of the left hand while unwinding. **B** The full-length is gently unwound and straightened before cutting. The scrub nurse does not pull hard or test the strand, but keeps a firm grasp on both ends to prevent the suture from snapping away and possibly becoming contaminated. **C** She or he folds the suture in half and cuts the loop.

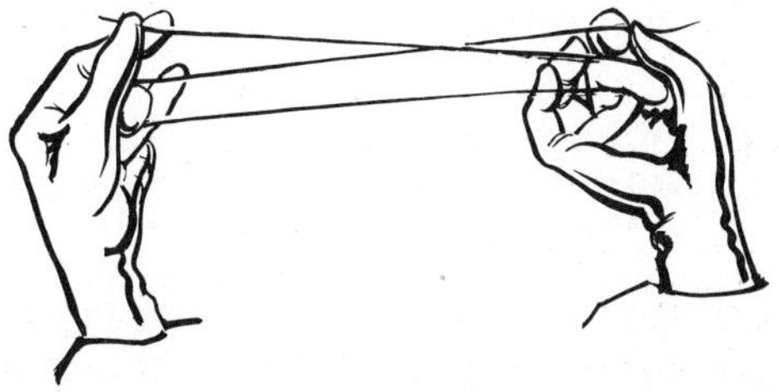

Figure 13-8 Scrub nurse preparing one-third length sutures. Pass one free end of the full-length strand from right to left hand, at the same time catching a loop around the third finger of right hand. Catching the other loop around the third finger of left hand while holding onto each end, adjust the suture to equal lengths (thirds), then cut each loop with scissors.

threading. These facilitate handling for the scrub nurse. They are dispensed individually from some primary packets or may be removed and placed in a fold of the suture book. Packets contain from 3 to 17 strands, depending on the material.

Swaged Needle-Suture Lengths are predetermined by the manufacturer; however, the surgeon has a wide variety of choices to meet all suturing needs. The scrub nurse must remember that a strand can be shortened but not extended. An appropriate length for the location of the tissue must be handed to the surgeon.

SURGICAL STAPLES

Stapling instruments were originally developed in Russia. They first became available in the United States in the 1960s. With these instruments, the surgeon can join tissue together with surgical staples.

Staples

1 They are made of nonreactive stainless steel. In internal tissue they form a shape like a capital letter B. This shape allows the staple to hold tissue together without crushing. Skin staples form a shape more like a rectangle over the incision.

2 They are supplied in presterilized, disposable cartridges that contain six or more staples. Quantities vary according to the instrument they fit. The number of cartridges needed varies with the procedure. The number of staples fired from the cartridge varies with the design of the instrument. Cartridges are color-coded by size of staples.

3 They are placed in the skin with a disposable skin stapler. This self-contained instrument, with an integral staple cartridge, is discarded after a single patient use.

Stapling Instruments

1. They are designed for stapling specific tissues, i.e., skin, fascia, bronchus, gastrointestinal tract, vessels, etc. The surgeon selects the correct instrument for the desired application.
2. They fire from the cartridge either a single staple or simultaneously one or two straight lines of multiple staples. A different instrument must be used for each type of firing.
   - **a** Skin stapler fires a single staple with each squeeze of the handle.
   - **b** Thoracoabdominal instruments place two straight, side-by-side staple lines that are 1 to 3 in. (2.5 to 8 cm) in length with 30, 55, or 90 staples, depending on the length of the jaws and the choice of cartridge.
   - **c** Gastrointestinal anastomosis instrument places two straight double lines of staples and simultaneously cuts the tissue between them.
   - **d** Ligating and dividing stapler doubly ligates and divides the tissue between the lines of staples.
3. They are manually operated mechanical instruments with many moving and detachable parts. The manufacturer's instructions for use and care must be followed to avoid technical failures. The scrub nurse is responsible for correctly assembling the instruments.
4. They should be cleaned in an ultrasonic cleaner and may be sterilized in steam or ethylene oxide gas, completely disassembled, according to the manufacturer's recommendations.

   NOTE. Preassembled, disposable stapling instruments eliminate assembling, cleaning, and sterilizing processes.

Advantages of Using Staples

1 This is a rapid method to ligate, anastomose, and approximate tissues. The time saved over conventional suturing techniques reduces total operating time, anesthesia time for the patient, and blood loss.

2 The healing of tissues may be accelerated because of minimal trauma and nonreactive nature of the stainless steel staples.

3 They produce an airtight, leakproof closure.

4 They can safely be used in many types of tissues and have a wide range of applications.

Disadvantages of Using Staples

1 The reusable instruments with separate cartridges of staples are expensive.

2 The instruments are not always reliable in their operation. They must be precisely aligned to fire accurately.

3 The consequences of an erroneous staple application are much more difficult to correct than those of manually placed sutures.

4 The surgeon must learn when and how to use the instruments; and the nursing personnel must learn how to care for them.

TISSUE ADHESIVES

Synthetic, glue-like adhesive substances that polymerize in contact with body tissues effect hemostasis and hold tissues together. Methyl methacrylate is used to augment fixation of pathologic fractures and to stabilize prosthetic devices in bone. Butyl cyanoacrylate may be used on friable tissue or highly vascular tissues, such as liver and spleen, to control bleeding and approximate tissues technically difficult to manage by other means, especially following massive resections or in traumatic injuries.

Methyl methacrylate is an acrylic, cement-like substance commonly referred to as *bone cement.* It is a drug supplied in two sterile components that must be mixed together immediately prior to use. One component is a colorless, highly volatile, flammable, liquid methyl methacrylate monomer in an ampul. This is a powerful lipid solvent so it must be handled carefully. The other component is a white powder mixture of polymethyl methacrylate, methyl methacrylate-styrene copolymer, and barium sulfate in a packet. The barium sulfate provides radiopacity to the substance. When the powder and liquid are mixed, an exothermic polymeric reaction forms a soft, pliable, dough-like mass. This reaction liberates heat as high as 110 °C (230 °F). As the reaction progresses, the substance becomes hard in a few minutes. The mixing and kneading of the entire contents of the liquid ampul and powder packet must be thorough and at least 4 minutes in duration. The substance must be adequately soft and pliable for application to bone. The completion of polymerization occurs in the patient. After it hardens, it holds a prosthesis firmly in a fixed position.

A hazard to operating room personnel has been reported in regard to the use of methyl methacrylate in the operating room. Some personnel have noticed dizzy spells, difficulty in breathing, nausea and vomiting, following the mixing of methyl methacrylate. The monomer and several of its ingredients are potent allergenic sensitizers when the vapor is inhaled. Experiments with volunteers suggest that inhalation of the vapor may have a temporary inhibitory effect on gastric motor function. Industrial inhalation-exposure levels have been recommended in America. Soviet workers have proposed levels of less than 12.5 ppm, finding that exposure over that level for longer than 20 minutes can lead to untoward systemic effects. The recommendation for ORs is to provide a suitable means of local exhaust that will collect the vapor at the source of mixing at the sterile field and will discharge it into the outside air or absorb the monomer on activated charcoal.

TISSUE REPAIR MATERIALS

Tissue deficiencies may require additional reinforcement or bridging material to obtain adequate wound healing. Sometimes the edges of the fascia, for example, cannot be brought together without excessive tension. In obese or elderly persons the fascia cannot withstand this tension because of weakness due to infiltration of fat. Biologic or synthetic mesh materials are used to fill congenital, traumatic, or acquired defects in fascia or a body wall and to reinforce the fascia, as in hernia repair.

Biologic Materials

Cargile Membrane A thin sheet of tissue obtained from the cecum of the ox. Cargile membrane is rarely used, although still commercially available in 4 by 6 in. (10 by 15 cm) size, to prevent adhesions after abdominal operations, for isolating ligations, and as a covering for packing in submucous nasal resections.

Fascia Lata Strips of fascia lata are obtained from the fibrous connective tissue that covers the thigh muscles of beef cattle. In lieu of commercial fascia lata—*a heterogenous graft*—the surgeon may strip a piece of fascia from the thigh of the patient—*an autogenous graft.* Fascia lata contains collagen. It increases the amount of tissue already present and becomes a living part of the tissue it supports. It is used to strengthen weakened fascial layers or to fill in defects in fascia. Since the advent of synthetic meshes, heterogenous strips $\frac{1}{4}$ by 8 in (6 mm by 20 cm) are used infrequently.

Synthetic Mesh

Polyester Fiber Mesh Polyester fiber mesh remains soft and pliable in tissue, but has limited elasticity. It is the least inert of the synthetic mesh materials. Potential complications of foreign-body tissue reaction are minimal, but it is not preferred in the presence of infection because of its multifilament construction. This mesh is machine-knitted by a process that interlocks each fiber juncture to prevent unraveling when cut. Nonsterile sheets are available in sizes 6 by 12 in. (15 by 30 cm) and 12 by 12 in. (30 by 30 cm).

Polypropylene Mesh Polypropylene is knitted into a mesh with high tensile strength and good elasticity. It will not unravel when cut. Because it is inert it may be used in the presence of infection.

It is available sterile in several sizes ranging from $2\frac{1}{2}$ by 4 in. (6 by 10 cm) to 9 by 14 in. (23 by 35 cm). If sufficient skin is not available to cover it, this mesh can be used as a body wall replacement and as a support for the viscera during healing by second intention.

Stainless Steel Mesh Available nonsterile in sheets 6 by 12 in. (15 by 30 cm), steel is the most inflexible and difficult of the meshes to handle. The sharp edges may puncture gloves. Use wire scissors, not dissecting scissors, to cut it. Steel is opaque to x-ray, which may be a disadvantage for the patient in later life. Also the mesh may fragment and cause patient discomfort.

Advantages of synthetic mesh:

1 It is easily cut to the desired size for the tissue defect.
2 It is easily sutured underneath the edges of tissue to create a smooth surface.
3 Fibrous tissue easily grows through the openings to incorporate the mesh into the tissue to maximize tensile strength.
4 Polyester fiber and stainless steel mesh can be steam-sterilized immediately prior to use. Polypropylene is supplied sterile, but also may be steam-sterilized.

NOTE. The melting point of polyester fiber is 250°F (121°C) so this mesh cannot be steam-sterilized at a higher temperature.

TISSUE REPLACEMENT MATERIALS

For centuries surgeons have sought materials to replace parts of anatomy. Tissue may be absent or distorted due to congenital deformity, traumatic injury, degenerative disease, or surgical resection. Replacement or substitution of tissue may be possible with biologic or synthetic prosthetic materials implanted into the body. A *prosthesis* is a permanent or temporary replacement for a missing or malfunctioning structure. Some implants replace vital structures, such as diseased heart valves and blood vessels. Devices, such as pacemakers, assist the function of vital organs. Other materials are used to repair or replace defects. Prosthetic materials implanted into the body must:

1 Be compatible with physiologic processes
2 Produce no or minimal tissue reaction
3 Be sterile so will not cause infection or become a culture medium
4 Be noncarcinogenic or other disease causative
5 Have viable and adequate tissue coverage, unless used as a biological dressing over denuded skin surfaces
6 Have adequate blood supply through or around them
7 Be stable so will not degenerate or change shape if used for permanent function
8 Contour or conform to normal tissue configuration as desired

Biologic Materials

The biologic materials are mentioned here, but detailed discussions of skin grafts and organ and tissue transplants will follow in other chapters.

Bone A bone graft affords structural support and a pattern for regrowth of bone within a skeletal defect. *Cancellous* bone is porous. Its porosity permits tissue fluid to reach deeper into it than into cortical bone, and thus most of the bone cells live. *Cortical* bone is used for bridging large defects in the skeleton, as it gives greater strength. It may be fixed in the recipient site by means of wire suture or screws.

While bone grafts become fixed to the recipient site, their main purpose is to stimulate new bone growth. *Autogenous bone,* which is obtained from the patient, usually is taken at the time of operation and may be obtained from the ilium or tibia. *Homogenous bone,* which is obtained from someone other than the patient, is stored in the bone bank until needed (refer to Chap. 20, p. 369). This bone is weaker than autogenous grafts, thus requiring a much longer time of immobilization. Homogenous bone is dead bone. The recipient bone regeneration is responsible for union with this type of bone graft. It may be desirable, however, to spare the patient the added operating time and trauma of removing an autogenous graft.

Bovine Heterografts Enzymatically treated bovine carotid artery heterografts are prepared commercially. These grafts are used for blood access in patients on hemodialysis who have poor blood vessels or in whom it is difficult to create either fistulas or shunts. Femoral arteriovenous bovine shunts can be punctured innumerable times with a low incidence of thrombus formation.

Collagen Collagen is used as a biomaterial in both its natural form, such as the bovine graft and the microcrystalline hemostatic powder, and restructured into membranes or films. Collagen can be altered by a variety of techniques to change its physical properties.

Organ Transplants Some whole body organs can be transplanted from one human to another. This is done in an effort to sustain life by compensating for physiological deficits or inadequate function of vital organs. Refer to Chapter 28 for complete discussion of transplantation.

Porcine Heterografts Pig (porcine) skin is used as a temporary biological dressing to cover large body surfaces denuded of skin. Biological dressings are needed over large skin defects, such as burns, until permanent skin grafting can be accomplished (see Chap. 25). Freeze-dried preparations of split-thickness pigskin are commercially available in sterile rolls of various sizes. These are soaked in sterile water or normal saline prior to use. Vascularization of the pigskin does not occur, but it adheres tightly while reepithelialization proceeds underneath it for as long as 2 weeks before it dries up and peels off spontaneously.

Tissue Transplants Skin and blood vessels are frequently transplanted from one part of the body to another. These are referred to as *autografts* since the patient is both donor and recipient. The transplanted tissue becomes a part of the living tissue in the recipient site. Refer to Chapter 25 for discussion of skin grafts and Chapter 21 for discussion of vascular grafts.

Some tissues can be transplanted from one person to another to restore function, such as the cornea, or provide support in structures, such as cartilage in nasal reconstruction. These are referred to as *allografts* or *homografts* (see Chap. 28).

Synthetic Materials

Inorganic substances are less than perfect for prostheses because they cannot unite with tissue. However, they can provide support, restore function, augment or restore body contour.

Metal Stainless steel, a cobalt alloy trade named Vitallium, and titanium are the metals used to manufacture prosthetic implants. Used primarily for stabilization or replacement of bone, metal implants must be strong enough to withstand stress of weight bearing or muscular action and must not corrode in body tissues. They are never reused due to a degree of weakening that comes with use. Refer to Chapter 20 for specific types and uses of metallic orthopaedic implants.

Special care must be taken in handling metal implants to protect the surface. A simple scratch on a metal implant can lead to corrosion in the body. It will be bathed continuously by weakly chloride body fluids. If corrosion begins, the implant may fail and have to be removed. It is very important, therefore, that all metal implants be protected from scratches. This can be accomplished by:

1 Wrapping each implant individually, or wrapping sets with each size implant in a separate compartment, for both storage and sterilization. Most prostheses come from the manufacturer in protective coverings or cases. Some of these are suitable for adequate sterilization with subsequent placement in the sterile field to minimize handling prior to implantation.
2 Preventing implants from coming in contact with other hard surfaces of metal or glass, either during storage and sterilization or on the instrument table.
3 Not handling or transferring an unprotected implant with any type of forceps.

Implants of one metal should not come in contact with those of another metal as an electrochemical reaction occurs between metals. Two different metals are not implanted in the same patient for this reason. Instruments used for insertion also should be of the same metal as the implant, e.g., a stainless steel screwdriver and screw.

Methyl Methacrylate A highly refined methyl methacrylate mixture can be molded and shaped to fit a defect in bone. When it hardens, this material looks and feels very much like bone. It is usually used to repair a skull defect (see Chap. 24, p. 435).

Polyester Fiber Polyester fibers woven or knitted into seamless cylinders are used to replace major arteries.

Polyethylene Struts Polyethylene tubing may be inserted into structures, such as fallopian tubes or ureters, to give support during healing or to bridge a defect in tissue continuity.

Silicone Silicone is one of the most inert of the synthetic polymers used for implantation into the body. It is used in many forms: as a gel, sponge, film, tubing, liquid, and preformed molded anatomic structures. A medical-grade silicone elastomer (Silastic) in one form or another is used in virtually every surgical specialty for tissue reconstruction or replacement.

Complete instructions for cleaning and sterilizing silicone implants before use are supplied by the manufacturer with each type of prosthesis. These instructions must be followed meticulously. After preparation, these implants are not handled with bare hands and care must be taken to ensure that they do not pick up lint and dust. Gloves worn during handling must be entirely free from powder. Skin oil, lint, dust, powder, and other surface contaminants can evoke foreign-body reactions around the implant in tissue.

Polytetrafluoroethylene (Teflon) Some prostheses or parts of prosthetic devices may be made of this synthetic polymer. Teflon may be woven into a fabric for arterial grafts, extruded into tubing for struts, or molded into a solid configuration for valves or joints. Its lubricity makes it a useful replacement for tissues when motion is desirable.

SKIN CLOSURE

In addition to sutures and staples, other materials may be used to hold skin edges in approximation.

Skin Clips

Clips made of noncorroding metal may be used to approximate skin edges. They tend to leave more scar than other methods of skin closure, but they may be applied quickly when time is a critical factor and cosmetic result is unimportant. They can be used in the presence of infection or drainage. A specially designed instrument is necessary to apply clips. Skin clips also may be used to secure stockinet or towels to the skin to isolate the incision, particularly on an extremity.

Skin Closure Strips

Strips of microporous polypropylene or nylon tape placed across the line of incision hold skin edges in approximation during healing. They may be used to close skin edges of superficial lacerations, as primary closure of skin layer in conjunction with a subcuticular suture, or in conjunction with interrupted skin sutures. Often they are used following early suture removal to support the wound during healing. A skin tackifier, such as tincture of benzoin, may be recommended by the manufacturer for assuring adhesion to skin.

Strips are available sterile in widths of $\frac{1}{8}$, $\frac{1}{4}$, and $\frac{1}{2}$ in. (3, 6, and 12.7 mm) and lengths from $1\frac{1}{2}$ to 4 in. (3.7 to 10 cm). They are ethylene oxide gas sterilized in peel-apart packets. Skin closure strips:

1 May be used in the emergency department on superficial lacerations and eliminate need for sutures that would require local anesthesia for placement with subsequent return of the patient for suture removal.

2 Eliminate foreign-body tissue reaction of suture material in skin.

3 Have enough porosity to permit adequate ventilation of clean or contaminated wounds.

4 Permit removal of sutures within 32 to 48 hours postoperatively. Crosshatch scarring and the possibility of infection are reduced when sutures are removed early. The skin closure strips provide long-term wound reinforcement and support.

5 Permit visibility of the healing wound so the surgeon can see how well the wound edges have coapted. Some strips are translucent; others have a color tone or opacity that does not afford this advantage.

6 Minimize skin irritation because they are hyporeactive.

7 Can be applied and removed rapidly.

8 Can be easily torn or cut to meet surgeon's exact length requirements.

DRUG AND MEDICAL DEVICE LEGISLATION

In 1906, the U.S. federal government enacted the Pure Food and Drug Act with the U.S. Department of Agriculture as the enforcing agency to assure the introduction of safe and sanitary foods to the public. The federal Food, Drug, and Cosmetic Act of 1938 extended regulation to include introduction of cosmetics and drugs as well as food, and, to a minimal extent, medical devices. The Food and Drug Administration (FDA), within the Department of Agriculture, became the enforcing agency with authority to implement a preclearance mechanism requiring drug manufacturers to provide evidence of safety before a new drug could be sold. Sutures were classified as drugs.

The Kefauver-Harris Drug Amendments of 1962 added strength to the new drug clearance procedures. Drug manufacturers must prove to the FDA the effectiveness as well as the safety of drugs prior to making them commercially available. These amendments established a mechanism for clinical investigations to evaluate the efficacy of drugs. Depending upon the nature of the drug, clinical studies often require several years before the FDA approves the commercial sale of a product.

The Medical Device Amendments of 1976 gave the FDA regulatory control over all medical devices (defined as any health care product that is not a drug), in addition to the FDA's previous regulatory control of drugs. All wound closure materials are classified as either drugs or devices under these amendments. Ethical manufacturers adhere to the guidelines, standards, and regulations of the FDA prior to release of a new drug or medical device.

Chapter 14

Economy, Work Simplification, and Safety

The 1972 amendments to the Social Security Act created the Professional Standards Review Organizations (PSROs) designed to involve health care practitioners in the ongoing review and evaluation of health care services. PSROs review health care provided to patients under Medicare, Medicaid, and Maternal and Child Health programs and make judgments concerning the medical necessity and quality of care. In addition, PSROs determine whether health care is provided at a level most economical and consistent with the patient's health care needs.

Cost control, one aspect of the PSRO legislation, is part of a comprehensive quality assurance program. The hospital's quality assurance program focuses on the improvement of practice. To assure quality, nursing care must be assessed in terms of outcome for the patient, actual care given, techniques and procedures used, supplies and equipment available, and efficiency within the organization.

A postoperative wound infection that prolongs hospitalization for the patient is expensive in time and money. If a consistent break in aseptic technique in the OR is identified as the cause and is corrected, this cost will be saved for other patients.

The OR staff must monitor the quality of care to determine what they are doing right, what they are doing wrong, and whether a less costly method can achieve the same or better quality nursing care. Efficiency is frequently referred to as the cost-benefit ratio. *Efficiency* is the attainment of quality reviewed in relationship of the manpower, facilities, supplies, and equipment to the appropriateness, acceptability, and cost to the patient. Quality assurance then becomes synonymous with cost control.

EFFICIENCY OF THE O.R. STAFF

Individuals working together coordinate their efforts to better accomplish the tasks necessary to achieve a common goal. In the OR suite, this common goal is to provide for the safety and welfare of each and every patient admitted through the doors. Efficiency, therefore, depends primarily upon individual effort and the working relationship between team members.

Each department takes on a personality from the individuals in it. This personality gives a reputation for good or otherwise, like an individual reputation. Unethical discussions, unprofessional conduct, lapses in sterile technique, carelessness in handling expensive equipment, breakage, or forgetfulness make impressions upon patients and visitors, who may take these as an index of the total department. They may carry these impressions to others outside the hospital. Constant vigilance is necessary. Pride in one's work and in the department as a whole leads to dissatisfaction with anything less than the very best.

Musts for OR Nurse and Technician

1 You must have initiative, energy, and stamina combined with honesty, dependability, and integrity.

2 You must have a responsive and pleasing personality. Make it a pleasure for others to work with you. It never hurts anyone to say "please" and "thank you." A spirit of cooperation will make any situation tolerable and will enhance efficiency.

3 You must have a positive attitude toward everyone with whom you work. In all work situations you will find individuals from different backgrounds with a divergence of life-styles. You must possess poise and graciousness, with a genuine willingness to be compassionate and understanding of individual differences. Being considerate will gain you the trust and respect of others and help ensure an efficient environment for patients.

4 You must have a sense of humor. Situations encountered in the OR are often difficult. The ability to keep one's sense of humor is a particular aid when dealing with tension.

5 You must have an open mind and flexibility. Changes in work schedules and procedures must be made when a need for change accommodates or improves patient care. You must be adaptable and able to demonstrate efficiency in all situations.

6 You must be willing to accept and profit from constructive criticism. One who can accept criticism without becoming defensive may prevent a minor situation from developing into a real difficulty. Keep a balanced perspective. Many times it is not the incident itself, but one's reaction to it that is so devastating. Constructive criticism should be given and received tactfully and kindly. Profit by it to improve your performance.

7 You must not go off duty and discuss incidents in the day's work. Operations, patients, surgeons, and the multitude of incidents involving them each day in the OR are not discussed outside the OR suite. To seek advice or to unburden yourself when problems arise, discuss your work situation with your instructor, the supervisor, or the head nurse before going off duty. Any unresolved problem will affect the quality of patient care either directly or indirectly.

8 You must be properly instructed in the use and care of equipment and supplies before being given the responsibility for them. Never be afraid to say "I do not know" or to ask questions. Learning is an active process. Go out to meet it, and be eager for new experiences.

9 You must know the policies and procedures and efficiently follow them in carrying out your work. Learn to do things right the first time and continue to do them that way. Many new things can be learned and much accomplished in the time wasted in correcting errors.

10 You must work rapidly. Learn to follow directions quickly and accurately to the smallest detail; carelessness or ignorance could cost the life or welfare of your patient. A change in diagnosis during operation may require an altogether different setup and a different procedure from the one anticipated. Emergencies will arise. You must be able to meet these situations quickly, calmly, and efficiently. You must know not only *what* to do in the basic situations, but also *why* you do it, to be able to exercise good judgment and to adapt to more radical situations.

11 You must be able to organize your work effectively, so that not a single minute is lost, not a motion superfluous. It is of the utmost importance to keep to a minimum the length of time a patient is under anesthesia. As the anesthesia time is prolonged, a greater burden is put on the patient's recovery. Also, the period of anxious concern is prolonged for the patient's family.

12 You must fit in and work smoothly as a member of a closely functioning team. An efficient, well-coordinated OR team is an absolute essential. Each member must anticipate not only his or her own needs but also those of the others. The surgeon must never be made to feel rushed by the OR team. Common interest in the goal provides teamwork in which all think and act as one unit. You must be an inconspicuous and highly efficient member of that team—inconspicuous through your alertness and anticipation and your smooth, precise, and quick actions.

13 You must anticipate the surgeon's needs and keep one step ahead. The surgeon's thought is distracted from the operation when handed the wrong instrument or when he or she must search through many to find the right one or wait for supplies. You must be alert in observation and have enough knowledge to use your imagination intelligently to read the surgeon's mind.

14 You must follow rigidly the rule that nothing is taken for granted. For example, you must know, not assume, that equipment is sterile. You must know and know that you know. While many sterile supplies are obtained commercially, some are packaged and sterilized in the OR suite or central service department. It is well to learn as much as you can about how all supplies are packaged and sterilized in order to supervise their use by others or to evaluate their level of quality and safety for the patient.

15 You must be responsible for all work assigned to you. Ask questions as necessary, and report work assignments as finished or unfinished. Your responsibility goes beyond your own assignments to those of the department as a whole. If the supervisor does not give you an additional assignment, look for ways to help others until all the work is finished. Do not waste time. Actual operations are only one part of the work in the operating room suite. Preparation and cleanup involve procedures with which you must become familiar.

TIME AND MOTION ECONOMY

Time Is Costly

Time is an important element in the OR. If time is wasted between operations, for example, the day's schedule is slowed down and later operations are delayed. The surgeons' time is wasted and they tend to come late, anticipating delays. The patients become more nervous waiting for their operations and more uncomfortable during the prolonged period without fluids.

Poor managers of time tend to become less efficient and thus drift into poor work habits. Your greatest ally is a little thing called *common sense.* Take time to stop and think. Is there a quicker, easier, or more efficient way of doing the job? Most work habits can be improved.

Records of time are necessary and important to determine efficiency—when the patient arrives, when the surgeon arrives, when the anesthetic is started, when the incision is made, when the incision is closed, when the patient leaves the room, cleanup time. Undue delays are identified and may be corrected. Thus the availability of time for further operations is increased.

You must be willing to take the time to study your existing situation in a methodical manner and gather the facts needed to support the desirability of alternative methods. Recognition that a problem exists is the first step toward solving a problem. Seek to develop more efficient and economical work methods.

Associations

Association is a great aid to memory and organization of work. The mention of one article brings to mind the others used with it. For instance, the scrub nurse knows a suture calls for a tissue forceps to the surgeon, needleholder to the assistant, then scissors.

Think of the order in which instruments and supplies are going to be needed and *do first things first,* e.g., prepare sutures for closing deep tissue layers before skin sutures.

Watch for and try to establish such associations. This is a good way to increase your efficiency. If surgeons must devote time and attention to details the nurses and technicians should know, they are distracted from their primary concerns. Time is wasted for all involved, including the patient.

To be proficient, you must know the organization of work and the relative importance of factors in accomplishing it. For example, if, as the patient is being prepped, the surgeon requests stainless steel retention sutures for closure instead of the usual sutures, the circulating nurse should realize there is plenty of time to get them after she completes other duties. She must tie the gowns, supervise the draping, adjust the Mayo stand and instrument table, focus the light, etc., to start the operation before getting the closure suture. When she gets the steel suture, association tells her to also get wire scissors and bumpers or bridges.

Motion Economy

Wasted motion is not only time-consuming, but also adds to physical fatigue. Fatigue is the result of body movement. Ten principles of motion economy can reduce fatigue from physical activity and improve your level of efficiency.

Motions Should Be Productive Once the steps in a procedure are learned, work to increase speed and manual dexterity in carrying them out. Avoid a hurried, rattled appearance. Rather make each movement count for some progress. Work quietly and quickly. Work as fast as possible without sacrificing accuracy and technique for speed.

The corollary to this principle is a place for everything and everything in its place. Keep an orderly work area to avoid fumbling and rehandling items. Arrange them properly and leave them there. This corollary is justification for standardization of procedures, such as a standardized instrument table setup, standardized stocking of supplies in cabinets or on carts, so that everything has a place and is in its place. Then you know instinctively where to put your hands on supplies when needed. A neat and orderly work area is one of the first requirements for productive motions. You should also consider the work flow so that minimal motions can be made to accomplish productive work.

Motions Should Be Simple Body movements should be confined to the lowest classification with which it is possible to perform work properly. Movements of the upper extremity are classified:

1 Class 1 involves the fingers. The knuckle provides the pivot for motion for such tasks as fingering through a card file, turning a set screw on an instrument, using a pair of scissors.

2 Class 2 involves both the hand and fingers. The wrist is the pivot for motion as in passing instruments, counting sponges, picking up or writing on an operative record.

3 Class 3 includes the forearm. Using the elbow as a pivot, more effort and time is expended in the third and succeeding classifications because the movements of any one class involve movements of all classes preceding it. It takes longer and more effort to turn the pages of a procedure book or patient's chart than to thumb through a file of surgeon's preference cards. The elbow pivots to open a peel-down package, unfold drapes, and unwrap small supplies.

4 Class 4 includes the upper arm. The shoulder pivot is used when opening a door, setting up the Mayo stand, and prepping a patient.

5 Class 5 adds the torso. The trunk bends or stretches to lift a patient, take supplies from a low shelf or drawer, reach to hang an IV bag, or bend to count the sponges in a kick bucket.

Upper extremity work should be arranged to reduce work to the lowest possible classification. Finger motion is the least fatiguing; shoulder motion is the most. The scrub nurse should position herself at the operating table so that she can use elbow, wrist, and finger motions. She should be positioned opposite the surgeon so that both can work with their elbows at their sides. This avoids prolonged shoulder motion for both of them.

It is quicker for the circulating nurse to stretch to hang an IV bag than to take time to use finger action to loosen the set screw on an IV standard, lower it with shoulder movement, hang the bag with elbow action, and repeat the sequence in reverse. However, stretching is more fatiguing. The more fatigued you get, the slower your motions become as the day progresses. Maybe you saved 30 seconds with the first patient of the day, but what happens to the last patient of the day? Time is lost because energy wanes.

Motions Should Be Curved Motions should go along curved rather than straight paths whenever possible. A circular motion to clean the flat surfaces of furniture is less fatiguing than straight push-and-pull strokes.

Motions Should Be Symmetrical Motions should be rhythmic and smooth flowing, and, when possible, both hands should be used symmetrically. A circular motion is less fatiguing, but damp cloths in both hands, going in opposing circles, will get flat surfaces cleaned even faster and easier.

Work Should Be within Grasp Range The work area should be arranged so that all materials are within grasp range to avoid changes in body position. Grasp range is within the radius from the pivot point of the elbow or shoulder, either horizontally or vertically. The minimum grasp range is within the radius of the arcs formed with only the forearms extended, using the elbows as the pivot points, on the horizontal plane (see Fig. 14-1).

The optimum grasp range is within the area where the left-hand and the right-hand arcs overlap. This is the area in which two-handed work, such as putting a needle in a needleholder, can be done most conveniently.

The maximum grasp range is within the arcs formed from the shoulder pivots. The overlapping of these arcs is the maximum extent at which two-handed work can be done within reach without changing body position.

The Mayo stand should be placed over the operating table at a height and in a position within

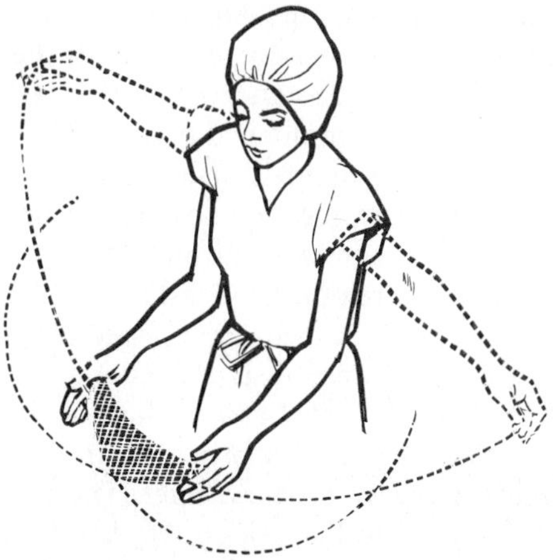

Figure 14-1 Grasp ranges. The minimum range is within the radius of the arcs formed with only the forearms extended, using elbows as pivotal points. The optimum range is within the area where arcs of hands overlap. The maximum range is within the arcs formed from the shoulder pivots.

the minimum and optimum grasp range of the scrub nurse. It must not rest on the patient, but it can be lowered to an inch or two above. The instrument table should be positioned as close to the horizontal plane within maximum grasp range as possible. Instruments or supplies requiring two-handed work should be placed on the Mayo stand and instrument table as close to the optimum grasp range as possible.

Hands Should Be Relieved of Work Hands should be relieved of any work that can be done more advantageously by other parts of the body. Many electrical instruments have foot pedals to facilitate operation.

Doors into the OR suite may be opened by stepping on a trigger mechanism or by passing an electric eye. Some people object to automatic doors due to the difficulty of holding them open if necessary. They are designed to adhere to this principle, however.

Injuries are sustained to the back, arms, or shoulders from lifting patients or equipment improperly. Lift with your legs. Bend your knees to get body weight under the load, and straighten legs to lift. A lifting frame or Davis roller helps relieve potential strain of moving unconscious or obese patients.

The Worker Should Be at Ease Tiring body motions, awkward or strained body posture should be avoided. During standing work, when the heels are together, constant muscular effort is required by the thigh muscles to maintain an erect posture. In contrast, when the heels are apart, the ligaments of the hips and knees support the body without effort. A wide stance while standing at the operating table for prolonged periods will be less fatiguing for the scrub nurse. The circulating nurse can stand in location to observe both the operation and the instrument table with both upper and lower extremities in a rest position. In this standing position the arms are clasped behind the back and the feet are in a wide stance. Weight bearing on only one foot causes additional strain.

This principle includes provision of a correct and comfortable work-place height. The operating table is adjusted to the best correct height for the surgeon. This may not be the most comfortable position for the other members of the sterile team. Team members should be able to stand erect with their arms comfortably relaxed from the shoulders, without stooping, and should not have to raise their hands above the level of their elbows for the majority of their work motions. Platforms, standing stools, may be needed to elevate the scrub nurse and/or the assistant surgeon to a feasible working height. Platforms should be long enough to allow a wide stance.

Correct posture in the sitting position is equally important. Your back is strongest when it is straight. When you sit, sit well back in the chair or on a stool and keep your body straight from hips to neck. Lean forward from the hips, not the shoulders or waist. This position puts the least strain on muscles, ligaments, and internal organs. Before and after the operation, the circulating and scrub nurses should rest in a sitting position between periods of standing. If work is to be done in a sitting position, the stool or chair should be adjusted to the correct height for the working surface.

Additional factors contribute to providing a comfortable working environment: ventilation, lighting, color, and noise. Lighting should be adequate; however, excessive glare produces fatigue. Illumination is the product of the light times the reflectance of the target. A bright, highly polished, mirror finish on an instrument tends to reflect light and can restrict the vision of the surgeon. Satin or dull-finished instruments eliminate glare and lessen the surgeon's eye strain. These instruments are made with varying degrees of dullness depending on the manufacturer. Tinted or Polaroid glasses may save the sterile team members from visual fatigue, but must not distort color of tissues.

Soft pastel colors, especially blues and green, are less reflective for linens and walls than white. Drapes with dark tones help reduce contrast between most tissues and the surrounding field. Some hospitals have a mural on a wall in the OR to enhance the visual effect of the environment, particularly if the OR suite is windowless.

Although attention is given to ventilation, lighting, and color, less attention is given to the design of the OR in terms of auditory effects. Some hospitals have piped-in music. Music can be relaxing for the patient awaiting operation or undergoing an operation under local anesthesia, and for personnel. However, it should be easily turned off in the OR at the request of the patient, surgeon, or anesthesiologist. It can be a distraction especially for the anesthesiologist who depends upon his hearing to aid him in monitoring the patient.

Noise can be irritating and potentially dangerous to patients and personnel. It can become intense enough to provoke peripheral vasoconstriction, dilatation of the pupils, and other subtle physiologic effects, as well as interfere with necessary communication and thereby provoke irritation.

The OR should be as quiet as possible except for the essential sounds of communication between team members directly concerned with the patient's care. When it is necessary to talk, do so in low voice. Conversation unrelated to the operation is out of place. Even during deep stages, an anesthetized patient does perceive noises and conversation that occur during the operation and may remember them. If a spinal or local anesthesia is used, remember that the patient can hear the conversation. Patients interpret anything they hear in terms of themselves, so all words must be guarded. Counts or requests for supplies must be done quietly, so the patient cannot hear.

The major sources of noise in the OR involve paper, gloves, objects wheeled across the floor, instruments striking one another, monitors, and high-pitched compressed-air instruments including suction. The scrub nurse must keep these sources and their effects in mind and avoid clattering instruments. Clamp off or kink a loop into suction tubing except while in actual use. The circulating nurse should keep all doors closed to shut out noise in the corridors, of water running in the scrub room, or of the sterilizer operating in the substerile room. Do not crush paper wrappings. Hold a bottle of solution inches, not feet, away from basin when pouring. Monitors with audible signals should be placed as far away from the patient's ears as possible, with the amplifier turned away from the patient.

Remember, working in a pleasantly quiet environment is less fatiguing with fewer psychologic and physiologic adverse effects, and greater efficiency on behalf of the patient.

Work Materials Should Be Prepositioned Supplies can be arranged for convenient use and minimal handling. Disposable or linen drapes are packaged in order of use so they do not need to be handled by the scrub nurse, except to move the stack to a corner of the instrument table, until ready to use. Instruments can be arranged in trays so all of them do not need to be removed until needed.

Economize time and effort by placing items on the instrument table and Mayo stand in the order in which they will be used, and put them in their proper places without rearranging them. Arrange the instruments on the Mayo stand in the position to hand to the surgeon or assistant to use. In passing an instrument, place it in the surgeon's hand in the position in which he is going to use it, so he will not need to make any readjustments (see Fig. 8-6, p. 140). Grasp it with the thumb and the first two fingers, far enough away from the handle so the surgeon can grasp it. Hand a needle in the needleholder the same way, supporting the suture so it does not drag, and having the needle pointing in the direction in which the surgeon will start to use it. Hand the thumb forceps so the surgeon can grasp the handle; do the same for retractors.

Gravity Should Be Used Scrub sponges or brush dispensers operate on the principle that gravity should be used whenever possible. Cabinets for smaller packages in the sterile supply room can be vertical and divided into appropriate-size slots. These can be filled from the top and dispensed from the bottom of each slot. This is convenient, saves space, and assures that older items are used first. Shelves for large, heavy packs can be made of rollers and slanted slightly to facilitate handling. Gravity-feed and drop-delivery installations eliminate or reduce motions. The quickest way to dispose of an object is to drop it. This may be the quickest way to break or contaminate it too, so the application of this principle requires good judgment.

Supplies Should Be Combined Items should serve two or more purposes whenever possible. Sterilizer indicator tape, for example, will serve a dual purpose: to hold the package closed and to tell you if it has been exposed to a sterilization process. And only inches, not a yard, of tape accomplishes the job.

Disposable kits and trays are purchased, or sets are made up of reusable items, so that all the supplies and materials needed for a procedure are combined into a single unit. This eliminates opening many separate packages.

A knife blade packet can be sterilized in the instrument tray with the knife handle. This eliminates a sterile transfer to the instrument table.

Put instruments that are sterilized in sets of various sizes, such as expensive prostheses, on a small sterile table or at one side of the instrument table. When the surgeon decides which size he or she needs, remove it from the set without contaminating the others, and thus save cleanup of those.

ECONOMICAL USE OF SUPPLIES AND EQUIPMENT

As the cost of supplies increases, OR personnel should be conscious of ways to eliminate wasteful practices. For example, throw away disposable items only. Avoid throwing away reusable ones. Continuous emphasis on cost reduction can reduce waste and result in economies of benefit to the hospital and ultimately to the patients.

The operating room suite is one of the most expensive departments of a hospital. Adequate linen, instruments, and other supplies are necessary for patient care. Dollars and cents cannot be the primary consideration. Beyond the point of safety, economy becomes a hazard. But supplies do not need to be used lavishly just because they are available. Remember the following principles:

"Just Enough Is Enough"

1 Keep the varieties and numbers of instruments and supplies needed for each operation to a minimum. If the procedure book and surgeon preference cards are kept up-to-date, articles no longer used are eliminated.

2 Do not pour an ounce of solution if a milliliter is needed. Pour just enough solution for a skin preparation according to the manufacturer's recommendation; it takes only a small amount. Do not unnecessarily open a bottle for a small amount if you know the remainder will not be used.

3 Follow procedures for draping to provide an adequate sterile field without wasting disposable draping material or overstocking launderable linen.

4 Do not open another packet of sutures for that last stitch. Usually a few leftover pieces are long enough to complete the closure.

5 Suction tubing, syringes, hypodermic needles, drains, catheters, extra linen, etc., are kept sterile. These supplies should be opened only as needed, not routinely "just in case" they might be needed.

6 Do not soak too much plaster when helping with cast applications. Keep just ahead of the surgeon. Watch him to see when he appears to be almost finished. Ask him if he wants more before soaking an extra one or two rolls of plaster.

7 Turn off lights when they are not needed.

Use Supplies and Equipment for Intended Use

1 Use table appliances according to procedure book for positioning and stabilizing patients. Do not use yards of adhesive tape for this.

2 Nonsterile gloves are available for nonsterile procedures in which the use of gloves is for hand protection. Open sterile gloves for sterile procedures only.

3 Use linen only as needed and for its intended purpose. If water runs over onto the floor, do not soak it up with good linen—use the wet-vacuum pickup or mop. But do not let it run over!

4 Do not use hemostats to clamp linen or tubing; that ruins both the hemostat and the tubing. Use a stopcock or special tubing clamp. Use a towel clip to anchor drapes.

5 Give the assistant surgeon a needleholder for pulling needles through the tissue for the surgeon. A hemostat can be ruined by using it for this purpose. A needle can be damaged.

6 Use wire scissors for wire, tissue scissors for tissue, and nurses' scissors for drains and dressings.

Handle All Supplies and Equipment Carefully to Avoid Damage and Breakage

1 Slip the patient's gown sleeve off before the intravenous transfusion is started preoperatively to avoid having to cut off a wet, soiled gown after the operation is completed.

2 Keep older supplies moving first so that items will not deteriorate or sterility become outdated.

3 Take special care to preserve the edges of sharp instruments.

4 Follow established procedures for the proper sterilization and care of instruments, electrical equipment, etc. If you are uncertain how to sterilize or care for any equipment, find out; do not ruin items by guessing. Items for ethylene oxide gas sterilization should be plainly tagged "for gas" to help avoid possibility of inadvertently putting them into the steam sterilizer.

5 Remove all tape from packages wrapped in linen. Tape must be removed and not merely torn open and left on the wrapper, as it will clog the washers in the laundry.

6 Do not handle adhesive with rubber gloves; it sticks to the gloves and tears them.

7 Check drapes to be certain instruments are not discarded in disposable drapes or sent to the laundry in linen drapes. At the end of the operation, the scrub nurse should search all working surfaces for instruments, needles, and equipment before discarding drapes and table covers. No instrument should be consigned to the laundry or trash!

8 Carry out safe and economical practices. Careless and accident-prone personnel should be eliminated from the department.

Carelessness Can Cause Infection

1 Avoid banging furniture against walls and doors. Stainless steel guards are used on corners and sides of door frames, wherever stretchers or tables are apt to bump them. These become a hazard if loosened. Chipped walls or doors can harbor microorganisms and interfere with effectiveness of housekeeping.

2 Avoid contamination of sterile supplies in transfer to the sterile field. Watch what you are doing when opening sterile packages. If in doubt about sterility, discard the item.

3 Thoroughly clean and properly sterilize instruments to avoid introduction of infection during the operation. A dirty instrument corrodes, does not function smoothly, and is difficult to sterilize.

4 Thoroughly clean all reusable items before sterilizing. The danger of cross infection in the reuse of cleanable, sterilizable items does not lie in the supplies themselves but in personnel practices in processing and handling them. If carelessness exists, many avenues for potential infection become a threat to the welfare of the patient.

5 Dispose of needles and knife blades safely so that housekeeping personnel or other staff members do not accidentally stick themselves or get cut. Hepatitis can be contracted from a contaminated needle or knife blade.

PROS AND CONS OF DISPOSABLES

A *disposable* is a product that is available when needed with complete assurance of safety and effectiveness and that is not salvaged after use. *It is used once and discarded.* The cost of adequately and safely processing supplies is high in most hospitals. This has led to the purchase of many disposable supplies for patient use. Some of these are "patient-charge" items, meaning that the cost of these items is added to the patient's bill. This requires specific and accurate records. It also requires evaluation of the advantages and disadvantages of disposable products to justify the cost to the patient.

Advantages of using disposables are:

1 When a sterile item is required, proper packaging and sterility must be assured. Sterility is guaranteed by reliable manufacturers as long as the integrity of their packages is maintained. Industry conforms to far more rigid standards of quality control than hospital conditions permit. All sterilized products are held in quarantine to establish negative results of bacteriological testing before they are distributed to hospitals.

2 One-patient-use items, such as catheters and gastric tubes, are aesthetically more acceptable to patients. More importantly, disposable products eliminate a potential source of cross contamination.

3 Items such as needles and safety razors assure more comfort for the patient because they are always new and sharp.

4 Standardized service at reduced cost per unit may be provided. Sponges are precounted and sterilized, for example. As usage increases, packs and trays become standardized.

5 Loss and breakage in reprocessing reusable items are eliminated.

6 Labor costs of processing supplies are reduced, particularly in the tedious, meticulous cleaning and packaging of small items, such as needles and syringes.

7 The need for expensive, mechanical cleaning equipment is reduced or eliminated.

Disadvantages of using disposables are:

1 Costly waste occurs if sterile items are contaminated or unnecessarily opened. Extreme care is needed in opening packages to maintain sterility. Handling must not cause wrappings to crack. Even though sterility of products from reliable manufacturers can be assured, their handling and storing in the hospital may pose a threat to the maintenance of this sterility.

2 Hospitals cannot be as flexible in complying with requests of individual doctors for special setups. No allowance is made for deviation from commercially supplied packs or trays. Procedures may need to be revised to conform to available items and sets.

3 If a defect is found in one package, it may extend throughout the total lot requiring replacement of the total supply on hand.

4 The circulating nurse may have to open an increased number of individually packaged items. Some disposable plastic products melt so they cannot be put into instrument sets before steam sterilization.

5 In event of disaster or a sudden increase in use, adequate inventory may not be readily available.

Many problems concerning economy, better use of personnel, storage, delivery, and disposal need to be evaluated by hospitals on an individual basis. Economy may or may not be shown with the use of disposables. Some considerations that can be argued pro or con include:

1 *Direct labor costs.* Some hospitals have saved money by reducing the labor force through conversion to as many total-disposable systems as possible, such as intravenous therapy, drapes, and special procedure trays. In some geographic areas,

efficient labor may be readily available at minimum wage so that disposables become more costly than labor. If professional personnel had been used for reprocessing supplies, disposables release nurses to give more care to patients and less time to "things."

2 *Storage.* Proper and safe storage facilities must be provided. Disposables may require more storage space or more frequent deliveries to maintain adequate inventories.

3 *Disposal.* Disposal may be an ecological problem. Someone must transport used items to an incinerator, compactor, or other safe waste-disposal area. Waste must not accumulate in the OR suite or in other hospital areas.

CARE AND HANDLING OF INSTRUMENTS

Surgical instruments are expensive and represent a major investment for every hospital. As operations have become more complicated and intricate, instruments have become more complex, more precise in design, and more delicate in structure. When abused, misused, or subjected to inadequate cleaning or rough handling, the life expectancy of even the finest quality instruments is reduced. Cost of repairs and replacements becomes unnecessarily high. With proper care, an instrument should have a life of 10 years or more. Instruments do, of course, deteriorate from normal usage. However, most damage and reduced life is caused by improper cleaning, processing, and handling.

Cleaning

1 Remove blood and organic debris as soon after use as possible to prevent drying on the surfaces or in the crevices. At the operating table, the scrub nurse wipes off the surfaces of instruments that will be used again with a moist sponge. Used instruments not needed again can be immersed in a sterile basin of sterile distilled water. Sterile saline is not used for soaking instruments. The sodium chloride in saline is corrosive.

2 Separate delicate small instruments and those with sharp or semisharp edges for special handling.

3 Disassemble all instruments with removable parts to expose all surfaces to detergent agent.

4 Open all hinged instruments to expose box locks and serrations.

5 Wash used and soiled instruments in a noncorrosive, low-sudsing, free-rinsing detergent solution. If they cannot be washed immediately after the operation is completed, they may be soaked for a short time in warm detergent solution.

> NOTE. The detergent must be compatible with the local water supply. Mineral content varies from one area to another. The strength of any solution increases when heated. Therefore, the detergent should be anionic or nonionic and have a pH as close to neutral as possible

6 Use a soft brush to clean serrations and box locks if manual washing is employed. Fine, delicate ophthalmic and microsurgery instruments should be washed by hand. A soft-bristled toothbrush may be used.

> NOTE. *Never* scrub surfaces with abrasive agents such as steel wool and scouring powders or pads. These will scratch and may remove the protective finish on the metal, increasing possibility of corrosion. The finish on stainless steel instruments protects the base metal from oxidation. Therefore, it is essential that the original finish be preserved.

7 Rinse instruments thoroughly with demineralized or distilled water after manual or ultrasonic cleaning to remove residual deposits and films.

8 Dry instruments completely before reassembling or storing. Instruments will corrode if they are stored with trapped moisture.

Processing

1 Inspect each instrument critically before and after each use for imperfections, cleanliness, and working condition. Each must be completely clean to ensure effective sterilization and proper function. Check hinged instruments for stiffness. Box locks and joints should work smoothly.

> NOTE. Stiff box locks and joints are usually caused by inadequate cleaning. Lubrication eases stiffness temporarily. Only a water-soluble lubricant can be used. Mineral oil, silicones, and machine oils are never used because they leave a residue that interferes with steam sterilization. Oiling any surgical instrument is a break in aseptic technique.

2 Test forceps for alignment. A forceps out of alignment can break during use. Close the jaws of the forceps slightly. If they overlap they are out of alignment. The teeth of forceps with serrated jaws should mesh perfectly. Hold the shanks in each hand, with the forceps open, and try to wiggle it. If the box lock has considerable play or is very loose, the forceps will not hold tissue securely. If a surgeon continues to use it, jaw misalignment will occur and the forceps' effectiveness is impaired.

3 Check ratchet teeth. Ratchets should close easily and hold firmly. Clamp the forceps on the first tooth only. Hold the instrument at the box lock. Tap the ratchet teeth lightly against a solid object. If the forceps springs open, it is faulty and should be repaired. Ratchet teeth are subject to friction and metal-to-metal wear by the constant strain of closing and opening. A forceps that will spring open when clamped on a blood vessel or duct is hazardous to the patient and an annoyance to the surgeon. The ratchets must hold.

4 Check the tension between the shanks. When the jaws touch, a clearance of $\frac{1}{16}$ to $\frac{1}{8}$ in. (1.5 to 3 mm) should be visible between the ratchet teeth of each shank. This clearance provides adequate tension at the jaws when closed.

5 Test needleholders for needle security. Clamp an appropriate-size needle in the jaws of the needleholder and lock on second ratchet tooth. If the needle can be turned easily by hand, the needleholder needs repair.

6 Test scissors for correctly ground and properly set blades. The blades should cut on the tips and glide over each other smoothly. Cut dissecting scissors through four layers of gauze at the tip of the blades; two layers if scissors are less than 4 in. (10 cm) in length. They should cut with a fine, smooth feel and a minimum of pressure.

7 Inspect edges of sharp and semisharp instruments, such as chisels, osteotomes, rongeurs, adenotomes, etc., for sharpness, chips or dents, and alignment.

8 Test penetration of cataract knives, keratomes, and other fine cutting instruments on a small kidskin drum. Slide the blade by gravity through the kidskin with the handle resting on the palm of your hand. The blade should penetrate the drum as though it were passing through butter. It should not stick or tear.

9 Check chrome-plated instruments for chips, sharp edges, and worn spots. Chipped plating may harbor debris. Sharp edges will damage tissue or tear gloves. Worn spots will corrode.

10 Flatten or straighten malleable instruments such as retractors, probes, etc.

11 Return unclean instruments to the cleaning area for ultrasonic cleaning.

12 Remove instruments in poor working condition from the sterile field or processing area. Instruments in poor working condition are a handicap to the surgeon and a hazard for the patient. Instruments should be repaired at the first sign of damage or malfunction. A place is usually designated in the OR suite for collection of instruments for repair. Do not allow a defective instrument to remain in circulation.

Handling

1 Know the name and use of each instrument.

2 Watch the sterile field for loose instruments. Remove them promptly after use to the Mayo stand or instrument table. The weight of instruments can injure the patient or cause postoperative discomfort. Keeping instruments off the field also decreases possibility of their falling to the floor.

3 Place used instruments, except sharps and delicate ones, into a tray or basin during or at the end of the operation. Careless dropping or throwing of instruments is absolutely prohibited.

General, Basic Operating Instruments

1 Hemostats, forceps, needleholders, retractors, etc., can be cleaned, assembled in trays, and sterilized together.

2 Heavier instruments always should be placed in the bottom of a tray with smaller, lightweight instruments on top.

3 Hand the surgeon the correct instrument to use for each particular task during the operation. Remember the principle, use for intended use only!

4 Instruments that must be marked for identification of ownership should be imprinted with an electro-etch device. A vibrating or impact-type marking tool breaks the finish on the instrument and can cause hairline cracks. Electro-etching should be put on the shank rather than the box lock to avoid box-lock fracture.

Sharp or Semisharp Instruments

1 Protect the edges of sharp instruments, such as scissors, knives, osteotomes, chisels, curettes, rongeurs, etc., during cleaning, sterilizing, and storing.

2 Sharp instruments must be kept separate from dull ones and demand respectful handling.

Microsurgical and Ophthalmic Instruments

1 Each delicate instrument must be separated from adjacent ones to prevent interlocking or crushing. Never pile them on top of each other. They are easily deformed.

2 Exact alignment of the teeth is an absolute necessity in fine-toothed forceps. The microscopic teeth are very easily bent.

3 Place instruments on a firm, flat surface for sorting and cleaning.

4 Sharp blades and tips should touch absolutely nothing, not even a towel. They must never touch another instrument or any part of a receptacle in which they are placed for storage or sterilization. Most instrument manufacturers supply special sterilization-storage racks so that the blades and tips remain suspended.

5 If the instrument has a protective guard, leave the guard on throughout sterilization and all handling until the surgeon is ready to use the instrument.

6 On the Mayo stand or instrument table, support the handles on a rolled towel or gauze sponge to keep the blades and tips suspended in midair.

7 The very small size of some instruments and their physical appearance (like fine wires) may cause the scrub nurse to mistake them for disposable equipment and they may be lost or discarded at end of operation. Avoid this.

Lensed Instruments

1 Never handle lensed instruments with forceps. A scratch on the instrument could cause injury to tissue or the mucous membrane lining of an orifice. Also, danger of dropping the instrument is greatly increased. The forceps could crush a telescope and ruin the optical system if held too tightly. Always handle sterile instruments wearing sterile gloves.

2 Never pile these delicate instruments one on top of another or mix them with other instruments.

3 Avoid rough handling, jarring, or bending of parts. Lay them on a towel to absorb the impact and to prevent wear on the sheath.

4 Check the light source for working order before use and after cleaning.

Air-powered Instruments

1 Be certain air exhaust is directed away from the sterile field.

2 Follow instructions for use, care, and sterilization recommended by the manufacturer.

3 Test instruments for working condition before surgeon is ready to use.

Electrical Instruments

1 Electrically powered instruments, such as saws, drills, dermatomes, nerve stimulators, etc., are potential explosion hazards in the OR. Most of the motors are designed to be explosionproof. All must have sparkproof connections. However, power switches should be off when plugging electrical cords into outlets.

2 Alert the anesthesiologist if electrical equipment will be used. He or she may change the anesthetic to eliminate explosive gases if a necessary electrical item must be used and it is potentially hazardous. These instruments should be used only with nonflammable anesthetic agents. Even so, connect the power-supply cord to the wall outlet before anesthetic gases are administered and do not remove during administration.

3 Do *not* immerse motor in liquid.

4 Follow the manufacturer's recommended methods of cleaning, lubricating, sterilizing, and using each piece of electrically powered equipment.

5 Check power cords and plugs for cracks or breaks and test for working condition before surgeon is ready to use instrument and the device is applied to the patient.

ELECTRICAL HAZARDS AND SAFEGUARDS

The OR is a location fraught with hazards for both patient and personnel, namely potential electrical shock, burns, fire, explosion, and mechanical injury. It is mandatory that the staff have knowledge of the equipment most often implicated in these incidents, the hazards involved in its use, and how accidents may occur. Each individual has a personal responsibility for ensuring a safe environment by correct handling of equipment and alertness to potentially hazardous situations.

Active interest in fire and explosions caused by anesthetic agents arose in 1925 with the use of ethylene gas. This was intensified in the following decade when cyclopropane anesthesia became popular. Since 1941 the United States government has issued information, recommendations, and regulations for the use of anesthetic agents. Also, reporting of every fire and explosion in an anesthetizing location to the National Fire Protection Association, United States Bureau of Mines, National Safety Council, and American Society of Anesthesiologists, Inc. provides valuable material for study and statistical analysis.

Medical-electronics safety is also a prime concern of hospital and industry personnel seeking safer patient care. Underlying this concern is the rapidly expanding use of electronic equipment in hospital procedures. The marketing and safety standards of medical electronic devices used in the operating room are also federally regulated. Standards of the Joint Commission on Accreditation of Hospitals must be met for hospital accreditation as well. Inadequately trained personnel, inappropriate design of suites, or malfunction of equipment that cause short-circuiting of devices such as heart monitors, defibrillators, and x-ray machines are responsible for the fatalities and near-fatalities that occur. Electrical safety in hospitals is neither a major problem nor a complicated one if personnel understand appropriate terminology and a few simple principles of electricity.

Definitions Pertaining to Safety Standards

Anesthetizing Location Any area of a hospital in which it is intended to administer any flammable or nonflammable inhalation anesthetic agents in the course of examination or treatment and shall include operating rooms, delivery rooms, emergency departments, and other *areas used for induction of anesthesia with flammable or nonflammable anesthetizing agents.*

Combustible Substance A flammable substance capable of reacting with oxygen to burn if ignited.

Conductive Materials Not only those materials that are commonly considered as electrically conductive, such as metals, but also that class of materials that, when tested in accordance with NFPA standard 56A, have a resistance to passage of electricity not exceeding 1,000,000 ohms. Such materials are required where electrostatic interconnection is necessary.[1]

Flammable Substance Any gas or liquid that will burn or is capable, when ignited, of maintaining combustion, including oxygen.

Grounding An equipotential system of conductors that establish a conducting connection, whether intentional or accidental, between an electrical circuit in equipment and earth or to some connecting body that serves in place of the earth to divert stray currents in the vicinity of the patient.

Hazardous Location The space extending 5 ft (1.5 m) above the floor during administration of a flammable anesthetic agent.

Isolated Power System An assembly of electrical devices that provides local isolated power, a single grounding point, and distinctive receptacles.

Leakage Current Any current not intended to be applied to a patient but that may be conveyed from exposed metal or other accessible parts of an appliance to ground.[1]

Line Isolation Monitor An instrument which continually checks the hazard current from an isolated circuit to ground.[2]

[1]From NFPA 56A, *Standard for the Use of Inhalation Anesthetics (Flammable and Nonflammable),* copyright 1973, National Fire Protection Association, Boston, Mass. Excerpted with permission.

[2]Ibid. Quoted with permission.

Macroshock Effect of large electric currents (milliamperes or larger) on the body.[2]

Microshock The effect of small electric currents (as low as 10 microamperes) on the body.[1]

Mixed Facility A hospital wherein flammable anesthetizing locations and nonflammable anesthetizing locations coexist within the same building, allowing interchange of personnel or equipment between flammable and nonflammable anesthetizing locations.[2]

Nonflammable Anesthetic Agent Inhalation agents that, because of their vapor pressure at 98.6°F (37°C) and at atmospheric pressure (760 mm Hg) cannot attain flammable concentrations when mixed with air, oxygen, or mixtures of oxygen and nitrous oxide.

Nonflammable Anesthetizing Location Any location used for, or intended for the *exclusive* use of, administration of nonflammable anesthetic agents.[3]

Patient Ground A terminal bus which serves as the single focus for grounding all electric devices serving an individual patient which are not connected by the power cord to the reference grounding point, and for grounding conductive furniture or equipment within reach of a patient or a person who may touch him.[2]

Concepts of Electrical Hazards

Areas within the OR suite are classified as flammable anesthetizing locations, nonflammable anesthetizing locations, and mixed facilities. This discussion is addressed primarily to *flammable anesthetizing locations,* those areas used or intended for the use of flammable anesthetic agents where static electricity is a potential hazard. Although these agents are rarely used, the following information incorporates the main components of the various groups of safety standards.

Electricity consists of three basic parameters:

1 *Voltage,* the driving force, forces electrons to move through material in one direction and causes current to flow.

2 *Current,* the rate of flow of electrons through a conductor.

3 *Resistance* is the measurement of the opposition to electron flow through a material. Electricity flows easily through conductors, i.e., metals and carbon. Flow is very difficult through insulators, i.e., rubber, plastic, glass. Insulators prevent equalization of potential differences. The

[3]Ibid. Adapted with permission.

resistance of the human body is more similar to a conductor than an insulator.

Electric Shock; Electrocution Electrocution occurs when an individual becomes the component that closes a circuit in which a lethal current may flow. Lethal levels may be attained by currents through the intact body via skin or by currents applied directly to the heart. Electric shock occurs when a current is large enough to stimulate the nervous system or large muscle masses, e.g., when the body becomes the connecting link between two points of an electrical system that are at different potentials. The physiological effect of shock may range from a mere tingling sensation to tissue necrosis, ventricular fibrillation, or death due to the electrical nature of sensory cells, nerves, or muscle that respond to electrical stimuli that originate intrinsically (within the body) or extrinsically (applied externally). Severity of the shock depends on the magnitude of current flow and path taken through the body. Two types of shock are commonly referred to:

Macroshock Shock in which the current flows through a relatively large surface of skin. It usually results from inadvertent contact of an individual with moderately high voltage sources and is expressed in milliamperes ($\frac{1}{1000}$ ampere). A current intensity of 1 to 5 amperes through the chest can cause severe burn at the point of contact. However, if the cardiac conduction system is involved, a current intensity of 50 to 100 milliamperes through the chest can cause ventricular fibrillation since the heart beat is electrically controlled. Macroshock occurs through the trunk of the body, with the current following many paths, each path carrying a fraction of the current. It may or may not be harmful depending on how much current flows through a susceptible heart along its path. Common sources of macroshock are electrical wiring failures allowing skin contact with a live wire or surface at full voltage. Never touch the victim, instrument, or surface with your bare hands in case of shock. Disconnect the power supply or use an insulating material to push the victim away from the source of electricity.

Microshock Shock occurring when current is applied to a very small contact area of skin. The development of medical techniques permitting application of electrical impulses directly to the heart muscle drew awareness of the extreme danger to the electrically sensitive patient who has externalized conductors, diagnostic catheters, or other direct electrical contact with the conduction system of the heart.

NOTE. Cardiac microshock is a potential hazard. Indwelling catheters filled with conductive fluid, probes inserted into the great vessels, and electrodes implanted about the heart multiply the potential for electrocution because they can be conductors of electricity. The external portion of a cardiac catheter generally consists of two parts: an inner conductor(s) of wires or conductive fluid and an outer insulating sheath. When there is a highly conductive pathway from outside the body to the great vessels and heart, small electric currents may cause ventricular fibrillation and cardiac arrest. When a shock has an internal route to the heart, it takes only one-thousandth as much electricity to be fatal as when the shock is transmitted through the surface of the skin. Microshock occurs only if the current from an exterior source flows through the cardiac catheter or conductor. The most important precaution to observe is to protect the exposed end of the cardiac conductor from contact with conductive surfaces, including your body. Always wear rubber or plastic gloves when handling the external end of a cardiac catheter or conductor. While the value of electronic devices in saving lives is unquestionable, the use of such equipment must not be allowed to cause needless death. Fibrillation and arrest may occur if the patient encounters an excess amount of accumulated small currents while connected to ground through implanted electronic devices or by contact with other grounded objects.

Electrical and Thermal Burns Electricity may cause burns by virtue of electric energy supplied by a defective system. In addition to monitors, high-powered equipment is hazardous. Current density effect is highly significant. Current is concentrated or of high density at the point of contact. This mechanism is utilized in some procedures and avoided in others.

Electrosurgical units can be dangerous. A high-frequency current is locally applied by the small active electrode to cut or coagulate tissue. The patient is protected by a patient ground plate that must be properly placed under the patient in contact with skin at a large fleshy area, not a bony prominence such as the sacrum. An electrical burn may be severe enough to require debridement. The plate provides a low current density pathway for the high-frequency current present at the active electrode back to the unit. Proper connections from the ground plate to the patient and ground plate to the unit are essential to prevent burns. Conductive surfaces must be capable of providing a return path for the current other than through the operating table or its attachments. If the return circuit of high-frequency equipment is faulty, the ground circuit may be completed through inadvertent contact with the metal parts or attachments of the operating table. If the ground area is small, the current passing through the exposed area of skin contact will be relatively intense, causing a burn to the patient. For example, one such contact point may be the thigh touching the leg stirrup in lithotomy position.

Surface burns can occur when battery-operated equipment, such as the peripheral nerve stimulator, is used with external electrodes. Tetanic stimuli should be limited to 1 or 2 seconds.

Other potential sources for burn include malfunctioning controls on heat-generating devices in contact with the patient, such as radio-frequency diathermy or hypo-hyperthermia machines. Factors such as the patient's nutritional state, the amount of body fat that acts as insulation, or the circulation in the body part in contact with the device influence individual reaction to a hazard.

Grounding

Grounding of all electrical equipment is essential for safety and prevention of stray leakage current. Grounding systems are designed to avoid the inadvertent passage of electric current through the patient by discharging any harmful potentials directly to the ground without including the patient in the circuit, thereby avoiding shock or burn. Electric power is brought into a hospital through two wires: *hot* and *neutral.* These wires transmit current to the three-wire outlets in the building. The third wire is the ground wire. When the cord from an electrical device is plugged into an outlet, the hot and neutral wires deliver the current. The ground wire is attached to a copper pipe driven into the ground at the point where power enters the building. An electrical connection to the ground provides a means for current to flow through the ground wire or any other conductive surface connected to the ground rather than going to the neutral wire. The copper ground wire is used to prevent the metal housings of electrical equipment from becoming electrically "hot." The ground wire within the three-wire power plug and cord connects the equipment (instrument) housing to the ground contact in the receptacle (wall outlet). This provides a constantly available return path for the current to the electrical source. If the insulation on wires is defective, such as broken or frayed cords or plugs, some current will leak or flow to other nearby conductors such as the equipment housing. When an instrument is grounded, leakage current returns through the ground wire to the earth, causing no damage. If the ground path is absent or broken, leakage current will seek another path to the ground.

Small, extraneous leakage currents can be prevented by proper grounding. Lack of grounding or use of defective electrical systems can cause microshock. This may occasion cardiac disturbances that lead to death or cause severe sparks that may be a source of ignition.

Equipotential Grounding System Current flows between points only when a voltage difference exists between them. Therefore, electric shock can be minimized by eliminating voltage differences. One system designed to do this is the equipotential grounding system, which maintains an equal potential or voltage between all conductive surfaces near the patient. To achieve equipotential grounding, all exposed conductive surfaces within 6 ft (2 m) of the patient are electrically connected to a single point that is itself connected by a copper conductor to the ground tie point at the electrical distribution center serving the area. Consequently, all exposed metal surfaces are electrically tied together and to the ground.

Isolation Power System Isolated power systems are used in hazardous locations such as operating rooms. A device, the isolation transformer, isolates the OR electrical circuits from the grounded circuits in the power mains; thus the isolated circuit does not include the ground in its pathway. The current seeks to flow only from one isolated line to the other. As a result, accidental grounding of persons in contact with the hot wire does not cause current to flow through the individual. A line isolation monitor checks the degree of isolation maintained by an isolated power system by continually measuring resistance and capacitance between the two isolated lines and ground. The meter reading is called the hazard index. The monitor, a wall-mounted meter, has an alarm that is activated at the 2-milliampere level. This warning system indicates when inadvertent grounding of the isolated circuits has occurred and alerts personnel to a dangerous situation. Since grounding can only take place when faulty equipment is plugged into ungrounded circuits, maximum safety is afforded by use of the isolation transformer. OR and obstetrical suite electrical circuits are required to be ungrounded circuits fed through isolation transformers. Permanently installed overhead operating lights and receptacles in anesthetizing locations are required to be supplied by ungrounded electrical circuits.

Static Electricity

Electrostatic spark is a common hazard everywhere and consists of high voltage and low ampere. Production of a spark is the major hazard. It develops from friction and accumulates on physical objects. When two static-bearing objects come in contact, the one bearing the higher potential discharges to the one with the lower potential. Air is a nonconductor. However, a high enough potential can overcome air resistance, jump the gap between it and a lower-potential object causing an arc across air gaps seen as a spark(s) from the heat thus generated. Sparks can ignite flammable materials or gases. Objects accumulate static in inverse proportion to their conductivity. The aim is to provide adequate channels for dissipation of static. Since the earth has a zero potential, a charge brought directly, or indirectly, through a conductor, into contact with it is discharged to the earth. A spark between two objects can occur only when there is no electrical path of good conductivity between them. If there is moderate conductivity, there is a tendency for gradual spread of charge over both objects so they come to the same potential. Generation of static electricity cannot be prevented absolutely because its intrinsic origins are present at every interface. For static electricity to be a source of ignition:

1 There must be an effective means of static generation.
2 There must be a means of accumulating the separate charges and maintaining a suitable difference of electrical potential.
3 There must be a spark discharge of adequate energy.
4 The spark must occur in an ignitable mixture.*

Explosion and Fire Hazards

While most hospitals have discontinued the use of flammable anesthetic agents, cyclopropane and ether are rarely used. They are highly flammable and/or explosive when mixed with air, oxygen, or nitrous oxide. Although oxygen and nitrous oxide are nonflammable gases, they support and accelerate combustion. Explosions may occur in hazardous locations or in anesthetizing locations. An explosion is the result of a combination of three factors:

1 A flammable gas, vapor, or liquid
2 A source of ignition
3 Oxygen (pure or in air) or some other substance providing oxygen such as nitrous oxide.

SAFEGUARDS AGAINST HAZARDS

To prevent disastrous consequences from the hazards encountered in the OR, regional, national, and federal guidelines, regulations, and laws must be adhered to.

Elimination of Elements of Combustion

Elimination of Explosive Agents

1 Use nonflammable agents.
2 Air-conditioning or ventilating systems aid in the prevention of pockets of gas in the room, although concentration of the agent around the anesthesia machine is not remarkedly reduced. Heavy gas can accumulate and channel along the floor for as far as 50 ft (15 m) in explosive concentration. Air streams can carry explosive concentrations of anesthetic to an ignition source.
3 Confining potentially explosive agents by use of the closed carbon dioxide absorption technique tends to restrict the region likely to be hazardous.

Elimination of Sources of Ignition

1 Electrostatic (incendiary) spark production is a major hazard. Precautions include the following:
   a Use conductive flooring in flammable anesthetizing locations, corridors and passageways adjacent thereto, in rooms connecting directly to anesthetizing locations such as scrub rooms and substerile rooms, and in storage locations for flammable anesthetic agents located in an operating room suite. A conductive floor shall meet the resistance provisions through its inherent conductive properties. The average resistance of the conductive floor shall be less than 1,000,000 ohms as measured between two electrodes placed 3 ft (1 m) apart at any points on the floor, and more than 25,000 ohms as measured between a ground connection and the electrodes placed on the floor. The resistance of conductive floors shall be initially tested prior to use and

*Excerpted with permission from NFPA 77, *Recommended Practice on Static Electricity,* copyright 1972, National Fire Protection Association, Boston, Mass.

thereafter measurements taken at intervals of not more than 1 month. A permanent record of readings is kept.*

b Assure electrical connection of the patient to the conductive floor, when flammable anesthetics are used, by provision of a 10-W impedance conductive strap in contact with the patient's skin, with one end of the strap fastened to the metal frame of the operating table. Mattresses and pillows are covered with conductive material.

c Discontinue administration of a flammable agent, when feasible, as soon as the ground monitor system indicates a warning. Following completion of the operation, the room in which the signal functioned is not used until the maintenance department corrects the electrical defect.

d Avoid contacting metals with force sufficient to produce percussion sparks.

e Use antistatic liners in kick buckets, and use caution in handling them.

f Cover all hair of patients, personnel, and visitors.

g Wear outer garments in the OR suite known to be antistatic in accordance with requirements of NFPA 56A. Hose and undergarments in which the entire garment is in close contact with the skin may be of synthetic material.

h Cover patient in the OR suite or other anesthetizing location with a cotton blanket. Woolen or synthetic blankets are not permitted.

i Wear shoes with soles and heels of conductive rubber or equivalent material. Conductive shoe covers should be worn in OR suites.

j Test conductivity. In hazardous areas, an instrument, known as a *calibrated ohmmeter,* is located at the entrance to the anesthetizing location and is used to measure the resistance of personnel and equipment.

k Maintain high relative humidity (weight of water vapor present); 60 percent is preferable, 50 percent is mandatory in anesthetizing locations. Moisture provides a relatively conductive medium, allowing static electricity to leak to earth as fast as it is generated. Sparks form more readily in low humidity.

l Do not move a patient from one area to another while a flammable anesthetic is being administered.

*Excerpted with permission from NFPA 56A, *Standard for the Use of Inhalation Anesthetics (Flammable and Nonflammable),* pp. 54ff, copyright 1973, National Fire Protection Association, Boston, Mass; for complete details see that standard, which is published by NFPA either as a separate pamphlet or in vol. 4 of the *National Fire Codes.*

m Avoid unnecessary motion in the area around the anesthesia equipment and the patient's head.

n Dissipate static charge. Anyone who must make contact with the patient or anesthesiologist does so by first touching the anesthesiologist's back or stool, the operating table, or the patient at least 2 ft (60 cm) from the face mask. This provides for the discharge of any charge in that person before he or she is close to the mask or machine. A stool with smooth rounded feet and bare metal top or conductive cushioning is recommended for grounding the anesthesiologist.

o Avoid friction on the reservoir bag of the anesthesia machine. Watch that drapes do not touch the bag or cover the machine.

p Use flammable agents only in flammable anesthetizing locations.

q Use explosionproof receptacles and attachment plugs that cannot be pulled apart accidentally. Grounding adaptor plugs and multiple-outlet plugs are prohibited. Cords should be rubber-coated and switches explosionproof.

2 Faulty electrical equipment may cause short circuit or electrocution.

a Particular care must be used with high-voltage equipment such as x-ray, electrosurgical unit, electronic monitoring devices.

b Hypo-hyperthermia machine must be at least 3 ft (1 m) away from anesthesia machine and both be adequately grounded.

c Electrosurgical unit should be located on the operator's side of the table as far as possible from the anesthesia machine and monitoring equipment. The power cable is not stretched across traffic lanes. If a flammable agent was employed for induction, even if followed by a nonflammable agent for maintenance, the electrosurgical unit should not be used on the neck, nasopharynx, and adjacent areas.*

d All electrical equipment, including a surgeon's personal property, must be inspected by the maintenance department prior to initial use.

3 Open flames and heated objects may cause fire or explosion. Minimum ignition temperatures of anesthetic agents in pure oxygen are all lower than in air.

a Flammable antiseptics or flammable fat solvents are not applied for preoperative preparation of the patient.

b Only approved photographic lighting equipment shall be used with suitable enclosures to

*National Fire Protection Association, *National Fire Codes,* vol. 15, p. 76C–45, 46, Boston, Mass., 1975.

prevent sparks and hot particles from falling into a hazardous area with occasional bursting of bulbs.

c Smoking is limited to dressing rooms and lounges with doors leading to corridors closed. Open flames and heated objects are prohibited in hazardous locations and corridors outside anesthetizing locations.

d Lights and sources of heat must be kept at least 4 ft (more than 1 m) away from the anesthesia machine or flammable agents.

4 Spontaneous combustion can be caused by a mixture of gases under high pressure or by oil or grease in contact with cylinders containing a flammable agent.

a Oil or grease is not used on oxygen valves or parts of anesthesia machines.

b Anesthesia machines, cylinders of compressed gas, and flammable liquid containers must be kept away from any source of heat and not touch each other.

5 Fire should be a matter of prime concern. Fires in oxygen-enriched atmospheres (OEA) are fundamentally different in character than those occurring in normal atmosphere. The fire-severity potential should be regarded as one of a high order, with extensive damage potential. The presence of flammable and combustible liquid vapors, gases, and particulate solids (dust) in OEA can result in ultrarapid combustion with explosive violence.*

Safeguards in Nonflammable Anesthetizing Locations Space precludes detailed listing but the requirements are less stringent than for flammable anesthetizing locations. Safeguards for the latter were included to cover dangers that might be present. The learner is referred to the bibliography for more information (see National Fire Codes 56A and 76B-T).

Nonflammable anesthetizing locations, whether located in a mixed facility or not, should be identified by prominently posted signs at all entrances to the operating room and within the location signifying the type of anesthetic permitted.

*National Fire Protection Association, *National Fire Codes,* vol. 14, p. 53M-75, Boston, Mass., 1976.

Chapter 15

Diagnostic Procedures

Diagnosis of pathologic disease, anomaly, or traumatic injury must be established prior to undertaking major operative procedures. Many modalities and techniques assist surgeons to assess each individual patient problem, to guide them through the operation, and to verify the results of surgical intervention. The term *diagnosis* refers to the art or the act of determining the nature of a patient's disease. Diagnostic procedures, as discussed in this chapter, include those procedures pertaining to establishment of or serving as evidence in diagnosis and treatment of surgical pathology. They will be classified as:

1 *Preoperative*—procedures performed prior to the patient coming to the OR suite or performed in the OR prior to incision
2 *Intraoperative*—procedures performed in the OR as a part of the operation
3 *Noninvasive*—techniques utilizing equipment placed on or near the patient's skin but outside body tissues
4 *Invasive*—techniques utilizing equipment placed into a body cavity or vessel and/or substances injected into body structures

Preoperative diagnostic procedures may be noninvasive or invasive; likewise intraoperative procedures utilize both techniques. OR nurses and technicians must be familiar with the modalities and the equipment necessary to assist with diagnostic procedures. Six broad categories of modalities are utilized in diagnosis:

1 *Radiology*—the branch of medicine that deals with x-rays, radioactive substances, and ionizing radiations for diagnosis and treatment, e.g., chest x-ray
2 *Pathology*—the branch of biological science that deals with the nature of disease through study of its causes, process, and effects, e.g., biopsy
3 *Endoscopy*—a visual examination of the interior of a body cavity or viscus, e.g., bronchoscopy
4 *Plethysmography*—the measurement of changes in volume of an extremity or organ caused by blood flow, e.g., oculoplethysmography
5 *Thermography*—a technique for recording infrared radiations spontaneously emanating from the body's surface, e.g., breast thermogram
6 *Ultrasound*—the use of ultrasonic energy for the purpose of studying alterations of anatomic structure, e.g, vascular disease

RADIOLOGY

Wilhelm Conrad Roentgen discovered x-rays in 1895. At first they were used mainly for localization of foreign bodies or visualization of fractures. *X-ray* is a high-energy electromagnetic wave capable of penetrating various thicknesses of solid substances and affecting photographic plates. X-rays are generated on a vacuum tube when high-velocity electrons from a heated filament strike a metal target (anode) causing it to emit x-rays. The photograph obtained by the use of x-rays may be referred to as an *x-ray film, roentgenogram, radiograph,* or other "-gram" name associated either with the specific technique used to obtain the photograph or the anatomic structures identified, e.g., mammogram. As the science of radiology has advanced, the diagnosis of disease in all surgical specialties has progressed. The treatment to be followed frequently is based upon radiologic findings.

Noninvasive Preoperative Studies

The following noninvasive radiologic studies are performed in the radiology department preoperatively. The surgeon may request that the x-ray films or radiographs be sent to the OR for reference during operation.

Chest X-Ray Most surgeons consider a chest x-ray an extension of the patient's history and physical examination, even though chest disease is not associated with the patient's clinical symptoms. Routine chest x-ray examination is part of the admission procedure for elective surgical patients in most hospitals to rule out unsuspected pulmonary disease that could be communicable or would contraindicate use of inhalation anesthetics. It is always a part of the diagnostic workup in patients with suspected or symptomatic pulmonary abnormalities.

Mammography A technique for projecting an x-ray image of the soft tissues of the breast, mammography has gained wide acceptance for early diagnosis of nonpalpable breast tumors. Three views of each breast are exposed to conventional x-rays. Tumors appear on the mammogram as opaque areas or occasionally as areas of punctate calcification.

Tomography An x-ray beam moves across the body in one direction, usually an arc, to photograph structures in a selected plane of tissue. The roentgenograms show detail of the structures within this single plane while blurring the images above and below the selected plane.

Computerized Tomography Special, complex, expensive equipment employs an x-ray beam in conjunction with a computer. Because the x-ray beam moves back and forth across the body to project cross-sectional images, the technique is referred to as *computerized tomography* (CT), *computerized axial tomography* (CAT), or simply *scanning.* It produces a highly contrasted, detailed study of normal and pathologic anatomy. The x-ray tube and photomultiplier detectors rotate slowly around the patient's head, chest, or body for 180° in a linear fashion along the vertical axis. The computer processes the data and constructs a picture on a cathode-ray tube in shades of gray (on a black and white monitor) or in colors that correspond to the density of tissue. Structures are identified by differences in density. This picture is photographed for a permanent record. The computer also prints out numerical density values related to the radiation-absorption coefficients of the substances in the area scanned. The radiologist uses this printout to determine whether a substance is fluid, blood, normal tissue, bone, air, or a pathologic lesion. Exact size and location of lesions in the brain and abdominal organs are identified. To assure proper utilization of this complex equipment, as well as to protect the patient from excessive or unnecessary radiation, the procedure is done under the supervision of a qualified radiologist.

Total-body Scanning Total-body scanning does not refer to computerized tomography but to a scanning procedure following intravenous injection of a radionuclide material (see p. 295). Uptake of the radionuclide within the tissues depends on blood flow. Therefore, the imaging procedure may by delayed for several hours after the dose is given, not because it takes long for the material to localize in a tumor or inflammatory lesion where the uptake is high, but rather because differentiation is achieved after washout from normal structures. Scanning may include the whole body or only those areas of specific interest. Total-body scanning includes identification of structures in the skeletal and vascular systems for diagnosis of pathology such as metastatic bone tumors or thrombotic vascular disease.

Xeroradiography The patient is positioned between an x-ray source and a photosensitive aluminum plate. The plate has an electrically charged selenium surface. The pattern of the charge remaining on the plate after exposure to the x-ray beam corresponds to the densities of the tissues and the amount of radiation absorbed. A negatively charged, blue toner powder is dusted on the plate. A pale blue and white image is transferred by photoconduction rapidly and permanently to a sheet of plastic-coated paper. Xeroradiography minimizes radiation exposure, is performed rapidly, and produces detailed images easier to interpret than x-ray film. It is used for diagnosis of breast disease, bone disorders, laryngeal disorders, to name a few anatomic structures, and for detection of foreign bodies in soft tissue.

X-Ray for Trauma In addition to being an aid in determining the extent of traumatic injury, x-rays may be entered as legal evidence in a court of law to establish injuries sustained by the patient or to justify medical care given. Conventional x-rays will show:

1 Fractures of bones
2 Presence and location of some kinds of foreign bodies, e.g., a bullet
3 Air or blood in the pleural cavity
4 Gas or fluid in the abdominal cavity
5 Outline of abdominal and chest organs and any deviation from normal size or location

Invasive Preoperative Studies

Invasive studies require the ingestion or injection of a radiolucent gas, a radiopaque contrast medium, or a radionuclide element prior to exposing the patient to radiation. The procedures that require injection of these substances must be performed under aseptic conditions using sterile equipment. Many hospitals have one or more rooms within the OR suite equipped for diagnostic as well as intraoperative radiologic procedures. In other hospitals, OR nursing personnel must go to the radiology department to assist with these preoperative diagnostic procedures.

Types of Equipment

Fixed X-Ray Equipment A fixed, overhead x-ray tube with housing may be mounted on a ceiling track for unrestricted movement of the x-ray beam into desired position over the patient. When not in use, it can be moved against a wall and retracted toward the ceiling. Some units are fixed to specially designed tables, such as the urological table for cystoscopic examinations (refer to Chap. 19). The controls are in an adjacent room or behind a lead shield. These are activated by the radiologist or radiology technician.

Portable X-Ray Machine An x-ray tube mounted on a portable generator of a nonexplosive design approved for use in hazardous locations may be moved from one room in the OR suite to another. It offers the advantages of flexibility in scheduling procedures and of availability when and where needed. However, it also has the disadvantage of being a source for cross contamination. All portable equipment must be thoroughly disinfected before being brought into a room and again after use. It should be stored within the OR suite between uses.

Cassette The lighttight holder for x-ray film is referred to as a *cassette.* The patient is positioned between the x-ray tube and the cassette. Holders for cassettes may be built into or attached to the operating table.

Processing Equipment Conventional x-ray equipment projects a black and white image on x-ray film that must be developed by a chemical process. Some OR suites have a darkroom where x-ray film is developed after exposure so that the surgeon can see the results of the study without excessive delay. Others have an automatic processor in which film can be developed in 90 seconds to 3 minutes.

Image Intensifier Rather than projecting the image of body structures on an x-ray film, the image intensifier converts the x-ray beam as it passes through the body into a fluoroscopic optical image projected onto a television screen or mirror. The clarity of this image is an aid in diagnosis particularly of vascular, neurologic, and bone disorders. The surgeon and radiologist can observe the progression of an injected substance as it moves through internal structures or the placement of a device into the body. When connected to other closed-circuit television facilities, the image can be transmitted to other rooms for teaching purposes. Also, the image can be filmed for a permanent record and for teaching. The monitoring screen may be ceiling-mounted above the operating table and thus save space in the OR, or it may be portable. A Bakelite (or other material capable of being penetrated by x-rays) table top must be attached to the lower end of the operating table and the foot section lowered so that the x-ray beam will fit under this table extension. The surgeon activates the image intensifier with a foot pedal.

Nursing Duties

1 Sterile technique of operative procedures in general applies also to invasive diagnostic procedures.
2 Each hospital has its own supply list for the procedures routinely performed. It is convenient to keep a stock of routine supplies on a portable cart if procedures are done in the radiology de-

partment. In general, the following items should be readily available:

a Sterile tray for the specific procedure
b Skin prep tray and solutions
c Intravenous administration sets and solutions
d Local anesthetic agents
e Radiopaque contrast material
f Sterile gowns, gloves, linen, and dressings
g Extra sterile syringes and needles
h Plastic tubing and catheters

As an element of risk is associated with some of these procedures, there should also be available:

i Stimulants
j Cardiac resuscitation equipment, including defibrillator

3 An explanation of the procedure must be given to patients to allay fears and assure their understanding of the value of the procedure in making a diagnosis. During the procedure, explanation should be given of the equipment being used and of the necessity to remain quiet while films are being taken.
4 Patients must be carefully observed during all procedures for any change in condition. Even if a procedure is done under local anesthesia, a stand-by anesthesiologist should be available to check vital signs.

Types of Invasive Studies The most common agents and some of the more commonly performed procedures are discussed. Each agent may have many more uses than described.

Radiolucent Gases Filtered room air, oxygen, nitrogen, carbon dioxide, or a combination of gases may be injected into body spaces or structures normally containing *fluid other than blood.* Gases are radiolucent, transparent to x-rays, so that gas-filled spaces appear less dense on x-ray film than surrounding tissues.

The first visualization of the ventricles of the brain was accidental and was reported by W. H. Luckett in 1913. The patient had sustained a skull fracture about 3 weeks previously, and x-rays showed the ventricles to be filled with air. Dr. Luckett explained that the patient in sneezing had forced air through the fracture lines and lacerated dura, thus filling the ventricles.

Walter E. Dandy first thought of replacing fluid in the ventricles with air and x-raying them. Since most lesions in the brain modify the size and shape of the ventricles, this would aid in localizing a lesion. In 1919, Dandy first injected air into the spinal canal to visualize the subarachnoid space. Modifications of his technique still are employed to determine appropriate neurosurgical access to brain lesions.

Pneumoencephalography is the study of the ventricular system of the brain following total or partial replacement of cerebrospinal fluid with gas. The procedure usually is performed in the radiology department. However, this invasive study has been supplanted by the noninvasive computerized axial tomography technique in most hospitals. Dilations, distortions in shape, and filling defects are interpreted for the differential diagnosis of tumor, hematoma, hydrocephalus, and other abnormalities in the flow of cerebrospinal fluid.

Ventriculography is the study of the ventricles following injection of gas directly into the lateral ventricles of the brain. It is used in preference to pneumoencephalography in patients with signs of increased intracranial pressure as a result of blockage of cerebrospinal fluid circulation. Ventricular needles or catheters may be inserted into one or both lateral ventricles through holes made in the skull. The ventricular needle has a blunt, tapered point that prevents injury to the brain as it is inserted into the ventricle. Openings on the side near the point permit removal of spinal fluid and injection of gas. If the patient is an infant whose suture lines in the skull are not yet closed, needles are inserted through these.

The entire procedure may be done in the operating room, or may begin in the OR, to drill the holes and insert the ventricular needles or an intraventricular catheter. The patient then may be transferred to the radiology department or diagnostic room within the OR suite. The indications for ventriculography are such that, if a lesion is identified, the diagnostic procedure may be followed immediately by operation due to the possibility of a further increase in intracranial pressure. If the patient is returned to the unit following the procedure, sterile ventricular needles should accompany the patient. If the intracranial pressure becomes too great after the gas injection, the needle can be inserted to remove the gas.

Arthrography is the study of a joint following the injection of gas into it. Conventional x-rays show only the bony structure of a joint. By injection of a gas, injury to the cartilage and ligaments may be visualized. A radiopaque, iodinated contrast medium also may be used for a double contrast study, particularly useful in knee arthrograms.

Radiopaque Contrast Media Agents composed of nonmetallic compounds or heavy metallic salts that do not permit passage of radiant energy are *radiopaque.* When exposed to x-ray, the lumina of body structures filled with these agents appear as dense areas. Radiopaque contrast media frequently used for the procedures described below include:

1 Cardiografin, for angiography
2 Hypaque, for arteriography, cardiography, cholangiography, intravenous pyelography, and venography
3 Renografin, for angiography, cystography, myelography, and pyelography
4 Angio-Conray, for arteriography
5 Dionosil, for bronchography
6 Barium sulfate, for gastrointestinal studies
7 Pantopaque, for myelography
8 Renovist, for cystography, retrograde pyelography, and ureterography

Most of these agents contain iodine. A history of sensitivity to iodine-related substances, such as seafood, or other allergies must be obtained before these agents are injected. A test dose of 1 or 2 ml may be given before the dose required for the x-ray study. The patient must be observed for allergic reaction throughout the procedure.

Egas Moniz, a Portuguese physician, was the first to do cerebral angiography in 1927. In 1929, Forssman, in Germany, catheterized the right atrium by passing a ureteral catheter into it through the veins of the right arm. He was not successful in his attempt to inject a radiopaque substance through the catheter to visualize the pulmonary vessels. In 1931, Moniz was able to visualize the right chambers of the heart and the pulmonary vessels using Forssman's technique. Poor visualization of areas and reaction of patients to the substance discouraged the pioneers in this procedure. However, by 1937 Robb and Steinberg had worked out the technique as it is used today, but enhanced by the advantages of more sophisticated equipment.

In 1935, the vertebral artery was first exposed and injected, and in 1949 it was first injected percutaneously. Although the latter technique is generally preferred, both methods are used for angiography.

Angiography is a comprehensive term for studies of the circulatory system following injection of radiopaque substance to permit visualization of a specific blood vessel system. These procedures are useful in the differential diagnosis of arteriovenous malformations, aneurysms, tumors, or vascular accidents due either to traumatic injury or acquired structural disease.

1 *Aortography* is the study of the aorta and its branches to determine the site and size of lesions within the aorta or its major branches such as the renal vascular system. A 7 in. (17.7 cm) x 15, 16, or 17 gauge needle may be inserted into the aorta through a translumbar approach with the patient in prone position. The more selective aortographic procedures are performed by positioning a catheter under direct fluoroscopic visualization via the femoral artery into a branch of the aorta.

2 *Arteriography* is the study of the arterial circulation of a specific vascular system. It is identified by reference to the major blood vessel to be injected: i.e., right or left carotid or vertebral arteriogram to study cerebral circulation; via right brachial artery to study coronary arteries of the myocardium; right or left femoral arteriogram to study circulation in a lower extremity. Various routes of entrance for a needle or intra-arterial catheter exist for injection of these major vessels.

3 *Cardiography* is the study of the chambers in the heart. A catheter is positioned under direct fluoroscopic visualization through one of the great vessels into the heart. Cardiography is done usually in conjunction with other cardiac catheterization procedures. *Cardiac catheterization* includes the recording of pressure measurements within the heart chambers and withdrawing blood samples for analysis (refer to Chap. 21, p. 391).

4 *Venography* is the study of veins to show inflow, filling, and emptying to determine venous blood flow and valve action.

Techniques and equipment to be used will vary according to the specific procedure, but all types of angiography have the following commonalities:

1 These procedures may be done under local or general anesthesia.
2 Access to the vessel to be injected with a radiopaque contrast medium may be made by percutaneous puncture or by a cutdown approach to the vessel. An intravenous drip is maintained on all patients when the latter approach is used.
   a Cannulated needles with or without a radiopaque plastic catheter, similar to the types used for intravenous infusions, may be used for percutaneous puncture. Cannulated needles used for these procedures have an obturator that remains in place until the contrast medium is injected to prevent backflow of blood. Long catheters have a guide wire to assist threading through the vessel.
   b Cournand needle has a curved flanged guard that contours to the body. It is particularly useful in carotid arteriography to hold the needle in position in the neck during injection.
   c Robb cannula is blunt with large lumen and a stopcock at the hub. It is inserted via a cutdown. It is used with a Robb syringe that also

has a large opening in the tip for fast injection.

d Sheldon needle has an occluded point with an opening at 90° to the lumen. When the vertebral artery is entered, a right-angle injection is made into the lumen of the artery.

3 The dosage of radiopaque contrast substances injected into blood vessels is computed for infants and children according to their weight. In adults the dose is measured so it can be repeated safely for more exposures if necessary. These radiopaque agents dissipate very rapidly in the bloodstream.

4 Radiopaque contrast material should be warmed to body temperature to prevent precipitation and to reduce viscosity.

5 If awake, the patient should be told to expect a feeling of warmth and possibly some pain when the contrast medium is injected.

6 Plastic tubing, 30 in. (76 cm) long with a syringe on one end and an adaptor on the other, is connected to the needle or catheter in the vessel to prevent jarring during pressure of injection and to keep the hands of the operator out of the x-ray beam.

7 Automatic, high-pressure injector may be used instead of injecting the contrast medium by hand. This device correlates injection and x-ray exposure. When an automatic injector is used, special high-pressure nylon tubing is used, since this does not pull apart with pressure. When this tubing is used, a stopcock is placed on the end for closing it off at the syringe connection, as nylon tubing cannot be clamped.

8 Automatic seriogram equipment takes rapid, multiple exposures while the contrast medium is in sufficient concentration to visualize the vessels. It can be set at $\frac{1}{2}$- to 2-second intervals to take multiple pictures in succession. Or a roll-film changer, like a movie camera, may be used. This can be set for multiple exposures per second also. These devices are used for angiography with the image intensifier.

Bronchography is a study of the tracheobronchial tree performed to aid in diagnosis of bronchiectasis, cancer, tuberculosis, and lung abscess or to detect a foreign body. The location of a lesion can be determined and operation planned accordingly. The procedure should be explained in detail to the patient, as cooperation is necessary to accomplish the desired result (refer to Chap. 23).

Gastrointestinal x-ray studies are performed to identify lesions in the mucosa of the gastrointestinal tract, such as an ulcer or tumor. Inflammatory lesions and partial or complete obstructions caused by a variety of lesions also may be identified. Barium sulfate either is swallowed by the patient or is instilled by enema to outline the lumen of the segments of the tract to be studied. These studies are done in the radiology department, but the surgeon often refers to the films during operation.

Myelography is a study performed to identify lesions in the spinal canal. It is helpful to determine if there is a filling defect and to localize it. There may be a spinal cord tumor or herniated nucleus pulposus. Some surgeons do not rely entirely on this method of diagnosis, as the patient's symptoms and signs are important in the final diagnosis.

Urography is a comprehensive term for radiological studies of the urinary tract. Most procedures are performed in the radiology department, but some are done in conjunction with cystoscopic examinations (refer to Chap. 19).

1 *Cystography* is the study of the bladder following instillation of a contrast medium. It is valuable in detecting ureterovesical reflux, a malfunction of the sphincter valves.

2 *Cystourethrography* is the study of the bladder and urethra to determine obstruction or abnormality in contour or position. The x-rays may be taken as the contrast medium is injected into the bladder or when the patient voids the material.

3 *Intravenous pyelography* is the study of the structures of the urinary tract and a study of kidney function. The contrast medium is introduced into the circulatory system by rapid intravenous injection or slow infusion IV drip. It is excreted through the kidneys. X-rays are taken at carefully timed intervals. If the medium is poorly excreted through the kidneys, the last film may be taken as many as 24 hours after injection of the contrast medium. Tomograms also may be taken while the contrast material is still in the urinary tract. These procedures are done in the radiology department rather than in the cystoscopy room.

4 *Retrograde pyelography* is the study of the shape and position of the kidneys and ureters. The contrast medium is injected through catheters placed in each ureter. This procedure is used to visualize the renal pelves and calyces.

5 *Ureterography* is the study of one or both ureters to identify position and patency of the lumina. Contrast medium is injected through ureteral catheters (refer to Chap. 19, p. 354).

6 *Urethrography* is a study of the contour and patency of the urethra. The contrast medium may be instilled into the bladder and the x-rays taken as the patient voids. The medium must flow well but be viscous enough to distend the urethra and give good detail of it on the x-ray. If the patient is anesthetized, a very viscous contrast medium is injected into the urethra and films taken. Because the urethra is quite short, the latter technique is of little value in the female patient.

Radionuclides Radioactive elements utilized in medicine are referred to as *radionuclides.* A *nuclide* is a stable nucleus of a chemical element, such as iodine, plus its orbiting electrons. A nuclide bombarded with radioactive particles becomes unstable and emits radiant energy; it becomes a *radionuclide.* Except for the emission of energy, the action of a radionuclide is the same in the body as its stable counterpart. Radionuclides that emit electromagnetic energy are used for diagnostic studies to trace the function and structure of most organs of the body. They may be given orally, intravenously, or by infusion. These agents may be used to visualize specific areas rather than radiopaque contrast media in some of the procedures previously described. They are particularly useful in studies of bone marrow, liver, spleen, biliary tract, thyroid, brain, urinary tract, and peripheral vascular system. Because they provide better quantification of arrival times for vascular perfusion above and below lesions, radionuclides may be a more accurate index of the functional significance of a lesion than other radiopaque contrast media.

Noninvasive Intraoperative Studies

Noninvasive x-rays are taken during operation most frequently to verify the position of a body structure, a metallic implant or instrument, or to identify the presence of a foreign body. The need for x-rays routinely can be anticipated and scheduled for:

1 Closed reduction of fractured bones, with or without internal fixation devices (refer to Chap. 20)
2 Open reduction of hip fractures and fractures of some other bones when internal fixation devices are implanted (refer to Chap. 20)
3 Stereotaxic neurosurgery to identify landmarks as instruments are introduced into the brain (refer to Chap. 24)

Unanticipated need for x-rays occurs when a sponge, needle, or instrument is unaccounted for at the time the final count is taken during wound closure. An x-ray will confirm whether the item is still in the patient. Unless the patient's condition demands immediate wound closure, an x-ray should be taken before closure is completed (refer to count procedures in Chap. 8).

Invasive Intraoperative Studies

The surgeon may wish to inject a radiopaque contrast medium into a blood vessel or other anatomic structure during operation to ascertain operative results prior to wound closure or to obtain further guidance for the operative procedure. Some operations are performed with the patient positioned on a fluoroscopic table equipped with an image intensifier for radiographic visualization of anatomic structures as the operation progresses. Examples of procedures that utilize radiologic control include, but are not limited to, the following:

Angiography Intraoperative studies often are essential to assess the results of vascular reconstruction. Angiography is one method of assessment to confirm the position and patency of an arterial or venous graft or the quality of a restored vessel lumen. Intraoperative angiography frequently is indicated for these assessments in the peripheral vessels of the extremities. After insertion of a bypass graft or endarterectomy, patency of the graft or vessel is checked by pulsations and also by arteriography (refer to Chap. 21 for further discussion of these operations).

Angiography also is utilized at the time of operation to identify the vascularity or exact location of some types of lesions in the extremities, brain, thoracic and abdominal cavities. After injection of the radiopaque contrast medium, radiological studies are made.

Cholangiography In addition to preoperative, diagnostic x-ray studies, some surgeons routinely request radiological studies in conjunction with cholecystectomy or cholelithotomy (refer to Chap. 17, p. 322) to identify gallstones in the biliary tract. Other surgeons selectively include cholangiography at the time of operation in patients in whom they suspect stones might be present or retained in the bile ducts. Conventional x-ray equipment or an image intensifier may be used for these intraoperative studies.

The basic difference between preoperative and intraoperative cholangiography is the site of administration of the radiopaque contrast medium. For preoperative invasive cholangiography, the contrast medium injected intravenously, through percutaneous venipuncture, is excreted by the liver into the bile ducts. During open operative procedures, the medium is injected directly into the bile ducts. When intraoperative cholangiography is scheduled, add to the usual sterile setup:

1 50-cc syringe
2 Radiopaque contrast medium, such as Hypaque
3 Radiopaque cholangiocath (a plastic catheter for insertion into the common or cystic duct)

All other precautions for patient and personnel safety must be observed.

Considerations for Patient Safety

1 The x-ray film cassette holder, sometimes called a bucky, must be properly positioned on the operating table under the area to be exposed to the x-ray beam. If the table does not have a built-in tunnel or compartment for the cassette, part of the mattress may be removed and the holder, a Bakelite or wooden frame, placed on the table in the appropriate section. A scout film may be taken after the patient is positioned, but before the operation begins, to check the position of the cassette.

2 The x-ray tube that will extend over the operative site must be free from dust. It should be damp-dusted with a disinfectant solution before the patient arrives and the operation begins. It may be covered with a sterile drape before moving it into the sterile field.

3 The draping towels may be sutured on rather than secured with towel clips, which might interfere with the view.

4 Aseptic technique must be maintained at all times. The scrub nurse covers the operative field with a sterile minor sheet to protect it from contamination while the x-ray tube is over it. The circulating nurse removes the sheet after the radiographs have been taken.

5 If a lateral x-ray film will be taken, as during fixation of a hip fracture, the lateral cassette holder may be positioned before the patient is draped and covered with the drape sheet. The circulating nurse raises the sheet for the radiology technician to place and remove the cassette. Or the holder may be left on the outside of the sterile drapes and covered with a sterile Mayo stand cover when ready to swing it into place for the lateral view.

6 The scrub nurse must enclose the cassette with a sterile cover if it must be placed within the sterile field. Disposable covers designed for this purpose are available or a Mayo stand cover may be used. Be certain gloved hands are well protected in a cuff of the cover while the circulating nurse places the cassette into it.

7 Radiopaque contrast medium used for injection must be sterile. The outside of ampuls or vials also must be sterile if they are placed on the sterile instrument table before withdrawing contents into a sterile syringe. Warm the radiopaque contrast medium to body temperature to overcome viscosity.

8 Remove all instruments, metallic or radiopaque items from the operative site.

9 The radiologist or radiology technician must be notified well in advance so that he or she is standing by when the surgeon is ready for the study. Delays waiting for the radiology personnel prolong the operation unnecessarily for the patient.

Protection from Radiation Although OR nursing personnel may assist with some of the invasive preoperative studies, all OR nurses and technicians are exposed to radiation during intraoperative studies and radiation therapy. The effect of radiation exposure is directly related to the amount and length of time of exposure. Radiation has the ability to modify molecules within body cells. Therefore, constant vigilance for personal safety and strict adherence to all hospital policies and procedures are essential to avoid excessive exposure to radiation (also see Chap. 27).

Radiation is measured in roentgens (R) and rads (the units of absorbed dose). The National Council on Radiation Protection and Measurements has formulated government standards for certification of x-ray equipment and for human exposure. Permissible doses of radiation are based on *units of equivalent dose,* the quantity that expresses all radiations on a common scale for the purpose of calculating their biological effects. The unit of equivalent dose is a REM (roentgen equivalent man). The maximum permissible dose for occupationally exposed persons over 18 years of age is 5 REMs per year. OR personnel rarely receive more than 2 or 3 REMs per year. However, the following precautions are taken to protect personnel:

1 Walls of rooms with fixed x-ray equipment are lined with lead to absorb emitted radiation.

2 Personnel should stand 6 ft (2 m) or more from the patient and out of the direct beam during exposure. Nonsterile team members should leave the room, and sterile team members should stand behind a lead screen if possible while x-rays are taken. Radiation from an x-ray tube is present only as long as the tube is energized. Automatic or manual collimators that confine the x-ray beam to precisely the size of the x-ray film or fluoroscopic screen are required for all equipment manufactured after August 1, 1974.

3 Lead-lined aprons and, if feasible, lead gloves should be worn during use of the image intensifier even though a lead shield is part of the installation. These aprons and gloves should be worn also by necessary attendant personnel while injecting a substance for an invasive study or holding a cassette in position.

PATHOLOGY

Clinical pathology is the use of laboratory methods to establish clinical diagnosis of the nature of disease. *Surgical pathology* is the study of alterations in body tissues removed by surgical intervention. Tissue or body fluid may be removed for clinical diagnosis before the surgeon proceeds with a definitive operation. Procedures to obtain specimens for pathologic examinations are always invasive.

Preoperative Pathologic Studies

Biopsy Tissue or body fluid removed for diagnosis is referred to as a *biopsy.* The surgeon performs the necessary procedure to obtain a biopsy prior to scheduling further surgical intervention. The pathologist confirms the diagnosis.

Aspiration Biopsy Body fluid is aspirated through a needle placed in a lesion that contains fluid such as a cyst or abscess.

Bone Marrow Biopsy Through a small skin incision or percutaneous puncture, a trocar puncture needle or aspiration needle is placed into bone, usually the sternun or iliac crest, to aspirate bone marrow.

Excision Biopsy Tissue is cut from the body. The surgeon may remove it through an incision in the skin or mucous membrane. This may be done through an endoscopic instrument. Localization of a lesion in soft tissue, such as the breast, to be incised through a skin incision may be guided by xeroradiography.

Percutaneous Needle Biopsy Tissue is obtained from an internal organ by means of a hollow needle inserted through the body wall. The percutaneous puncture into the lesion may be guided by angiography under image intensification or ultrasound. Special needles are used; some types are disposable.

1 *Dorsey cannula* resembles a ventricular needle except it is a bit larger and the end is open. It is used, sometimes through a burr hole, to remove a biopsy of brain tissue.

2 *Franklin-Silverman* biopsy needle is used for obtaining biopsy specimens of thyroid, liver, kidney, prostate, and other organs. It consists of a 14 gauge, thin-wall outer cannula with a beveled obturator. It has an inner split needle that fits into the outer cannula and protrudes beyond the end of it. The distal tips of this split needle are grooved inside. They enter the tissue and close on the specimen and trap it as the inner split needle is withdrawn.

NOTE. Slight bleeding may follow liver biopsy. Prothrombin time is checked. This method of biopsy is not used if patient has any blood abnormality.

Intraoperative Pathological Studies

Tissue or fluid specimens may be removed immediately prior to or during operation for pathologic examination to determine further therapy.

Cultures Frank pus is removed from an abscess and may be encountered in other known or suspected areas of infection. Drainage is cultured to enable the surgeon to effectively prescribe antibiotics. (Refer to Chap. 8 for the procedure for handling culture specimens during operation.)

Frozen Section A frozen section is a special preparation and examination of tissue to determine whether it is malignant and whether regional nodes are involved. When the surgeon removes a piece of tissue and wants an immediate diagnosis, the pathologist comes to the OR suite to do the frozen section. The circulating nurse should alert the pathologist that his or her services will be needed. The frozen section takes only a few minutes. If malignancy is present and the individual situation indicates, the surgeon proceeds with a radical resection of the affected organ or body area.

NOTE. The specimen should be placed on a towel before the circulating nurse gives it to the pathologist. Never allow a counted sponge or instrument to leave the room during operation.

Surgical Specimens All tissue removed during operation is sent to the pathology laboratory for verification of diagnosis. (Refer to Chap. 8 for care of tissue specimens.)

ENDOSCOPY

Endoscopy is a combined form of two Greek words, *endon* and *skopein*: *endon* meaning "inside," *skopein* meaning "to examine." *Endoscopy,* as the term is used in medicine, is a visual examination of the interior of a body cavity, hollow organ, or structure with an *endoscope,* an instrument designed for direct visual inspection. The endoscope usually is inserted into a natural body orifice, i.e., the mouth, anus, or urethra. It may be inserted through a small skin incision and/or trocar puncture, as through the abdominal or vaginal wall. An endoscopic procedure is designated by the anatomic structure to be visualized. The endoscope likewise is named for the anatomic area it is designed to visualize, e.g., an ophthalmo*scope* is used for ophthalmo*scopy.* From head to foot, nearly every area of the body can be visualized with an endoscope.

Ophthalmoscopy: direct and indirect examination of the eye
Otoscopy: auditory canal and tympanic membrane
Nasopharyngoscopy: nasopharynx
Antroscopy: maxillary sinus
Laryngoscopy: direct visualization of the larynx (Indirect laryngoscopy is an examination with a laryngeal mirror.)
Bronchoscopy: tracheobronchial tree
Mediastinoscopy: mediastinal spaces in the chest cavity
Pleuroscopy: pleural cavity
Thoracoscopy: pleural surfaces
Esophagoscopy: esophagus
Gastroscopy: stomach
Duodenoscopy: duodenum
Jejunoscopy: jejunum
Colonoscopy: colon from ileocecal valve to anus
Sigmoidoscopy: sigmoid colon and rectum
Proctoscopy: rectum and anal canal
Anoscopy: lower rectum and anal canal
Choledochoscopy: common bile duct
Nephroscopy: renal pelvis
Peritoneoscopy: within peritoneal cavity for visualization of abdominal and pelvic organs
Laparoscopy: through abdominal wall for visualization of abdominal organs, but usually the female pelvic organs
Culdoscopy: through the vaginal wall into the retrouterine space for visualization of female pelvic tissues, especially the ovaries
Hysteroscopy: uterus
Colposcopy: vagina and cervix
Cystoscopy: urinary bladder
Urethroscopy: urethra
Arthroscopy: a joint, usually the knee
Vascular endoscopy: arterial or venous lumen

All the above procedures are invasive, except ophthalmoscopy, because the scope is placed into a body orifice or cavity.

Design of Endoscopes

Although the sizes and shapes vary according to specific uses, all endoscopes have similar working elements.

Viewing Sheath (Scope) The surgeon views anatomic structures through a round- or oval-shaped sheath. Diameter varies from 5 mm or less of the arthroscope to 22 mm of an anoscope. Length must be appropriate to reach the desired structure. The scope may be rigid or flexible.

Rigid Scopes These are either hollow sheaths that permit viewing through them in a forward direction only, such as laryngoscopes, or a sheath with an eyepiece and telescopic lens system that permits viewing in a variety of directions, such as cystoscopes. Most rigid scopes are metal. Disposable plastic anoscopes and otoscope sheaths are available.

Flexible Scopes These have a dial adjuster that contours the lensed tip into and around anatomic curvatures to permit visualization of all surfaces of the wall of a structure, as within the hollow organs of the gastrointestinal tract viewed through a flexible gastroscope or colonoscope. The sheath of these instruments is made of plastic material.

Light Source Illumination within the body cavity is essential for visual acuity. The light source may be through a fiberoptic bundle or from an incandescent light bulb.

Fiberoptic Lighting This is an improved lighting system that illuminates body cavities including those that cannot be seen with other light sources. Light is conducted through a bundle of thousands of coated glass fibers encased in a plastic sheath. Each fiber is drawn from optical glass into a strand 10 to 70 microns in diameter that is coated to minimize loss of light by reflection. Light entering one end of the fiber is transmitted by refraction through its entire length. The light produced through the bundle of fibers is nonglaring and evenly distributed on the area to be visualized. Although it is of high intensity, the light is cool, even though a minimum rise of temperature in the tissues exposed to it may occur.

Bulbs Bulbs screw into the fitting either at the end of a removable light carrier or at the end of the built-in lens system. Electric current is conducted through a single-filament wire to illuminate the tiny incandescent light bulb. When changing bulb, put a bit of wax on the threads to seal bulb socket from moisture to prevent short circuits. Fiberoptic lighting has replaced bulbs in most endoscopes and prevents this hazard.

Power Source Electric current must be transmitted to the light source connected to the fiberoptic bundle or to the light bulb. The electric current is entirely external to the patient with fiberoptic lighting. Current flows through a power cord attached to the endoscope inserted into the patient and through the instrument to the light bulb at the distal end of the light carrier or sheath. The power source may or may not be connected to the electrical system in the room.

Projection Lamp This has a light bulb that provides an intense light source, similar to a film projector, for transmission of light through a fiberoptic bundle to the distal end of the scope. Usually a portable, compact, self-contained unit, the intensity of the light may be regulated from 400 footcandles (fc) to as much as 5200 fc in some illuminators. The bulb must be positioned securely in its socket so that its output focuses on the center of the fiberoptic bundle. If it is not properly positioned, the light output will not be of maximum value.

Battery Box With one or more sets of dry-cell batteries, this may be used as the power source for light bulbs. The batteries may be recharged in some units, but eventually they must be replaced. A battery provides a good source of current, is safe, and can be used in conjunction with other electrical equipment.

Rheostat This is a resistor for regulating flow of current from the electrical system. Rapidly introduced high voltage may burn out the delicate filament in the light bulb. The rheostat reduces the electrical potential and allows gradual increase of current to the desired brightness of the light. However, safety precautions must be observed when using this power source to prevent shock to the patient and operator. Rheostats that cannot be grounded should not be used. Also, they cannot be used when the cutting current of the electrosurgical unit is in use. The cutting current will not work if another piece of equipment is on the same circuit.

Accessories Accessories such as suction tubes, snares, biopsy forceps, grasping forceps, electrosurgical tips, sponge carriers, etc. are used in conjunction with endoscopes. These can be passed through channels in the endoscope to remove fluid or tissue, coagulate bleeding vessels, inject fluid or gas to distend cavities, etc. Lensed scopes may be equipped with a still or motion picture camera so organs or lesions can be photographed during the procedure. Some rigid scopes have an obturator, a blunt-tipped rod placed through the lumen of the scope, to permit smooth insertion of the instrument as into the anus. The accessories that will be needed will be determined by the type of endoscope and the purpose of the procedure.

Preoperative Endoscopy

Diagnostic endoscopy frequently is performed in conjunction with radiologic studies or to obtain specimens for pathologic examination. A radiolucent or radiopaque contrast material may be injected through the endoscope or an accessory prior to radiologic studies. Fluid and secretions may be withdrawn for culture or chemical analysis. Biopsies are frequently obtained. Direct visualization alone may confirm presence or absence of a suspected lesion or abnormal condition. Endoscopic diagnosis often provides the information necessary to proceed with open operation or results in cancellation of anticipated operation.

Intraoperative Endoscopy

Vascular endoscopy and visualization of other vessels, such as the biliary and hepatic ducts, following either removal or bypass of an obstruction, confirm the patency of the vessel before completion of the operation. Colonoscopy may be performed intraoperatively to locate soft, nonpalpable tumor masses that must be removed transabdominally. Flexible fiberscopes are used for these procedures.

Minor treatments are performed through endoscopes without subjecting the patient to open operation. Removal of a foreign body, excision of a small tumor or polyp, application of a medication, aspiration of fluid, permanent hemostasis of bleeding, ligation of a structure are examples of therapeutic procedures. Electrosurgery, cryosurgery, and the carbon dioxide laser beam may be used through an endoscope to destroy or remove tissue.

Considerations for Patient Safety

1 History of allergies and previous drug reactions must be obtained. This history should include allergy to fish if a radiopaque contrast medium containing iodine will be injected for radiologic study in conjunction with endoscopy.
2 The patient must be observed for signs and symptoms of reaction to drugs. Endoscopy is frequently performed with the use of sedatives and a topical or local anesthetic agent or no anesthesia at all. The patient is awake during

these procedures. Psychotropic drugs such as diazepam (Valium) and narcotics such as meperidine hydrochloride (Demerol) may be administered intravenously as an adjunct to other preoperative sedation to produce relaxation and cooperation during the procedure and amnesia afterward. Respiratory depression and transient hypotension can occur. Antagonistic drugs should be available to reverse narcotic depression.

3 A topical agent frequently is applied to the nasal or oral and pharyngeal mucosa prior to introduction of an endoscope into the tracheobronchial tree or gastrointestinal tract. Refer to Chapter 9 for reactions to topical and local anesthetic agents.

4 Teeth and gums must be protected if the endoscope is introduced through the mouth. Dentures are removed. A mouthpiece is inserted.

5 Two major complications of endoscopy are:

a *Perforation.* This is a constant cause for concern when rigid scopes are used. Flexible fibroscopes have decreased this danger, but it remains a potential complication.

b *Bleeding.* Bleeding can occur from a biopsy site, pedicle of a polyp, or other area where tissue has been cut.

Some hospitals require the patient to sign a consent for operation prior to an endoscopic procedure in the event a complication develops.

6 Hydrogen and methane gases are normally present in the colon. These gases must be flushed out with carbon dioxide before electrosurgery through the colonoscope to avoid possibility of explosion within the colon.

7 Extreme care must be taken to observe patients after endoscopies for effects of respiratory or circulatory distress due to trauma or medication. Many endoscopic procedures are performed on ambulatory outpatients. They must not leave the hospital until vital signs are stable and side effects have passed.

8 Two major electrical hazards associated with endoscopy are:

a *Improperly grounded electrical equipment.* If you expect the surgeon will use the electrosurgical unit, place the inactive electrode with adequate skin contact to allow conduction of electric current.

b *Unsuspected current leaks.* Corrosion or accumulation of soil can inhibit flow of current across the screw fitting between the light carrier and bulb. Current can leak through the instrument to the patient. Ideally, endoscopes should not contain electrically conductive elements or metals that can corrode. Corrosion can be caused by repeated exposure to body fluids, hard water, or chemical agents.

Electrical systems used with endoscopy must conform with the standards and be subjected to routine maintenance procedures prescribed by the National Fire Protection Association code for electrical safety.

9 Power sources and lights should be tested before each use and they should be kept in working order.

10 The heat generated from the projection lamp of a fiberoptic illuminator must be dissipated. It should not be enclosed in drapes because the heat could set them afire. If the unit contains a fan for heat regulation, the direction of air flow must be away from the patient and the sterile field to minimize airborne contamination. A flammable anesthetic agent must not be used when fiberoptics is the method of lighting for any piece of equipment.

11 Endoscopes must be smooth, with no nicks on the surface. Do not handle metal endoscopes with metal lifting forceps that can scratch the sheaths. They should be handled only with the hands, usually gloved.

12 Not all endoscopic procedures are performed as sterile procedures; some are termed *surgically clean.* When an endoscope is introduced into the gastrointestinal tract through the mouth or anus, which normally harbor resident and transient microorganisms, the procedure may not be considered sterile. However, every patient must be protected from cross infection. Endoscopes and their accessories must be thoroughly cleaned and terminally sterilized after use, although sterility is not maintained between and during some patient uses.

13 The endoscope and all accessories *must be sterile,* regardless of point of entry, if body tissue will be incised or excised. This principle of patient safety requires control of scheduling endoscopic procedures so that sterile instruments are available.

Nursing Duties

1 Often only a circulating nurse assists the surgeon with an endoscopic procedure. The nurse sets up the supplies and equipment, as much as possible, before the patient and surgeon arrive. Consult the procedure book. Remember sterility must be maintained for a sterile procedure.

2 Explain the procedure if the patient does not understand it. It is important that the patient know the reasons for any discomfort that may be experienced so that symptoms of discomfort will be recognized as normal.

3 Explain the position and need for it before positioning the patient. The position the patient must assume during the procedure is often uncomfortable.

4 Drape the patient properly to prevent unnecessary exposure.

5 Divert the patient's attention as much as possible during the procedure. The patient may complain of pain more than is justified as a way of expressing displeasure at the invasion of the endoscope or position required during the procedure. The nurse should stay with the patient to offer reassurance and emotional support. Suggest that slow, deep breaths may help relaxation and lessen the discomfort. Soft music may help the patient relax. The surgeon may allow the patient to watch the procedure through a viewing attachment on the endoscope. The nurse evaluates the patient's level of discomfort and informs the surgeon of unusual reactions.

6 The surgeon usually wants the room in semidarkness, but not so dark that the patient's skin color and condition cannot be observed. A dimmer on the room light is helpful.

7 Be sure you can identify the different scopes and their accessories. Know how to assemble and handle them. When passing the suction tube or biopsy forceps, the nurse or assistant should place the tip directly at the lumen of the scope so that the surgeon can grasp the shaft and insert it without moving eyes from the scope.

8 Endoscopic instruments are delicate and expensive. Care must be taken not to drop them. Fiberoptic bundles are glass, so do not kink or bend them.

Care of Endoscopes

Cleaning Clean all parts of endoscope as soon as possible after use while organic debris is still moist. Mucus, blood, feces, and protein-type residue can become trapped in the channels of the scope. This is difficult to remove if it becomes dry and may render the scope useless.

Wash endoscopes in warm, never hot, water and a mild, nonresidue liquid-detergent solution. Use a pipestem cleaner or small brush to clean inside lumen of all channels. The stopcocks on some scopes must be thoroughly cleaned, too, as dirty ones will stick. Open them to clean; never force them but loosen them with a drop of solvent or lubricant.

Particular attention must be paid to the cleanliness of lenses or viewing will be obstructed. Debris can be carefully removed from around the lens with a fine toothpick. Special lens paper is used on the lens itself. Lensed instruments cannot be cleaned with any substance containing alcohol as it dissolves the cement around the lens.

Rinse thoroughly and dry well. If scopes are to be sterilized in ethylene oxide gas, they must be thoroughly dry. Gas combines with water on items that are damp to form ethyl glycol (refer to Chap. 5, p. 102). Use cotton on a wire stylet, or a pipestem cleaner, or force air through channels to dry inside them.

All endoscopic equipment must be terminally sterilized.

Sterilization After cleaning, place each endoscope with all its parts *disassembled* in a well-padded perforated tray of convenient size. Some endoscopes, such as an arthroscope, are supplied in a perforated case lined with foam cut to fit each disassembled part. Wrap the tray or fitted case for sterilization. Instruments should be packaged immediately and sent to be steam- or ethylene oxide gas-sterilized.

Some parts of endoscopes can be safely steam-sterilized, and therefore should be. Hollow, rigid metal sheaths, such as a sigmoidoscope, can be terminally steam-sterilized after use, but then may be stored to keep it clean rather than sterile for a surgically clean procedure.

Parts with lenses and some fiberoptic carriers, such as a colonoscope, cannot be steam-sterilized. High temperature and moisture will soften the cement holding the lenses or fiberoptic fibers in place. The flexible shafts of some accessory instruments, such as biopsy forceps, erode when steam-sterilized. These parts should be sterilized in ethylene oxide gas or soaked in activated glutaraldehyde solution for *10 hours* if ethylene oxide is not available.

During ethylene oxide sterilization of a fiberoptic lighting system, the manufacturer may recommend that the pressure not exceed 5 lb. Follow manufacturer's instructions for handling, using, cleaning, and sterilizing these items.

Aeration is necessary following ethylene oxide sterilization if any part of the endoscope is nonmetallic, such as the Bakelite eyepiece of a lensed instrument. EO is a vesicant if it comes in contact with the skin. It also can cause eye irritation. To avoid discomfort for the surgeon and patient, *parts that could retain residual gas must be aerated.*

If endoscopes and accessories are immersed for 10 hours in activated glutaraldehyde solution, use a plastic tray without a towel in the bottom. Prolonged use of a stainless steel tray may create an electrolytic action between the metals and can cause metallic deposits on the instruments. Solution must be well rinsed from scopes and all accessories before they are used to prevent tissue irritation.

Disinfection When necessary to immediately reuse an endoscope that cannot be steam-sterilized, wash in nonresidue liquid-detergent solution, rinse, dry, and immerse in activated glutaraldehyde solution for a minimum of *10 minutes. Remember this is disinfection, not sterilization.* Instruments that will be used inside a body cavity, such as the laparoscope, must be sterile. Double standards in the practice of sterile technique do not exist. The same principles apply in all procedures, diagnostic or intraoperative.

Storage If not immediately wrapped for sterilization and storage, endoscopes are terminally sterilized, preferably, or at least disinfected before returning them to their respective storage cabinets. Store clean, unwrapped instruments on a soft material like plastic sheeting or foam. Towels hold a residual of laundry detergent that can cause tarnish on metal.

PLETHYSMOGRAPHY

Pressure-sensitive instruments placed on an organ or around an extremity record variations in the volume and pressure of blood passing through the tissues. Tracings reflect pulse-wave impulses transmitted from moving currents within the arteries or veins. A quantitative, noninvasive, diagnostic technique, plethysmography does not provide anatomic information regarding exact location, extent, or characteristics of vascular disease.

Oculoplethysmography

The instrument is placed on each eyeball to record pulse waves in the eye emanating from the cerebrovascular system for diagnosis of cerebral vascular obstruction. Sometimes the carotid arteries are compressed momentarily for comparative pressure evaluations in both eyes.

Strain Gauge Plethysmography

Pneumatic cuffs are placed snugly around both thighs, calves, ankles, and/or great toes. An electronically calibrated strain gauge attached to the plethysmograph and pulse-volume recorder is secured around each foot. Each cuff is inflated in sequence to measure changes in blood flow and systolic pressures in the lower extremities. Changes in blood-flow volume are measured by changes in circumference of the calf, foot, or toe. Systolic pressure is noted when the strain gauge registers a change in volume on a pen recorder. The test is usually done before and repeated after exercise. This test provides an index of peripheral vascular resistance in the lower extremities due to venous thrombosis, varicose veins, or arteriosclerotic disease.

THERMOGRAPHY

An infrared detector measures heat emission from the skin surface and produces a *thermogram,* a photographic record of the skin's heat pattern. Body heat is produced by cellular metabolism, distributed by blood and lymph, and emitted through the skin by infrared energy. Altered metabolism or blood supply in tissues shows up on the thermogram as variations in skin temperature over the area scanned by the detector. A camera with a wide-angle lens converts the infrared rays into electronic video signals. Either a color or black and white image is projected onto a television display screen and/or photographic film. Dr. Ray Lawson of Montreal first used thermography in 1956 to detect breast cancer. Cancer in the breast usually generates an exothermic heat reaction of 2°C (4 or 5°F), detectable on the thermogram as a hotter area than surrounding breast tissue or a benign breast lesion. Thermography has valuable uses in addition to being a supplementary screening procedure to diagnose breast tumors. It is used to evaluate peripheral vascular disease, acute abdominal inflammatory diseases such as appendicitis, and depth of burns.

ULTRASOUND

Vibrating high-frequency sound waves, beyond the hearing capability of the human ear, can detect alterations in anatomic structures or hemodynamic properties within the body. The basic component of any diagnostic ultrasound system is its specialized transducer, which is a piezo-electrical crystal. The transducer converts electric impulses to ultrasonic waves at a frequency greater than 1 million cycles per second. These ultrasonic frequencies are transmitted into tissues through the transducer placed on the skin. A water-soluble gel is applied to the skin to maintain airtight contact between skin and transducer because ultrasonic waves do not travel well through air. A portion of the transmitted ultrasonic waves is reflected back to a separate receiving crystal. The transducer is held on the skin long enough to obtain a graphic recording of the reflected high-frequency sound waves. Connected to a microprocessing computer, uniform imaging of a wide range of body tissues is possible. Ultrasound is not effective in the presence of bone or gases in the gastrointestinal tract. Whether used as a preoperative or intraoperative diagnostic technique, ultrasound is a rapid, painless, noninvasive procedure. It distinguishes between fluid-filled and solid masses.

Preoperative Studies

Alterations in Anatomic Structure Ultrasonic frequencies are reflected when the beam reaches target anatomic structures of different density and acoustical impedance. The reflected signal is picked up by the transducer/receiver as an echo. The intensity of the returning echo is determined not only by the angle formed between the ultrasound beam and the reflecting surface of the anatomic structure, but also by the acoustic properties of that surface. The resulting echo is described in terms of time and intensity. The echo can be displayed on a sonarscope, a cathode-ray oscilloscope, for immediate interpretation of movements and dimensions of structures, and recorded on film to provide a permanent record known as an *echogram.* Ultrasound is a useful adjunct to other procedures in the diagnosis of:

1 Space occupying lesions in the brain. The echoencephalogram will show a shift of the brain due to tumor.

2 Lesions in the breast, thyroid, and parathyroid glands, and in abdominal or pelvic organs. Ultrasound can distinguish between a cystic and a solid tumor mass in the kidney, pancreas, ovary, and uterus.

3 Emboli, either blood or fat. This is particularly useful in the early diagnosis of pulmonary embolism. Fat embolus syndrome can develop following long bone fractures.

4 Fetal maturation. Fetal head size is an aid in determination of fetal maturation. This can be measured by ultrasound prior to an elective caesarean section or to determine need for caesarean section because the head is too large for vaginal delivery.

5 Cardiac defects. Structural defects, insufficient valvular movement, and blood-flow volumes within the heart chambers and myocardium can be detected. This diagnostic technique is known as *echocardiography.*

Hemodynamic Properties of the Peripheral Vascular System Blood-flow velocity and pressure measurements are possible with ultrasound because moving blood cells produce a sufficient interface with surrounding vessels to independently reflect high-frequency sound waves. The Doppler ultrasonic velocity detector emits a beam of 5 to 10 megahertz ultrasound that is directed through the skin into the bloodstream. A portion of the transmitted ultrasound is reflected from moving particles in the blood. Known as the *Doppler effect,* the reflected sound wave changes in frequency because the source of the sound is in motion. This shift in frequency is proportional to blood-flow velocity. Originally introduced for use in detecting obstruction in arterial blood flow, the Doppler instrument is used extensively to locate and evaluate blood-flow patterns in peripheral arterial and venous diseases or defects.

1 *Arterial disease.* Detection of altered hemodynamics in arterial flow is significant in diagnosis of obstructive or occlusive arterial lesions. For example, the Doppler instrument will indicate regions in the neck where carotid artery blood flow to the brain is obstructed by atherosclerosis. Operation can be performed to remove or bypass the obstruction to avoid the patient suffering a cerebral vascular accident (stroke). It also may help the surgeon determine the appropriate level of lower extremity amputation for ischemia caused by peripheral arterial occlusive disease.

2 *Venous disease.* Occlusion of superficial or deep veins and presence of incompetent valves can be located and identified by sounds made by the flow of blood through the peripheral venous system. The Doppler instrument can qualitatively demonstrate the abnormal venous hemodynamics in patients with varicose veins and thrombotic disease. This information helps the surgeon plan surgical intervention.

Intraoperative Uses

Air Embolus The Doppler instrument can be used to monitor patients during open-heart surgery or operations on the great vessels in the chest to detect the escape of air into the circulation. Air entering an artery to the brain (cerebral air embolism) may cause brain damage or death. By detecting an air embolism at the time it occurs, therapy can be initiated immediately.

Percutaneous Puncture Direction and depth of needle punctures to locate lesions in various abdominal organs, such as pancreatic cyst, can be determined by following the ultrasound beam continuously visualized on the sonarscope. The echo from the tip of the needle is easily visible on the scope when the lesion is entered. These procedures are performed to obtain pathological specimens for diagnosis.

Chapter 16

Microsurgery

Microscopy, the use of the microscope, has been an essential modality in scientific investigation for centuries. From it has evolved *microsurgery,* the performance of operative procedures while directly viewing the operating field under magnification. Because the operating microscope affords surgeons greater visual acuity of small structures, microsurgical techniques are utilized in every surgical specialty.

The concept of microsurgery of course was antedated by the invention and refinement of the microscope, which produces enlarged images of objects too small to be seen unaided.

HISTORICAL INTRODUCTION

The invention and refinement of methods of magnification became a serious pursuit in the sixteenth and subsequent centuries. Names like Janssen and van Leeuwenhoek identify pioneers whose contributions to the development of microscopes assisted in the adoption of the germ theory. Objects as small as bacteria could be seen only through a light microscope, as viruses can be seen only through the more recently developed electron microscopes.

In the latter part of the seventeenth century, Huygens took van Leeuwenhoek's simple single-lens instrument one step further by inventing the simple, effective two-lens eyepiece widely used in modern times. Microscope design and elimination of color distortion were advanced by numerous other experimenters, among them Joseph Jackson Lister, the father of the English surgeon who introduced antiseptic surgery. The elder Lister perfected the achromatic lens and improved the compound microscope to eliminate color aberrations. The achromatic lens projects images practically free from extraneous color or the rainbow effect, which had been a problem. Ernst Abbe, in the nineteenth century, did further work with color-corrected lenses and eyepieces.

The basic system for modern binocular eyepieces was devised in 1902. Ophthalmologists were the first to use the stereoscopic microscope in clinical examination to magnify objects in three dimensions. Ordinary laboratory microscopes employ a light source that is transmitted to the observer's eye through the object being examined. In contrast, the ophthalmic biomicroscope, commonly referred to as a *slit lamp,* utilizes incident light. This form of light is directed from the observation side of the microscope. It is thus possible to focus both the illuminating light and the observation lens in the same plane to achieve better depth perception or stereoscopic viewing. Stereopsis is basically achieved through binocular viewing so that each eye has a slightly different positional view of the object under examination. The observer's brain then combines the two dissimilar images taken from points of view a little distance apart, thus producing a perception of solidity and depth.

Ophthalmologists perform minor procedures such as removal of extraocular foreign bodies under the slit lamp. The principles employed in the biomicroscope eventually led to the development of the operating microscopes presently used for many operative procedures. These are being continually and vastly improved in structure and function.

ADVANTAGES OF MICROSURGERY

Microsurgery provides unique advantages in the restoration of wholeness and function of the body, such as restitution of hearing, vision, tactile sensation, and circulation. It is utilized in many surgical specialties, improving the precision of already established operations as well as permitting the successful performance of procedures previously not possible. For example, blood vessels less than 3 mm in exterior diameter can be sutured. In general, microsurgery allows:

1 Dissection and repair of fine structures through precision of technique by better visualization.
2 Adaptation of operative procedures to individual patient requirements. Variation in anatomical landmarks is more distinct with magnification.
3 Diminution of operative trauma and complications because of safer dissection.
4 Superior focal lighting of the operative field, particularly in deep areas.

DESCRIPTION OF OPERATING MICROSCOPE

One must understand the parts and their functions, but it is also helpful to know the classifications of the operating microscopes to comprehend their use. They may be classified individually according to the type of lens systems used, or by the source of illumination.

Lens Systems

The simplest instrument, like van Leeuwenhoek's, consists of a single lens with relatively high magnification. Examples are the simple magnifying glass or the jeweler's lens. The *magnifying power* is the ratio of the size of the image produced on the viewer's retina by the instrument to the size of the retinal image when the object is viewed without optical aid. Surgeons requiring lesser magnification than that provided by the microscope employ an operating loupe, commonly a simple magnifying lens. This device magnifies approximately 2X. It attaches to a headband or to the surgeon's spectacles. *Loupe surgery is not microsurgery,* as it terminates where microsurgery begins.

Compound microscopes use two or more lens systems or several lenses grouped in one unit. Examples are the laboratory light microscope and the electron microscope. These instruments consist fundamentally of an objective lens, which is the lens system nearest the object to be viewed, and an eyepiece or ocular. The objective has a short focal length and forms an enlarged image that becomes the object of the second lens system, which is the ocular in the light microscope and the projector lens in the electron microscope. Since these microscopes are not used for operating, they will not be discussed further.

The operating microscope is a compound binocular instrument. Interchangeable objective lenses combined with interchangeable eyepieces allow a wide range of magnification and working distances adjustable to the surgeon's needs.

Source of Illumination

The operating microscope employs light waves for illumination. These waves are bent as they pass through the microscope so that the image seen by the viewer's eye is magnified. In order to create a distinct image, adjacent images must be separated. An indistinct image remains unclear no matter how many times it is magnified. The ability to discern detail by focusing images is known as *resolving power.* The ability to enlarge an image is known as *magnifying power.* The shorter the wavelength of the illumination source, the greater the resolving power.

Basically, various operating microscopes incorporate the same essential components, which are the mounting system, optical system, controls for magnification and focus, illumination system, electrical system, and accessories (see Fig. 16-1A and B).

Mounting Systems

The stability of the microscope during operation is of paramount importance. Stability is provided and the microscope system supported by the mounting system. The body or optical portion of the instrument is mounted on a vertical column

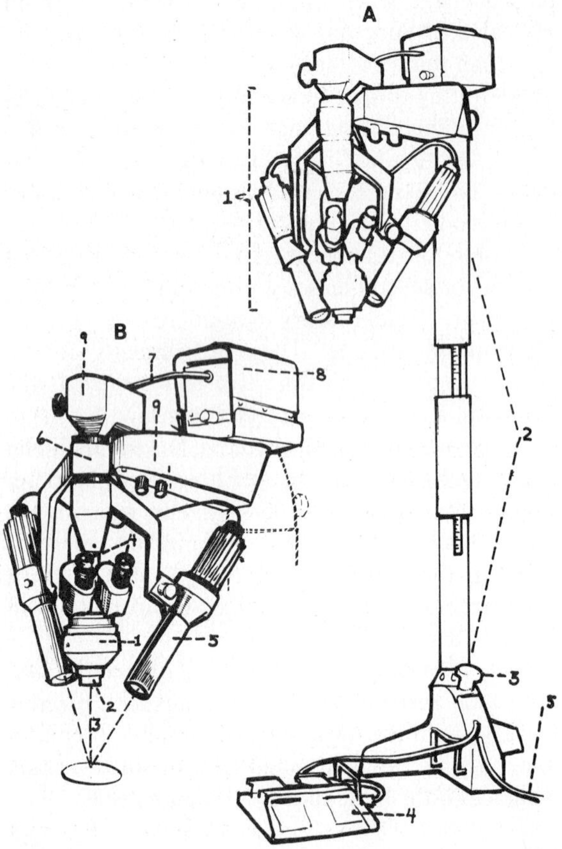

Figure 16-1 (A and B) Floor-mounted operating microscope (Edward Weck & Co, Inc.). **A** (1) optical portion, (2) vertical column, (3) brake knob, (4) foot control, (5) power cord. **B** Microscope detail. (1) body with zoom mechanism, (2) objective lens, (3) working distance, (4) oculars, (5) paraxial illuminator, (6) coaxial illuminator, (7) fiberoptic cable, (8) fiberoptic light source, (9) support arms.

that may be supported by the floor, ceiling, wall, or attachment to the operating table. The body of the microscope is attached to the column by a hinged arm and a central pivot. The mounting permits positioning of the microscope as desired. It may be adjusted horizontally or vertically, rotated on its axis, and tilted at different angles. The microscope can be aimed in any direction. During operation the objective is aimed at the principal site of the operative procedure.

The floor and ceiling mounting systems are the most popular and versatile. All microscopes must have a locking mechanism to immobilize the body, the optical portion, over the operative field.

Floor The base of the vertical support rests on the floor. The base has retractable casters for ease in moving the entire instrument. However, when lowered to working position, the base is locked into position (see Fig. 16-1A).

Ceiling This mount, subdivided into fixed and track-mounted models, provides freer floor space. The fixed unit is suspended from a telescoping column attached directly to the ceiling. The vertical support of the track-mounted unit is suspended from a ceiling rail along which it can be moved out of the way to a wall or cabinet when not in use (see Fig. 16-2). It is advantageous to retract the unit up away from the operating table during anesthesia administration and to position and focus the microscope after the patient is anesthetized. A ceiling-mounted instrument is operated by a control panel on a wall (on-off switch) and by foot controls for focusing, magnifying, raising, and lowering.

A ceiling mount is generally very stable but it is only as stable as the supporting ceiling. Mechanical devices adjacent to the OR, such as air-conditioning units, may cause vibration. The microscope *must* be vibration-free. A ceiling mount permits the same flexibility of positioning as a floor mount.

Wall The microscope is bracketed by a flexible arm to a stable wall. The swing-arm extension permits proper positioning.

Operating Table Smaller microscopes may be mounted on the framework of the table. This system has many disadvantages so is not popular.

Optical System

Components The heart of the optical system is the *body,* which contains the *objective lens* (lens closest to the object). The *head* or *binocular oculars* (eyepieces) through which the surgeon looks are physically and optically attached to the body. The optical combination of the objective

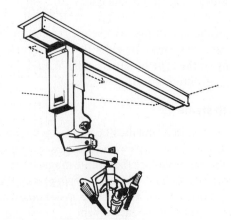

Figure 16-2 Ceiling-track-mounted microscope.

lens and the oculars determines the magnification of the microscope. (See Fig. 16-1B.)

Objective lenses are available from the manufacturer in various focal lengths ranging from 100 to 400 mm, with intervening increases by 25-mm increments. The 400-mm lens provides the greatest magnification. The designation of the objective lens enumerates the *working distance,* which may be defined as the distance from the lens to the operating field. For example, a 200-mm lens will be in focus at a working distance of 200 mm or approximately 8 in. (20 cm).

The oculars serve as magnifying glasses that are used to examine the real image formed by the objective. Most objectives are achromatic so that true color of tissues can be viewed in sharper detail. The binocular arrangement provides stereoscopic viewing.

Magnification The ability of the microscope to magnify depends on the design and quality of the parts in addition to the resolving power. The total magnification is computed by multiplying the enlarging power of the objective lens by that of the lenses of the oculars. The depth of the field, which is the vertical dimension within which objects are seen in clear focus, decreases with increase in magnification or power. Likewise, the width of the field of view narrows as the power of magnification increases. For example, at 20X magnification the field of view narrows to 10 mm, less than 12.7 mm ($\frac{1}{2}$ in.). It is difficult for the surgeon's hand to remain within such a field no matter how steady the hand.

Vertical viewing of the operative field is extremely important, particularly in higher magnification ranges. It allows the surgeon more effective use of the increasingly limited depth of field at higher powers.

In more complex microscopes a third set of lenses is interposed between the oculars and the objective lens to provide additional magnification in variable degrees as desired by the surgeon. A continuously variable system of magnification, for increasing or decreasing images, is possible with a *zoom lens.* The faster, easier to handle zoom is preferred by most surgeons to the simpler turret magnifier that manually changes magnification by fixed increments. The zoom is usually operated by a foot control that permits the surgeon to change the magnification without removing the hands from the operative field. The popular range of magnification in the zoom microscope is from 3.5X to 20X magnification. At 3.5X, the depth of the field is 2.5 mm or about $\frac{1}{10}$ in.; at 20X the depth is 1 mm or about $\frac{1}{25}$ in. Some microscopes magnify to 40 times. Practically speaking, magnifications greater than 20X are difficult to employ.

Focus Focusing is accomplished by a foot-controlled motor that raises and lowers the body of the microscope to the desired distance from the object to be viewed. Some microscopes divide the focusing into gross and fine.

Illumination Systems

There are two basic sources of illumination in the operating microscope. The intensity of illumination can be varied by controls mounted on the support arm of the microscope body.

Paraxial Illuminators One or more light tubes or paraxial illuminators contain incandescent bulbs and focusing lenses. The illuminators are attached to the mounting of the body of the microscope in a position so as to illuminate the field of view. The light is focused to coincide with the working distance of the microscope.

One of the paraxial illuminators may be equipped with a diaphragm containing a variable-width slit aperture. This device permits a narrow beam of light to be brought to focus on the objective field. This slit image assists the surgeon in defining depth perception, i.e., in ascertaining the relative distance of objects within the field (which are closer, which are farther).

Coaxial Illuminators The second source, usually fiberoptic, is transmitted through the optical system of the microscope body. This type of illumination is called *coaxial* because it illuminates the same area in the same focus as the viewing or objective field of the microscope. The fiberoptic system provides intense, though cool, light that protects the patient's tissues and the optics of the microscope from excessive heat. If a fiberoptic system is not used for coaxial illumination, a heat-absorbing filter must be interposed in the illumination system. Direct heat from a high-intensity source can damage and even burn tissues.

Electrical System

The same precautions are observed with the operating microscope as with any electrical equipment in the OR. Switches and wall interlocks should be explosionproof. Circuits must be protected from overload by breaker relays and fuses. All light controls preferably should be in the off position when the power plug is inserted or removed from the wall outlet to avoid short-circuiting or sparking. A red pilot light illuminates on the control panel when the electric power is on.

Optical Accessories

A number of optical accessories are available, including observation and photographic equipment (see Figs. 16-3 and 16-4).

Assistant's Binoculars A separate body with nonmotorized, hand-controlled zoom can be attached to the right or left side of the main microscope body for use by the assistant. This mechanism can be focused in the same plane as the surgeon's oculars. However, its field of view does not coincide exactly with that of the surgeon. This can be rectified by using a *beam splitter,* which takes the image from one of the surgeon's oculars and transmits it through an observer tube, thereby providing the assistant with an identical image of the surgeon's view. This is particularly important in critical areas where a difference of 1 or 2 mm is crucial.

Broadfield Viewing Lens Attached to the front of the body of the surgeon's ocular, this lens is a low-power magnifying glass used for grasping needles or getting an overall view of the field adjacent to the objective (see Fig. 16-4).

X-Y Attachment An automated mechanism, this provides a precision method of controlling small movements of the microscope in the field of view.

Still Photographic, Motion Picture, and Television Cameras Such devices may be attached to the beam splitter, permitting filming of the operative procedure. Their output is highly useful in assisting, teaching, and research.

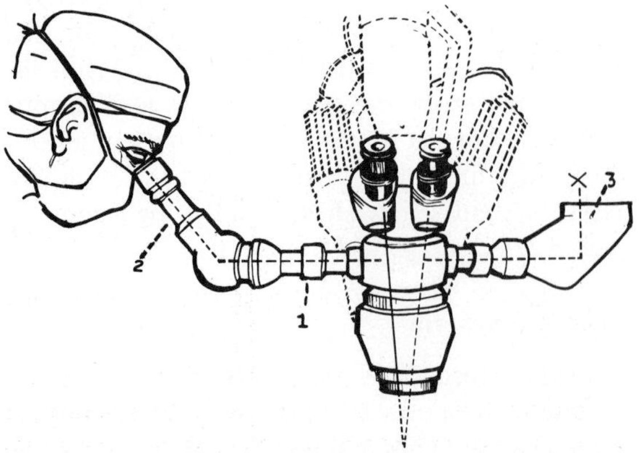

Figure 16-3 Microscope accessories. (1) beam splitter attachment, (2) observer tube, (3) camera attachment.

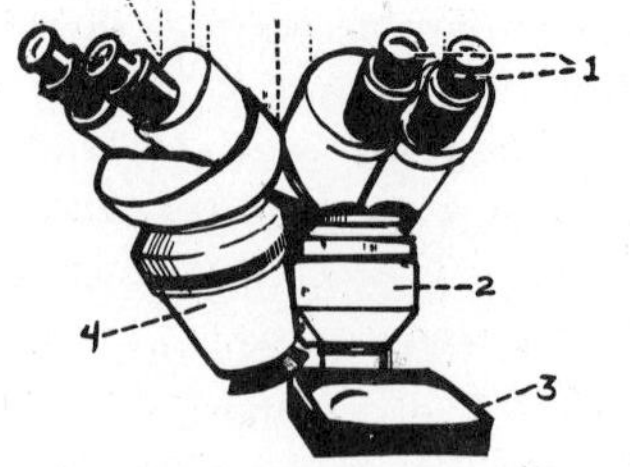

Figure 16-4 Surgeon's microscope on the right with assistant's attached microscope on the left. (1) oculars, (2) body with motorized zoom mechanism, (3) broadfield viewing lens, (4) body with manual zoom mechanism.

Remote Foot Controls

Simple microscopes are manually operated. However, it is more convenient for the surgeon to utilize foot-controlled, motorized functions such as focus, zoom, and tilt. Foot controls may be activated by switches of the push-button type, heel-to-toe, or side-to-side motion. The number of switches corresponds to the number of motor-controlled functions. There may be additional foot switches for the camera or other non-microscope associated equipment such as cryosurgical or bipolar electrosurgical units. Switches may be separated by a vertical bar to prevent inadvertent contact. The bar also serves as a foot rest for the surgeon.

Personal preference plays an important role in a surgeon's selection of an operating microscope. Hospital equipment committees should consult members of the various surgical departments before purchasing this expensive equipment.

MICROSCOPE DRAPE

The microscope is covered by a sterile drape to permit the surgeon to position it and to adjust the optics. Sterile drapes for the microscope may be made of reusable material or disposable plastic, which is heat-resistant, entirely lint-free, and transparent. Disposable drapes are available with and without observer arms. The entire working mechanism of the microscope may be encased in a sterile cover, allowing any part to be touched by sterile gloves.

Ideally, draping the entire microscope permits it to be brought into the sterile field. The scrub nurse pulls the drape over the body and extended arms while the circulating nurse helps guide the drape toward the vertical column and secures it. A sterile towel is placed around the vertical column adjacent to the sterile field. Sterile rubber bands secure the drape to the oculars. They must be removed before the drape is removed. If not heat-resistant, a plastic drape covering the overall instrument may cause heat buildup beneath that can damage the microscope. A heat guard may be applied over the light source or heat evacuated by an opening in the top of the drape.

Just the parts to be touched by sterile team members may be covered with sterile handle covers made of metal, silicone, or plastic. These parts include the oculars, illuminating tubes, light switches, and adjustment buttons or regulators for focus and zoom, if not controlled by the foot pedal. Covers are sterilized and replaced between patients.

Since the assistant has a separate ocular system, it also must have sterile ocular covers as well as a cover for the wand that manually controls the zoom. In some microscopes metal tubes that screw over the illuminators serve as handles for adjustment.

CARE OF MICROSCOPE

Persons responsible for the microscope should consult the manufacturer's manual. Any malfunction should be reported to the OR supervisor or appropriate person who can arrange for repair service. Nevertheless, a few points in care warrant mention.

1 Lenses should be cleaned according to the manufacturer's recommendation only, to avoid scratching or damage to the antireflective lens coating.
2 When changing the oculars, care must be taken to avoid dropping the lens.
3 Both hands should be used for attaching observation tubes.
4 Openings into the microscope body for attachment of ancillary devices such as the observer tube should be closed with covers provided by the manufacturer, when not in use, to prevent accumulation of dust.
5 Careful storage is important, i.e., away from traffic but close to areas where used.
  a The microscope should be enclosed in an antistatic plastic cover when not in use to keep it free of dust. Attachments also are kept dust-free.
  b Lenses and viewing tubes should be protected.
6 The microscope should be damp-dusted before use.
  a External surfaces, *except the lenses,* are wiped with a clean cloth saturated with detergent-disinfectant solution.
  b Casters or wheels should be clean to reduce contamination and prevent interference with mobility.

TECHNIQUE OF MICROSURGERY

All things look considerably different under magnification. Tissues not otherwise visible can be manipulated. The use of microsurgical instrumentation and techniques is an entirely new experience. It does not consist of adapting formerly learned conventional methods to use under the microscope. The techniques themselves for handling instruments, sutures, and tissues are different, i.e., infinitely more complex, precise, and time-consuming because of the meticulous skill involved. Coordination must be adapted to work with minute materials in a field of altered perception and position.

Groundwork for proficiency and facility in employment of the operating microscope should include liberal amounts of time spent by the surgeon in special instruction and laboratory practice under relaxed conditions. This entails practice in movements and manipulation of instruments and suture materials under various magnifications. Mastery is achieved only by practice, repeated performance, and dedication to the task. Pride in workmanship is attained by perfection of these techniques, which is the ultimate realization of Halsted's principles. Therefore, healing literally becomes practically free of undesirable tissue reactions.

Divergence from tactile-manual to vision-oriented techniques requires of the surgeon and assistants maximum attention to detail, as well as diverse judgments. A surgeon who does not use an operating microscope may not realize how much potential visualization of detail he is being denied. *The microscope provides a more limited, although more readily visible, operative field.*

The most common maneuvers utilized in placing and manipulating instruments, making an incision with a scissors, and tying sutures involve a combination of several basic movements:

1 *Compression-decompression*—to close scissors and forceps (The handle spring on micro-instruments permits them to open.)
2 *Rotation*—to insert a needle, to cut, to extract, to engage or disengage
3 *Push-pull, direct or linear*—to incise with a razor knife

The surgeon also must be able to maintain a steady stationary position such as is necessary during remote activation of equipment such as a cryosurgical unit. It is advisable that surgeons do no manual labor for at least a day prior to operating. Very little tremor is tolerable in microsurgery.

MICROSURGICAL INSTRUMENTATION

The cliché that a carpenter is no better than his tools indeed has validity in the present context because of the performance standards required for microsurgery. The improved results of operative intervention utilizing microsurgical techniques are due in no small measure to the miniaturized precision instrumentation developed in association with the performance of more delicate procedures. Microsurgeons work with manufacturers to develop appropriate instruments, suture materials, and needles. Many surgeons invest a considerable sum of money to purchase the instruments of their choice. Whether owned by the surgeon or the hospital, microinstruments require exacting care to maintain desired function.

Instruments are designed to conform to the surgeon's hand movements under the microscope. They must permit secure grasp, ease of holding and manipulation, and fulfillment of their intended purpose. They are shaped so as not to obscure the limited field of view. While these factors are important criteria for any instrument, they are especially vital for microinstruments. Conventional instruments, once considered delicate, appear mammoth beneath a microscope. They are much too large and cumbersome for use in microsurgery. Upon perfecting microsurgical techniques, many surgeons wonder how they ever operated with standard instruments.

As microsurgical techniques differ from conventional operative techniques, so do the instruments. They are extremely fine, delicate, and miniature enough to handle in the very small working area. Manipulation becomes more difficult with increased size or bulk and weight. Like technique, instruments too are constantly being improved. Everyone assisting in or setting up for microsurgical procedures must learn and know the identification and functions of these unique instruments. Design is coincident to function.

Handles

These are designed for secure and comfortable grasp with diameter similar to that of a pen or pencil. Minimal diameter between fingers facilitates feel and accuracy of manipulation. Double-handled instruments (scissors, needleholders) have a somewhat larger diameter than single-handled ones (razor knife). The shape of the handle is important to manipulation. For example, instruments rotated between the fingers when in use, such as needleholders, must be turned easily. Their handles therefore are rounded or six-sided like a pencil. Those not rotated have finger grips or are flattened, e.g., tying forceps.

Handles must be long enough for comfort in the working position but must not extend above the hand in order to avoid contact with the unsterile objective. Therefore, the maximum length of many microsurgical instruments is about 100 mm (4 in.). Gripping surfaces should be functionally located on the instrument to prevent fingers from slipping during manipulation. These surfaces serve as a guide to accurate finger positioning. The gripping area may be six-sided, round, knurled, or flat serrated. Surfaces are finished carefully to avoid snagging sutures or drapes.

Springs and Hinges

Many instruments, particularly scissors and some needleholders, have spring handles that return the tips of the instruments to open position between cutting or grasping functions. The distance from hinge to tip will vary according to function of the instrument. Proper spring tension easily can be ruined by mishandling. Ring-handled instruments are not practical in microsurgery.

Instrument Shape

Microsurgical instruments are shorter than standard instruments and often angulated for convenience of approach and avoidance of obstruction of the operative field.

Instrument Tip

The teeth of some tissue forceps may be as small as $\frac{1}{10}$ mm ($\frac{1}{250}$ in.) in diameter. Therefore, many tips are barely visible to the unaided eye. Nontoothed tying forceps must have perfect apposition of the grasping surfaces to handle microsutures. The suture must be grasped firmly but without trauma, often from a slippery surface. Other smooth forceps are used on friable tissues. Scissor blades may be sharp or blunt, long or short, straight or angulated.

Instrument tips have minimal separation compatible with their function. The increased finger pressure and movement necessary to close wider tips is undesirable because it may induce tremor.

Surface

Finishes of portions of instruments that are exposed to light in the field are deliberately dulled during manufacture to reduce glare from light reflection, which is both annoying and tiring to the surgeon. Oblique lighting, incorporated in microscopes, reduces reflectivity.

Material

Microsurgical instruments are made of stainless steel or titanium. Titanium alloy is considerably stronger yet lighter in weight than stainless steel. Some are malleable for desired angling; some are disposable. All are extremely vulnerable to abuse.

Instrument Use

Appropriate instrumentation is used for specific types of procedures. While all surgical instruments are structured for a definitive use, function of microinstruments is even more restricted. The reason is that tissue can be severely injured by use of an improper or imperfect instrument. Instruments too can be damaged by use on inappropriate tissue. They therefore must not be used for varying manipulations.

Primary usage includes cutting (knives and scissors), exposure (spatulas and retractors), gross and fine fixation (forceps), suture manipulation (tying and suturing), and needle manipulation (suturing).

Knives The edges of razor, diamond, and dissecting knives have different degrees of sharpness and varying thickness of blades appropriate to the cutting function of each, i.e., to make a penetrating or a slicing incision. A clean cut is desired to minimize trauma and tissue destruction.

Scissors Like knives, scissors are designed to make a specific type of incision related to plane as well as to thickness. Examples are vertical, horizontal, or a special configuration such as curved or two-planed. Use is governed by hinging and blade relationship. Scissors are hinged to cut vertically or obliquely. Cutting is usually done by the distal part of the blades for better control. Some scissors come in pairs with right and left curves. This is true of some ophthalmic scissors where it is essential that the blade with the blunt point be inside the eye to avoid inadvertent trauma. Team members must know how to tell the difference. Often the part number inscribed by the manufacturer on the handle will be an even number for a right-hand instrument and an odd number for a left-hand one. Available as straight or curved, microsurgical scissors have a spring-type handle.

Spatulas and Retractors These instruments are used to draw tissue back for better exposure or protection of the tissue itself.

Forceps Straight and curved forceps may be toothed or smooth. These instruments have light spring action and minimal tip separation. Toothed forceps are used for grasping tissue and never for grasping needles or sutures. Special, extremely delicate, smooth forceps are used for tying delicate ligatures and sutures. For stability of grasp and avoidance of injury to the suture strand, the forceps tips must be absolutely parallel.

Needleholders These vary as to locale of use. Some have spring handles. *They should be used to hold only minute microsurgical needles so as not to ruin alignment.* The instrument should be lightweight yet strong and short enough to stay within the working distance.

Handles are round to permit easy rotation between the fingers. While a lock on a needleholder may cause the tips to jerk when engaged or released, some instruments have a holding catch for use in deep wounds to prevent loss of small needles. Needleholders held closed by finger pressure rather than a catch firmly hold a needle shaft yet permit easy adjustment of needle position.

Microsurgical needleholders are only for suturing, not ligating, because the very fine suture materials would break if tied with a needleholder.

Clamps Mosquito hemostats and various clamps are used for vascular occlusion and for approximation of edges of tissues such as nerves and vessels. Crushing of the vessels must be avoided.

Care of Microsurgical Instruments

The reader should review Chapter 14, p. 281. The following points are mentioned for emphasis:

1 Microinstruments are more susceptible to damage than standard instruments. Edges very easily are dulled and fine tips bent or broken. They should be cleaned in an ultrasonic unit, separated in racks so they are not in contact with each other. They should never remain wet for long periods of time, which is conducive to corrosion and discoloration. Rather, they should be dried by hot-air blower, never a towel. It is advisable to check tips with a magnifying glass after cleaning, to detect any damage.

2 Ethylene oxide is the sterilization method of choice. Steam sterilization is also used.

3 Tip-protecting covers or instrument-protecting plastic sleeves are made of material that does not melt or deform with heat. These guards should be left on the instruments until actual use. When instruments are in use, extreme caution is necessary not to catch the tips on any object that could bend them.

4 Instrument sets are secured in holders in boxes for protection when not in use.

SUTURES AND NEEDLES

The reader should review Chapter 13, for the same basic information applies to microsurgery. However, microsurgical closure is unique in that the smallest sizes of sutures and needles manufactured are used. Microsurgical suture sizes range from 8-0 to 11-0, as small as 45 to 18 microns in diameter. Because of the minute size, proportionately small needles are swaged to the suture. Single or double arm, one or two needles respectively, are available. Suture lengths are designated in both inches and centimeters on the packet.

Suture materials include synthetic absorbable and nonabsorbable polymers. A strand of the material is finer than a human hair. Packets provide ready access to the needle. When in use, the needle should always be kept in view in the operative field since a strand may easily be lost from view as well as difficult to pick up. Also, the surgeon should inspect the strand for damage while passing it through the tissue to be sure the holding power *in situ* is not threatened. It is safest and easiest for the scrub nurse to handle and keep these sutures on a white or light-colored, nonslipping surface. White suture towels are used in some hospitals.

Stainless steel microsurgical needles are measured in mils of wire diameter and millimeters in length. An advantage of swaged needles is the uniform diameter and sharpness of each one. Needles that do not penetrate through tissues easily cause damage. In general, to achieve deep placement in tissue, the needle is short and sharply curved. Less curvature is required for more superficial suturing. Straight needles may be preferred for some tissues.

Various methods of arming a needle in the needleholder are preferred by surgeons. Some microsurgeons want the scrub nurse to hold the open suture packet under the accessory magnifier so that they may grasp the needle with the needleholder themselves. The nurse then gently removes the packet away from the strand. Or, the nurse may remove the suture from the packet, letting the needle rest on the back or side of one hand. The surgeon grasps the needle lightly but firmly in the needleholder. The nurse then releases the strand, which is taken into the operative field. Any readjustment of the position of the needle is done by the surgeon under the microscope (refer to Figs. 22-4 and 22-5 in Chap. 22).

A main principle of operative technique, closure of an incision with the least trauma to produce minimal fibrosis and scarring, is enhanced by use of the very small suture-needle combinations. Fine sutures can be placed closely together to yield a firm, even, apposition line and anatomically secure wound. The integrity of the sutures compensates for minimal scar tissue in supporting the wound. Use of the zoom microscope facilitates tying and cutting sutures.

SPONGES

Suitably small sponges and patties of lint-free material such as compressed cellulose are used to accommodate the operative field. Lint readily is visible under the microscope.

GENERAL CONSIDERATIONS OF MICROSURGERY

Preparation of Patient

The patient is prepared as for a standard operative procedure.

Anesthesia If general anesthesia is to be administered, the patient is anesthetized and intubated prior to prepping and draping. Also, the anesthesiologist should be informed in advance of the surgeon's intention to use the microscope. This is especially pertinent in ophthalmic procedures where patient or eye movements under light anesthesia during operation can result in disaster. In addition, the anesthesiologist's position in relation to the patient must be considered to allow room for the microscope. The anesthesiologist should be aware of the fact that microsurgical procedures take somewhat longer time, e.g., suturing.

If local anesthesia is to be used, the operative area is prepped and draped before injection is made. With local anesthesia it is important as always to adequately instruct the patient. He or she should also be sedated but not disoriented. Many patients sleep during the procedure. The patient should be encouraged to relax, and instructed to lie quietly and to tell the anesthesiologist or circulating nurse of any desire to move. The patient's awakening with a startle reflex or moving unexpectedly is especially hazardous in microsurgery where the surgeon's mobility and field of view are limited. If the patient jerks or turns, he or she literally may move out of the surgeon's hands and often out of the view of the operative field. This can be catastrophic. Therefore, the patient *must* be closely monitored by the anesthesiologist or circulating nurse. Both persons must be intrinsically familiar with the operative procedure so as to thoughtfully and safely guide the patient through the procedure.

Preparation of Team

The increased operating time that is needed for the use of the operating microscope can be minimized by adequate preparation and assistance. Each team member should thoroughly understand the microscope and every facet of microsurgical techniques.

Team members can be kept up-to-date by inservice explanation of new instruments and demonstration of the microscope. It is extremely helpful as well as contributory to understanding if the surgeon shows the nurses and technicians anatomical structures and instruments through the microscope. In this way they can mentally visualize what the surgeon sees. A comparison of microinstruments with standard instruments under the microscope is always a revelation. A television monitor is a great advantage in providing the scrub nurse and anesthesiologist continuous observation of the operative procedure. All members must be completely familiar with the instrumentation. Not only are instruments then properly cared for, but even more importantly, operating time is reduced.

Need for Stability

A vital factor for successful microsurgery is stability of the operative field, the microscope, and the surgeon's hands. It is mandatory that these be adequately supported as a shift of even 1 mm ($\frac{1}{25}$ in.) can alter the operative field, particularly at higher magnifications.

The complete microsurgical unit consists of the operating table with the patient, the microscope, and the surgeon's chair. They must be functionally positioned in relation to each other so that major adjustments need not be made during operation. The surgeon and the circulating nurse should check that all components are properly placed before the incision is made.

Patient The patient must be positioned comfortably and safely with the operating table locked in position. The operative site is immobilized if possible.

Microscope

Floor Mount The base should be properly positioned in relation to the operating table before anesthesia is administered or the patient prepped. To maintain balance and control, gently push (don't pull) the instrument when moving it. The brake should be released or casters activated before moving. The arms should be folded close to the column with all attachments locked into place. Cords should be out of the way. Observation tubes should not be used as handles. Never use force in moving the microscope or in applying attachments. Check the problem instead. A floor-based microscope with column support is placed to the left of a right-handed surgeon. The base should not interfere with the foot controls or power cables. It must be clear of any table attachments as well.

The assistant's oculars and/or observer tubes can be moved to either side. These units are also heavy so should be placed on the appropriate side of the microscope, right or left, before the operative procedure begins.

As a safety factor, the base must not be moved when the instrument is over the patient because it is top-heavy. Gross adjustments, such as height of the microscope in relation to the operative field and focus, are made with the microscope swung away from the patient. Operating table height, chair, and armrest heights are adjusted at the same time gross adjustments are made. Fine focusing and adjustments are done after the microscope is in position for operating. The assistant's microscope is adjusted to the same focus as that of the surgeon. During prepping and draping, the instrument is rotated out of position, then back over the operative area for the procedure.

Since the surgeon and assistant frequently sit for microsurgical procedures, the height of the operating table must permit them adequate knee room to operate foot pedals.

Ceiling Mount The vertical support has a fail-safe mechanism, a memory stop that can be preset for a preselected operating table height. This setting should be checked and adjusted for each table-position change. The mechanism is a safety factor to prevent accidental lowering of the microscope at high speed too close to the patient. High-speed lowering should be done away from the patient until the memory stop is reached. As with the floor-mounted instrument, gross adjustments are never made over the patient. Fine adjustment and focusing are done after the microscope is over the operative field.

Operating Chair The value of a good microscope is obviated without proper ancillary equipment. Support of the surgeon's arm must be continuous from shoulder to hand to give stability and to minimize tremor, especially in fine finger movements. A detachable, sterile wrist support may be affixed to the operating table.

A chair with hydraulic foot controls for raising or lowering it provides the necessary forearm support by means of attached armrests. These are individually draped. Mayo stand covers are convenient. The armrests can be moved independently to a variety of levels and positions. They must be secured in the desired position. The surgeon must be in a comfortable position to work.

Special Features of Microsurgery

While a stabilized situation is crucial to microsurgery, a second fundamental necessity is the need for the surgeon to keep the eyes on the field of view through the microscope at all times. Looking away from the field then requires readjustment of vision to the field. Faultless team cooperation and coordination prevents the surgeon's distraction from the operative site.

The Mayo stand and instrument table should be placed convenient to the surgeon's hand so he or she does not have to look around the microscope. If handing instruments, place one in position for use and guide the hand toward the wound so the surgeon may keep his or her eyes on the field. Necessary instruments are placed on the Mayo stand in anticipated order of use. The surgeon or nurse should replace them in the original position, not touching each other. Instrument holders are available for keeping the tips in the air.

Special awareness of potential for contamination of the operative field by the microscope or the surgeon, whose attention is centered on a very small area, is needed.

Nurses' Duties

All duties for a standard procedure are applicable.

Additional Duties: Circulating Nurse

1 Know how to care for and position the microscope. A checklist to verify the functioning of various parts prior to operation is helpful.
   - **a** Check that all knobs are secured after the microscope is in operative position.
   - **b** Take special care of power cables to prevent accidental breakage by heavy equipment; be sure that cords are properly rolled for storage.
   - **c** Check electrical connections for proper fit or wire fraying.
   - **d** Take special care of lenses to prevent breakage and fingerprinting.
   - **e** Extra lamp bulbs and fuses for the microscope should be on hand. The nurse must know where they are stored and how to change them. It is advisable to check bulbs periodically to avoid necessity for replacement during a procedure. New bulbs should be inserted if a long procedure is anticipated.
   - **f** Properly store the microscope and accessories.

3 See that foot pedals are always in a convenient position so that the surgeon does not have to search for them.

Scrub Nurse

1 Assist efficiently but never put hands in the operative field unless requested to do so.

2 Set up Mayo stand and instrument table without touching tips of instruments.

3 Keep debris (blood, mucus, or suture ends) from tips of instruments. Wipe them gently on a nonfibrous sponge or lint-free gauze.

4 Understand the need for slow dissection at times. Do not let attention stray; watch television monitor if available.

Joseph Lister stated that success is attention to detail. That is the essence of microsurgery as practiced in the surgical specialties. Residency programs include education and training in microsurgical techniques, the techniques of the present and the future.

Chapter 17

General Surgery

INTRODUCTION

The earliest time in which surgical procedures were done is not known, but in 5702 B.C. an Egyptian physician put into writing his knowledge of anatomy.

The Greeks were noted for their written records concerning bowel obstruction, hernias, and amputations. Gastric ulcers were recorded as early as the fourth century B.C. Hippocrates was recognized as the medical authority for 2000 years.

Revolutionary discoveries by Semmelweis, Pasteur, and Lister marked the beginning of present-day aseptic surgery. The introduction of surgical specialties was the outgrowth of increased knowledge of etiology of disease and specialized treatment of all parts of the body. *General surgery,* the basis for all specialties, decreased in breadth as specialization increased. The parts of anatomy not specifically delegated to the specialists have remained in the realm of the general surgeon. The scope of this specialty is not clearly delineated as disciplines often overlap; however, this chapter will focus on procedures commonly categorized as general surgery.

SPECIAL FEATURES OF GENERAL SURGERY

Frequently, the operation performed depends on the biopsy and frozen section report at the time of operation and while the patient is still under anesthesia. Although the patient has been informed preoperatively of any anticipated procedure, the unknown factor is cause for much apprehension. The operating room nurse must convey sincere concern.

1 Malignant lesions account for a large percentage of surgical interventions, especially in operations of the breast, thyroid, and gastrointestinal tract. Operability of the lesion sometimes may be determined only after thorough exploration at operation.
2 Frequently the nurse must be prepared with two draping and instrument setups depending on the diagnosis established after the operation begins. Anticipated equipment and supplies must be available without delay.
3 Positioning and draping of the patient in a general surgical procedure is as varied as the operations. Ingenuity often is required of the nurse to position the patient safely since the surgeon may have alternatives for positions and incisions in a given procedure. Extra pillows, padding, and accessory positioning aids must be available. Elastic bandages may be used to wrap the legs.
4 All types of anesthesia may be administered. Occasionally none is needed.
5 Instrumentation is quite varied and suited to function in an anatomical area. For example,

gastrointestinal procedures require the addition of crushing clamps used to occlude the intestinal lumen before resection, and rubber-shod clamps to protect delicate tissues. Included in all procedures are instruments for exposing, dissecting, grasping, holding, clamping, occluding, and suturing.

Various lengths of umbilical tape, hernia tape, or Vesseloops may be placed around vessels to retract them. Vesseloops are thin strips of disposable radiopaque material that are nontraumatic to blood vessels, nerves, and ureters.

6 A number of general operative procedures are adaptable to ambulatory surgery while others are extremely extensive.
7 The electrosurgical unit frequently is used.
8 In abdominal and pelvic procedures:
   a Indwelling or ureteral catheters often are inserted preoperatively.
   b A nasogastric tube frequently is passed before or during the operation.
   c After the abdominal cavity is entered, single, free 4 by 4 sponges should be removed from the field. They are used only folded and secured on a sponge stick. Wet or dry tapes (laparotomy packs) are used in the abdominal cavity. A small dissector always is clamped in a forceps before handing to the surgeon.
   d Suction always must be available and immediately ready to use before the peritoneum is incised, especially in biliary or intestinal procedures or when fluid or blood may be anticipated in the peritoneal cavity.
   e Before resecting the gastrointestinal or biliary tract, lap packs are used to isolate the area to prevent contamination of the peritoneal cavity.
   f A drain may be exteriorized through the incision or a stab wound in the adjacent abdominal wall prior to closure.
   g Contaminated items such as those used to anastomose intestinal segments are placed in a discard basin on the sterile field. Only the outside of the basin is touched.
   h The wound often is irrigated prior to closure to remove blood and debris.
   i Retention sutures may be used to give additional strength to wound closure (refer to Chap. 13).
9 Assorted sizes of drains, tubes, drainage bags, and wound-suction apparatus should be available.
10 Irrigating solutions should be at body temperature before using. All radiopaque dyes, anticoagulants, and solutions on the instrument table must be clearly labeled to avoid any error in administration.
11 Blood loss and urinary output frequently are recorded.

NECK PROCEDURES

It is convenient to classify operations by anatomical location. The head, face, and parts of the neck belong to other specialities, but general surgery claims the thyroid, parathyroid, cervical and scalene node areas.

Thyroid Procedures

The *thyroid gland,* located in the anterior aspect of the neck, is composed of two lobes that lie on either side of the trachea and are united by a narrow band, the isthmus. The *thyroid hormone* controls rate of body metabolism and may influence physical and mental growth.

Hyperthyroidism (Grave's disease), hypothyroidism, and an enlarged gland (goiter) are the main disorders of the thyroid. Drugs, radioactive iodine, and/or surgical resection are used to treat hyperthyroidism. This disease, rare in elderly patients or the very young, affects females more frequently than males. Replacement of the thyroid hormone with drug therapy is specific treatment for hypothyroidism. Oral administration of thyroid extract or iodine may reduce glandular size, but frequently surgical excision is necessary.

Thyroid Biopsy A Vim-Silverman needle biopsy or an excisional biopsy may be performed to aid in establishing a diagnosis of thyroiditis and differentiation between nodular goiter and carcinoma.

Subtotal Thyroidectomy The usual operation for hyperthyroidism is removal of approximately five-sixths of the thyroid gland. This procedure generally relieves symptoms permanently, as the remaining thyroid tissue secretes sufficient hormone for normal function.

Thyroid Lobectomy The removal of a lobe of the thyroid is adapted especially for toxic diffuse goiter, which is usually benign. In case of malignant growth, the lobe and the lymph nodes in the neck that drain into the involved area may be dissected. Care must be exercised not to damage the recurrent laryngeal nerve and parathyroid glands that lie in close proximity because trauma can result in temporary or permanent laryngeal paralysis. Voice disturbance with hoarseness occurs with paralysis of one vocal cord.

Substernal Intrathoracic Thyroidectomy Goiters invading the substernal and intrathoracic regions occur less frequently, but their size and location often cause tracheal obstruction. The sternum may have to be split to remove a large adherent intrathoracic goiter.

Postoperative complications of thyroid and associated procedures include hemorrhage, edema of the glottis, injury to the recurrent laryngeal nerve, tetany, and acute thyrotoxicosis. A tracheotomy set (refer to Chap. 23) must remain at the patient's bedside postoperatively per hospital routine or until released by the surgeon, usually for at least 24 hours, in case of respiratory obstruction.

Thyroglossal Duct Procedures

Thyroglossal Duct Cystectomy Excision of a thyroglossal cyst requires removal of the entire cystic sac and a portion of the hyoid bone.

Parathyroid Gland Procedures

Parathyroidectomy The *parathyroids,* the four or more small endocrine glands attached to or within the thyroid, regulate metabolism of calcium in the body. Diseased glands are surgically excised; however, resection of all parathyroid tissue may cause severe tetany.

Cervical and Scalene Node Procedures

Biopsy Cervical and/or scalene nodes are biopsied for diagnosis of metastatic extension of cancer or tuberculosis into these lymphatic nodes. The procedure also may be performed by thoracic surgeons.

BREAST PROCEDURES

Operative procedures performed on the breasts may be carried out in the presence of disease or because of other physical and psychological determinants. The *mammary glands* are bilateral organs lying in the superficial fascia of the pectoral area. They are attached to the underlying muscles by loose areolar tissue. The breasts extend from the border of the sternum to the anterior axillary line and from approximately the first to the seventh rib. General surgery on the breast includes diagnostic procedures and those performed for known pathology. Diagnostic techniques, continually improving, include mammography, xeroradiography, and thermography, as well as the traditional tissue biopsy. Self-examination by the patient plays an important role in detection of potential breast problems.

It is generally agreed that the desired operative procedure should be determined on an individual basis after careful diagnostic studies and histologic diagnosis. Size, location, and type of diseased tissue or stage of malignancy are important considerations. No single operation is suitable for all patients.

Incision and Drainage

Surgical opening of an inflamed and suppurative area of the breast is most frequently carried out because of infections in the lactating breast. The cavity usually is irrigated and the wound packed and allowed to heal by granulation. The causative organism often is staphylococcus and consequently the patient may be placed on isolation precautions.

Biopsy of the Breast

In order to determine the exact nature of a mass in the breast, tissue is removed for histologic examination. Until proven benign, all breast masses are considered malignant. A *needle biopsy,* a type of incisional biopsy, is done by inserting a large bore needle attached to a syringe into the mass and withdrawing a core of suspected tissue for cytological examination. Any retrieved fluid is also sent to pathology. If an *incisional biopsy* is performed, the mass is incised and only a portion is removed. An *excisional biopsy* consists of removal of the entire mass. Biopsy is carried out for the presence of a tumor mass detected by palpation, x-ray diagnostic studies, skin changes such as dimpling, and nipple discharge. Excisional biopsy usually is the procedure of choice as it permits examination of the whole mass and avoids entering the lesion with accompanying risk of seeding or implantation of malignant cells. A Penrose drain may be inserted. This also may be referred to as *lumpectomy* (wide excisional biopsy).

A patient may be scheduled for breast biopsy and frozen section done while the patient is anesthetized. In these patients, the surgeon usually intends to proceed directly with the indicated surgery if the results of the section warrant it. Preoperatively, the surgeon discusses with the patient the possible findings and treatment and the patient agrees to definitive operation. When a patient has a biopsy and immediate extended operation, two separate prepping, draping, and instrument sets are necessary. Individual hospitals may vary in their routine setup.

Partial Mastectomy

This procedure is recommended only for patients with small, peripherally located lesions and consists of removal of the entire tumor mass along with at least 2.5 cm (1 in.) of surrounding nondiseased tissue.

Subcutaneous Mastectomy (Adenomammectomy)

This procedure may be performed for patients with chronic cystic mastitis who have had multiple previous biopsies, patients with multiple fibroadenomas or hyperplastic duct changes, and patients with central tumors of the breast that are noninvasive in origin. Removal of all breast tissue is carried out with the overlying skin and nipple remaining intact. A prosthesis may be inserted at the time of operation, depending on the surgeon's decision.

Simple Mastectomy (Total Mastectomy)

In this procedure, the entire breast is removed but without lymph node dissection. Simple mastectomy may be performed if the malignancy is confined to breast tissue with negative nodes, as a palliative measure for an advanced ulcerated malignancy, or to remove extensive benign disease. Skin grafting may be necessary if primary closure of skin flaps would create unacceptable tension. Skin flaps then are loosely approximated and grafts taken from the thigh are applied to the remaining defect.

Modified Radical Mastectomy

This usually is done for localized, small malignant lesions. The term *modified* encompasses various techniques but all include removal of the entire breast (total mastectomy). In addition, all axillary lymph nodes are resected. The underlying major pectoral muscle is left in place. The minor pectoralis muscle may or may not be removed.

Radical Mastectomy

Radical mastectomy is performed for larger, infiltrating cancers to control the spread of malignant disease. Following a positive tissue biopsy, the entire involved breast is removed along with axillary lymph nodes, the pectoral muscles, and all adjacent tissues. During operation, skin flaps and extensive exposed tissue are covered with moist packs for protection. The chest wall and axilla are irrigated before closure.

Extended Radical Mastectomy (Urban Procedure)

This procedure is indicated when malignant disease is present in the medial quadrant or subareolar tissue, as it tends to spread to the internal mammary lymph nodes. Cancer is a disease that grows deeply as well as laterally. The involved breast is removed en bloc along with the underlying pectoral muscles, axillary contents, and the upper internal mammary (*mediastinal*) lymph node chain. This procedure is more difficult than classical radical mastectomy.

Considerations for Female Breast Procedures

Patients for breast procedures are placed in supine position with the involved side close to the edge of the table and the arm on the affected side extended on an armrest. General anesthesia usually is preferred, as local infiltrate may obscure the tumor or the patient may become agitated by positive findings.

Because of the vascularity of breast tissue, mastectomy patients should be watched carefully for excessive bleeding. A compression dressing usually is applied in the OR. A closed-wound suction system may be inserted depending on the amount of tissue resected, to remove extravasation of blood and serum and prevent necrosis of skin flaps.

Patients who have undergone mastectomy frequently are referred by the surgeons to the "Reach to Recovery" rehabilitative program. Under this program, extremely effective volunteers who have had mastectomies visit the patients and share information with them, as well as give encouragement.

Reduction of the Male Breast

This procedure is carried out for *gynecomastia,* a pathologic lesion consisting of bilateral or unilateral enlargement of the male breast. It occurs primarily after the age of 40 or during puberty and usually is related to alterations in normal hormonal balance. All subareolar fibroglandular tissue is removed, followed by reconstruction of the resultant defect.

OPERATIVE ABDOMINAL INCISIONS

Surgical opening of the abdominal wall and entering of the peritoneal cavity is called *laparotomy.*

Various types of incisions are used but each follows essentially the same technique. The exact position of incision is determined before the surgeon begins. The skin and subcutaneous tissue are incised and blood vessels ligated. Fascia covers the muscles anteriorly and posteriorly. The anterior fascia is incised and each muscle layer is separated, and/or divided, with bleeding vessels ligated. The layers are retracted. The peritoneum is the thin serous membrane lining the interior of the abdominal cavity (*parietal peritoneum*) and surrounding the organs (*visceral peritoneum*). It lies beneath the posterior fascia. Both posterior fascia and peritoneum may be cut at the same time, thus exposing the contents of the abdominal cavity (refer to Fig. 17-1).

All incisions incorporate with varying degrees of success certain characteristics that include:

1 Ease and speed of entry into the abdominal cavity
2 Maximum exposure
3 Minimum trauma
4 Least postoperative discomfort
5 Maximum postoperative wound strength

The surgeon chooses the most suitable incision for the procedure to be performed.

Types of Incisions

The two main factors governing incisions are direction and location. Incisions may be vertical, horizontal, or oblique, in various areas of the torso (see Fig. 17-2). The following incisions are applicable to abdominal or pelvic procedures.

Paramedian Incision This is a vertical incision about 4 cm (approximately 2 in.) lateral to the midline on either side, in the upper or lower abdomen. After the skin and subcutaneous tissue are incised, the rectus sheath is split vertically and muscle retracted laterally. This incision allows quick entry into the abdominal cavity with excellent exposure, limits trauma, avoids nerve injury, is easily extended, and gives a firm closure. Examples of use: right upper, biliary tract or pancreas; left lower, resection of sigmoid colon.

Longitudinal Midline Incision This incision can be upper abdominal, lower abdominal, or a combination of both going around the umbilicus. Depending on the length of the incision, it begins in the epigastrium at the level of the xiphoid process and may extend vertically to the suprapubic region. After incision of the peritoneum, the falciform ligament of the liver is divided. *Upper*

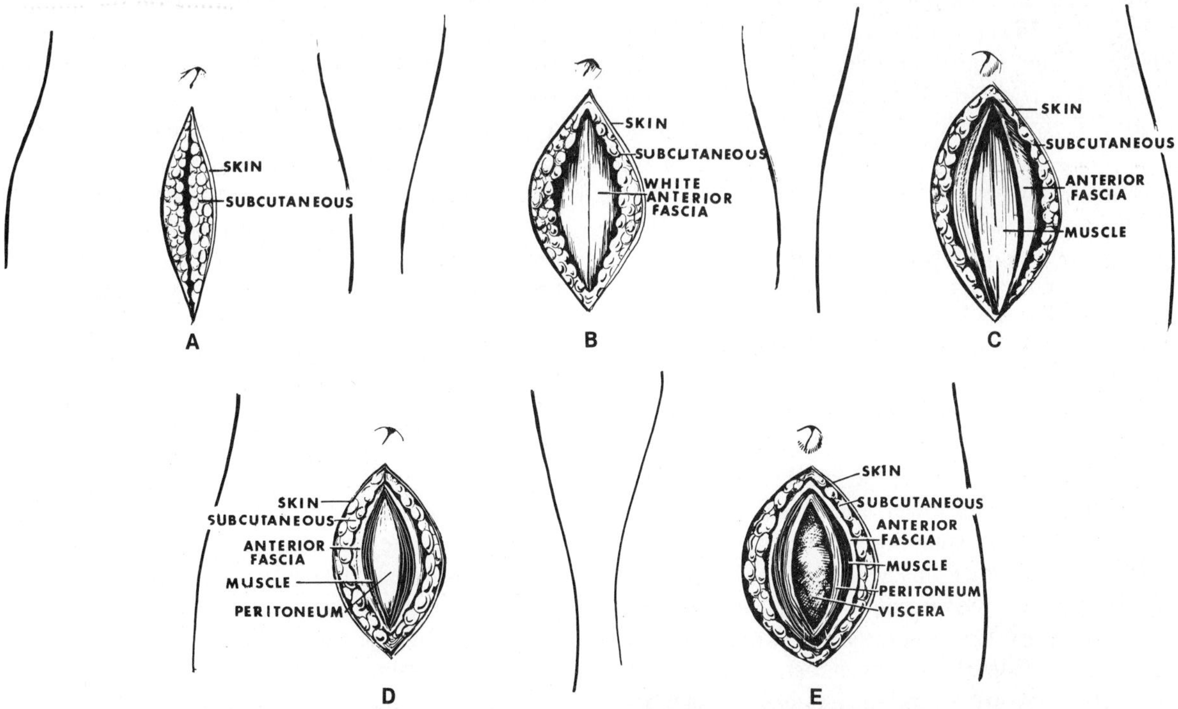

Figure 17-1 (A, B, C, D, and E) Dissecting tissue layers of the abdomen. **A** Subcutaneous (yellow). **B** Anterior fascia (white). **C** Muscle (red). **D** Skin through muscle dissected. Thin white peritoneum presenting for dissection. **E** Opened peritoneum with viscera beneath.

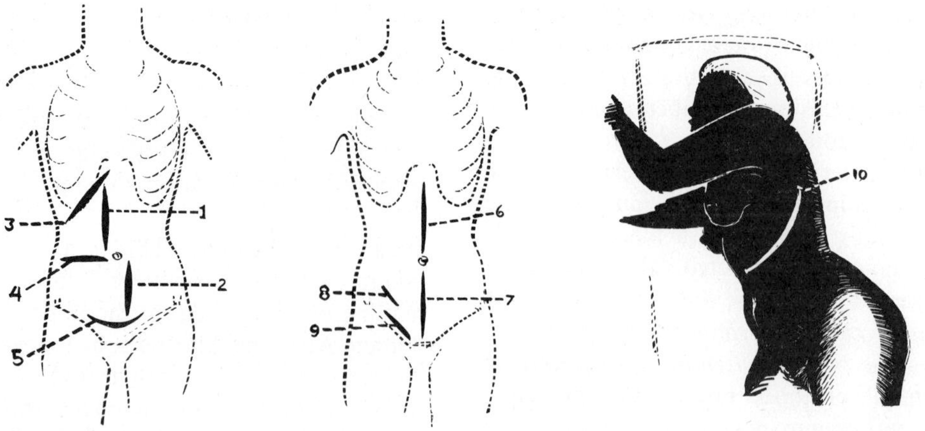

Figure 17-2 Abdominal incisions. (1) right upper paramedian, (2) left lower paramedian, (3) right subcostal, upper quadrant oblique, (4) right midline transverse, (5) Pfannenstiel, (6) upper longitudinal midline, (7) lower longitudinal midline, (8) McBurney's, (9) right inguinal, lower oblique, (10) left thoracoabdominal.

midline incision offers excellent exposure of upper abdominal contents and rapid entry but is not a strong incision and may disrupt. The *lower midline incision* provides exposure of pelvic organs, and rapid entry. It is not as strong as paramedian incision. Examples of use: upper for gastrectomy; lower for intestinal resection.

Subcostal, Upper Quadrant Oblique Incision A right or left oblique incision begins in the epigastrium, and extends laterally and obliquely just below the lower costal margin. It continues through the rectus muscle, which is either retracted or transversely divided. Although the incision affords limited exposure except for upper abdominal viscera, cosmetically it provides good results since it follows the skin lines and produces limited nerve damage. It is a strong incision postoperatively, although a painful one. Examples of use: biliary procedures, splenectomy; or, bilateral incisions joining in the midline are used for stomach and/or pancreas procedures.

McBurney's Incision The area just below the umbilicus and 4 cm (about 2 in.) medial from the anterior superior iliac spine marks McBurney's point in the right lower quadrant. A muscle-splitting incision extending through the fibers of the external oblique muscle is made. The incision is deepened and the internal oblique and transversalis muscles are split, retracted, and the peritoneum entered. This is a fast, easy incision although exposure is limited. Example of use: appendectomy.

Thoracoabdominal Incision With patient in lateral position, either a right or left incision begins at a point midway between the xiphoid and the umbilicus and extends across the abdomen to the seventh or eighth costal interspace, and along the interspace into the thorax. The rectus, oblique, serratus, and intrathoracic muscles are divided in the line of incision down to the peritoneum and pleura. This converts the pleural and peritoneal cavities into one main cavity, thus allowing excellent exposure for the upper end of the stomach and lower end of the esophagus. Examples of use: esophagectomy, repair of hiatus hernia.

Midabdominal Transverse Incision This incision starts on either the right or left side slightly above or below the umbilicus. It may be carried laterally to the lumbar region between the ribs and crest of the ilium. Intercostal nerves are protected by cutting the posterior rectus sheath and peritoneum in the direction of the divided muscle fibers. Advantages are rapid incision, easy extension, provision for retroperitoneal approach and secure postoperative wound. Examples of use: choledochojejunostomy or transverse colostomy.

Pfannenstiel Incision This is a curved, transverse incision across the lower abdomen within the hairline of the pubis. The rectus fascia is severed transversely and the muscles separated. The peritoneum is incised vertically in the midline. This lower transverse incision provides good exposure and strong closure for pelvic procedures. Example of use: abdominal hysterectomy.

Inguinal Incision, Lower Oblique An oblique incision of the right or left inguinal region, it extends from the pubic tubercle to the anterior crest of the ilium, slightly above and parallel to the inguinal crease. Incision of the external oblique fascia gives access to the cremaster muscle, inguinal canal, and cord structures. Example of use: inguinal herniorrhapy.

Wound Closure

Closure is done in reverse order of incision. Each layer is closed with interrupted or continuous sutures (see Fig. 17-3). Separation of tissues produced by failure to approximate wound edges closely results in dead space, which delays healing. Absorbable material is usually used for peritoneal closure. Either absorbable or nonabsorbable material is used on the muscle and fascia. If the subcutaneous tissue is thick, it may be necessary to place a few absorbable sutures in the layer. The skin edges are approximated with nonabsorbable suture, skin clips, or skin staples. Sometimes the suture line is supported by retention or stay sutures.

BILIARY TRACT PROCEDURES

The *gallbladder* is located in a fossa on the undersurface of the right lobe of the liver. It is a thin-walled sac with a normal capacity of about 50 to 60 ml of bile. Bile, which is secreted by the hepatic cells, enters the intrahepatic bile ducts and progresses to the common bile duct. When not needed for digestion, bile is diverted through the cystic duct into the gallbladder where it is stored. When needed, the gallbladder contracts, emptying bile into the cystic duct from which it flows to the common bile duct, and on into the duodenum. *Gallstones,* concretions of elements in bile, may be found in the gallbladder or any portion of the hepatic duct system. Incidence of stones or calculi increases with age, and is more prevalent in women. Roentgenographic studies, including oral and intravenous cholecystography, are used for visualization of the gallbladder in primary evaluation of patients with biliary symptoms. Acute or chronic inflammation, common duct stone (*choledocholithiasis*), carcinoma, or congenital absence of the bile ducts (*biliary atresia*) are the most common indications for operation. Obstructive jaundice, potentially fatal, may be a sign of ductal cholelithiasis or the presence of a neoplasm. Cause of the jaundice must be determined and the condition relieved to spare the patient irreversible progressive liver damage.

Cholecystostomy

This is operative formation of an opening into the gallbladder to permit drainage and to avoid rupture. It usually is done under local anesthesia in patients whose general condition prohibits a prolonged procedure. A purse-string suture is placed in the fundus and the gallbladder decompressed

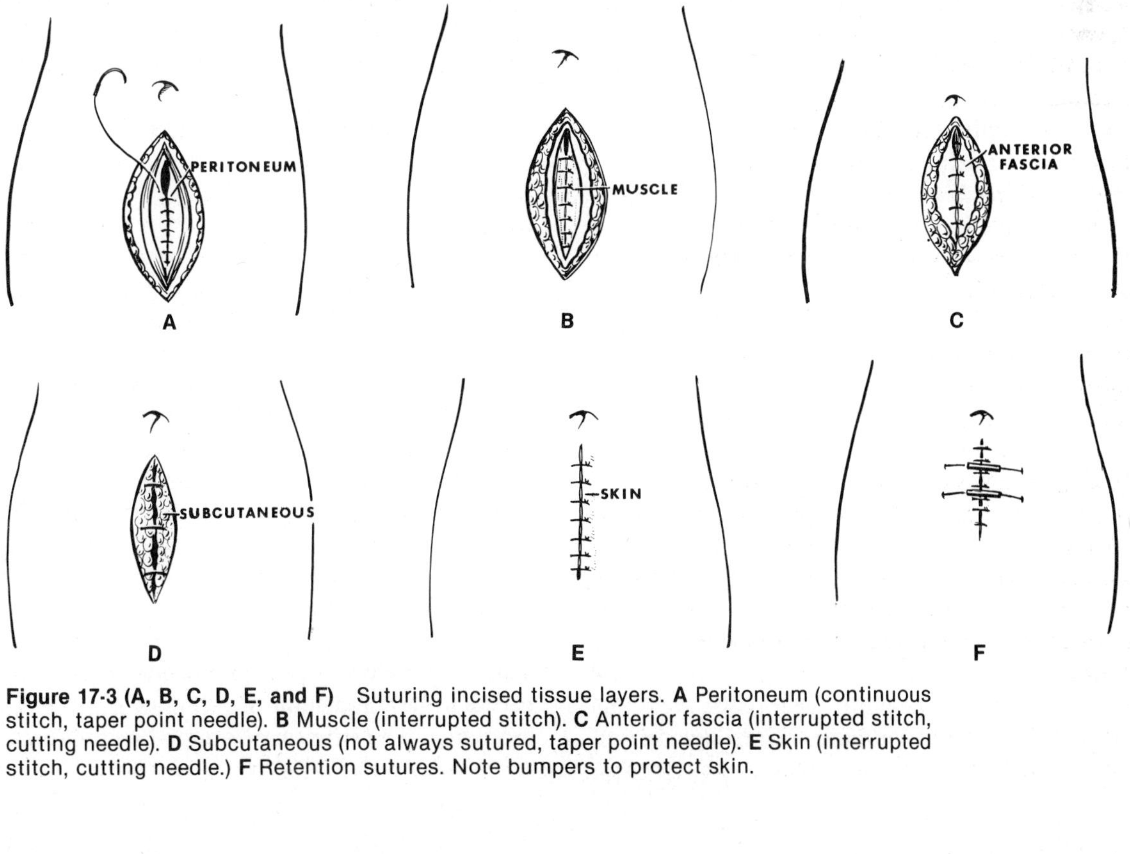

Figure 17-3 (A, B, C, D, E, and F) Suturing incised tissue layers. **A** Peritoneum (continuous stitch, taper point needle). **B** Muscle (interrupted stitch). **C** Anterior fascia (interrupted stitch, cutting needle). **D** Subcutaneous (not always sutured, taper point needle). **E** Skin (interrupted stitch, cutting needle.) **F** Retention sutures. Note bumpers to protect skin.

and aspirated by insertion inside the purse-string of a trocar with attached suction. After removal of the contaminated trocar, the opening is enlarged to permit insertion of a stone forceps or spoon and removal of any calculi. A drainage catheter is placed in the opening and the purse-string closed around it. The catheter may be secured with additional suture and the fundus of the gallbladder sutured to the abdominal wall to reduce the hazard of bile leakage. A Penrose drain is placed in the abdominal cavity and the wound closed. A specimen of the aspirated fluid is sent for culture.

Cholecystectomy

Removal of the gallbladder is the most common operation performed on the biliary tract. It is done to relieve gastrointestinal distress common in patients with acute or chronic cholecystitis with or without calculi. Also, it removes a source of recurrent sepsis.

Supine position is used with the gallbladder rest elevated. The table may be tilted slightly so that abdominal contents tend to gravitate downward away from the operative area. The gallbladder usually is reached through a right subcostal or right paramedian incision.

Following exploration of the abdominal cavity, laparotomy packs are used to wall off surrounding organs from the gallbladder. Infected contents must not be spilled into the peritoneal cavity, to prevent peritonitis. No attempt is made to remove the gallbladder until biliary tract structures are identified accurately. These include the cystic duct, cystic artery, hepatic ducts, and common bile duct. *Operative cholangiograms,* injection of radiopaque solution into the cystic duct or into a tube placed in the common duct, frequently are done intraoperatively to permit identification and removal of overlooked stones. The x-ray department is notified in advance if cholangiography is anticipated. Scout films should be taken when the patient is initially positioned on the operating table.

Concomitant *exploration of the common duct* often is done during cholecystectomy. Curved stone forceps, small malleable scoops, dilators of various sizes, and Fogarty balloon-tipped catheters are useful in clearing ducts of stones to prevent their lodging in the duct, with subsequent obstructive jaundice. *Intraoperative biliary endoscopy* by use of the choledochoscope gives image transmission and illumination allowing the surgeon visual guidance in exploring the biliary system. After the scope is introduced into the common duct, a flexible stone forceps or a Fogarty biliary catheter may be inserted through the instrument channel to allow manipulation of the stone under direct vision. A biopsy forceps may be inserted to obtain a tissue sample.

Blunt dissection with dry dissector sponges is used to separate adhesions caused by previous inflammation. If the gallbladder is tightly distended, it may be aspirated before removal. After palpation of the ducts for stones, and ligation and division of the cystic duct and artery, the gallbladder is removed. Penrose drains and/or T-tubes (in ducts) usually are inserted and brought out through the incision or stab wound to the right of the incision. Complications of cholecystectomy include hemorrhage and injury to the common duct.

Choledochostomy; Choledochotomy

Choledochostomy is drainage of the common bile duct through the abdominal wall. A T-tube is used for drainage. *Choledochotomy* is incision of the common bile duct for exploration and removal of stones. Intraoperative cholangiography may be performed before and after exploration and/or stone removal. The duct is irrigated after removal of calculi. Patency of the duct and of the ampulla of Vater is investigated. If a neoplasm is found during exploration, resectability is determined. However, many tumors of the liver or pancreas are inoperable. A T-tube is placed in the common duct and a Penrose drain inserted before abdominal closure if a cholecystectomy also is performed.

Cholecystoduodenostomy; Cholecystojejunostomy

These procedures are done to relieve an obstruction in the distal end of the common duct. They establish continuity, by anastomosis, between the gallbladder and duodenum or gallbladder and jejunum. Careful evaluation precedes operation. These are bypass procedures to avoid further obstructive jaundice.

Common causes of obstruction are calculi, stricture of the duct, or neoplasms of the duct, ampulla of Vater, or pancreas.

Choledochoduodenostomy; Choledochojejunostomy

These procedures are side-to-side anastomoses between the duodenum or jejunum and the common duct. They are carried out when the surgeon is not totally satisfied that all stones have been removed or is concerned about the possibility of subsequent reexploration.

LIVER PROCEDURES

The *liver* is the largest gland in the body and is divided into left and right segments or lobes. It is located in the upper right abdominal cavity beneath the diaphragm. The stomach, duodenum, and hepatic flexure of the colon lie directly beneath the liver. A tough fibrous sheath, *Glisson's capsule,* completely covers the organ. The tissue within the capsule is very friable and vascular. The hepatic artery, a branch of the celiac axis, maintains the arterial supply. Blood from the stomach, intestine, spleen, and pancreas is carried to the liver by the portal vein and its branches.

The many functions of the liver include forming and secreting bile, which aids digestion, transforming glucose into glycogen, which it stores, and helping to regulate blood volume. The liver is vital in metabolic function of the body. This organ has remarkable regenerative capacity and up to 80 percent may be resected with little or no alteration in hepatic function. Liver function tests are used to assess degree of functional impairment and evaluate liver activity and reserve. Most of these tests involve taking a series of blood samples from the patient for specific studies. Ascites may result from impaired liver function. The most frequent surgical interventions include:

Liver Needle Biopsy

A needle biopsy may be done to help establish diagnosis of hepatic disease. Since the procedure is done under local anesthesia, during explanation the patient must be instructed to take several deep breaths and to hold the breath and remain absolutely still while the needle is inserted. Failure of patient cooperation can cause needle penetration of the diaphragm or liver injury resulting in hemorrhage, a serious complication. Leakage of bile into the abdominal cavity may produce chemical peritonitis, an additional hazard. After prep and local anesthesia, with the patient supine, a Silverman biopsy needle is introduced into the liver via intercostal (transthoracic) or subcostal (transabdominal) route. After insertion, the needle is rotated, thus separating a fragment of tissue about 1 to 4 cm ($\frac{1}{2}$ to $1\frac{1}{2}$ in.) in length. The needle is withdrawn, the specimen removed and sent to pathology. As soon as the needle is removed, the patient is told to resume normal breathing and is assisted in turning onto the right side to compress the chest wall at the penetration site to prevent bile or blood seepage.

Drainage of Subphrenic and Subhepatic Abscesses

Abscesses in and about the liver may be caused by a variety of pyogenic microorganisms, secondary amebic types, or as secondary infections from abdominal organs. They generally are treated by incision and drainage. Care must be taken to avoid contamination of the pleural or peritoneal cavity. Location of the abscess determines approach, i.e., transpleural, subpleural, transperitoneal, or retroperitoneal.

Hepatic Resection

Indications for right or left hepatic lobectomy or wedge resection include metastatic or primary carcinoma or severe lacerations of the liver caused by trauma. Lacerations may cause intraperitoneal hemorrhage and shock.

The abdominal cavity is entered through a right subcostal incision that is extended through the seventh or eighth interspace. Or, a right upper abdominal vertical incision is used for laceration, to permit incision extension if necessary, and for exploration. It is necessary to divide the appropriate ligamentous attachments and ligate the anatomical veins and arteries before rotating the liver forward and segmentally excising the diseased or injured portion.

Liver tissue is very friable and hemostatic substances often are used to control bleeding. Prevention or arrest of hemorrhage is a prime concern. Large, blunt, noncutting needles are used to suture the organ. Drains usually are placed in the wound and brought out through the incision or adjacent drain sites. Equipment for blood replacement, portal pressure measurement, and thoracotomy drainage should be readily available.

SPLENIC PROCEDURES

The highly vascular *spleen* is located in the upper left abdominal cavity, protected by the lower portion of the rib cage, and lies beneath the dome of the diaphragm. The capsule of the spleen is covered with peritoneum and held in place by numerous suspensory ligaments. The splenic artery furnishes the arterial blood supply. The splenic vein drains into the portal system. As the largest lymphatic organ of the body, it has an intimate role in the immunologic defenses of the body and acts as a blood reservoir. The spleen has several functions, chiefly concerned with formation of blood elements. Roentgenographic examination and radionuclide scanning provide information in regard to diagnostic problems.

Splenectomy

The most common cause for removal is *hypersplenism* (overactivity that causes reduction in the circulating quantity of red cells, white cells, platelets, or a combination of them). Splenectomies frequently are scheduled at specific times since these patients often require administration of whole blood immediately prior to operation. Often the patients also are on steroid treatment and provisions must be made to maintain therapy during the operation and postoperatively. Traumatic ruptures, tumors, or accessory spleens also may be cause for operative intervention. Splenic rupture requires immediate operation to prevent fatal hemorrhage.

A left rectus paramedian or subcostal incision is used to enter the peritoneal cavity. The spleen is displaced medially by careful manual manipulation and the splenorenal, splenocolic, and gastrosplenic ligaments are ligated and divided. Great care must be exercised in ligating the splenic artery and vein as frequently these vessels are very friable. Hemorrhage is the principal hazard encountered intraoperatively. After removal of the spleen, careful inspection for bleeding from the splenic pedicle and retroperitoneal space is essential before closure. A drain, exteriorized through a stab wound, may be inserted in the left subdiaphragmatic space in patients with extensive trauma.

PANCREATIC PROCEDURES

The *pancreas* is both endocrine and exocrine gland. Islets of Langerhans comprise the endocrine division and secrete insulin and glucagon, hormones essential to carbohydrate metabolism and storage of calories. Acini and the ducts leading from them constitute the exocrine portion that secretes pancreatic juice into the duodenum. Pancreatic juice neutralizes stomach acid and loss of it results in severe impairment of digestion and foodstuff absorption.

The pancreas lies transversely across the posterior wall of the upper abdomen behind the stomach. The head or right extremity is attached to the duodenum and the tail or left extremity is in close proximity to the spleen.

Disorders of the pancreas generally include acute and chronic inflammation, cysts, and tumors. Accuracy of diagnosis in pancreatic problems is difficult, but evaluation by roentgenography, ultrasound, and scanning has led to significant improvement in planning operative treatment.

Pancreatitis most often is associated with gallstones or alcoholism. Corrective biliary tract operations usually alleviate gallstone pancreatitis.

Pancreaticojejunostomy

This may be performed for relief of pain associated with chronic alcoholic pancreatitis and pseudocysts of the pancreas. There are several types of procedures for drainage of obstructed ducts or pseudocysts. These involve anastomosing a loop of the jejunum to the pancreatic duct. Hemorrhage or leakage of bile are complications to be avoided.

Pancreaticoduodenectomy (Whipple Operation)

This extensive procedure is performed for patients with carcinoma of the head of the pancreas or ampulla of Vater. A gastrointestinal setup is used. The abdominal cavity is exposed through one of several possible anterior incisions, but usually a long right paramedian incision is made. The abdominal and pelvic cavities are explored for distant metastases. Since many vital structures and organs are involved in resecting the diseased portion of the pancreas, careful dissection of the vessels is emphasized to prevent hemorrhage, which complicates the procedure. Structures removed include part of the pancreas, the distal part of the stomach, and the duodenum. Several methods of reconstructing the digestive tract are possible but all include anastomosis of the pancreatic duct, common bile duct, stomach, and jejunum. Watertight seal of all anastomoses is essential to prevent peritonitis or pancreatitis. Drains are inserted.

Postoperatively, the most common complications are shock, hemorrhage, renal failure, and pancreatic or biliary fistula. If a fistula should occur, wound suction is continued until the fistula closes. Generally, it will close spontaneously if adequate nutrition and electrolyte balance are maintained.

Improvements in pre- and postoperative care

and refinement of technical details have increased the survival rate of this potentially hazardous radical operation.

GASTRIC PROCEDURES

The *stomach,* a hollow muscular organ, is situated in the upper left abdomen between the esophagus and duodenum. Anatomically it is divided into the fundus, body, and pyloric antrum. The two borders of the stomach, the *lesser* and *greater curvatures,* are important surgically because of their relation to the major vascular and lymphatic systems supplying the stomach. A double fold of peritoneum attached to the lesser and greater curvatures loosely covers the intestines. The autonomic nervous supply by the vagus nerve controls reflex activities of movement and secretions of the alimentary canal and is significant in the rhythmic relaxation of the pyloric sphincter.

Food entering the stomach must be reduced to a semiliquid consistency to pass through the duodenum and small intestine. Interference of gastric activity or muscular contractions results in gastrointestinal complaints. Abdominal pain, nausea, vomiting, hemorrhage, and dyspepsia are the major problems. Some diseases such as cancer may not produce symptoms until the condition is far advanced.

Operation is indicated when the presence of disease is established following laboratory tests such as gastric analysis, gastroscopy, and/or radiographic studies.

Separation of instruments used for resection and anastomosis, and abdominal closure is essential. Two distinct setups may be used, but the single setup, most commonly used, consists of identifying and using only selected instruments and supplies for resection, anastomosis, and abdominal closure, and discarding contaminated instruments and equipment from the field after use. Acid secretions from the resection site are very irritating and may cause peritonitis. Gloves are changed before closure, and in some hospitals gowns also may be changed.

It is necessary to have a variety of gastrointestinal tubes available in the OR for irrigation and aspiration. Electrosurgery frequently is used. Intestinal forceps jaws should be protected with soft rubber tubing to reduce tissue trauma. Stapling devices used to mechanically suture tissue are preferred by some surgeons. Warm saline is always required in abdominal procedures for laparotomy packs and irrigation.

Gastrointestinal Surgery and Metabolism

The advances of surgical management of patients with gastrointestinal problems has lessened the mortality rate, although treatment may be palliative rather than curative. Extensive diagnostic studies are done prior to operation unless it is an emergency situation such as acute perforation of a peptic ulcer.

Interference with the gastrointestinal tract affects its functioning and specific deficiencies may result from gastrointestinal surgery, depending on the site and extent. Massive resection of the small intestine can produce long-term nutritional problems, such as weight loss and malabsorption of most nutrients, thus endangering compatibility with life. Metabolic bone disease may follow gastric surgery, due to poor absorption of calcium and vitamin D. Patients who have undergone extensive gastric operation should have periodic nutritional evaluation. Biochemical tests monitor nutritional status. These include serum proteins, albumin/globulin determination and ratio, and blood urea nitrogen. Body weight is significant also. If caloric intake is inadequate, protein is converted to carbohydrate for energy and protein synthesis then suffers.

The *dumping syndrome* may be experienced by patients shortly after eating following gastric surgery. This complication occurs because of rapid emptying of food and fluids into the jejunum. It is characterized by nausea, vomiting, sensations of weakness and dizziness, pallor, sweating, palpitations, and diarrhea. It usually subsides within 6 months to a year.

Gastric Procedures

Gastroscopy This is the passage of a fiberoptic scope via the mouth into the stomach. The operator is able to visually inspect the walls of the stomach and sometimes remove a tissue specimen, thus allowing differential diagnosis.

Total Gastrectomy The entire stomach is excised through a bilateral subcostal, long transrectus, or thoracoabdominal incision. This procedure is done for malignant lesions in the stomach. The operation necessitates reconstruction of esophagointestinal continuity by establishing an anastomosis between a loop of the jejunum and the esophagus. Leakage at the site of the anastomosis leads to peritonitis. Frequently, gastric carcinomas are inoperable due to extended metastases to the liver and surrounding tissues. The type of operation performed is determined after thorough exploration of the abdominal cavity by the surgeon.

Partial Gastrectomy, Billroth I-II, Subtotal Gastrectomy The presence of a benign or malignant lesion located in the pyloric half of the stomach requires removal of the lower half to two-thirds of the stomach. In patients with peptic or duodenal ulcer, the operation relieves pain, bleeding, vomiting, weight loss, and limits gastric acidity. The peritoneal cavity is entered through a right paramedian abdominal incision and a variety of operations may be used to reestablish gastrointestinal continuity. Anastomosing the remaining portion of the stomach to the duodenum, gastroduodenostomy (Billroth I) or to a loop of the jejunum, gastrojejunostomy (Billroth II) frequently are done.

The most common modifications of the Billroth I method include the Schoemaker and the von Haberer-Finney techniques. The Schoemaker operation involves end-to-end anastomosis of the stomach and duodenum after the lesser curvature of the stomach is sutured to make the anastomosis site the same size as the duodenum. With the von Haberer-Finney method, the lateral wall of the duodenum is brought up to the stomach so the entire end of the stomach is open for direct anastomosis.

The popular Billroth II modifications include Polya and Hofmeister techniques. These involve variations of end-to-side gastrojejunostomy.

Gastrostomy The establishment of a temporary or permanent opening in the stomach is indicated to serve as a feeding tube when a patient cannot tolerate major operation or the lesion is inoperable. It may be used in patients with extensive esophageal lesion. Through a small upper left abdominal or midline incision the stomach is exposed and a catheter or tube inserted into the anterior gastric wall. It is held in place with a purse-string suture. Foleys and various mushroom catheters frequently are used. Related procedures include:

Vagotomy and Pyloroplasty Chronic peptic ulcers and gastric ulcers that do not respond to medical treatment cause patients severe pain and difficulty in eating and sleeping. A combination vagotomy and pyloroplasty may be recommended since it interrupts vagal impulses, thus lowering gastric hydrochloric acid production and hastens gastric emptying. *Vagotomy* is division of the vagus nerve; *pyloroplasty* is enlarging the pyloric opening. Vagotomy with gastroenterostomy or vagotomy and antrectomy may be selected depending on the individual case. Offering conservative operative therapy as compared to gastrectomy, these procedures have decreased operative risk.

INTESTINAL PROCEDURES

The intestines is an inclusive term referring to the continuous muscular tube of the bowel, which extends from the lower end of the stomach to the rectum. Food and products of digestion pass through this section of the alimentary canal during the processes of digestion, absorption, and elimination of waste products. Anatomically, the intestines are divided into the small (upper) and large (lower) intestine, with subdivisions of each.

The small intestine extends from the pylorus to the ileocecal valve. The three sections include the *duodenum* or proximal portion, the *jejunum* or middle section, and the *ileum* or distal portion that joins the large intestine. The *ileocecal valve,* a sphincter muscle, prevents return of material that has been discharged to the large intestine.

The large intestine or *colon* extends from the ileum to the rectum and is generally divided into ascending, transverse, descending, and sigmoid colon. A blind pouch, the *cecum,* is formed where the large intestine joins the small intestine.

The *mesentery,* a peritoneal fold, attaches the small and large intestines to the posterior abdominal wall, and contains the blood vessels that nourish the intestines.

Inflammation, intestinal obstruction, and disruption in absorption and motility are disorders that may lead to surgical intervention. Etiology of the disorder determines the operative procedure.

Resection of Small Intestine

Certain tumors, strangulation from adhesions, volvulus, obstruction, and regional ileitis usually are treated by resection of the involved segment. An abdominal incision is made over the suspected or known site of pathology. After exposure, clamps are placed above and below the diseased segment of the bowel and mesentery to avoid spillage. The involved area is resected. An end-to-end, end-to-side, or side-to-side anastomosis is done to restore continuity. Variations of this technique are used for other related problems of the small intestine such as extensive perforation.

NOTE. Bowel strangulation and obstruction necessitate immediate operation to prevent necrosis, peritonitis, and death.

Jejunoileal Bypass

Intestinal bypass procedures have been developed to treat the morbidly obese patient. Variations of the procedure simply bypass a portion of the intestinal tract, thus causing derangement of normal bowel continuity. This in turn produces a malabsorption state initiating weight loss. The procedure most frequently performed is the jejunoileal bypass. The Wise (modified Scott) method anastomoses the proximal jejunum end-to-end to the distal ileum.

Persons who weigh more than 100 lb over ideal weight, have no serious disease, and have failed to lose weight despite years of medical treatment are potential candidates for this procedure.

The physical size of the patient presents special needs in transporting, positioning, instrumentation, and psychological support.

Diarrhea, fluid and electrolyte imbalance, and liver changes are the most common postoperative complications.

Hemicolectomy, Transverse Colectomy, Anterior Resection, Total Colectomy

Various operations may be performed to remove a diseased segment of the colon. Colitis, diverticulitis, obstruction, and neoplasms are the most frequent reasons for operative intervention. There are numerous opinions regarding effective surgical management, but fundamentally all involve opening the abdomen, walling off the peritoneal cavity, incising and clamping at the points where resection is to be carried out, and finally reestablishing continuity by anastomosis. The separate instrument technique must be employed in intestinal procedures.

Bowel procedures are major ones requiring pre- and postoperative supportive care of the patient. Specifically, this care includes preoperative administration of intestinal antibiotics, bowel-cleansing methods, and diet restrictions. Postoperatively, nasogastric tubes inserted before operation remain in place until partial healing of the anastomosis occurs and effective peristalsis returns. Fluid and electrolyte balance must be maintained.

Intestinal Stomas

An intestinal *-ostomy* is a surgically created opening, stoma, from a portion of the bowel to the exterior, via the abdominal wall. The procedure is:

1 To divert intestinal contents so as to permit healing of inflamed bowel

2 To decompress pressure caused by an obstructive lesion or to bypass the obstruction, such as a benign or malignant tumor

The type and level of the lesion determine whether an ileostomy, cecostomy, or colostomy is indicated. The opening may be permanent or temporary, depending on the etiology and course of the disease or obstruction. In patients with a temporary stoma, intestinal continuity is reestablished following healing by closure of the opening in the bowel and anastomosis of the previously resected ends. Following combined abdominoperineal resection for rectal carcinoma, a permanent colostomy in the sigmoid colon forms an artificial anus. A collection device for fecal material is not needed after a patient's bowel evacuation becomes regulated.

Patient acceptance of these procedures is as varied as an individual's emotional reactions. Each patient requires a rehabilitation plan based on personal needs. These plans should include care of collection device, maintenance of skin integrity, proper diet, odor control, and comfortable concealing clothing. Patient participation is an integral part of preparation for self-care and enhances self-confidence.

Ileostomy This procedure is performed for a condition such as chronic ulcerative colitis, or following removal of the colon (*colectomy*). The proximal end of the transected ileum is externalized through the abdominal wall. The liquid or semisolid discharge is collected in an ileostomy bag. The skin around the stoma requires special care, such as use of karaya gum, to prevent excoriation and irritation.

Cecostomy This operation creates an opening between the cecum and lower right side of the abdomen. It may be performed as an emergency decompression prior to subsequent colon resection.

Colostomy This procedure establishes an opening from some portion of the colon to the exterior, thus creating an artificial anus. It is performed at a more distant level than the previous procedures, either in the transverse or descending colon. Either a double-barreled or loop colostomy may be performed. In the *double-barreled colostomy,* the transverse colon is divided and both ends are brought out to the margins of the skin incision. The proximal stoma serves as an outlet for stool while the distal opening leads to the nonfunctioning bowel. In the *loop-colostomy* method, a loop of transverse colon is brought out onto the abdominal wall and a glass rod is placed under the loop to hold it out on the exterior abdominal wall. A short length of rubber tubing is connected to each end to stabilize the rod in position. The peritoneum is closed and the wound around the colostomy sutured. Some surgeons prefer to leave an intestinal clamp in place. This is exteriorized until the stoma is opened and then removed.

Appendectomy

Appendicitis can occur at any age but is seen most frequently in adolescents and young adults. It may sometimes imitate many other conditions such as pneumonia, ruptured ovarian cyst, or ureteral calculus. Some appendices are retrocecal, making diagnosis more obscure. Classical symptoms of early appendicitis include right lower quadrant pain, rebound tenderness, nausea, and moderate temperature and white blood count elevation.

Emergency operative removal of an acutely inflamed vermiform appendix is necessary to prevent progression to gangrene and perforation of friable tissue, with subsequent peritonitis. A right lower quadrant, muscle-splitting incision is made over McBurney's point. Suction must be readily available. The blood supply is ligated and severed. A crushing clamp is applied to the appendiceal base, which is then ligated and severed from the cecum. Following amputation, the surgeon may elect to cauterize the stump with phenol and alcohol to reduce contamination or invert the stump into the cecum as a purse-string suture is tightened around the stump, or do both. Since the intestinal tract is laden with bacteria, a culture generally is taken in case of future infection.

Drainage is indicated in the presence of an abscess, rupture of the appendix, or any gross contamination of the wound.

Usually appendectomy is an uncomplicated procedure with rapid convalescence unless life-threatening peritonitis results.

COLORECTAL PROCEDURES

Colorectal carcinoma is one of the most common abdominal malignancies. It affects approximately 100,000 persons annually with females having the highest incidence. Almost two out of three who die of it might be saved by early diagnosis and prompt treatment. Surgical resection of the carcinoma is the treatment of choice; however, electrocoagulation and cryosurgery have been proven valuable in elderly or high-risk patients who have low-lying rectal cancers.

Various procedures aid diagnosis and are performed in patients with bowel or rectal bleeding, chronic diarrhea, or history of polyps and/or carcinoma of the colon. These procedures routinely are done before rectal or colorectal surgery. Serial guaiac stool tests are valuable in testing for occult blood. Barium enema, which frequently follows endoscopy, provides complete radiographic study of the colon. Some therapeutic procedures also may be accomplished through endoscopes.

Sigmoidoscopy

This is direct visual inspection of sigmoid and rectal lumens by means of a rigid lighted endoscope, usually fiberoptic.

The patient is carefully prepared preoperatively with enemas. Knee-chest or Kraske position allows the sigmoid colon to fall forward into the abdomen. Sims or lithotomy position may be used for an extremely obese or extremely ill patient. The surgeon may inflate air to better visualize the mucosal walls. This causes a feeling of desire to defecate, which necessitates reassurance of the patient.

Colonoscopy

This provides visual inspection of the lining of the entire colon. The scope is flexible and consists of two channels, one for suctioning and one for operating. Although valuable to confirm or amplify x-ray findings, colonoscopy is not a replacement for barium enema. Its greatest use is for survey of the cancer-prone colon, especially search for and excision of polyps. Other indications are for study of inflammatory bowel or diverticular disease, passage of blood in the feces (hemochezia), change in bowel habits, preoperative screen prior to colostomy closure, confirmation of x-ray findings, and followup of patients who had intestinal procedures performed.

Preparation consists of clear liquids for 48 hours, castor oil at bedtime, and saline enemas until clear the morning of the procedure. Lateral position is used, and the scope introduced through the anus.

Contraindications are the precariously ill or uncooperative patient. If perforation is likely, relative contraindications may include acute, severe, or radiation inflammatory disease or complete obstruction.

Among the complications are electrical burn during polypectomy, tear or perforation of the colon by tip pressure, tear of the liver or the spleen by air pressure, tear of diverticuli by introduction of air into them.

Polypectomy

This often is performed through a sigmoidoscope or colonoscope. However, in some patients polyps are excised or the involved segment of colon removed by abdominal approach, although the development of colonoscopy has reduced need for laparotomy.

Many surgeons and pathologists believe that every mucosal polyp in the terminal colon is a potential malignancy and should be removed. Intestinal polyps may be single or multiple. Although benign and often of familial tendency, they frequently undergo malignant changes. Polyps easily are excised at the base. If they are pedunculated, they are cauterized and retrieved. Electrocoagulation of the base provides hemostasis. These patients are followed for the remainder of their lives as adenomatous polyps, common in the colon, are prone to become malignant.

Abdominoperineal Resection

This is an extensive procedure for mainly rectal, but sometimes lower sigmoid or anal canal carcinoma. Preoperative preparation is meticulous for verification of the diagnosis, search for metastases, and optimal condition of the patient. Prior to operation, a Levin or Miller-Abbott tube is inserted, ureteral catheters often are inserted, and an indwelling bladder catheter is attached to a closed-drainage system.

Two approaches, abdominal and perineal, are required, necessitating prep and drape of both areas. After resection of the sigmoid, contaminated instruments are removed from the field, as the colon is a reservoir of bacteria. Two sets of instruments are necessary. With the patient in Trendelenburg position, the peritoneal cavity is entered through a lower abdominal incision. Preliminary exploration is done to seek metastases. If the tumor is resectable, the sigmoid colon is mobilized, clamped, and divided. Using the proximal end of the sigmoid, a permanent colostomy is created. The sigmoid is externalized through a stab wound in the left lower quadrant and a clamp placed on the colostomy to maintain its position. The mesentery may be sutured to the abdominal wall to prevent internal hernias. The distal end of the sigmoid is tied to prevent contamination, and placed deep in the presacral space for ultimate removal. The pelvic floor is reperitonealized and the abdomen closed. Dressings are placed on the abdominal incision and the colostomy.

The second phase of the operation is closure of the anus with a purse-string suture to prevent contamination, and removal of the anus, rectum, rectosigmoid, surrounding nodes and lymphatics through a perineal incision. Drains are placed and the perineum closed.

When the abdominal and perineal procedures are done simultaneously, two teams are employed. The patient is initially positioned supine in modified lithotomy position. This approach reduces operating time and blood loss and provides simultaneous exposure of abdominal and perineal fields.

Patients must be carefully monitored to prevent hypovolemic shock because of the great amount of blood loss from vascular areas and length of the procedure.

ANORECTAL PROCEDURES

Hemorrhoids, abscesses, fissures, and fistulas are frequently indications for surgical intervention. The anal region is well supplied with nerves and these procedures often cause much discomfort. Patients also are sensitive and embarrassed because of the operative site. Following rectal surgery, patients may have initial difficulty voiding and usually experience considerable pain, requiring medication and sitz baths.

Anoscopy, Proctoscopy, Sigmoidoscopy

These diagnostic procedures are used to visually examine the mucosa of the anus, rectum, and sigmoid. Sigmoidoscopy is routinely done before rectal surgery and in routine physical examination. Fiberoptic equipment has aided in early detection of tumors, polyps, and ulcerations.

Hemorrhoidectomy

This is surgical excision and ligation of varicosities of the veins of the anus and rectum that do not respond to conservative treatment. Hemorrhoids are classified as *internal* (occurring above the internal sphincter) or *external* (appearing outside the external sphincter). Often both types are present in the patient. External hemorrhoids cause pruritis and pain. The internal type frequently bleed and may become thrombosed and edematous. Rectal bleeding cannot be assumed to be from hemorrhoids, but requires thorough investigation to rule out gastrointestinal disease.

The usual procedure consists of dilating the sphincter, ligating the hemorrhoidal pedicle with suture ligatures, and excising each hemorrhoidal mass. The electrosurgical or cryosurgical unit may be employed. Kraske position usually is used, with the patient's buttocks retracted by hemorrhoid straps fastened to the edges of the operating table. Petrolatum gauze packing is inserted in the anal canal, or a compression dressing and perineal binder are applied at completion of operation.

Incision and Drainage of Anal Abscess

Localized infection in the tissues around the anus results in abscess formation. Early incision and drainage are essential to prevent the infection from spreading.

Fistulotomy/Fistulectomy

Formation of a fistula-in-ano often results following incision and drainage or spontaneous drainage of an abscess. The fistulous tract may be opened to allow drainage and healing by granulation, or the tract may be excised. Injection of a dye or use of a probe and grooved director aid in identifying the tract.

Fissurectomy

This operation is necessary when a benign ulcerative lesion occurs in the lining of the anal canal. The anus is dilated and the infected tissue excised. Fecal incontinence due to damage to the anal sphincter is a potential complication the surgeon tries to avoid.

Treatment of Rectal Tumors

Surgeons prefer to study a small rectal cancer under anesthesia (often caudal) and not hasten into a radical operation, since many such cancers are amenable to local treatment using an operating endoscope and microsurgical technique. Electrosurgical cutting and coagulation can be combined to leave a treatment crater, sweeping away a superficial cancer. The cutting loop is used to sweep or comb the tumor back and forth; needle coagulation is used for depth and penetrates the tumor to destroy tissue. For electrosection, the lesion should be small, mobile, polypoid, and posterior, with no palpable rectal lymph nodes.

Protocol includes external radiation therapy, electrocoagulation, and reevaluation in 6 weeks. Sometimes interstitial radiation therapy is used for small anorectal squamous-cell carcinoma.

EXCISION OF PILONIDAL CYST AND SINUS

A painful, draining cyst with fistulous tract(s) may occur in soft tissues of the sacrococcygeal region. When they become infected, drainage is necessary to relieve pain, swelling, and suppuration. The cyst and sinus tracts must be *excised* or *marsupialized* to prevent recurrence. Marsupialization is the suturing of the cyst walls to the edges of the wound, following evacuation, to permit the packed cavity to close by granulation. Surgical judgment determines whether primary closure or healing by granulation is chosen. A compression dressing is applied.

HERNIA PROCEDURES

A *hernia* is the protrusion of an organ or part of an organ through a defect in supporting structures that normally contain it. A hernia may be congenital, acquired, or traumatic. The majority of hernias occur in the inguinal or femoral region; however, umbilical, ventral, and hiatus hernias do occur.

Usually a hernia is composed of a covering (the sac), the hernial contents, and an aperture, but in some locations the covering or sac is absent.

When hernial contents can be returned to the normal cavity by manipulation, the hernia is called *reducible.* If the hernial contents cannot be reduced, it is called *irreducible* or *incarcerated.* Bowel present in an incarcerated hernia may not only lack adequate blood supply but may also become obstructed. This is referred to as a *strangulated* hernia. Immediate operation is necessary to prevent necrosis of the strangulated bowel.

Inguinal Herniorrhaphy (Hernioplasty)

Repair of inguinal hernias involves two types, indirect and direct.

Indirect The peritoneal sac containing intestine, protrudes through the internal inguinal ring and passes down the inguinal canal. It may descend all the way into the scrotum. Indirect inguinal hernia, more common in males, represents a congenital defect.

Direct This operation is used to repair a weakness of the fascial floor of the inguinal canal. The hernia protrudes through the abdominal wall in the region between the rectus abdominis muscle, inguinal ligament, and inferior epigastric artery. This hernia is the most difficult type to repair and appears more frequently in men. An acquired weakness of the lower abdominal wall, a direct inguinal hernia often results from straining, such as heavy lifting, chronic coughing, or straining to urinate or defecate. Prompt operative repair avoids possible discomfort and threat of later complications.

Femoral Herniorrhaphy

This procedure involves repairing the defect in the transversalis fascia as well as removing the peritoneal sac protruding through the femoral ring. Normally, the transversalis fascia is attached to Cooper's ligament, which prevents the peritoneum from reaching the femoral ring. To repair this defect it is necessary to reconstruct the posterior wall and close the femoral ring. These hernias appear more frequently in women.

Umbilical Herniorrhaphy

Repair of an umbilical hernia consists of closing the peritoneal opening and uniting the fascia above and below the defect to reconstruct the abdominal wall surrounding the umbilicus. This type of hernia, seen most frequently in children, represents a congenital defect of protrusion of peritoneum through the umbilical ring. It also may be acquired by women following childbirth.

Ventral (Incisional) Herniorrhaphy

Impaired healing of a previous operative incision, usually a vertical abdominal one, may cause incisional hernia. Often the result of weakening of abdominal fascia, projections of peritoneum carrying segments of bowel protrude through fascial perforations. It is necessary to reunite the tissue layers to close the defect.

After excising the old scar, the peritoneal sac is opened, the hernia reduced, and the layers firmly closed. If existing tissue is not sufficient for repair, synthetic mesh may be used to reinforce the repair.

Incisional hernias are sometimes the aftermath of postoperative hematoma, infection, or undue strain.

Hiatus (Diaphragmatic) Herniorrhaphy

A hiatus hernia results when a portion of the stomach protrudes through the hiatus of the diaphragm. The *hiatus* is the opening for the esophagus through the *diaphragm,* which is the chief muscle of respiration. A weakening in the hiatus permits violation of the muscular partition between abdomen and chest.

Symptoms largely are due to inflammation and ulceration of the adjacent esophagus, caused by reflux of gastric juices from the herniated stomach. Symptoms include pain, blood loss, and difficulty in swallowing (*dysphagia*). Diagnosis is made by radiologic and endoscopic studies.

Surgical treatment is appropriate when medical therapy fails to alleviate the problem. Operative approach may be via the abdomen or chest, or thoracoabdominal. Each offers certain advantages. However, the better view of the hiatal region afforded by opening the thorax favors this approach. Repair of hiatus hernia frequently is performed by a thoracic surgeon utilizing thoracic routines, such as chest-tube insertion and underwater-seal drainage (refer to Chaps. 12 and 21).

LIGATION AND STRIPPING OF VEINS

When the valves of the veins fail to function normally, the increased back pressure of blood in the veins causes them to become dilated, tortuous, or elongated (varicose veins). Pain and secondary complications such as thrombophlebitis and varicose ulcers from venous stasis may follow. It is believed that there is a familial tendency toward varicosities, which afflict both men and women. Habitual long periods of standing, repeated pregnancies, and obesity are other predisposing factors.

Operative treatment consists of ligating the great saphenous vein at the femoral junction. The vein then is excised in toto with the aid of a stripping device, additional incisions being made along its course from groin to ankle as required to excise affected tributaries. Preoperatively, the surgeon may wish to mark with an indelible marker areas of varicosity for incision.

Following closure of the incisions and dressing applications, the full length of the leg is wrapped in cotton elastic bandages for compression.

Postoperatively, it is important to stimulate circulation and prevent venous thrombosis by early ambulation.

AMPUTATION OF EXTREMITIES

Amputation is the total or partial removal of any extremity. Necessity for amputation is associated most frequently with massive trauma, presence of malignant tumor, extensive infection, and vascular insufficiency.

In preparing a patient for a lower extremity amputation, expose both legs for comparison before the skin preparation in addition to checking the chart. *Be absolutely certain the correct leg is prepared.*

Many lower extremity amputations are done under spinal anethesia. See that the specimen is never, at any time, within the patient's sight. Follow hospital policy in regard to patient's permission for disposal of an extremity.

Two types of amputation generally are performed, *open* (*guillotine*) and *closed.*

The guillotine operation, rarely performed, is regarded as an emergency procedure. Tissues are cut circularly with the bone transected higher to allow soft tissues to cover the bone end. Blood vessels and nerve endings are ligated, but the wound is left open. The operation frequently is followed by prolonged drainage and healing, muscle and skin retraction, and excessive granulation tissue. A second operation often is required for final repair. Patients who are severely ill or toxic, or experience severe trauma, such as an extremity caught under an immovable object, are candidates for this operation.

The conventional flap or closed type of amputation is more desirable. Constructing curved skin and fascial flaps prior to amputating the bone allows for deep and superficial fascia to be approximated over the bone end before loose skin closure. Drainage by catheter or suction apparatus may or may not be required. The wound usually heals in about 2 weeks.

Amputations of the Lower Extremity

Amputations of the lower extremity are classified as above the knee (AK), below the knee (BK), toe, transphalangeal, transmetatarsal, and Syme amputation. The level of amputation is determined by the patient's general health, vascular status, and rehabilitative potential.

AK Amputation This involves the lower third of the thigh, and is selected when gangrene or arterial insufficiency extends above the level of the malleoli. Mid-thigh amputation involves circular incision over the distal femur, creating large anterior and posterior skin flaps, transecting fasciae and muscles. Vessels and nerves such as the femoral and sciatic, respectively, are ligated and severed. Sharp bone edges of the stump are smoothed by filing and the wound well irrigated with sterile saline before closure of tissue layers. Hemostasis is important to prevent massive hemorrhage or painful hematoma. Depending on surgeon's preference, drains may be used. A noncompressive dressing is applied. A longer time is required for rehabilitation than after BK amputation since AK is a more extensive procedure. A prosthesis generally is fitted 4 to 6 weeks after amputation.

BK Amputation This transects the middle third of the leg and provides for more functional prosthesis fitting and reduction of phantom limb pain. It permits a more natural gait. An immediate postoperative prosthesis (IPOP) can be applied in the operating room. The IPOP dressing requires a stump sock, felt and lamb's wool for padding, twill Y straps that are attached to a fitted corset, and a rigid plaster dressing. This dressing not only protects the stump, but aids in controlling the weight placed on it. The prosthesis is metal and provides a pull on the stump. The pylon (foot) may be attached before the patient returns to the unit. However, if the patient is obese or debilitated, weight bearing may be delayed several days.

Toe, Transphalangeal, and Transmetatarsal Amputations These are generally performed for gangrene and osteomyelitis.

Syme Amputation This is usually performed for trauma and involves the distal part of the foot. The amputation is above the ankle joint. The skin of the heel is used for the flap.

Hip Disarticulation and Hemipelvectomy These are radical procedures involving total removal of a posterior extremity including the hipbone. They are indicated for malignant bone or soft tissue tumors and extensive traumatic injuries. These operations most often are performed by orthopaedic surgeons. Specialized prosthetic devices are available to permit ambulation.

Amputations of the Upper Extremity

Amputations in the Hand Such amputations usually result from trauma and include part or all of the distal phalanges of the digits. Attention should be directed to keep the hand as a working unit when one or more fingers are removed. In any event, every effort should be made to save the thumb, since the smallest stump is better than a prosthesis.

Forearm and Forequarter Amputation Wrist, elbow, and humerus disarticulations are radical procedures performed for malignant tumors or extensive trauma.

Rehabilitation

Postoperative considerations of any amputation include control of bleeding and phantom limb sensations, stump care, immediate fitting and functional terminal prosthesis, exercises to prevent flexion contractures, and ambulation or use of a hand or arm.

The loss of an extremity involves major adjustment psychologically and physically. The rehabilitative process, so important, often is affected by the emotional reactions of the amputee. Patients with an early postoperative prosthesis have a more positive outlook about their loss. Being able to walk the first postoperative day or soon thereafter (which will depend on the surgeon's orders for the weight-bearing program in the case of a leg amputee) boosts morale. This in turn aids in ambulation.

The combined efforts of patient, family, and interdisciplinary professional personnel are needed for successful rehabilitation.

Refer to Chapter 28 for discussion of replantation of traumatically severed extremities.

Chapter 18

Gynecology

Gynecology, commonly referred to as "gyn," is the science of diseases of the female reproductive organs. Gynecological surgery also includes certain problems of the female genitourinary tract.

HISTORICAL DEVELOPMENT

Ancient interest in diseases of women is attested to by recordings in the Egyptian *Ebers papyrus* dating from the sixteenth century B.C. Treatises on gynecology included therapeutic agents. Hippocrates was familiar with the use of gynecological instruments centuries later. During the Greco-Roman period, Galen, Celsus, and Soranus of Ephesus dealt with gynecological conditions. The writings of Soranus, who practiced in Rome in the second century A.D., were regarded as authority for 1500 years. During that time, removal of a prolapsed uterus by cautery was a suggested procedure. Writers on gynecology in the fourth and fifth centuries A.D. merely compiled the work of predecessors. Practice remained bound by ancient authority and tradition and even regressed during the medieval period. It was not until the Renaissance that new interest developed in medicine, as in the fine arts. In 1566, Caspar Wolf of Switzerland issued a large encyclopedia of gynecology entitled *Gynecia.*

Reports by Hendrik van Roonhuze (seventeenth century) on extrauterine pregnancy, uterine rupture, and vesicovaginal fistula are regarded as the first writings on operative gynecology that have modern connotation. In the following century, practitioners advocated treatment of ovarian cysts by tapping or excision. Retroversion of the uterus and removal of extrauterine pregnancy were also described.

Operative gynecology became an independent specialty in the early nineteenth century with the works of Ephraim McDowell and James Sims. In 1809, McDowell removed an ovarian cyst by abdominal approach and the patient survived for 31 years. Sims became famous for treating vesicovaginal fistulas. A limited variety of gynecological procedures such as oophorectomy and salpingectomy were developed by succeeding pioneers. The first successful vaginal hysterectomy was performed in 1818.

Early gynecologists had to fight public prejudice against exposure of the female organs for examination. Clergy, midwives, and some physicians as well were among those attempting to deter such practice. Examination of organs by speculum was a notable advance. The progress of surgery in general, which followed development of antisepsis and anesthesia, eventually overcame opposition.

Because of their anatomical and physiological relationships, clinical gynecology and obstetrics combined into a single specialty. The American Board of Obstetrics and Gynecology was established in 1930. However, some surgeons limit their practice to one or the other area.

Obstetricians and gynecologists were influential in introducing the concept of periodic health examination on a large scale. Obstetricians aim to protect the pregnant woman and unborn fetus from unnecessary complications. The intent of gynecologists is to discover and treat pelvic disease, especially carcinoma, in early stages. This discussion is limited to gynecology.

ANATOMY AND PHYSIOLOGY

The genitourinary system comprises the organs, glands, secretions, and other elements of reproduction. Its components are both external and internal organs (see Fig. 18-1). A review of anatomy and physiology of the female reproductive system will help the learner comprehend surgical therapy.

External Genitalia

Vulva is a collective term for the female external genitalia. This sensitive, delicate area is highly vascular, with an extensive lymph supply and rich cutaneous sensory innervation. The vulva includes:

Labia Majora These are two large folds or lips containing sebaceous and sweat glands imbedded in fatty tissue covered by skin. They join together anteriorly in a fatty pad, the *mons veneris,* which overlies the pubic bone. Sebaceous secretions of the labia lubricate the proximal area. The labia majora atrophy after menopause, making the labia minora more prominent.

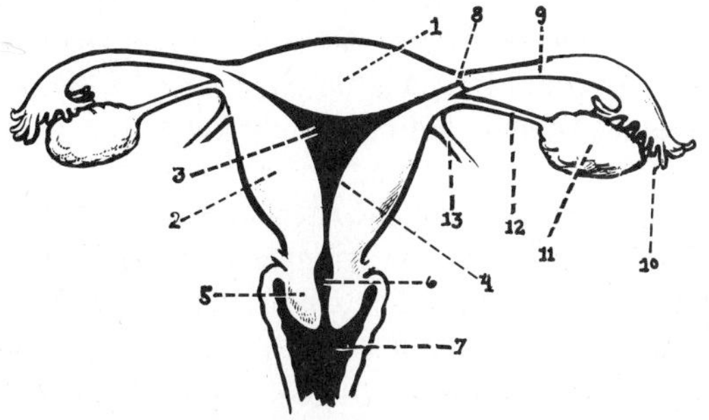

Figure 18-1 Female reproductive system. (1) uterine fundus, (2) corpus uteri, (3) uterine cavity, (4) endometrium, (5) cervix, (6) endocervical canal, (7) vagina, (8) cornu, (9) fallopian tube, (10) fimbria, (11) ovary, (12) ovarian ligament, (13) round ligament.

Labia Minora These small lips, lying within the labia majora, are flat folds of connective tissue containing sebaceous glands. Anteriorly these labia split into two parts. One part passes over the clitoris to form the protective prepuce or foreskin. The other passes under the clitoris to shape a *frenulum* or fold of mucous membrane. Posteriorly they join across the midline to form the *fourchette* or fold of skin just inside the posterior vulvar commissure.

Clitoris This erectile organ is the female homologue of the penis. The mucous membrane covering the glans contains many nerve endings. The urethra opens just below the clitoris.

Vestibule This is the space, or shallow elliptical depression below the clitoris, enclosed by the labia minora. The fourchette bounds it posteriorly. Opening into the vestibule are four canals: the urethra, the vagina, and the bilateral ducts from the Bartholin's glands.

Bartholin's glands These small bilateral glands lie deep in the posterior third of the labia majora, within the bulbocavernosus muscle. The mucous secretion is a coital lubricant.

Hymen This is a thin vascularized connective tissue membrane that surrounds and may partially or completely occlude the vaginal orifice. It varies individually in thickness and elasticity. The central aperture permits passage of menstrual flow and vaginal secretions.

Perineum This is a diamond-shaped wedge of fibromuscular tissue between the vagina and the anus. It is divided by a transverse septum into an anterior urogenital triangle and a posterior anal triangle. It consists of the perineal body and perineal musculature. With the fibers of six muscles converging at its central point, the perineum forms the base of the pelvic floor and helps support the posterior vaginal wall. These muscles are the bulbocavernosus (vaginal sphincter), the two superficial transverse perineal, the two levator ani, and the external anal sphincter. The levators ani are the largest and, in contrast to the other superficial muscles, are deep. The most important muscles in the pelvis, the levators ani (pelvic diaphragm) form a hammock-type suspension from anterior to posterior pelvic wall, beneath the pelvic viscera. These muscles retain the organs within the pelvis by offering resistance to repeated increases in intra-abdominal pressure, such as coughing, respiration, bearing down in labor, and straining at stool.

Internal Genital Organs

The internal organs lie within the pelvic cavity, protected by the bony pelvis. Bones and ligaments form the pelvic outlet. The dilated cervix of the uterus and the vagina constitute the birth canal.

Vagina The vagina is a thin-walled, fibromuscular tube extending from the vestibule obliquely backward and upward to the uterus, where the cervix projects into the top of the anterior wall. Constituting a copulatory and parturient canal, the vagina is capable of great distention. The bladder lies anteriorly to it, the rectum posteriorly.

The vagina is lined with mucous membrane and contains glands that produce a cleansing acid secretion.

The anterior vaginal wall is shorter than the posterior. The upper third of the posterior wall is covered by peritoneum reflected onto the rectum. Normally the anterior and posterior walls relax and are in contact. However, the lateral walls remain rigid due to the pull of the muscles and therefore are in close contact with pelvic tissues.

A rich venous plexus in the muscular walls makes the organ highly vascular. Uterine and vaginal arteries supplying the area are branches of the internal iliac artery. Branches of the vaginal artery extend to the external genitalia and the adjacent bladder and rectum. Lymphatic drainage is extensive. The upper two-thirds of the vagina drains into the external and internal iliac nodes, the lower third into the superficial inguinal nodes.

The *vault,* dome or upper part of the vagina, is divided into four *fornices* or arches (see Fig. 18-2). During digital pelvic examination, the gynecologist can palpate pelvic contents through the thin walls of the vault.

The anterior fornix, in front of the cervix, is adjacent to the base of the bladder and distal ends of the ureters.

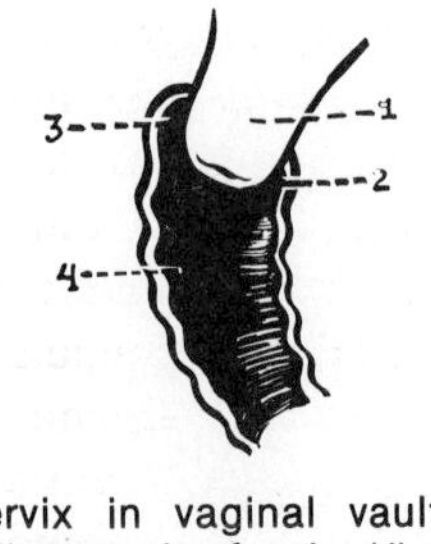

Figure 18-2 Cervix in vaginal vault. (1) cervix, (2) anterior fornix, (3) posterior fornix, (4) vagina.

The *pouch of Douglas* (retrouterine cul-de-sac) directly behind the larger posterior fornix lies behind the cervix. This pouch separates the back of the uterus from the rectum. It is bounded anteriorly by the uterine peritoneal covering, which continues down to cap the posterior vaginal fornix, and posteriorly by the anterior wall of the rectum. Lateral boundaries are the uterosacral ligaments, as they embrace the lower third of the rectum in their course. The floor of the pouch, about 7 cm above the anus, is formed by the reflection of the peritoneum from the rectum to the upper vagina and uterus. The posterior fornix is the route of entry for a number of diagnostic or operative procedures because the pouch of Douglas, the lowest part of the peritoneal cavity, is separated from the vagina only by the thin vaginal wall and peritoneum of the fornix.

The lateral fornices lie on either side of the cervix, in contact with anterior and posterior sheets of the broad ligaments surrounding the uterus. Proximal structures are the uterine artery, ureters, fallopian tubes, ovaries, and sigmoid colon.

Uterus The uterus is the organ of gestation that receives and holds the fertilized ovum during development of the fetus and expels it during childbirth.

Resembling an inverted pear in shape, this hollow muscular organ is situated in the bony pelvis. It lies between the bladder anteriorly and the sigmoid colon posteriorly. By a slight constriction it is divided into a wider upper part, the body or *corpus uteri,* and a narrower lower part, the *cervix uteri* or neck. The corpus meets the cervix at the *internal os.* Peritoneum covers the corpus externally; the endometrium lines it internally. This mucous membrane is uniquely adapted to receive and sustain the fertilized ovum. The *fundus* or domelike portion of the uterus lies above the uterine cavity.

The *uterine cavity,* flattened from front to back, is roughly triangular in shape in the nonpregnant female. The upper lateral angles extend out toward the openings of the fallopian tubes, which enter through the uterine walls at the *cornua.* The apex of the triangle is directed downward to the cervix. The cavity within the cervix, the *endocervical canal,* narrows to a slit at the end where the cervix communicates with the vagina via the *external os.* The corpus and cervix are considered individually in relation to disease and therapy because they differ in structure and function.

As the incubator and nurturer of the developing

embryo, the uterus is capable of expansion. Much of the bulk of the corpus consists of involuntary muscle, the *myometrium,* composed of three layers. The inner layer prevents reflux of menstrual flow into the tubes and peritoneal cavity, which could result in endometriosis. It also contributes to the competency of the internal os sphincter to prevent premature expulsion of the fetus. The middle layer encloses large blood vessels. These muscle fibers act as living ligatures for hemostasis after delivery. The outer layer has expulsive action, ejecting menstrual flow and clots, aborted embryo, or the baby at term.

Usually the uterus lies bent forward at a right angle to the vagina and resting on the bladder. While the cervix is anchored laterally by ligaments, the fundus may pivot about the cardinal ligaments widely in an anterior-posterior plane. Mobility rather than position is the criterion for normality.

Fallopian Tubes (Salpinges) These small, hollow, musculomembranous tubes, sometimes called *oviducts,* run bilaterally like arms from each side of the upper part of the uterus to the ovaries. Near each ovary, the open end of each tube expands into the *infundibulum,* the edges of which are divided into *fimbriae,* fingerlike projections that are thought to sweep up the *ovum* (the female reproductive cell) as it is expelled from the ovary. Fertilization of the ovum by the sperm takes place in one tube. Within the tube are ciliated cells that move the fertilized egg toward the uterus. The lumen of the tube becomes very narrow where it penetrates the uterine wall to reach the uterine cavity.

Contractions in the muscular walls change shape and position of the tubes. At ovulation they move the fimbriated ends into close apposition with the ovarian surfaces.

Ovaries The ovaries are oval-shaped and lie in a shallow peritoneal fossa on the lateral pelvic walls from which they are suspended by the infundibulopelvic ligaments. They are attached to the posterior layer of the broad ligament by the *mesovarium,* a peritoneal fold, and to the uterus by the *ovarian ligament,* a fibromuscular cord.

The ovaries give rise to the ova and are the counterpart of the male testes. Every ovary consists of a center of cells and vessels surrounded by the *cortex,* the main portion, which contains the stroma or fibrous framework in which the ovarian follicles are imbedded. Of the approximately 200,000 primordial follicles present at birth, less than 400 are likely to produce a mature ovum (*graafian follicle*) during the reproductive years. A serous covering derived from peritoneum surrounds the ovaries.

In addition to containing the ova, the ovaries, which atrophy after menopause, produce female sex hormones.

The ureters lie immediately behind the ovaries.

Muscles and Ligaments Muscles and ligaments support the uterus and fallopian tubes in normal position in the center of the pelvic cavity.

Broad Ligaments or Mesosalpinges These are composed of a broad double sheet of peritoneum extending from each lateral surface of the uterus outward to the pelvic wall. Between these two layers of peritoneum are a number of important structures, such as the fallopian tubes enclosed in the free upper border with the tubal ostia opening directly into the peritoneal cavity.

Round Ligaments These are round muscular bands that extend from the anterior surface of the lateral borders of the fundus to the labia majora. They run beneath the peritoneum of the anterior sheet of the broad ligament down, outward, and forward through the inguinal canal to the labia.

Cardinal Ligaments The lower portion of the broad ligaments, these are attached to the lateral vaginal fornices and supravaginal portion of the cervix. They act as a supportive pivot.

Uterosacral Ligaments These are peritoneal folds containing connective tissue and involuntary muscle. They arise on each side from the posterior wall of the uterus at the level of the internal os, pass backward around the rectum, and insert on the sacrum at the level of the second sacral vertebra. Their course describes an archlike curve with concavity toward the midline. They pull on the cervix to keep the uterus anteverted and, through the cervix, the vagina in position as well.

Physiology

The function of the female reproductive organs is to conceive, nurture, and produce offspring. The development and function of these organs are influenced by the hormonal secretions of the ovaries, adrenals, thyroid, and pituitary. The organs also affect sex characteristics.

The physiological cycle prepares the womb for the fertilized ovum. Hormone production stimulates the endometrium and breasts, resulting in thickening and increased blood supply.

Each month during the years from puberty to menopause, one of the ovaries produces on its surface a follicle from within. When the matured graafian follicle ruptures, it discharges the enclosed ovum, which enters the fallopian tube at the fimbriated end. The process of maturation and discharge of the egg is called *ovulation,* a fertile period that lasts several days. Changes in cervical mucus and vaginal epithelium also accompany ovulation. Union of the ovum with a viable mature male germ cell (*spermatozoon*), which has ascended to the fallopian tube from the vagina, results in *fertilization.* The fertilized ovum normally proceeds to the cornu of the uterus where it enters to implant in the endometrium. Pregnancy has occurred.

Menstruation is the end result of lack of fertilization. It is the periodic discharge of blood, mucus, disintegrated ovum, and uterine mucosa formed during the cycle. Duration of the menstrual period varies, but the average is 3 to 5 days. The amount of blood lost varies greatly. The menstrual cycle, the time between the onset of each period, is approximately 28 days in length. Regularity of menstruation can be disturbed by disease conditions and emotions in addition to onset of pregnancy. This physiological cycle continuously recurs throughout the reproductive life of the woman.

SPECIAL FEATURES OF GYNECOLOGIC SURGERY

Operative techniques discussed in the previous chapter apply to gynecologic surgery. Diagnostic and operative procedures may be carried out through a vaginal or abdominal approach, or the two approaches may be combined. Each requires a different position, and different preparation, drapes, and setup. The discussion of diagnostic and operative procedures is combined because a number of procedures may be done in one operation. In both vaginal and abdominopelvic procedures:

1 The patient is catheterized in the OR unless she has an indwelling catheter. Frequently, a Foley catheter is inserted in the OR to prevent the bladder from becoming distended during operation, and to record urinary output. The circulating nurse should check the collection bag regularly and report any blood that could indicate injury to the bladder or ureters.

2 Spinal or (more commonly) general anesthesia is used.

3 Early ambulation and use of antiembolic stockings are especially important in pelvic surgery because deep major vessels are in the operative field and lithotomy position slows circulation. Postoperative thrombosis is a serious complication.

4 The electrosurgical unit frequently is employed. The unipolar unit has cutting and coagulating current at the option of the operator. Bipolar forceps pinpoint hemostasis of small bleeders without effect on adjacent tissue. Current passes only from tip to tip and not into surrounding tissue.

5 Various drains such as Penrose or closed-wound suction drainage may be used to prevent hematoma or serum accumulation.

Vaginal Approach

1 Vaginal procedures generally are performed with the patient in lithotomy position.

2 Instrumentation includes implements of sufficient length for use within the vaginal canal and uterine cavity, e.g., long curved dressing forceps for insertion of vaginal packing. In addition to cutting, holding, and clamping instruments, vaginal setups include *D&C (dilation and curettage) instruments:*

- Posterior retractor
- Weighted posterior retractor
- Narrow lateral Heaney retractors
- Single- and double-toothed tenaculi
- Jacobs tenaculum
- Uterine sound
- Graduated dilators
- Goodell dilator
- Sharp and blunt, large and small uterine curettes
- Sponge forceps
- Polyp and biopsy forceps
- Uterine dressing forceps

3 Sponges should be secured on a sponge forceps in deep areas. Long narrow gauze pads with tape on the end are used for packing off abdominal viscera in vaginal procedures. Sponge and instrument counts are very important in these procedures.

4 Vaginal packing is inserted following certain procedures. Antibiotic cream may be applied to the packing during insertion. The packing should be recorded on the patient's chart and removed at the surgeon's order.

5 At completion of operation, a belt is placed on the patient to hold the perineal pad in place postoperatively.

6 The cryosurgical unit may be used in vaginal work to remove hypertrophied tissue or certain benign neoplasms.

7 The laser is occasionally used in patients with cervical dysplasia. It is said to permit selective destruction of large areas of vaginal epithelium without injury to adjacent tissue or excessive scarring, a possible cause of vaginal and cervical stenosis. It also minimizes blood loss by sealing as it coagulates.

Abdominal Approach

1 Supine or Trendelenburg position is used for abdominopelvic procedures. The preparation and drapes are the same as for abdominal laparotomy.

2 When there is a large abdominal mass or the pelvic organs are pushed from their normal relationships, ureteral catheters may be inserted prior to operation to permit easy identification of the ureters in proximity to or within the dissecting area. Inadvertent severing of ureters during operation greatly increases postoperative morbidity and mortality if the injury is not detected and corrected.

3 Instrumentation includes basic laparotomy setup with the addition of long instruments for deep manipulations within the pelvis. Some surgeons prefer a double Mayo stand with instruments for superficial work on one and supplies for deeper areas on the other.

Combined Vaginal-Abdominal Approach

If vaginal surgery as well as abdominal is indicated, a combined procedure is planned. For example, the patient may be scheduled as prep vault, vaginal plastic, abdominal hysterectomy. In such instances the vaginal procedure is performed first. Then the patient is removed from lithotomy position and the abdominal prep and operation carried out.

1 Because of the hazard of infection, separate sterile setups are used for vaginal and abdominal procedures performed concurrently.

2 Vaginal preparation precedes exploratory pelvic laparotomy in readiness for the unexpected, or for D&C scheduled to precede an abdominal operation. A separate sterile prep table is used for the external genitalia and vagina. Another sterile setup is used for the abdominal prep.

DIAGNOSTIC TECHNIQUES

The gynecologist employs both noninvasive and invasive diagnostic techniques. Some are performed as office or ambulatory procedures, especially those using the vaginal approach.

Pelvic examination includes inspection and palpation of external genitalia, bimanual abdominovaginal and abdominorectal palpation of the uterus, fallopian tubes, and ovaries, and speculum examination of the vagina and cervix. This inspection is augmented by a cytologic study of smears of cervical and endocervical tissue obtained by scrapings. The purpose of this screening technique is to detect both premalignant lesions that are not yet clinically obvious but have a high rate of cure, or frank invasive cancer. The *Papanicolaou smear* has facilitated a significant increase in diagnosis of patients with cervical cancer at incipient stages. Characteristic cellular changes in cervical epithelial cells may be identified. Cytologic aspiration from within the endocervical canal may reveal unsuspected carcinoma of the endometrium, tubes, or ovaries as well as occult cervical cancer.

Schiller's test involves staining the vaginal vault and cervical squamous epithelium with an iodine (Lugol's) solution. The glycogen in normal epithelium takes up the iodine. Abnormal tissues, with little or no glycogen, do not stain brown and therefore pinpoint sites for biopsy. Abnormal cytology is an indication for further evaluation by histological tissue study. These methods will be discussed in association with operative procedures relating to the anatomical area involved.

Biopsy of Cervix

Cervical cancer may not present symptoms in the early stage and may progress to invasion before discovery. Intermenstrual (*spotting*) or postmenopausal bleeding may be the first visible sign. The condition may be suspected by cytologic examination or visual inspection, but diagnosis must be made by biopsy. Methods that may be used are:

Punch Biopsy Removal of small pieces of tissue with a cervical biopsy forceps may be a simple ambulatory procedure. If cervical polyp is diagnosed, it easily can be removed. If malignancy is diagnosed, hospitalization is necessary for continued study and treatment.

Colposcopy This allows directed precision biopsy, which may obviate conization (see p. 340). Multiple specimens may be taken from the cervix and vagina for histological examination and diagnosis. The illumination and binocular magnification afforded by the colpomicroscope, focused on the cervix, permit study of abnormal epithelium on the *ectocervix* (portion of cervix that protrudes into the vagina), the lower part of the cervical canal, and the vagina. Wiping the cervix with 3% acetic acid eradicates mucus and facilitates view of the surface and vasculature. Endocervical curettage also may be performed.

Excisional Biopsy Resection of tissue is the most common method of biopsy of cervical dysplasia. Only knife biopsy provides tissue for pathological study.

Cone Biopsy/Conization of the Cervix Colposcopic examination and directed biopsy have obviated cervical conization in some instances. However, patients diagnosed by Papanicolaou smear as having cervical dysplasia or intraepithelial carcinoma of the cervix may require conization to rule in or out invasive carcinoma. The biopsy is taken with a scalpel or cervitome (*cold knife conization*) so as to include the squamo-columnar junctions of the ectocervix and tapered to include the endocervical canal to the level of the internal os. Hemostasis is secured by sutures. Multiple blocks and sections are examined by the pathologist to rule on invasive disease.

NOTE. Uterine cancer consists of two entities: cervical cancer and endometrial cancer. These differ by age groups, types, and consequences. Cancer of the cervix appears most often in association with coitus at an early age, multiple partners, nonbarrier contraceptives, poor sexual hygiene, herpes infection, or chronically infected cervices. Prompt early treatment of cervical malignancy yields an excellent rate of cure.

Each form of therapy for cancer has certain advantages and limitations. Factors affecting response to treatment are host factors, clinical stage of malignancy, histological grade of malignancy, and the therapy employed. Pretreatment workup is extensive for all modes of therapy.

Pelvic Endoscopy

Pelvic endoscopy is an established part of the gynecologist's diagnostic and therapeutic armamentarium. It permits detailed intraperitoneal inspection of pelvic organs without laparotomy. The procedure is not without danger, however, and requires an experienced operator, careful patient selection, and adequate anesthesia. Two methods are employed, culdoscopy by vaginal approach and laparoscopy by abdominal approach. Endoscopic inspection of the abdominal cavity, introduced in 1902, has become a frequently employed procedure since the advent of fiberoptic illumination.

Culdoscopy This is a direct visualization of pelvic organs and adjacent structures through a culdoscope introduced into the peritoneal cavity via the posterior vaginal fornix and the pouch of Douglas. It is useful in patients where laparoscopy is contraindicated or unavailable but contraindicated in patients with fixation of organs adjacent to the cul-de-sac, e.g., large pelvic tumors, pelvic inflammatory disease (PID), or endometriosis.

Indications are unexplained pelvic pain, questionable pelvic masses, ovarian disorders, or infertility.

Local or caudal anesthesia is used, with the patient in knee-chest position. Inadvertent perforation of the bowel or rectum is a major hazard. Vaginal preparation and empty bowel and rectum are prerequisites to the procedure. With the posterior lip of the cervix held by a tenaculum and retracted anteriorly, the uterus is elevated while counterpressure is applied to the posterior vaginal wall by speculum. This maneuver stretches the posterior vaginal fornix while a trocar and cannula penetrate the thin wall and enter the pelvis between the uterosacral ligaments. When the trocar is removed with the cannula in place, air enters the cul-de-sac due to the negative intra-abdominal pressure produced by knee-chest position. Air displaces the bowel and the scope may be inserted through the cannula.

To check for tubal patency, an aqueous solution of dye such as methylene blue or indigo carmine in saline can be instilled via a cervical Foley catheter and the dye observed dripping from the fimbrial end of the tube. Or, if obstruction is present, the nature of the block may be demonstrated.

At completion of the procedure, the culdoscope is removed. Before the cannula is removed, the operating table is straightened and the patient flattened while as much air as possible is evacuated by hand pressure on the abdomen. Some surgeons place a suture in the puncture site.

Laparoscopy Laparoscopy is insertion of a fiberoptic laparoscope into the peritoneal cavity for diagnostic and/or therapeutic purposes. It permits direct observation and selective biopsy of pelvic and upper abdominal organs and peritoneal surfaces. This technique is used to diagnose ectopic pregnancy, inspect the ovaries for evidence of follicular activity, visualize pelvic masses, and determine etiology of pain, infertility, endocrinopathies, or amenorrhea. It can often obviate the need for laparotomy. Pelvic diseases such as endometriosis, adhesions, and tubal occlusions may be identified. Operative procedures such as tubal sterilization by electrocoagulation with/without division or partial resection, placement of a metal clip or silicone ring on the tube, biopsy, or lysis of adhesions can be performed. Because it allows a view of the anterior surface of the uterus, bladder, and cul-de-sac, laparoscopy is preferred to culdoscopy in many patients.

Usually general anesthesia by intubation is administered. Vaginal prep, catheterization, and D&C often are performed first. A special cannula or catheter may be inserted into the cervix for instillation of a dye solution to observe tubal patency and for manipulation of the uterus to afford greater visibility. The vaginal area is covered with a sterile drape and, with the patient in modified lithotomy position (stirrups adjusted so the legs are at a 45° angle to the axis of the operating table), the abdomen is prepped and draped as for laparotomy. A combined sheet (double fenestration) also may be used.

Insertion of the scope is prefaced by adequate adominal distention produced by the creation of pneumoperitoneum. The subumbilical midline area is most commonly used if no scars, with possible adherent viscera beneath, are present. This area is preferred because it has no abdominal wall vessels that might be injured. The firm attachment of fascia to peritoneum facilitates entry. However, great care must be taken to avoid injury to the great vessels or intra-abdominal organs.

To produce pneumoperitoneum, a Verres needle is introduced percutaneously into the peritoneal cavity. This needle has an outer sharp trocar with an inner blunt hollow retractable cannula or a stylet with a spring at its base. The needle also has a two-way stopcock at the base for control of gas flow. A plastic tube with adaptor to fit the needle hub connects to the carbon dioxide insufflation apparatus. The gas is slowly introduced into the cavity under controlled flow and pressure. The volume injected varies according to need, but overdistention must be avoided to prevent complications.

After insufflation, the valve is closed and the patient placed in Trendelenburg position. A small subumbilical incision is made in the anterior abdominal wall and through it the trocar and cannula (sleeve) are introduced into the peritoneal cavity via puncture. The sharp tip must be carefully guided to avoid inadvertent perforations. The trocar is removed and the scope of the same caliber is inserted through the sleeve, which remains in the cavity. The fiberoptic cable is connected to the light source and the gas tube reconnected to the cannula.

Although operating scopes permit insertion of accessory instruments, these may be introduced through a second small incision in the lower abdomen. Another, smaller trocar and cannula are inserted into the peritoneal cavity under direct vision through the laparoscope, which offers good transillumination for the puncture when the room lights are dimmed. After removal of the trocar, an operating instrument is inserted through the cannula. Accessory instruments include calibrated metal probe for assessment of organ size or distance between organs, insulated electrosurgical unit electrodes for unipolar or bipolar cautery and coagulation, aspirating tube, and biopsy forceps.

At completion of operation, the accessory instrument and cannula are removed. Hemostasis is surveyed and the scope removed from the primary puncture site. The valve of its sleeve is opened to allow escape of intraperitoneal gas while gentle pressure is applied to the adomen. The skin incisions are sutured and a small dressing applied.

While numerous complications have been reported, the most common ones are perforation of a hollow viscus such as the intestine, hemorrhage from a punctured vessel or a biopsy site, gas embolism from intravascular injection, and burns of the abdominal wall and bowel.

NOTE. 1. Laparoscopy is a sterile procedure and only adequately sterilized, *not disinfected,* equipment should be used.
2. The patient requires close monitoring by the anesthesiologist because increased intra-abdominal pressure may lead to cardiovascular disturbances from vagal reflex due to stretching of the peritoneum, retention of carbon dioxide, or compression of the inferior vena cava.
3. Fogging of the distal lens of the optic by intraperitoneal temperature and moisture can be prevented by warming the tip of the scope in warm towels or saline prior to use.
4. Carbon dioxide is used as the insufflation medium because it is nontoxic, highly soluble in blood, and rapidly absorbed from the peritoneal cavity.

Hysteroscopy This is direct inspection of the uterus by means of a fiberoptic hysteroscope to diagnose or treat intrauterine disease. It may be used to supplement curettage of the uterine cavity. Adequate dilation of the cavity is a prerequisite for careful viewing of endometrial surfaces. To provide distention, 5% glucose in water, carbon dioxide, or viscid dextran solution is used.

Hysteroscopy is not widely performed because of the availability of other diagnostic methods and its own disadvantages. These disadvantages include the need for extensive training in the method, the danger of tumor cell dissemination in the presence of malignancy, and the obscuration of the visual field by bleeding.

Culdocentesis and Posterior Colpotomy

Culdocentesis This is performed by the insertion of a spinal needle into the cul-de-sac for aspiration of any fluid, blood, or pus collected there.

Colpotomy This is a transverse incision made through the posterior vaginal fornix into the posterior cul-de-sac to facilitate diagnosis by intraperitoneal palpation, inspection of pelvic organs, or determination of free fluid, blood, or pus in the pouch of Douglas. Pus from a pelvic abscess or blood, possibly a sign of ectopic pregnancy or ruptured ovarian cyst, is evacuated. The tubes and ovaries are inspected and, if they are normal, the incision is closed. A drain may be inserted. Some operative therapy can be performed through the incision although exposure and visualization are limited. An involved tube or ovary sometimes is removed through the vagina. Sterilization procedures by tubal ligation may be carried out by this approach.

Uterotubal Insufflation (Rubin's Test)

In addition to hysterosalpingography and pelvic endoscopy, uterotubal insufflation is a valuable diagnostic aid in the study of infertility. It is done to test the patency of the fallopian tubes. The test preferably is done prior to ovulation, so as not to interfere with potential fertilization.

After vaginal prep, a uterine sound is passed to discover depth of the cervical canal. A special cannula with airtight seal is inserted into the cervicouterine canal, the seal adjusted, and the cannula connected to an insufflation apparatus. Carbon dioxide is introduced slowly under controlled flow. Resistance to flow—back pressure—is measured on a mercury manometer. A relationship exists between stenosis and the pressure required to force gas into the tubes. The manometer is watched closely for fluctuations in pressure, which indicate tubal patency. A sudden drop in pressure after initial rise to about 100 mm of mercury suggests patency of one or both tubes as gas flows out of them into the peritoneal cavity. In a normal test, as flow slowly continues, the pressure fluctuates between 40 and 80 mm of mercury, reflecting tubal peristalsis.

Sudden, sharp, transient shoulder pain when the patient sits up, after conclusion of the procedure, is characteristic of a positive test. This is referred pain due to irritation from subdiaphragmatic carbon dioxide before total absorption from the peritoneal cavity. If pain is delayed, the tubes may be patent but ascent of gas retarded by intra-abdominal adhesions. The test may be therapeutic in relieving minor obstructions.

Contraindications include genital tract infection, possible pregnancy, or any uterine bleeding because of danger of gas embolism. To prevent embolism, a Rubin's test should precede, never follow, a D&C (see p. 345).

Hysterosalpingography

Radiologic investigation of the uterus and tubes may afford further evaluation of infertility following repeated negative Rubin's tests. The tip of a catheter is inserted into the cervical canal and a water-soluble radiopaque dye instilled. The contrast medium ascends into the corpus uteri and tubes and yields information about structure and function.

VULVAR PROCEDURES

Benign growths, although rare, mainly consist of fatty and fibrous tumors. These are excised if large. Suspicious lesions should be removed for pathological examination. Cancerous lesions may be multicentric, with the majority found on the labia majora, a lesser percentage on the labia minora, vestibule, clitoris, and posterior commissure. Vaginal smears should be taken to determine presence of metastatic growth to the vaginal wall. Treatment depends on the size of the primary lesion, the involvement of nodes, and the extent of metastasis. Mutilative procedures require emotional adjustment to the permanent change. Therapeutic procedures include:

Excision of the Lesion Wide local excision of only the lesion may be done if there is a single, well-localized area with no premalignant changes elsewhere.

Simple Vulvectomy without Node Dissection This is performed for premalignant lesions and early cancer of limited penetration (*microinvasive cancer*). The labia majora and minora, part of the mons veneris, hymenal ring, including the clitoris may be removed. Occasionally the clitoris and perianal region are spared if the lesion is small. Incision must be wide to avoid local recurrence.

Total Vulvectomy Basal cell carcinoma usually does not metastasize but often is locally extensive and prone to recur. Treatment consists of wide total vulvectomy also without node dissection.

Radical Vulvectomy with Bilateral Inguino-Femoral (Groin) Lymphadenectomy This procedure usually is done in one stage and is mandatory for large invasive vulvar cancers. Resection lines may vary depending on location and size of the lesion. Since the procedure involves adbominal and perineal dissection, both areas, including the thighs to the knees, are prepped. Structures generally removed include all from the anterior surface of the pubis to the perianal region posteriorly, with wide lateral excision beyond the vulva, to fascial depth. More specifically, these include large areas of abdominal and groin skin, labia majora and minora, the mons, clitoris, Bartholin's and periurethral glands, superficial and sometimes deep inguino-femoral lymph nodes, and portions of the saphenous veins. In early cancers with no superficial node involvement, the deep pelvic node dissection may be avoided. If the urethra and anus are involved, or they are near the tumor, they are removed also. Anal involvement may require a colostomy. Involvement of the vagina may require resection of part of the vagina.

Lymphadenectomy is carried out en bloc with the patient in supine position. Suction drains are inserted and inguinal incisions closed. The patient then is placed in lithotomy position for vulvectomy. Reconstruction of the pelvic floor and vaginal walls may be necessary. Vaginal packing is inserted and suction drainage used postoperatively to avoid fluid collection beneath skin flaps. Postoperative care emphasizes open wound management for prevention of infection.

Marsupialization of Bartholin Cyst or Abscess The cyst enlarges as secretions accumulate. Obstruction may be postinflammatory and the cyst prone to secondary infection or abscess formation. Marsupialization establishes drainage from within the vagina by creation of a new enlarged ductal opening. The cyst is incised linearly in the region of the normal opening, evacuated, and the edges of the vaginal mucosa and cyst wall are sutured together to produce epithelization. After epithelization no cyst recurrence can occur.

VAGINAL PROCEDURES

Biopsy of Adenosis Lesion This type of benign epithelial tumor should be biopsied and studied histologically to rule out adenocarcinoma. Vaginal adenosis and gross cervical abnormalities such as collar or hood as well as clear cell adenocarcinoma of the vagina have occurred in female offspring of women who received diethylstilbestrol (DES) or similar synthetic estrogen during the first trimester of pregnancy to avoid miscarriage.

Vaginectomy Vaginectomy (partial or complete) is performed for carcinoma *in situ* or carcinoma of the vagina. Vaginoplasty is necessary for reconstruction. External radiation and radium application (refer to Chap. 27), with possible eventual pelvic exenteration (p. 348), is the treatment for advanced invasive malignancy. The proximity of the bladder and rectum makes therapy difficult.

Radical vaginal or abdominal hysterectomy and vaginectomy with extraperitoneal lymphadenectomy sometimes are combined for carcinoma of the upper and middle thirds of the vagina if the bladder or rectum is not involved.

Procedures for Repair of Pelvic Outlet Injury to the muscles and fascia of the perineum and/or genital tract, usually during childbirth, may result in extensive vaginal relaxation. Manifestation of perineal herniae may be delayed until later years when generalized loss of elastic tissue develops. Moderate to severe degrees of herniation of viscera require surgical intervention to restore pelvic floor integrity and sphincter competency. It has been said that competent obstetrics is preventive gynecology. Vaginal plastic procedures for genital prolapse consist of narrowing and reconstructing the damaged pelvic floor. The repair procedures are:

1 *Anterior colporrhaphy.* This is performed for prolapse of the anterior vaginal wall, to repair *urethrocystocele,* which is herniation of the bladder into the vaginal canal. With the patient in lithotomy position, the wall is incised and a strip of redundant vaginal mucosa excised, extent depending on severity of prolapse. The bladder is dissected free from the vaginal septum and returned to normal position by suturing the pubocervical ligaments beneath it. Approximation of the pubococcygeus muscles provides further suburethral support. The vaginal wall is closed by sutures. By improving support to the bladder neck region, restoring the posterior urethrovesical angle, and narrowing the urethral opening, stress incontinence (urinary loss with strain) is relieved. The operation also prevents the recurrent cystitis that accompanies retention of urine due to a cystocele hanging below the bladder neck.

2 *Posterior colpoperineorrhaphy.* Repair of the posterior vaginal wall for *rectocele,* a herniation of the rectum into the vagina, consists of triangular excision of redundant vaginal mucosa and separation of the vagina from the rectum. Support is reestablished by suturing together the rectovaginal fascia, as well as the levator ani, as high as possible. Perineal muscles are reconstructed to restore continuity of support. A lacerated perineum may also be sutured. The operation relieves fecal incontinence and/or constipation.

3 *Repair of enterocele.* An abnormally deep hernial sac may contain a segment of intestine, referred to as *enterocele* or cul-de-sac hernia. Repair consists of opening the hernial sac, reducing its contents, excising the sac, closing the aperture or weakness that allowed the sac to descend into the rectovaginal septum, and strengthening the normal anatomical coverings. Approximation of uterosacral ligaments and the levator ani in the midline removes the cul-de-sac defect.

4 *Repair of prolapsed uterus or procidentia.* There are various operations for correction and restoration of support. In complete prolapse both cervix and uterine body protrude through the vaginal aperture and the vaginal canal is inverted. Bleeding ulceration of exposed tissue may occur. Often cystocele and rectocele are present, and are simultaneously repaired. Correction of prolapse anteverts the uterus and shortens an elongated cervix and the cardinal ligaments. Most patients, however, are treated by vaginal hysterectomy.

5 *Colpocleisis (Le Fort operation)* obliterates the vagina by denuding and approximating the anterior and posterior walls. Colpocleisis is generally reserved for elderly patients or those who are a poor operative risk.

NOTE. 1. Insertion of a vaginal pessary to support a retrodisplaced or prolapsing uterus is utilized in women who are poor operative risks. 2. Vaginal hysterectomy (p. 346) is done for severe prolapse, prolapse accompanied by stress incontinence, and when childbearing is no longer desired.

Procedures for Repair of Genital Fistulas These fistulas are abnormal communications between a part of the genital canal and either the urinary or intestinal tract. Various dye tests, cystoscopy, and pyelography help pinpoint a urinary tract fistula. Injury during parturition, operative trama (especially radical procedures for cancer), penetrating extension of cervical carcinoma, and radiation necrosis are common etiologic factors.

1 *Repair of vesicovaginal fistula.* The most common type, this fistula is between the bladder and vagina. A small opening permits seepage of urine, although the patient may void normally. Total incontinence may result from a large fistulous aperture and cause irritation of vagina, vulva, and thighs. Through vaginal approach the anterior vaginal wall is dissected free. The fistula to the bladder is closed and the bladder to vagina attachment reestablished.

2 *Repair of ureterovaginal fistula.* This fistula is between the ureter and vagina; its repair depends on location. If the fistula is near the junction of the ureter and bladder, the ureter can be divided above the defect and reimplanted in the bladder. If the fistula is not proximal to the bladder, it can be excised and the severed ureteral ends anastomosed. Occasionally a nephrectomy on the involved side is necessary.

3 *Repair of urethrovaginal fistula.* This fistula is between the urethra and vagina; repair consists of layered closure. If the neck of the bladder is involved, the area must be reconstructed. This may include transplant of the bulbocavernosus muscle.

4 *Repair of rectovaginal fistula* This fistula between the rectum and vagina may follow episiotomy, obstetrical perineal lacerations, vaginal surgery such as culdoscopy, or rectal surgery such as hemorrhoidectomy. Fecal incontinence and fecal material in the vagina are characteristic, although the anal sphincter is intact. Preoperative bowel preparation, including prophylactic antibiotic therapy, is important because of the contaminated operative area. A temporary colostomy may be advisable before the operation to divert the infective fecal stream from the repair site.

Using a vaginal approach, a plastic repair of the perineum is done. Scar tissue and the fistulous tract are excised and the edges of the perineal muscles and fascia are approximated.

Cervix

Treatment of the abnormal cervix should be preceded by tests to rule out early malignant change. Operative treatment of the cervix involves a number of procedures.

Electrocautery The cervix may be cauterized to treat chronic inflammation and/or leukorrhea.

Conization This modality is employed therapeutically for chronic inflammation and for precancerous lesions in women of child-bearing age.

Amputation The cervix may be amputated to remove an intraepithelial cancer. However, because this procedure leaves the corpus uteri, which may become cancerous, some surgeons prefer total hysterectomy to cervical amputation.

Treatment of Cervical Cancer Refer to Chapter 27 for discussion of internal and external radiation therapy. If surgery is contemplated, pelvic lymphangiography is included in the preoperative workup. Operative treatment is discussed under the appropriate procedures.

Cerclage This procedure is employed when a diagnosis of incompetent cervix has been made by eliciting a history of rapid, painless, second- or early third-trimester spontaneous abortions in apparently normal pregnancies. The procedure is preferably elective in patients with typical history and is performed after the sixteenth week of pregnancy. Occasionally the operation may be performed as an emergency in a patient with dilating cervix and bulging membranes as long as the membranes have not ruptured or premature labor has not begun. Treatment consists of purse-string suture of the incompetent cervix. This operation may be performed in the nonpregnant patient with such a diagnosis.

Shirodkar Procedure A small incision is made in the anterior vaginal mucosa at the level of the bladder reflexion and at the posterior cervico-cul-de-sac junction. A tunnel under the cervical mucosa is then made to join the anterior and posterior incisions. Using an aneurysm needle, a synthetic polyester ribbon is placed around the internal os and tied, and the knot secured by a suture. The mucosal incisions are closed. At term, the patient is usually delivered by cesarean section. The operation is not indicated in the presence of bleeding, premature rupture of the membranes, or premature labor.

Uterus

Examination under Anesthesia Bimanual examination of the pelvis with the patient in lithotomy position and relaxed from anesthesia allows more thorough inspection, especially in women experiencing pain, nervous tension, or obesity. This examination should precede every gynecological operative procedure, since it allows the size, outline, consistency, position, and mobility of the uterus, tubes, and ovaries to be assessed accurately. The examination also helps the surgeon determine the stage of malignancy and whether or not a lesion is resectable. It is a routine prelude to vaginal and abdominal operations. In patients for laparotomy, the vaginal vault is prepped and examination performed prior to the abdominal preparation.

Dilation and Curettage (D&C) The most frequently performed gynecologic operation, dilation of the cervix and curettage is done for diagnostic and/or therapeutic purposes. Sometimes both are accomplished by the same operation. Fractional curettage specimens differentiate between the endocervix and the endometrium of the corpus, which helps locate a lesion. The main purpose of D&C is to establish the etiology of abnormal uterine bleeding so the gynecologist can plan definitive treatment. The procedure is mandatory in women with postmenopausal bleeding or symptoms suggestive of endometrial cancer, even when cytological smears are negative. It may be performed in infertility studies, or to confirm preoperative diagnosis before amputation of the cervix or hysterectomy. Therapeutic applications are to relieve dysmenorrhea by cervical dilation only, to remove polyps or benign endometrial pathology, to remove residual tissue and arrest bleeding following incomplete abortion, or for voluntary or therapeutic abortion before the thirteenth week. A regional paracervical block or general anesthesia is required.

Schiller's test of the cervix utilizing Lugol's solution usually precedes D&C. Then, with the anterior lip of the cervix held in a tenaculum and the posterior vaginal wall retracted, a small curette is introduced into the endocervical canal, which is scraped from the internal to the external os. The specimen is put into a container. The scraping precedes cervical dilation to avoid dislodging tissue from above. A uterine sound then is introduced into the uterus and the length and direction of the intrauterine cavity determined. It is important that the surgeon know the shape and position of the uterus to avoid perforation and injury to it and to other pelvic organs, the primary complications. Dilators are then passed through the cervix and internal os to permit insertion of a curette into the uterine cavity for curettage of the endometrium. Submucous fibroids are usually discernible as the curette passes over them. The endometrial curettage specimen is kept separate from the endocervical one. Both specimens are sent to pathology for histological examination. Exploration of the fundus with a polyp forceps generally extracts any polyps that are present in the endometrium. The cervix may be biopsied if indicated by the Schiller's test in association with D&C.

NOTE. 1. Separate instruments should be used for fractional curettage specimens.
2. Following incomplete abortion, it is vital to remove all retained products of conception to prevent infection, especially anaerobic, which may proceed to septic shock (see Chap. 29). The removed tissue is sent for culture and pathologic examination.

Suction Curettage (Dilation and Evacuation, D&E) Suction curettage is the aspiration of intrauterine contents performed for termination of pregnancy in the first trimester or for early incomplete spontaneous abortion. Cervical dilation is adjusted to the cannula necessary for this simple procedure. A vacuum aspirator-cannula is connected by tubing to an electric vacuum pump. The specimen is collected in the vacuum bottle. D&C setup is used.

Disposble equipment for ambulatory diagnostic suction curettage not requiring dilation or anesthesia is commercially available.

Vaginal Hysterectomy (Standard) Vaginal hysterectomy is performed for severe uterine prolapse, prolapse accompanied by stress incontinence, and occasionally for sterilization of patients with pelvic relaxation or history of myomata, irregular uterine bleeding, or treated premalignant lesion.

The uterus is removed through the vagina, with incision of the vaginal wall and the pelvic cavity. D&C should be done prior to hysterectomy. Urinary incontinence, enterocele, and/or rectocele may be simultaneously repaired by anterior and posterior colporrhaphies and with reconstruction of the pelvic floor. Advantages of the procedure include restoration of normal anatomic relationships and preservation of vaginal function. The ovaries are not usually removed. Contraindications are immobility of pelvic organs, a large uterus, or pathology such as ovarian mass.

The vaginal wall is incised anteriorly and the bladder separated from the cervix. The incision is continued around the cervix. The peritoneal cavity is entered through the posterior cul-de-sac and the anterior uterovesical pouch. Ligaments supporting the uterus and uterine vessels are ligated and cut. The fundus is delivered, the upper pedicles sutured, the uterus removed, and the peritoneum closed. Suturing the cardinal and uterosacral ligaments together and to the vaginal vault supports the vault and prevents prolapse of the vagina.

Radical Vaginal Hysterectomy (Schauta Operation) An operative approach to early carcinoma of the cervix, this procedure does not permit pelvic lymph node dissection but is useful in selective patients, e.g., obese patients. It consists of vaginal removal of the uterus, upper third of the vagina, parametria, fallopian tubes, and ovaries. Damage to the ureters or bladder is a potential complication.

ABDOMINAL PROCEDURES

The abdominal approach is used for fixed or enlarged uterus, exploration, inflammatory disease, and most malignant lesions of the uterus, fallopian tubes, and ovaries. This approach permits inspection of pelvic and abdominal organs as well as lymph glands for biopsy or treatment.

Abdominal Cavity

Exploratory Pelvic Laparotomy ("Lap") This is performed for diagnosis but may be followed immediately by a therapeutic procedure such as hysterectomy. Significant pelvic pain, uterine bleeding, or pelvic mass are frequent indications for differential diagnosis from abdominal disease.

NOTE. The appendix may be removed incidentally unless the patient's condition precludes the procedure.

Uterus

Abdominal Hysterectomy This is removal of the uterus through abdominal incision and opening of the peritoneal cavity. The most frequent indication is leiomyofibroma, commonly known as benign fibroids or myomas. The most common gynecologic tumors, fibroids are composed of muscle and fibrous connective tissue. They may be single or multiple and most often are present in the wall of the uterus. Some may be attached by pedicle and hang into the uterine cavity or the peritoneal cavity. Fibroids, which are usually slow-growing, are treated conservatively if small and presenting no problems. The tumor ceases to grow at menopause. If symptoms such as menometrorrhagia, bladder or bowel pressure, pelvic discomfort, or rapid tumor growth develop, operative treatment is essential. Differential diagnosis includes dysfunctional bleeding due to disturbed endocrine function, tubal or ovarian masses, and pelvic malignancy.

In addition to the above indications, hysterectomy is performed for extensive endometriosis and for cervical or uterine malignancy.

Various types of hysterectomy are:

1 *Supracervical (subtotal, partial hysterectomy).* Rarely performed, this procedure involves removal of the corpus uteri only and is reserved for poor-risk patients or difficult operations in which total hysterectomy would increase morbidity or mortality. Leaving the cervix subjects the patient to risk of possible future cervical cancer. The operation may also be performed in disseminated ovarian carcinoma with removal of the primary ovarian tumor. Reduction of the total mass facilitates radiation therapy.

2 *Total hysterectomy.* The entire uterus, the corpus uteri and cervix uteri, is resected. If normal, the ovaries are preserved whenever possible in patients under 45 years of age.

After vaginal and abdominal preparation, the abdominal peritoneal cavity is entered through a vertical midline or horizontal Pfannenstiel incision. Vertical incision facilitates exploration. The patient is placed in deep Trendelenburg position. Incision through the uterine peritoneum is carried laterally. Abdominal organs are retracted and protected with warm saline laparotomy packs. The fallopian tubes and the round and broad ligaments are clamped, cut, and ligated. The ovaries, when not removed, are suspended to avoid adherence to the vaginal vault. With the uterus forward, the posterior sheets of the broad ligaments are incised, the ureters identified, and uterine vessels and uterosacral ligaments clamped, divided, and sutured. All uterine-supporting ligaments must be divided and ligated. The bladder is mobilized from the cervix and vagina, the vaginal vault incised, and the cervix dissected from the vagina. After the uterus is removed, the connective tissue ligaments are anchored to the vagina. The vaginal mucosa and muscular wall are approximated by sutures, and the bladder, vault, and rectum (pelvic floor) reperitonealized or covered with peritoneum. Abdominal layers are closed as for laparotomy.

NOTE. When the surgeon is closing the vaginal vault following removal of the uterus, the needle, suture, needleholder, and all instruments used on the cervix and vagina are considered contaminated. The scrub nurse holds the specimen basin to receive them and does not touch them. Separate instruments are used for abdominal closure.

3 *Wide cuff hysterectomy.* This is removal of the total uterus and a generous cuff of the vagina. Surgeons employ this procedure for cervical carcinoma *in situ* or early stromal invasion (microinvasion) if invasion is less than 5 mm and no tumor cells appear within lymphatic or vascular channels. Preservation of ovaries depends mainly on the patient's age.

4 *Radical hysterectomy with pelvic node dissection (radical Wertheim operation).* This may be performed for early stages of invasive cervical cancer. It involves wide removal of paracervical, parametrial, and uterosacral tissues, and at least the upper third of the vaginal canal. Bilateral pelvic lymph nodes and channels surrounding the external iliac artery and vein, hypogastric artery and vein, and obturator fossae are also dissected and removed.

NOTE. Some surgeons perform a *modified Wertheim operation* for microinvasive carcinoma. This is somewhat less extensive than the radical procedure and may omit lymphadenectomy.

5 *Total hysterectomy and bilateral salpingo-oophorectomy.* This procedure is used for endometrial, tubal, or ovarian cancer. Fallopian tubes and ovaries are removed along with the uterus.

NOTE. Endometrial malignancy, which is increasing in incidence, is essentially a disease of peri- or postmenopausal years. It is characterized by intermittent spotting between periods or after menopause, or steady bleeding. Postmenopausal bleeding is considered to be due to cancer until proven otherwise. Most patients are treated by preoperative radiation.

Complications of hysterectomy include injury to the ureters with possible fistula formation or renal failure, injury to the bladder or bowel with fistula formation, or massive hemorrhage from damage to major vessels.

Medical, psychosocial, and sexual impacts on the patient must be considered when contemplating hysterectomy. Medically the procedure may be lifesaving in patients with malignancy or severe hemorrhage. The gynecologist has an obligation to consider the individual patient's attitudes when more than one mode of therapy is available as an alternative to hysterectomy.

Signaling as it does the end of the patient's reproductive potential, hysterectomy may cause psychological stress and a sense of incompleteness, even though sexual responsiveness is not dependent on the uterus. Patients whose families are complete, however, often feel relief at the thought of no unanticipated pregnancy.

Myomectomy Single or multiple fibroid tumors can be removed from the uterine wall in premenopausal women who may still desire pregnancy. The operation is especially adaptable to pedunculated tumors, which may become necrotic from interference with blood supply. Removal of large submucous fibroids may require opening the uterus.

Pelvic Exenteration This is an ultraradical procedure for invasive carcinoma that is not performed for palliation but only when there is a possibility of cure. The extent of the disease determines the amount of exenteration. In *anterior exenteration,* the reproductive organs, distal part of the ureters, bladder, and vagina are removed. This modification is performed for cancer of the cervix, vagina, or vulva with extension to the bladder. The ureters are diverted to an ileal conduit while the bowel remains intact. *Posterior exenteration* removes the reproductive organs, sigmoid colon, and rectum. It is done for cervical carcinoma involving the rectum, or advanced rectal carcinoma involving the uterus and posterior vaginal wall. The urinary system remains intact; fecal diversion is by colostomy. *Total or complete exenteration,* rarely performed, involves en bloc dissection of the bladder, reproductive organs, perineum, rectum, and pelvic lymph nodes. These mutilative operations change structure, function, body image, and sex life and must be preceded by intensive physical and psychological preoperative preparation.

Numerous complications may occur involving any major system. Anesthesia and operating times are long, and blood replacement essential. Multiple stoma and gross pelvic defect with much dead space predispose to infection; therefore wound drainage is used.

Fallopian Tubes

Tubal Ligation Frequently performed by laparoscopy, tubal ligation by open abdominal approach may be done alone, in conjunction with other indicated abdominal surgery, or in cases where previous operations interfere with laparoscopic technique. Ligation may be performed through a small horizontal incision in the pubic hairline area. This is referred to as *minilaparotomy.* In some patients, tubal ligation (Pomeroy type) and occlusion techniques may be reversible by subsequent reparative operation.

Tuboplasty This procedure may restore fertility by removal of occlusion in the fallopian tube. Although tubal patency may be restored, function may remain abnormal, limiting the chance of successful uterine pregnancy and increasing the risk of tubal pregnancy. The procedures, dependent on the site of obstruction, are tubal resection and anastomosis, cornual resection and replantation, and fimbrioplasty. These are microsurgical techniques.

Salpingectomy/Salpingo-Oophorectomy Acute tubal infections may be diagnosed by laparoscopy. Operative treatment is indicated when a pelvic function such as salpingitis does not respond to antibiotic therapy. Removal of large tubo-ovarian abscesses is essential to prevent rupture and dissemination of pus in the abdominal cavity. *Salpingectomy* (removal of a fallopian tube) is often performed in association with partial or total removal of the corresponding ovary. It is then referred to as *salpingo-oophorectomy.* The procedures may be uni- or bilateral. Indications are:

1 Extensive damage to the tube and ovary such as chronic tubo-ovarian abscess from repeated pelvic inflammatory infections. Since this is a bilateral disease, it is often treated by total abdominal hysterectomy (TAH) and bilateral salpingo-oophorectomy (BSO).

2 Ectopic pregnancy. This is life-threatening, and must be diagnosed early. Treatment consists of removal of the affected tube. Removal of the associated ovary depends on the extent of damage. In more advanced stages, rupture and hemorrhage result in extensive trauma to the tube and mesosalpinx. *This is a gynecologic emergency.* The patient often is in severe shock from excessive bleeding; immediate operation and blood replacement are imperative. Symptoms of tubal pregnancy are abdominal pain and menstrual irregularity. Diagnosis usually is made by detecting the presence of blood in the cul-de-sac by aspiration (culdocentesis).

3 Primary adenocarcinoma of the tube. Total hysterectomy and bilateral salpingo-oophorectomy are performed.

Salpingostomy This is an incision of the fallopian tube. It may be performed to evacuate an early small tubal pregnancy and preserve the tube in a woman desiring children. The involved portion of the tube is resected and the ends anastomosed using a polyethylene splinting catheter. If the pregnancy is in the cornual region, and other portions of the tube are normal, cornual resection and tubal replantation are done. Salpingostomy is also performed for infectious occlusion of the fimbriated ends of the tubes.

Ovaries

Ovarian pain usually is referred to the lower abdomen just above either groin, making differential diagnosis from abdominal disease pertinent. Ovarian mass due to cyst or tumor requires exploration for evaluation. Ovarian tumors may be benign or malignant, cystic or solid. Some secrete hormones. Cysts are by far the most frequent. Cysts may simulate abdominal disorder or ruptured ectopic pregnancy. Pelvic endoscopy assists diagnosis. The cyst may rupture, causing massive bleeding necessitating laparotomy.

Genuine neoplastic cysts such as dermoid (the most common) persist and increase in size. Dermoid cysts are encapsulated and often contain embryonal remnants. Rupture or leakage of their content is very irritating to the peritoneal cavity.

Cysts of considerable size or solid tumors, even if asymptomatic, should be removed as a precaution because they may degenerate into malignancy, increase in size, or lead to twisting of the pedicle. The type of operation depends on type of cyst, age of the patient, and importance of preserving pregnancy potential.

Oophorocystectomy, Cystoophorectomy, Ovarian Cystectomy (Removal of Ovarian Cyst) Many benign ovarian cysts and tumors are treated by local excision with preservation of the ovary. Immediately after removal, the surgeon incises the cyst for examination to determine its character, since gross appearance as well as frozen section is important. If there is reasonable assurance that the lesion is benign, removal of only the cyst or resection of a diseased portion, e.g., endometrioma, is justified, with preservation of normal tissue.

Oophorectomy (Removal of an Ovary) The most frequent indications are benign ovarian tumors. Many gynecologists believe that cystadenomas and all solid benign ovarian tumors should be treated by unilateral salpingo-oophorectomy because of the difficulty of clean dissection and the questionable assurance of their benign nature. In postmenopausal women, both ovaries, the tubes, and the uterus are removed to avoid future cancer.

If there is a strong probability or proof of malignancy in any ovarian cyst or mass, total hysterectomy and bilateral salpingo-oophorectomy usually are performed, regardless of age. The extent of operation is determined by the lesion. In malignant tumors, a differentiation is made between primary and metastatic ovarian cancer, which influences treatment (see Chap. 27).

Incision or Biopsy This is performed as indicated for diagnosis. Sometimes when a benign cyst is found in one ovary at laparotomy, the gynecologist carefully transects the other ovary to rule out any small neoplasm.

Muscles and Ligaments

Urinary stress incontinence may be corrected abdominally by suspending the bladder. Sometimes it is treated by a combined abdominoperineal procedure. Differential diagnosis from fistulas, bladder neuropathies, and primary lesions may be established by cystoscopy or urethrocystography.

Marshall-Marchetti Vesicourethral Suspension This operation is done by extraperitoneal abdominal approach through the prevesical space. After mobilization, the urethra and bladder neck are suspended to the posterior surface of the pubis by sutures placed through the anterior vaginal wall on each side of the urethra and then through the retropubic periosteum. Sutures also may be placed adjacent to the bladder neck and through the rectus muscle fascia to prevent descent of the bladder neck. Marshall-Marchetti suspension is the most effective procedure for correction of stress incontinence. The operation may be performed in conjunction with other pelvic surgery. Variations of the procedure have been devised.

SEX REASSIGNMENT

Sex transformation (gender transformation) is an established phenomenon in modern society. The patient shows an anxious desire to change from one physical status to another. A sex change, however, requires a stable personality, psychiatric counseling for feasibility, and careful preparation and support. While the majority of transformations are from male to female (see Chap. 19), female to male cross-gender is also possible in satisfactory candidates; however, the management of this change is more complex. A treatment schedule of hormonal substitution, i.e., androgens (male hormone) in the female patient, is begun well in advance of the operation.

In a one-stage procedure, bilateral subcutaneous mastectomy, total abdominal hysterectomy, and bilateral oophorectomy are performed. Three additional stages are necessary to complete transformation. These are:

1 Urethral reconstruction, to the tip of the enlarged clitoris
2 Transfer of the labia for penile lengthening and scrotal reconstruction
3 Prosthetic testical implantation

An understanding, nonjudgmental, unembarrassed attitude on the part of health care personnel can help the patient adjust mentally, as well as recover physically, after the radical change.

Chapter 19

Urology

"Urology is that branch of medicine and surgery concerned with the study, diagnosis, and treatment of abnormalities and diseases of the urogenital tract of the male and the urinary tract of the female. The practice of urology involves, aside from routine diagnostic and surgical work, special knowledge and skills in the treatment of pediatric urologic problems, infections of the urinary tract, infertility and sterility, male sexual problems, renal dialysis and renal transplantation, renal hypertension, endocrine problems as they relate to the adrenal, testes and prostate, and cancer immunology and therapy. Because of shared responsibility in patient care with pediatricians, internists, nephrologists, endocrinologists, surgeons, and chemotherapists, close association with specialists in these disciplines is essential."*

DEVELOPMENT OF UROLOGY

Writings that date back to 3000 B.C. tell of urinary diseases. The earliest known specimen of a bladder stone was found in the grave of an Egyptian dating back to 4000 B.C. Around 2000 B.C. people in India are known to have suffered from bladder stones. Removal of a stone from the bladder through an incision is one of the earliest known operations. It was often performed by itinerant lithotomists, who flourished from the time of Hippocrates to the early eighteenth century. Hippocrates wrote that he did not remove stones, but left them for those trained for such work. For centuries this operation was not considered a part of surgery.

While enlarged prostates were noted in the time of Hippocrates, the attempts to remove part of them perineally during lithotomy or to tunnel through them with a sharp instrument were extremely dangerous.

Urethral sounds were found in the ruins of Pompeii, as were bronze catheters, buried there since 79 A.D. Metal catheters were used until the invention of rubber ones in the late nineteenth century.

The first urologists were mainly venereologists and "instrumenteurs" of the urethra. Although physicians sought to visualize the interior of the bladder, the first attempts at cystoscopy were not made until the early nineteenth century. However, the source of light was a candle or lamp and the instruments were inadequate. In 1876, Nitze, an Austrian, developed an instrument that is the basis of our modern cystoscope. Only after the incandescent lamp was invented and an optical system was devised could an efficient instrument be

*Definition of the American Board of Urology.

made. Improvements started about 1878, and the precise instruments of today have evolved since that time, making possible the conservative treatment of many conditions of the urinary tract.

Urologists have contributed to the evolution of medicine in general. Swick's development of intravenous pyelography is the foundation of modern angiography. Huggins opened a new vista to oncology when he identified that prostatic cancer was not fully autonomous. The use of antibacterial drugs by urologists freed all physicians from time-consuming treatment of venereal disease. Urology has been and continues to be a supporting speciality within medicine and surgery and is interdependent with other specialties.

SPECIAL FEATURES OF UROLOGY

The largest portion of the practice of urology is surgical—and this portion is expanding. The basic principles and techniques of surgery previously discussed apply to operations in the genitourinary tract.

The genitourinary tract is sometimes referred to as the *GU* tract. Open operation is performed only after conservative treatment fails or examination of the GU tract confirms a condition that does not yield to this treatment. Fortunately, the majority of urologic conditions can be diagnosed and treated conservatively through a urologic endoscope and its accessories. The urologist performs open operations to repair, revise, reconstruct, or remove organs when a congenital or acquired condition will not respond to conservative therapy. Obstructive and neuromuscular disorders are common problems of the urinary tract.

The majority of patients seen by urologists are in the preadolescent and older age groups. Congenital and common pediatric problems are discussed in Chapter 26. Discussion here will focus on adult problems. Most of these occur in men over 50 with prostatic disease. Among middle-aged patients, renal calculus disease and tumors in the urinary tract are most commonly diagnosed. All these conditions may cause obstruction and subsequent infection in the kidneys, ureters, or bladder.

COMMON OPERATIONS IN URINARY TRACT

Kidney

Definitive renal operations are justified for management of renal neoplasms, large cystic lesions that compromise renal function or induce obstruction, inflammatory diseases that necessitate drainage, or renal vascular disease. The kidney usually is approached posteriorly with the patient in a lateral position elevated on the kidney rest. A flank incision is made parallel to and just below or over the eleventh and twelfth ribs. Sections of the ribs may be removed. Operations include:

Nephrectomy Removal of a kidney is indicated when tumor, chronic degenerative disease, or severe traumatic injury has produced irreparable damage to renal cells and absence of renal function.

Nephrectomy also is performed in the OR on a living donor (unilateral) or cadaver (bilateral) to harvest a kidney(s) for transplantation. Meticulous dissection is necessary to free the kidney, its blood vessels, and the ureter with minimal trauma. The ureter is dissected free and transected while the renal blood supply remains intact to assure adequate urinary output. This operative procedure may last much longer than the usual nephrectomy.

Bilateral nephrectomy may be indicated for a pretransplant patient who is maintained on chronic hemodialysis (see p. 353) but who has prolonged, severe hypertension. Following kidney transplantation, if rejection is uncontrollable, the patient may require transplant nephrectomy and return to chronic hemodialysis. This is less likely following transplant from a live donor than from a cadaver. Transplantation is discussed in Chapter 28.

Partial or Heminephrectomy Partial excision may be sufficient when one pole has been destroyed by localized disease but the remainder of the kidney is functional.

Nephrolithotomy or Pyelolithotomy Stone fragment or a large staghorn renal calculus that does not dislodge from the calices or renal pelvis may have to be removed through an open incision. A nephroscope may be used during the operation for direct visual examination of the nephrons to locate and remove residual calculi.

Removal of branched or multiple renal calculi is difficult. Preservation of renal function is the primary objective of lithotomy operations. Localized hypothermia provides the surgeon with a bloodless operative field and extends the period of time in which the renal artery may safely be clamped without loss of renal function during search for and extraction of calculi.

Nephrostomy or Pyelostomy An incision through the renal parenchyma or into the renal pelvis may be necessary to establish temporary or permanent drainage when an obstruction prevents flow of urine from the kidney. A tube placed in the kidney exits through the skin. A cutaneous nephrostomy tube may be used to drain a kidney postoperatively during healing following renal reconstruction or revascularization. Silastic tubes placed internally through a cystoscope eliminate the need for open operation for temporary urinary diversion.

Pyeloplasty Revision or reconstruction of the renal pelvis is performed to relieve an anatomic obstruction in the flow of urine by creating a larger outlet from the renal pelvis into the ureter. This may be done to repair or excise damaged tissue so that kidney function will be restored without a partial or total nephrectomy.

Renal Hemodialysis *Hemodialysis* is the process of removing waste products from the blood of a patient in renal failure by diffusion through the semipermeable membrane of a *dialyzer* (artificial kidney machine). This treatment modality alleviates the acute manifestations of uremia and controls many of the chronic long-term complications of end-stage renal disease. Grossly undernourished and anemic patients with severe electrolyte imbalances must be adequately stabilized by hemodialysis prior to kidney transplantation. Some patients will remain on periodic weekly dialysis the remainder of their lives. Therefore, patients undergoing chronic dialysis must have a means of dialysis access established. This may be:

External Arteriovenous Shunt Shunts can be placed in either an arm or leg. The Quinton-Scribner shunt, the oldest and simplest device, consists of two Teflon tips attached to Silastic tubing. One tip is placed in the artery and the other in a nearby vein. Tubing from each tip is exteriorized through a subcutaneous tunnel to the skin and connected together. Blood flows from the artery to the vein between periods of dialysis. Variations and modifications of this basic external shunt may be used. Each provides ready access to the patient's circulation for hemodialysis. Clotting and infection are potential problems that must be avoided. Needles must never be inserted into the Silastic tubing. Blood samples must be obtained for blood-gas analysis under strict aseptic conditions.

Subcutaneous Arteriovenous Fistula An anastomosis, usually between the radial artery and the cephalic vein in the forearm, creates an arterialized peripheral vein that permits dialyzer connections to be made by venipuncture. Needles are placed in the venous limb of the fistula for blood outflow and return. Saphenous vein grafts may be used in either the arm or thigh to create an arteriovenous fistula.

Bovine Heterograft A segment of sterile processed bovine carotid artery is a biologically acceptable graft material that may be used to create an arteriovenous fistula in either the forearm or thigh. These grafts tolerate repeated venipuncture well. They are prepackaged sterile and handled much like a human artery. They can be inserted under local anesthesia.

Patients with chronic renal failure can tolerate extensive operative procedures with minimal complications. Their management in the OR must include strict attention to maintenance of a patent dialysis access shunt or fistula, careful monitoring of fluid and electrolyte balance, and avoidance of postoperative infections. Even after kidney transplantation, the patient may require postoperative dialysis, so the access must remain patent during and after operation.

Renal Revascularization Stenotic lesions of the renal arteries are the predominant etiology in surgically correctable forms of hypertension. Renovascular reconstructive procedures are designed to improve blood flow through the stenotic area to the kidney or to bypass the stenotic area. Revascularization procedures may have a dual purpose: to correct hypertension and to preserve renal function. The patient is in supine position for these procedures as the renal arteries are approached through an abdominal incision.

In Situ Vascular Reconstructive Techniques Renal artery obstruction most often occurs from atherosclerotic stenosis at the origin of the renal artery or fibromuscular dysplasia (abnormal development) confined to the main renal artery. The obstruction is most often resected and replaced by an aortorenal-saphenous vein bypass graft. A reversed segment of proximal saphenous vein, gently distended and irrigated, is anastomosed first to the aorta and then to the renal artery. Prosthetic woven Dacron grafts may be used rather than an autogenous vein graft for renal artery bypass combined with distal aortic replacement (see Chap. 21 for discussion of vascular grafts).

Segmental resection of diseased arterial segments with primary end-to-end anastomosis may be performed. However, thromboendarterectomy (see Chap. 21, p. 396) is more frequently performed than the latter procedure. All these procedures may be performed bilaterally or as staged bilateral renal artery reconstructions.

Ex Vivo Extracorporeal Kidney Surgery When stenotic disease or other obstructive lesion extends into the branches of the renal artery, *in situ* reconstruction may be difficult, hazardous, or impossible. In these patients, temporary nephrectomy with microvascular repair followed by autotransplantation of the kidney may be performed. Referred to as *workbench surgery,* the kidney is completely mobilized from the retroperitoneal space. If one kidney is to be reconstructed, the ureter can remain intact and the reconstruction performed on a sterile bench placed over the patient's lower abdomen. For bilateral reconstruction, one kidney is detached from the ureter to permit complete removal from the abdomen. A second team works on the contralateral kidney while the first is reconstructed at an adjacent dissecting bench.

Extracorporeal perfusion is necessary for renal preservation during reconstruction. This may be accomplished either with simple cold storage in saline slush, or with perfusion of cold Ringer's lactate or other hyperosmolar solution by gravity flow, or with a continuous hypothermic perfusion through a Belzer pump machine.

The kidney may be autotransplanted into the patient's groin or pelvis. This procedure may be used for revascularization of the kidney, removal of renal tumors or calculi, or repair of injuries of the ureter.

Traumatic Injury If the kidney is ruptured or injured by blunt trauma, bullet or stab wound, fatal or near-fatal hemorrhage may be associated with the accident. This requires immediate operation. The surgeon makes every effort to save kidney tissue and ureter. A Foley catheter is inserted to keep an output record as well as to check for the presence of hematuria, pre- and postoperatively. Gross hematuria preoperatively usually points to injury of the bladder or urethra. Kidney damage may be diagnosed by presence of blood seen microscopically.

Ureter

The ureters are the vital anatomic structures for the flow of urine produced in the kidneys to the bladder. An obstruction to urinary flow must be corrected or diverted. The ureters may be approached either through a cystoscope or through open incision.

Complete Cystoscopy *Complete cystoscopy* implies that the procedure extends beyond the bladder into the ureters. This procedure may be performed for:

1 Drainage of the renal pelvis for differential diagnosis or renal function

2 Insertion of ureteral catheters to provide constant drainage for one or both kidneys or to outline the ureters during a difficult pelvic operation

3 Insertion of a ureteral stent for internal drainage of an obstructed ureter

4 Dilation of a stricture in the ureter

5 Manipulation and removal of ureteral calculus

6 Ureteral meatotomy to enlarge the opening of one or both ureteral orifices into the bladder

The endoscopic instruments introduced into the urinary bladder are discussed later in this chapter. Only accessories used for diagnostic or therapeutic procedures within the ureters are mentioned here. These include:

Ureteral Catheters Made of flexible woven nylon or other plastic material, ureteral catheters range in caliber from size 3 to 14 French and are about 30 in. (76 cm) long. Sterile, prepackaged, disposable catheters are available. Most are radiopaque so that they can be visualized on x-ray.

The urologist visualizes the ureteral orifice through the cystoscope. The catheter is then inserted through the instrument and introduced into the ureter. The catheter has graduated markings in centimeters so the urologist can judge the distance the catheter has been inserted into the ureter. The urologist will request the size and style of catheter tip best suited for the intended purpose. The most commonly used tips are:

1 *Whistle tips.* These are used for drainage, as ureteral markers, or for injection of radiopaque contrast medium for retrograde pyelography (refer to Chap. 15, p. 294). The largest sizes are used to dilate the ureters to facilitate passage of a calculus.

2 *Olive tips.* These may be used in the same way as whistle tips.

3 *Round tips.* These may be preferred for drainage.

4 *Flexible filiform tips.* These may be used to bypass an obstruction for drainage.

5 *Blassuchi curved tips.* These may be preferred to bypass a ureteral stricture more easily than straight tips.

6 *Braasch bulb, whistle tips.* These are used to dilate the ureter or to inject contrast medium for a ureterogram (refer to Chap. 15, p. 294).

7 *Acorn or cone tips.* These may be preferred for a ureterogram.

8 *Garceau tapered tips.* These are used to dilate the ureter.

NOTE. If left indwelling to provide drainage, ureteral catheters must be attached to a sterile closed urinary-drainage system. Since they are smaller in diameter than the standard urinary-drainage catheter, an adaptor must be used. This may be a small rubber tip or nipple placed on one end of a straight connector or both ends of a Y connector. The catheters are put through the hole in the tips. The other end of the connector is attached to the constant-drainage system with a piece of sterile tubing.

A separate drainage system for each catheter may be desired by the urologist. Each drainage container must be labeled to identify the right and left ureteral catheters.

Ureteral Stent Catheter The Gibbons silicone indwelling stent catheter is inserted for long-term drainage in a wide variety of benign and malignant diseases causing ureteral obstruction. The stent is passed through the cystoscope over a ureteral catheter used as a guide. When the catheter guide is withdrawn, the stent remains fixed in the ureter for internal urinary drainage through the obstructed area.

Basket-type Stone Dislodgers (Stone Baskets) Flexible-shaft instruments are used in removal of ureteral calculi. These are inserted into the ureter through the cystoscope in the same manner as ureteral catheters. Several types of stone baskets are available, including the Dormia, Johnson, Levant, and Lomac. These have a fine wire or nylon basket that can be expanded through the shaft to ensnare a calculus located in the lower third of the ureter.

Stone baskets must be cleaned promptly after use in a nonresidue liquid-detergent solution to remove debris. Removable parts must be disassembled. Debris should be brushed *away* from the junction of basket and shaft with a small soft brush. During cleaning, inspection of the basket wires is critical. If they are cracked or broken at the end closest to the shaft, the basket may be passed into the ureter but it cannot be withdrawn without trauma.

Cutaneous Ureterostomy Diversion of urinary flow into the bladder can be accomplished by bringing the end of the ureter closest to the bladder through the abdominal wall to the skin. Ureterostomy can be performed unilaterally or bilaterally with a single cutaneous stoma for permanent diversion or a double-loop stoma for temporary diversion. The patient must be fitted postoperatively with an appliance for the collection of urine directly from the ureter to the exterior of the body. This procedure may be performed as a temporary emergency measure following trauma to the bladder, such as a ruptured bladder.

Ureteroenterocutaneous Loops Bilateral transplantation of the ureters for permanent urinary diversion is performed when neoplasms, congenital anomalies, chronic infection, trauma, or other etiology impairs bladder function. The ureters are implanted into the intestinal wall, or more commonly into an isolated segment or loop of the intestine. This loop becomes a conduit for urinary flow.

Ileal Conduit This is the procedure most frequently performed. The ureters are anastomosed to an isolated (6- to 10-cm) segment of the terminal ileum, near its proximal end. The distal end is everted and sutured to a predetermined stoma site on the skin. The stoma is usually located on the right side of the abdomen, below the waist. A urinary collection appliance is secured over the stoma before the patient leaves the OR.

Ureterosigmoidostomy or Ureteroileosigmoidostomy This is preferred by some surgeons because the external stoma of an ileal conduit creates the psychological stress of altered body image for the patient. The ureters may be anastomosed to the sigmoid colon. The ureteroileosigmoidostomy operation implants the ureters into an isolated segment of the ileum anastomosed to the sigmoid colon. Urine diverted into the colon may cause physiologic complications; however, the patient retains an intact body image.

Ureterolithotomy If a calculus fails to pass spontaneously through the ureter or cannot be removed with a stone basket, open operation may be necessary. The patient is positioned for a lateral flank incision below the twelfth rib if the calculus is high in the ureter near the kidney. An abdominal incision is used to reach one in the lower segment near the bladder. When exposed, the ureter will be dilated proximal to the calculus and collapsed distal to it. The surgeon makes a small incision directly over the calculus and extracts it from the ureter with a stone forceps.

Ureteroneocystostomy Implantation of the ureters into the bladder wall can be performed to relocate the ureters into a different site for correction of ureterovesical reflux, to reestablish urinary flow following temporary diversion, or to establish urinary flow from renal transplant following bilateral nephrectomy and ureterectomy.

Ureteroureterostomy Anastomosis of two segments of one ureter usually is performed to reestablish ureteral continuity following traumatic injury. A ureteral catheter may be inserted as a stent and the ureter sutured over it. This procedure or *transureteroureterostomy* anastomosis may be indicated to bypass a ureteral stricture or to eliminate ureteral reflux that also may be the result of trauma to a ureter. Injury to a ureter can occur as a complication of pelvic or abdominal operations, as well as from external penetrating wounds. Ideally, a transureteral anastomosis can be made 2 to 4 cm above the pelvic brim since ureters are close at this point and the recipient ureter has a straight course into the bladder.

Bladder

The bladder may be opened through a suprapubic incision when a neoplasm, calculus, obstruction of the bladder neck, or traumatic injury is not amenable to treatment through the cystoscope. Diagnosis usually is established through direct visualization prior to operation.

Cystectomy Total or partial removal of the bladder and adjacent structures usually is performed to excise a carcinoma within the bladder wall. If a urinary diversion procedure (previously described) has not been performed prior to removal of the bladder, transplantation of the ureters into the skin or into the intestinal tract for urinary drainage is required at the time of cystectomy.

Cystolithotomy and Litholapaxy Calculi usually can be removed from the bladder through the urethra. Crushing a urinary calculus in the bladder with a lithotrite is referred to as *litholapaxy* or *lithotrity.* A lithotrite, introduced into the bladder through the urethra, is used to pulverize and remove calculi. This may be an instrument with hinged jaws or an ultrasound lithotriptor, or an electrohydraulic lithotrite. The electrohydraulic lithotrite generates energy shock waves at the tip of a flexible probe inserted through a cystoscope. With either instrument a telescope enables the urologist to work under vision. The stone fragments are irrigated from the bladder.

If a litholapaxy is unsuccessful or contraindicated, the removal of a calculus by incision into the bladder may be necessary. This operation is a *cystolithotomy.*

Following removal, urinary calculi should be placed in a dry container and sent to pathology for chemical analysis.

Cystometrogram A cystometrogram may be done to measure voiding pressure within the bladder to determine muscular tone and to check nerve supply. A calibrated recording tidal irrigator cystometer is used. When 350 ml of solution are put into the bladder, the patient should feel a desire to void. Carbon dioxide gas is used with some electronic transducers or radio pressure gauges. Normal maximum capacity is 500 ml. Normal pressure is 40 to 50 ml of water. If the problem is neurogenic, cystometric findings are not higher than normal. If the problem is a hypertonic bladder, they are higher than normal.

Cystoscopy *Cystoscopy* is a visual examination of the interior walls and contents of the bladder. The term is used broadly as various procedures may be carried out in conjunction with it by using especially designed instruments through the cystoscope.

Plain cystoscopy is a routine examination of the bladder. Complete cystoscopy and litholapaxy have been previously described. In conjunction with plain cystoscopy, the following other procedures may be performed within the bladder.

1 Biopsy of tumor with a flexible-shaft biopsy forceps to obtain specimens

2 Cystogram for diagnostic x-ray studies (refer to Chap. 15, p. 294) after injection of contrast medium into the bladder

3 Fulgeration of a tumor by use of an electrode (see p. 363)

4 Resection of or incision into a bladder neck obstruction with electrosurgical equipment (refer to resectoscope on p. 363)

5 Removal of foreign body with flexible-shaft foreign-body forceps

6 Insertion of radon seeds (refer to Chap. 27)

Cystostomy Urinary drainage from the bladder may be provided via a catheter inserted through a suprapubic incision into the bladder. If the bladder or urethra is injured due to trauma associated with bony and soft tissue injuries of the pelvis, the bladder may be drained with a catheter placed above the pubic arch. This method of drainage also is preferred following some ureteral, bladder, prostatic, and urethral operations to decrease tension on sutures and to ensure a patent route for urinary drainage. The most commonly used catheters for cystostomy drainage are:

1 Foley, 30-cc balloon, French size 20, 22, or 24.

2 Foley, 5-cc balloon, French size 24, three-way irrigating catheter. The third lumen can be used for continuous irrigation.

These suprapubic catheters are connected to a sterile closed constant-drainage system before the patient leaves the OR.

Cystotomy An incision into the urinary bladder through a suprapubic incision may be performed to repair a bladder laceration or rupture due to trauma. The bladder also is incised to perform a Y-V plasty to relieve a stricture or contracture of the bladder neck by broadening the outlet of the bladder into the urethra.

Urethra

The urethra funtions as the outlet for urine to pass from the bladder. Obstruction or dysfunction of the urethra may cause urinary retention or incontinence. Enlargement of the prostate may cause obstruction. Gonorrhea, other disease processes, or traumatic injury may cause a stricture. Problems associated with congenital displacement of the urethra are discussed in Chapter 26.

Perineal Urethrostomy When indwelling or intermittent urethral catheterization is contraindicated in the male patient with an obstructed or traumatized urethra, urinary drainage from the bladder may be established through a perineal incision. An indwelling catheter is inserted into the bladder through an incision into the membranous urethra.

Urethral Dilatation Periodic dilatation may be necessary for weeks to years following an infection or trauma that has caused a stricture of the urethra. Either woven filiforms and followers, bougies, or metal sounds are used. If the latter are preferred by the urologist, curved metal sounds are used to dilate a male urethra; straight sounds are used on females.

Urethroplasty Reestablishment of continuity without stricture is the ultimate objective following traumatic urethral injury, usually associated with pelvic fracture in men. Scrotal-inlay urethroplasty or other method of urethral reconstruction usually is delayed until the extent of the injury can be fully evaluated by urethrograms. A suprapubic cystostomy catheter, inserted as an emergency measure, can maintain urinary drainage for several weeks to months. Insertion of a urethral catheter into a ruptured urethra in the immediate posttraumatic period can produce periurethral infection, stricture, and other irreparable damage.

Urethrotomy An Otis urethrotome may be used to cut into a urethral stricture. After this instrument is passed into the urethra, the blade is released to cut the stricture. If a specimen of the urethra is to be taken for biopsy, a rigid biopsy forceps is used through a cystourethroscope.

ENDOCRINE GLANDS

Two pairs of glands in the endocrine system are of primary interest to the urologist: the adrenals in both sexes and the testes in the male.

Adrenal Glands

The adrenal glands secrete substances that help regulate fluid and electrolyte balance, influence metabolism and sexual organs, and assist the body in coping with stress. These glands are located in the retroperitoneal spaces immediately above the superior pole of each kidney. Total or partial excision of one or both adrenal(s) usually is performed by the urologist. However, in some hospitals, this operation has become the province of endocrinologic surgical specialists.

Adrenalectomy may be indicated for the removal of a benign, malignant, or metastatic tumor within the adrenal medulla, or to eliminate adrenal hormonal secretions. The adrenal glands are a rich source of estrogens. Bilateral adrenalectomy may be performed as supplemental treatment of advanced prostatic or breast cancer to reduce the hormonal environment within the body. Estrogens may stimulate recurrence or metastasis from prostatic or breast cancer.

For a unilateral adrenalectomy, the adrenal gland usually is approached posteriorly through a lateral incision into the retroperitoneal space. The surgeon may prefer a posterior approach also for a bilateral adrenalectomy with the patient placed in a modified prone position for bilateral incisions. Other surgeons prefer an anterior thoracoabdominal or transabdominal incision into the retroperitoneal space with the patient in supine position. The circulating nurse must verify with the surgeon the preferred position before the patient is positioned, prepped, and draped. The thoracoabdominal incision may be preferred to extend the incision across the costal margin into the eighth or ninth intercostal space for exposure and exploration of the extra-adrenal paraganglion system, depending on the preoperative diagnosis.

Testes

The *testes* are the pair of male reproductive glands suspended in the scrotum that, after sexual maturity, are the source of spermatozoa. They also secrete hormones that influence growth and development, sexual activity, and secondary sex characteristics. When both testes are excised, the castrated patient becomes sterile and deficient in male hormones.

Bilateral orchiectomy usually is performed as adjunctive therapy in patients with prostatic cancer to alter the hormonal environment. Control of the disease following this relatively simple procedure is attempted before the urologist considers adrenalectomy. Psychological preparation is important to help the patient accept sterilization and other body changes, such as breast enlargement, which may occur as a result of alteration in the hormonal system.

Bilateral oblique incisions in the inguinal canals extend into the upper anterior surface of the scrotum over the testes. Following ligation of the spermatic cords at the external or internal inguinal rings, the testes are removed from the scrotum. Silicone rubber prostheses may be implanted in the scrotal sac to improve the cosmetic appearance or for the psychological rehabilitation of the patient.

MALE REPRODUCTIVE ORGANS

Testes

The testes are both hormonal glands and male reproductive organs. Disorders in or around one (or both) testis that inhibit sexual activity, reproductive capability, or cause discomfort in the scrotum may necessitate an operative procedure.

Unilateral Orchiectomy Removal of one testis does not sterilize the patient. This procedure may be performed (unilaterally as described for bilateral orchiectomy) to remove a testicular tumor, or may be indicated following traumatic injury or infection.

Hydrocelectomy A *hydrocele* is an accumulation of fluid in the sac of the tunica vaginalis of the testis. Through an anterior incision into the scrotum, the hydrocele sac is dissected away from the testis and removed from the scrotum.

Scrotal-Testicular Trauma A scrotal-testicular injury may require exploration to ligate bleeding vessels or to insert a Penrose drain. Infection is apt to occur following a penetrating wound so the extraperitoneal spaces in the scrotum must be drained thoroughly.

Varicocele Ligation Dilatation of the spermatic veins of the pampiniform plexus of the spermatic cord can cause a soft, elastic, often uncomfortable swelling in the scrotum. This condition, known as *varicocele,* occurs more frequently on the left side. It can cause loss in testicular mass and a decrease of sperm density associated with male infertility. Ligation of the spermatic vein can improve the sperm count if the testis has not atrophied.

The spermatic vein is ligated above the inguinal canal lateral to the inferior epigastric vessels or in the retroperitoneal space lateral to the iliac artery. In the latter approach, a transverse abdominal incision starts at the anterior superior iliac spine and extends toward the lateral aspect of the rectus abdominis muscle. The hemiscrotum must be manually emptied of all blood before the vein is ligated or the varicocele may persist postoperatively.

Vas Deferens

The *vas deferentia* are the small, fibromuscular excretory ducts that carry sperm upward through the spermatic cords from the epididymides lying along the upper portion of each testis, to the seminal vesicles, the pouchlike glands in front of the urinary bladder near the prostate gland. Interruption of or obstruction to the vas deferens inhibits normal spermatogenesis.

Vasectomy Elective bilateral vasectomy is an established method of male sterilization. This is usually performed as an ambulatory surgical procedure. A segment of each vas deferens is removed. The cut ends are either ligated with suture or clips, or fulgerated by coagulating the epithelium of the lumen, depending on the preference of the urologist. Techniques vary, but all patients should be informed that spontaneous regeneration of a severed vas deferens does occur in a small percentage of patients.

Vasovasostomy Recannulization of the vas deferens for restoration of fertility requires a nonobstructed anastomosis. The tough, 2-mm outer diameter with an inner diameter of 1 mm or less at the distal end, plus dilatation of the proximal end, make precise anastomosis under the operating microscope preferable to nonmicrosurgical techniques in which it is difficult to see the lumen of the vas deferens on the distal side. One-layer anastomosis and splinting techniques for vasectomy reversal often result in a stricture caused by scarring within the lumen of the vas deferens that inhibits the passage of sperm. After a scrotal incision is made to expose the vas deferens above and below the site of previous ligation, the two ends are cut to excise the scar tissue and to open the lumen. Under magnification of the operating microscope, interrupted sutures are placed in the mucosal lining of the lumen to create a fluid-tight, nonstrictured anastomosis. The muscularis is approximated separately. Sperm counts return to normal soon after operation.

Prostate Gland

A musculoglandular organ encased in a fibrous capsule, the *prostate gland* surrounds the posterior urethra at the bladder neck. It is divided into five lobes. Normal function of this gland provides secretions to the seminal fluid for sperm mobility during ejaculation.

Though this gland normally weighs 20 g, it will enlarge to some degree in most men by the time they reach age 50. Enlargement of the prostate gland can cause obstruction of the urethra. Difficulty in voiding most often brings patients with prostatic disease to a urologist. The entire gland or one or more lobes can be enucleated from its capsule transurethrally. Prostatectomy also can be performed through a suprapubic or retropubic abdominal incision or a perineal incision. A radical prostatectomy, performed through a retropubic abdominal or perineal incision, includes extirpation of the prostate, periprostatic tissue, seminal vesicles, and vas ampullae en bloc. The approach and procedure depend on the urologist's preference for removing the pathology. Carcinoma of the prostate is the second most common cancer in all males and the most common in men over 50 years of age. Benign prostatic hypertrophy (BPH) also is a common indication for prostatectomy in males over 50.

Transurethral Prostatectomy A *resectoscope* (refer to p. 363) is introduced into the prostatic urethra. Transurethral resection (TUR) of the prostate refers to electroresection or cryosurgical removal of all or part of the glandular tissue within the prostatic capsule. BPH of glands under 50 g in size are the usual indication for TUR. This approach is not without potential complications of impotence and urinary incontinence. The technique is one of the most difficult for the urologist to master.

If cryosurgery is used, continuous rectal palpation is required and unit temperature must be monitored continuously. This is a rapid technique with only slight blood loss, particularly useful for poor-risk patients. However, there is danger of freezing too widely, with slough into the bladder. Tissue may slough much later with delayed hemorrhage.

Following a TUR, the urologist may insert a three-way 30-cc Foley catheter. The third lumen provides a means for continuous irrigation of the bladder for a time postoperatively to prevent formation of clots in the bladder.

Suprapubic Prostatectomy The suprapubic approach is limited almost exclusively to removal of a large benign hypertrophied gland over 50 g. Through a midline vertical incision above the symphysis pubis, the superior bladder wall is opened to expose the prostatic urethra. The prostatic lobes are enucleated with a finger inserted through an incision into the mucosa of the urethra. This procedure may be termed *transvesicocapsular prostatectomy* because the prostatic capsule is approached through the bladder. Hemostatic agents usually are packed into the extremely vascular prostatic fossa to help control bleeding. Pressure from the Foley catheter balloon inserted after closure of the urethra also helps obtain hemostasis. A cystostomy tube is inserted to facilitate urinary drainage from the bladder during the healing process.

Retropubic Prostatectomy The prostate gland is exposed below the bladder neck through a vertical or transverse abdominal incision above the symphysis pubis. The gland is removed through an incision in the prostatic capsule; this is a *transcapsular prostatectomy.* The periprostatic tissue, seminal vesicles, and vas ampullae also may be excised if the operation is performed for carcinoma but there is no evidence of spread beyond the prostatic capsule. This latter radical procedure may be carried out as a second stage following either a diagnostic transurethral or suprapubic prostatectomy.

Perineal Prostatectomy With the patient in an extreme lithotomy position, the perineum affords the most direct open operative approach to the prostate through a relatively avascular field. The urologist incises the perineum above the anal sphincter and dissects the rectum from the posterior surface of the prostate, or dissection may be carried out between the external anal sphincter and the rectum. The perineal approach may be used to enucleate the prostate gland from its capsule or for total prostatovesiculectomy. The latter radical procedure includes removal of the entire prostate gland, its capsule, the seminal vesicles, and a portion of the bladder. The classical radical perineal prostatectomy may be the urologist's operation of choice to reduce morbidity from early or advanced prostatic carcinoma.

Pelvic Lymphadenectomy Through a lower abdominal incision into the extraperitoneal space, lymph nodes are dissected bilaterally from the iliac vessels, the obturator spaces, and the hypogastric vessels. These nodes may be examined by frozen section to detect early and subtle metastases from prostatic carcinoma. If several positive nodes are present, the patient is unlikely to benefit from radical prostatectomy. If nodes are negative, the urologist may proceed with a radical retropubic prostatectomy. Pelvic lymphadenectomy also may be done as a staged procedure prior to radical perineal prostatectomy.

Penis

The *penis* is the male organ of copulation. Because it contains the urethra, a deviation or malformation in structure may affect the normal urinary flow from the bladder. Operations to repair congenital anomalies of the penis and circumcision are discussed in Chapter 26 because these procedures usually are performed during infancy and childhood. In the adult, however, erectile impotency frequently brings the patient to the urologist. The etiology of impotence can be classified as *organic* or *psychogenic.* Patients must be thoroughly evaluated and properly selected for surgical therapy.

Implantation of a penile prosthesis can enable some impotent men to achieve a satisfactory return of sexual activity. Penile prosthetic implants are of two types: one is rigid and the other is an inflatable hydraulic device.

1 The Small-Carrion rigid prosthesis consists of two partially sponge-filled silicone rods inserted into the corpus cavernosum on the left and right sides of the penis, usually through a vertical incision in the perineum underneath the scrotum. The suitable-size prosthesis is selected from lengths available measuring from 12 to 19 cm (5 to $7\frac{1}{2}$ in.). The prosthesis maintains an erectile penis.

2 The Scott inflatable hydraulic device is inserted through a midline incision extending from the base of the penis to a point midway between the symphysis pubis and the umbilicus. Silicone elastic cylinders, filled with frozen sterile distilled water, are placed inside the penis. Tubing connected to these cylinders at the base of the penis is brought into the left inguinal canal, into the prevesical space, into the right inguinal canal, and connected to tubing from the pump-release mechanism placed in the scrotum. A reservoir is placed in the prevesical space. Tubing from this reservoir is also connected to the pump-release mechanism. To achieve erection of the penis, the patient squeezes the pump in the scrotum.

Transsexual Surgery

Transsexual surgery is the only cure for a patient who is psychologically possessed with the desire to physically and emotionally become a member of the opposite sex. This type of surgery presents extreme challenges to the urologist and gynecologist. Operative techniques have been developed to eliminate the obvious external genitalia of a male by dissection of penile structures, shortening of the urethra, and removal of the testes. The penile and scrotal skin are preserved for construction of a pseudofemale vaginal orifice. This procedure is done as the final stage following change of secondary sexual characteristics by hormonal or surgical therapy to produce breast enlargement, suppression of beard and body hair, redistribution of adipose tissue, voice change, and removal of pronounced thyroid cartilage (the Adam's apple). This final stage of transsexual surgery, from male to female, creates a vagina by inverting the hollow penis into the hypogastrium between the new urethral orifice and the rectum. Because the nerve endings from the penis are intact, the newly constructed vagina is capable of experiencing orgasm postoperatively. The prostate and seminal vesicles are retained so that orgasm with emission is possible. The scrotal skin forms the labia.

UROLOGIC ENDOSCOPY

Cystoscopic and other conservative urologic procedures are performed in an especially designed and equipped area, often referred to as the *cysto room* or *suite.* This may be within the OR suite or in the urology clinic. X-ray control booths and developing units are adjacent to or within the area. Because x-ray procedures are frequently performed, the walls and doors of the room must be lead-lined.

All safety regulations apply in the cysto room just as they do elsewhere in the OR suite, to protect the welfare of the patients and personnel. All lighted instruments and electrical equipment should be checked for proper function before and after each use. Personnel who must remain in the room with the patient while x-rays are taken should wear lead aprons. Patients should be protected with gonadal shields whenever feasible.

Proper OR attire is worn by all personnel entering the room. Most urologists don a conductive water-repellent apron before scrubbing, unless sterile water-repellent gowns are provided. The urologist wears sterile gown and gloves. Procedures performed in the cysto room must maintain a sterile field. Adherence to all the principles of aseptic technique is mandatory to prevent nosocomial urinary tract infection.

Preparation of the Patient

1 The patient should be encouraged to drink fluids before coming to the cysto room, unless the procedure will be done under general or regional anesthesia. Fluids ensure a rapid collection of urine specimens from the kidneys.
2 Frequently procedures are done without anesthesia, with topical agents, or with local infiltration anesthesia. The patient should be reassured that the procedure usually can be performed with only mild discomfort. Respect the patient's modesty, and try to avoid embarrassing him or her.
3 The patient is assisted into lithotomy position with knees resting in padded knee supports. Pads avoid undue pressure in the popliteal spaces.
4 The drainage pan is pulled out of the lower break of the urologic table after the patient's legs are positioned on the knee supports and the foot of the table is lowered.

   NOTE. The urologic table differs from the standard operating table in that it must provide an x-ray unit with a film cassette holder, a drainage pan, and knee supports. Some tables are equipped with hydraulic or electrical controls to adjust height and tilt, tray attachments for the light source and electrosurgical unit, and hooks for irrigating solution containers.

5 The pubic region, external genitalia, and perineum are mechanically cleansed with an antiseptic agent according to the routine skin-preparation procedure (refer to Chap. 11). Warm the solution before applying it to an unanesthetized patient.
6 Topical anesthetic agents are applied to the urethra at the end of the prep procedure. A viscous liquid preparation of lidocaine hydrochloride, 1 or 2%, may be used. This medium remains in the urethra rather than flowing into the bladder.
   a *For female.* The female urethra is most sensitive at the meatus. Thus, a small sterile cotton applicator dipped into the anesthetic agent and placed with the cotton tip in the meatus is sufficient. It is removed when the urologist is ready to introduce an instrument.
   b *For male.* A syringe or bottle with a rubber acorn tip or nozzle is used for intraurethral insertion. The agent is injected into the urethra and the penis compressed with a penile clamp for a few minutes to retain the drug.
7 A sterile stainless steel filter screen is placed over the drainage pan. The patient is draped as for other perineal procedures in lithotomy position. The urologist may want to have access to the rectum. A disposable O'Connor sheet is used. This has a synthetic rubber rectal sheath

that protects the finger during rectal palpation. The perineal sheet has two fenestrations: one exposes the genitalia; the other fits over the screen on the drainage pan. A gauze filter is incorporated into this latter fenestration in a disposable cystoscopy drape.

The urologist may prefer to wear a sterile disposable plastic apron over his or her gown. Attached to the table, this provides a sterile field from the urologic table to the urologist's shoulders. A receptor kit that attaches to the apron eliminates the need for the drainage pan. Tissue specimens are collected as irrigating fluid passes through a collecting basket.

Urologic Endoscopes

Urologic endoscopic instruments and catheters are available in sizes to suit infants, children, and adults. Size of these instruments and catheters is measured on the French scale: the diameter in millimeters multiplied by 3. Ureteral catheters are available in sizes 3 to 14 French, as described on page 354. The smallest is 1 mm in diameter times 3, or 3 French.

Specific endoscopic equipment is required to perform all the procedures under the broad term *cystoscopies.* All urologic endoscopes have the same basic components as follows:

Sheath The hollow sheath may be concave, convex, or straight in configuration at the distal end inserted into the urethra. The other end has a stopcock attachment for irrigation. Sizes range from 11 French for infants to 30 French for adults. Within the sheath, space is provided to accommodate instruments for work in the bladder or urethra. Other instruments and catheters can be inserted through the sheath into the ureters and kidneys for purposes of diagnosis or treatment as previously described.

Obturator The stainless steel obturator, inserted into the sheath, occludes the opening and facilitates introduction into the urethra without trauma to the mucosal lining.

Telescope Telescopes are complex precision optical systems. Each telescope contains multiple, finely ground optical lenses. The newest optical system has a series of 10 rod-shaped relay lenses that relay the image from the distal end inside the bladder or urethra to the ocular of the urologist. Five additional rod-shaped elements, known as *field lenses,* are between each pair of relay lenses. Properly spaced throughout the length of the telescope, the lenses give an undistorted clear vision at the desired angle with some magnification. Telescopes are costly, delicate instruments and must be handled gently at all times. The optical systems provide several angles of vision:

1 Direct forward vision is useful for ureteral catheterization.

2 Right angle is most suitable for viewing the entire bladder.

3 Lateral, which deviates 70° but includes right angle in line of vision, is used for wide-angle viewing within the bladder.

4 Foroblique, which is a forward vision with an oblique view somewhat in front of right angle, is used to examine the urethra.

5 Retrospective, which provides an approximate 55° angle of retrograde vision, is used to inspect the bladder neck.

All telescopes are made of stainless steel with a Bakelite ocular. Some have operating or working elements incorporated into the telescopic instrument.

Light The light source may be either a fiberoptic bundle or an incandescent bulb (refer to Chap. 15). This may be an integral part of the sheath or the telescope. A cord connects the instrument to the fiberoptic light projector, a rheostat, or battery. Fiberoptics have largely replaced incandescent lamps.

Types of Urologic Endoscopes While many different urologic endoscopes and accessories are in use, only the ones most commonly used are described.

Brown-Buerger Cystoscope The stainless steel sheaths range in size from 14 to 26 French. Size 21 French is used most frequently in adults with a right-angle examination telescope for routine inspection of the bladder. Size 24 or 26 French is used to accommodate larger instruments and catheters that cannot be used through size 21. The sheath contains the light carrier.

A Brown-Buerger cystoscope set usually consists of two sheaths, one concave and one convex, each with its own obturator, and two or three right-angle telescopes. Along with the basic examination telescope, the set may have a combination operating and double catheterizing telescope, known as a *convertible telescope,* or the operating and double catheterizing functions may be in separate telescopes. The convertible, operating, and catheterizing telescopes have a small deflectable lever on the distal end to aid in directing ureteral catheters or flexible stone baskets into the ureters. All corresponding parts of each set must be of the same French size.

McCarthy Panendoscope The stainless steel sheaths range in size from 14 to 30 French. These are used most frequently with the foroblique telescope for viewing the urethra. Other telescopes are available for bladder visualization. The telescopes are interchangeable with all sizes of sheaths. A bridge assembly is required to fit the telescope properly to the sheath. The light is supplied through the telescope.

Wappler Cystourethroscope This instrument combines the functions of the Brown-Buerger cystoscope and the McCarthy panendoscope. The stainless steel sheaths range in size from 17 to 24 French. The foroblique and lateral telescopes, which also supply the light, are interchangeable with all sheaths. A visual obturator may be used to permit visualization and irrigation during introduction of the sheath into the urethra.

NOTE. Verify with the urologist the type and size of the available endoscopes preferred for examination and/or treatment prior to placing the instrumentation on the sterile instrument table.

Resectoscope The resectoscope uses electric energy to excise tissue from the bladder, urethra, or prostate. The components of this instrument include the sheath, obturator, telescope, working element, and cutting electrode. The sheath, usually 28 French, must be made of Bakelite or fiberglass to prevent short circuit of the electric current. If the short beak post sheath is used with a wide-angle telescope, a Timberlake obturator must be used to introduce the sheath into the urethra.

The working element of the resectoscope, inserted through the sheath, has a channel for the telescope and cutting electrode. The types of working elements differ by the method in which the cutting electrode moves.

1 The *Iglesias* resectoscope uses a thumb control on a leaf spring-lock mechanism. The working element can be adapted for simultaneous irrigation and suction to control hydraulic pressure in the bladder.
2 The *Nesbit* resectoscope uses a thumb control on a spring.
3 The *Baumrucker* resectoscope uses finger control on a sliding mechanism.
4 The *Stern-McCarthy* resectoscope uses a rack and pinion to move the loop forward and back. This requires two hands.

The cutting electrode is the most critical component of a resectoscope. Because it must both cut and coagulate tissue, the electrode must be stabilized in the working element so that it retracts properly into the sheath after each cut. The electrode has a cutting loop from which electric current is passed through the tissue, an insulated fork, an insulated stem, and the contact that is inserted into the working element. Several loop sizes are available; the stem is usually color-coded by size. The loop size corresponds to the French size of the sheath. The electrode is malleable; therefore, it must be checked before use to be certain the insulation is intact and the loop is not broken. Electric current is applied only when the loop is engaged in tissue and inactivated after a cut is completed. The sheath can be charred if electric current is maintained after the cutting loop has been retracted into it.

Conductive lubricants must never be used on the sheath. They may provide a pathway for the electric current. Cleanliness of the sheath and all other components is essential to proper function.

Electrodes

In addition to the cutting loops used with the resectoscope primarily for transurethral resections, other types of electrodes are used in the bladder. These are inserted through the operating telescope of the Brown-Buerger cystoscope or Wappler cystourethroscope. They are used mainly for fulgeration of bladder tumors, coagulation of bladder vessels to control bleeding following biopsy, and ureteral meatotomy. More electric current is needed when working in solution, as in the bladder, than in air. The power control settings on the electrosurgical unit should be as low as possible, however. All precautions and safeguards for the use and care of electrosurgical equipment apply to urologic procedures (refer to Chap. 14).

Irrigating Equipment

Continuous irrigation of the bladder is necessary during a cystoscopy to:

1 Distend the bladder walls so the urologist can visualize them
2 Wash out blood, bits of resected tissue, or stone fragments to permit continuous visibility and collection of specimens

A sterile disposable closed irrigating system is preferred because it prevents airborne contamination of the solution. However, a Valentine irrigator may still be in use in some hospitals. This is a large glass container, open at the top.

Two to four or more liters of sterile irrigating solution may be needed for a single examination. Ten to twelve liters are needed for a TUR. Disposable tandem sets may be used to connect several containers together. Tandem sets allow for a continuous flow and for replacement of containers without interruption of flow. Sterile disposable irrigating tubing is connected to the irrigating solution container before hanging it on a hook on the urologic table, in the ceiling, or on a stand placed beside the table. The solution container should be at a level $2\frac{1}{2}$ ft (.75 m) above the table: a lower level decreases flow; a higher level increases hydraulic pressure with consequent fluid absorption by the patient's tissues. The tubing should be filled with solution before it is attached to the sheath of the cystoscope or resectoscope. The plastic tubing from the container to the instrument is for individual patient use only.

Sterile isosmotic irrigating solutions that are nonhemolytic and nonelectrolytic are generally preferred by most urologists. However, sterile distilled water may be used for observation procedures. If a sufficient amount enters the circulation through open blood vessels during a TUR, water may hemolyze red blood cells. As much as 3 to 6 liters of solution may be absorbed during a transurethral prostatectomy. The minerals in water or saline act as a conductor and disperse the current when the electrosurgical unit is used.

Isosmotic solutions of 1.5% glycine, an amino acid, or sorbitol, an inert sugar, premixed in distilled water are commercially available in 1.5- and 3-liter containers. A glycine solution, Urogate or Uromatic, is more commonly used for TUR.

During the procedure, the flow of solution into the endoscope is controlled by the stopcock on the sheath where the tubing attaches. Rubber tips or nipples are used to seal other openings on the instrument to prevent escape of solution during a procedure. The openings through which catheters or instruments are to be inserted are closed with tips containing a hole. The accessory can be inserted through this hole with the seal maintained.

When the urologist wishes, the irrigating solution flows away from the instrument into the drainage pan through the filter screen. The solution drains from the pan, through tubing, into a collecting bucket that is emptied after each patient use. Some cysto rooms have floor drains. These may be a source of environmental contamination unless cleaned thoroughly. If large quantities of solution are used, observe the level of drainage into the bucket to avoid overflow on the floor or around the foot pedal of the electrosurgical unit.

Evacuators

Evacuators may be used to irrigate the bladder and to aspirate stone fragments, blood clots, or resected tissue. The two most commonly used types are the Ellik and Toomey.

Ellik This is a double bowl-shaped glass evacuator containing a trap for fragments so they cannot be washed back into the sheath of the endoscope while irrigating with pressure on the rubber-bulb attachment.

Toomey This is a syringe-type evacuator with a wide opening into the barrel. It may be used with any endoscope sheath. A metal adaptor permits its use with a catheter.

Care and Preventive Maintenance

1 Adequate sterilization is mandatory; therefore, all endoscopes and reusable accessories must be free of debris and residue.
   - **a** Disassemble all parts and open all outlets.
   - **b** Clean all parts in a warm nonresidue liquid-detergent solution, rinse in clean water, and dry thoroughly.
   - **c** Clean the interior of sheaths and openings with a soft brush.
   - **d** Wipe lenses gently with a soft, dry cloth.

2 Place endoscopes on a towel, to act as padding, in the sink, on countertops, and in trays to protect them from hard surfaces during handling and storage.

3 In cleaning the inside of a sheath or telescope, take care not to break the glass window over the light. These windows should be inspected each time the endoscopes are used, as the urethra may be lacerated by a broken window.

4 Check function of all moving parts, clarity of vision through telescopes, and patency of channels through instruments and catheters.

5 Keep sets of sounds, bougies, and filiforms and followers together so that the urologist will have a complete range of sizes readily accessible.

6 After cleaning, wrap items for sterilization. Flexible instruments should be protected by a rigid container.

7 Clean, dry stone baskets may be sealed in a peel-open package and sterilized in ethylene oxide

gas. Retractable stone baskets must be sterilized in the open position.

8 The principles and methods of sterilization discussed in Chapter 5 apply to urologic instrumentation. Steam-sterilizable items should be steam-sterilized. However, with the exception of nylon and rubber catheters and bougies and nonflexible stainless steel instruments that do not have lenses, urologic endoscopes and accessories must be sterilized in ethylene oxide gas or activated glutaraldehyde solution. All items should be sterilized after cleaning and then placed in sterile storage. Aeration following ethylene oxide sterilization is essential for Bakelite parts of endoscopes, woven and synthetic materials.

Chapter 20

Orthopaedics

Orthopaedics is derived from two Greek words: *ortho* (straight) and *pais* (child). Orthopaedics, as the name implies, began with the treatment of crippled children by means of rest, braces, and exercises. As a contemporary surgical specialty, it is "that branch of surgery especially concerned with the preservation and restoration of the functions of the skeletal system, its articulations and associated structures."* Diseases and disabilities affecting the neuromusculoskeletal system cause loss of function and impair the activity of many individuals. The increasing age of the population has added numbers to those suffering from these diseases and disabilities. Congenital deformities of the musculoskeletal system are frequent. Conservative, noninvasive methods are nearly always used first, but patient care must be individualized to restore both form and function.

DEVELOPMENT OF ORTHOPAEDICS

Records tell of the treatment of fractures in Egypt 4500 years ago. Mummies have been found with splints still in place. Some of these were made from the bark of trees; others were strips of linen impregnated with a glue-like substance. Egyptian mummies and murals show evidence of crippling diseases. One drawing, over 800 years old, shows a man using a crutch.

Hippocrates described scoliosis, congenital dislocation of the hip, clubfoot, and tuberculosis. His writings included the accumulated knowledge of past centuries, so no doubt many of the treatment methods he advocated date back beyond his time. Almost all the principles of treating fractures currently followed are included in his book *On Fractures.* He discussed the use of traction, countertraction, bandages, splints, and treatment of compound fractures. He used mixtures of gelatinous substances and clay to coat the bandages. He recognized the necessity of immobilizing the joint above and below the fracture. He described the proper position of fixing joints for the best possible future function. He wrote that exercise strengthens but inactivity wastes an immobilized part. He advocated mobilization of fractures as much as possible, to prevent atrophy. For centuries much of the material in the books of Hippocrates was ignored or forgotten, then rediscovered.

Galen described the muscles of the body and their function as a motor system directed by the brain through nerves. He named the spinal deformities still known as lordosis, scoliosis, and kyphosis.

*American Board of Orthopaedic Surgery.

In the sixteenth century, Paré described appliances to support or correct orthopaedic conditions. He wrote a book on dislocations. His description of fractures of the spine was the beginning of modern spinal surgery.

Modern orthopaedic surgery began to evolve in the eighteenth century. The earliest known institute for treatment of skeletal deformities was founded in Switzerland in 1790. The development of orthopaedic surgery has been enhanced by expenditures of governments and societies for the care of the crippled and disabled, and by the growth of hospitals and rehabilitation centers.

Lewis Sayre was appointed to the first orthopaedic professorship in an American medical school in 1861 when the Bellevue Hospital Medical College opened in New York City. Of the orthopaedic surgeons in the late nineteenth century, no one contributed more to the development of the specialty than Charles Fayette Taylor (1827–1899). His investigations in *kinesipathy* (movement cure) and surgical mechanics contributed to the undertaking of exercise and rest in the treatment of musculoskeletal disorders. Fundamental concepts of these and other early teachers have not changed; their methods of treatment have changed as new knowledge has been gained and materials have been improved. Knowledge of skeletal tissue led orthopaedists to attempt operations of tendons and joints. An increased knowledge of bone regeneration, the concept of aseptic technique, the discovery of x-ray, the introduction of sulfonamides and antibiotics, the development of instrumentation and appliances all have contributed to the advancement of orthopaedic surgery.

The multidisciplinary approaches of physics and biology created a surge of interest in neuromusculoskeletal science and technology for orthopaedic surgery. Attempts were made in the 1950s to replace the components of the hip joint. In 1959, John Charnley suggested in England that methyl methacrylate, used in dentistry, might be used to hold prosthetic components in place. The field of biomechanics really began to develop, however, when Charnley introduced the low-friction torque prosthesis for total hip replacement in 1962. Since then biomechanics has revolutionized orthopaedic surgery.

SPECIAL FEATURES OF ORTHOPAEDIC SURGERY

The orthopaedic surgeon, also referred to as an *orthopaedist* or *orthopod,* attempts to restore the mechanical function of the body. Operations may be performed to correct congenital deformities (refer to Chap. 26), reconstruct or eradicate degenerative disease processes, or repair traumatic injuries. The orthopaedist is basically concerned with the bones, ligaments, tendons, muscles, and capsule tissues of the extremities, including the shoulder and hip joints, and the vertebral column. A large percentage of the operations involve contaminated wounds or tissues highly susceptible to infection. An infection in bone may remain for life or may cause loss of an extremity. Therefore, meticulous attention to aseptic technique is critical in all orthopaedic procedures. Some additional points that apply specifically to orthopaedic surgery are discussed here.

Instrumentation

Each orthopaedic operation must have the correct instrumentation for *that* particular bone, joint, tendon, or other structures the orthopaedist will encounter. An instrument used on a hip procedure is not appropriate for a hand. Orthopaedic instruments are heavy, often large and bulky, but also delicate. Each instrument has a specific purpose and requires special care and handling. Orthopaedic instruments can be divided into categories by functional design.

Exposing Instruments It is necessary to expose a bone or joint for many procedures. Special retractors and elevators are used.

1 Retractors are contoured to fit around the bone or joint without cutting or tearing muscles.

2 Periosteal elevators are semisharp instruments used to strip the periosteum from the bone without destroying its ability to regenerate new bone.

Grasping Instruments These are required to hold, manipulate, or retract bone. Bone-holding forceps should be selected appropriately for the size of the bone in the operative field. Bone hooks are used for retraction and leverage. Heavy clamps are needed to hold smaller bones or to grasp the capsule, such as a meniscus clamp.

Cutting Instruments These are used to remove soft tissue around bone, to cut into, cut apart, or cut out portions of bone, or to smooth jagged edges of bone. The orthopaedist's armamentarium includes osteotomes, gouges, chisels, curettes, rongeurs, reamers, bone-cutting forceps, meniscitomes, rasps, files, drills, and saws. These have sharp edges. Take extra care not to nick or damage cutting edges by protecting them on the instrument table and during cleaning, sterilizing, and storing. Fitted sterilizable racks, trays, or canvas cases are used to keep sets together by sizes, e.g., osteotomes, gouges, chisels, and curettes, as well as to protect the cutting edges.

NOTE. Cutting instruments must be kept sharpened. Osteotomes, chisels, gouges, and meniscitomes can be sharpened by OR personnel with hand-held hones or a honing machine designed for this purpose. Most manufacturers provide a service for sharpening and repairing instruments. Curettes, rongeurs, and reamers should be returned for sharpening. Small drill bits and saw blades usually are discarded when dulled.

Power-driven Cutting Instruments These instruments increase the speed and decrease the fatigue of manually driven drills, saws, reamers, and rongeurs. The power source may be electricity from direct current or a battery, or compressed dry nitrogen.

1 *Electrical saws and drills* that are explosion-proof should be used. Observe rules for use of electrical equipment (refer to Chap. 14).

2 *Air-powered instruments* use compressed nitrogen either piped into the OR or in a cylinder on a stable carrier. The pressure must be set and monitored by the operating pressure gauge of the regulator. The instruments are small, lightweight, and easy to handle for pinpoint accuracy at high speed, free of vibration.

These instruments offer precision in drilling, cutting, shaping, and beveling bone. Blood loss from bone is reduced by the tiny particles packed into the cut surface. The instrument may have rotary, reciprocating, or oscillating action. Rotary movement is used to drill holes or insert screws, wires, or pins. Reciprocating movement, a cutting action from front to back, and oscillating cutting action from side to side are used to cut or remove bone. Some instruments have a combination of movements and can be changed from one to the other. In some the change may be made by adjusting the chuck forward or backward and locking it in the desired position. Power instruments are not used without some inherent dangers.

1 Heat generated can damage bone cells. Air-powered instruments cause minimal heating by comparison with electrical instruments because they operate at a faster, higher speed. When using electrical saws or drills, the orthopaedist usually has the assistant drip saline solution on the area from a bulb syringe, to cool the bone and wash away particles. Care must be used so the syringe does not touch the blade, especially if it is glass. Plastic bulb syringes are less hazardous.

2 Normal tissue, including the orthopaedist's or assistant's finger, can be caught in a rapidly spinning drill or oscillating saw unless carefully controlled. The instrument may cut more than desired. When a power instrument is being used, particularly with rotating movement, all team members are very careful to keep their hands away from the blade.

3 Disconnect a direct-current electrical instrument from its power source when not in use so a team member cannot inadvertently activate it. Some electrical saws and drills are activated by a foot pedal. As an added protection, set the instrument and attachments on a small sterile table, alone, when not in use. Air-powered instruments have fingertip controls. The safety slide should be set in position to prevent inadvertent activation until ready for use.

4 Always handle and store the electrical power cord or air hose with care. A broken cord can short-circuit the instrument. A broken hose under pressure can whip out of control possibly injuring the patient or personnel. Always inspect cord or hose prior to use.

5 Always be certain attachments and blades are completely seated and locked in the handle before activating power.

6 Always operate, clean, and sterilize power instruments according to the manufacturer's manual with directions for use and care.

Implant-related Instruments These include drivers, clamps, and retractors used for inserting, securing, or removing fixation and prosthetic implants. Each type of implant requires its own instrumentation. As stated in Chapter 13, instruments used for insertion or extraction of metallic implants must be of the same metal as the implant to prevent galvanic reaction.

Items Used Frequently

Although not used in every orthopaedic procedure, the items discussed are handled frequently.

Bone Grafts When necessary to remove a piece of bone from one part of the skeletal system to reinforce another bone, a separate small sterile table may be prepared for the instrumentation required for the donor site. If the recipient area is potentially contaminated, as in Pott's disease or tuberculosis of a joint, the donor site must be kept free from possible contamination from the recipient site. Autogenous cancellous bone is obtained from the crest of the ilium, cortical bone from the tibia.

Bone Bank Allografts Bone may be fresh frozen and preserved for use as needed to fill a bone defect. This is especially useful when autogenous bone is not available in sufficient quantity, or the orthopaedist deems it undesirable to subject the patient to a secondary incision or the added operating time required to remove bone for an autogenous graft. Bone, such as a rib or femoral head, may be salvaged from patients free from malignancy or infection for a homogenous graft into another person. Autogenous bone may be preserved following operation by storage in the bone bank for subsequent grafting into the same patient. Bone may be stored for as long as 6 months. To preserve bone, the following procedures usually are carried out:

1 A small piece of the bone is put into a sterile petri dish for culture. This is done during the operation by one of the sterile team members. The culture is sent to the bacteriologist.

2 This person may cut the bone into convenient sizes, if necessary, to put each piece into the inner part of a sterile double-plastic container. The smaller inside container is placed on the sterile table when the bone is used, so must not be contaminated during preparation of the bone.

3 The bone specimens are put into the freezer on a shelf labeled "not ready for use." Each container has a card attached. When the culture report comes back from the laboratory, it is recorded on the card.

4 All specimens with negative culture reports are labeled "sterile," and then are transferred to the compartment in the freezer labeled "ready for use."

5 Any bone that has a positive culture or any bone obtained from a source under nonsterile conditions is packaged in double-plastic covers, with a glass bead inside the covers with each specimen. These bones are shipped in dry ice to a center equipped to sterilize them by irradiation. The glass bead is an indicator and turns dark with sterilization.

6 When the packages of bone are returned from the sterilization center, one piece from the lot is sent for a culture. A card is placed on each package indicating the lot number. Each lot is held on the "unsterile shelf" in the freezer until the negative culture report is received and recorded.

7 When the bone is used, the card is completed with the patient's name and operation. This is kept as a part of the patient's permanent record.

Bone Cement Methyl methacrylate powder and liquid components are mixed at the instrument table immediately prior to insertion into the intramedullary canal of a long bone, the shaft of a bone, or the socket of a joint. Bone cement is used to reinforce fixation of some prosthetic implants or to increase strength of fixation implants. Follow the manufacturer's instructions for handling this material and avoid excessive exposure to vapors (refer to Chap. 13, p. 267). Also avoid getting lipid solvent on gloves; it can diffuse through latex to cause an allergic dermatitis.

Bone Wax Used for hemostasis in bone, bone wax is put on the instrument table and opened as requested. Check the orthopaedist's preference card before opening packet.

Casts and Braces A cast or brace is a means of obtaining external fixation of a fracture or a part following tendon repair, arthrodesis, or other type of operation. It is the means of putting a part at rest or attempting to correct an injury or abnormality. Cast application in the OR is discussed in detail later in this chapter.

Cast Room Casts are applied in the cast room, sometimes referred to as the *plaster room*. Many closed, noninvasive procedures are performed here, particularly those requiring general or regional anesthesia, when a cast room is located within the OR suite. This frees the OR for open, invasive operations. It also keeps plaster dust from the individual operating rooms, an important aspect of aseptic environmental control. Following open operation, the patient can be wheeled on the operating table into the cast room for application of a cast, if the patient is not endangered, while the nursing personnel prepare the OR for the next patient.

Clean-Air System Special care must be used to carry out strict asepsis. Infection is the most serious, dreaded, and costly complication of orthopaedic surgery. Many orthopaedists, therefore, prefer to operate within a clean-air system, especially for total joint-replacement procedures. Laminar airflow, as described in Chapter 4, probably is used more frequently by orthopaedic surgeons than by any other surgical specialists.

Fixation and Prosthetic Implants Fixation and prosthetic implants are used to temporarily stabilize or permanently replace bone, joints, or tendons. They are made of stainless steel 316L, cobalt or titanium alloys, silicone, polyester covered with silicone, polyethylene or polytetrafluoroethylene. Due to the high cost of these implants, the inventory is kept as low as possible, yet large enough to ensure their availability when needed. These expensive implants usually are patient-charge items. After measurements are taken in the operative field, the correct size, shape, and design is selected from the sets available to assure handling only the one to be used without touching others. An infection around a fixation or prosthetic implant may require its removal, often resulting in permanent deformity or disability.

Orthopaedic Table An orthopaedic table, often referred to as the *fracture table,* is used for many operations requiring traction, image intensification or conventional x-ray control, and/or cast application. The many available attachments make possible any desired position and traction on any part of the body. The table can be raised, tilted laterally, put into Trendelenburg or reverse Trendelenburg position. The attachments are designed not only for stabilizing the patient in the desired position, but also for exerting traction to help reduce a fracture, and for providing the means of evaluating the diagnosis or therapy by radiologic control. Bakelite, a material that does not interfere with the view in radiographic studies, is used for attachments that might otherwise obscure the radiologic findings.

Essential standard component attachments on all models of orthopaedic tables include three-section patient body supports, lateral body brace, sacral rest, and traction apparatus. Optional accessories are available to accommodate the need for the types of procedures performed and the model of the table. When the orthopaedic table will be used:

1 Consult the surgeon's preference card, procedure book, and the manufacturer's manual for attachments needed for each desired position.

2 Assemble the necessary attachments. Pad all parts of the table and attachments to prevent pressure on joints, sacrum, and perineum.

3 Attach the standard components and accessories to the table frame so all is in readiness for positioning the patient when the orthopaedist arrives. The patient may be anesthetized before positioning is completed.

Nerve Stimulator The nerve stimulator is used occasionally to verify neural tissue when doing a partial nerve resection to control spastic muscles. When the popliteal nerve, for example, is given a slight shock with it, the foot jerks. Both direct electric current and disposable battery-operated stimulators are available.

Sutures Ligaments, tendons, periosteum, and joint capsules are very fibrous tissues. They are primarily tough, stringy collagen and contain few cells and blood vessels. As a result, they heal slower than vascular tissues. Nonabsorbable materials are generally used to suture ligaments, tendons, and muscles involved in the movement of the bony structure of the body. Absorbable suture is generally preferred to suture periosteum. Check the surgeon's preference card before opening suture packets.

X-Ray Control Conventional x-ray equipment and image intensifiers frequently are used during orthopaedic procedures. The considerations for patient safety and personnel protection described in Chapter 15 apply to the use of radiologic control for invasive or noninvasive orthopaedic procedures performed in the OR suite. Special positioning and draping techniques may be necessary, especially when an image intensifier is used.

Often both anterior-posterior (AP) and lateral views are necessary to assess the alignment of a bone or to determine the position of a fixation or prosthetic implant. X-rays document the work of the orthopaedist.

Special Considerations

1 Although unit beds and wheeled equipment should not enter the OR suite, in the interest of the patient's comfort and safety this rule is relaxed for some orthopaedic patients, such as patients in traction apparatus. Beds, frames, and stretchers can be decontaminated in the exchange area.

2 A cast should be removed preoperatively in the cast room. If the OR suite does not have a cast room, a cast may be precut in the patient's room and then removed in the OR. Cover sterile tables with a large sterile sheet while cast is being completely removed to prevent airborne contamination from plaster dust.

3 Positioning on the orthopaedic table for some operations requires an extra amount of activity. When possible, it is well to position these patients in the cast room before transporting them into the OR, and thus avoid dispersing lint and microorganisms into the air to settle on sterile tables.

EXTREMITIES

Although the instrumentation may vary by size of the structures involved, basic techniques apply to handling both upper and lower extremities.

General Considerations

1 A sterile irrigating pan is placed under an extremity to catch the solution if an open wound is to be cleansed, irrigated, and debrided, as for compound fracture (refer to Chap. 11, p. 225).

2 A tourniquet usually is used during operation on or below the elbow and knee. This provides a field free of blood, and thus the surgeon can more readily see fine structures (refer to discussion of tourniquets in Chap. 12).

The tourniquet cuff is applied before the extremity is prepped. However, *it is not inflated* until the draping is completed. Remember ischemia time is a critical factor in patient safety. Remind the orthopaedist after the first 45 minutes and every 15 minutes thereafter, throughout tourniquet application.

An Esmarch bandage may be applied before the pneumatic tourniquet is inflated to force blood from the extremity.

3 An extremity is always held up for skin preparation. See that the area under it is dry before draping (see Chap. 11). Prevent prep solution from running under tourniquet.

4 A self-adhering plastic drape may be used as the first drape applied. It may be impossible to adequately drape with self-adhering plastic drapes or fenestrated sheets. If the extremity must be manipulated during the operation, the entire circumference must be draped. A split sheet may be used.

5 Stockinet may be used over the self-adhering plastic drape or to cover the skin. This is cut with nurses' scissors over the line of incision. The cut edges may be secured over the skin edges with skin clips if a plastic drape is not used. A medicine cup is a handy receptacle for these clips after removal. The scrub nurse holds this at the field to receive the clips as the orthopaedist removes them.

6 A self-adhering plastic drape eliminates the need for either stockinet and metallic skin clips or towels and towel clips that might interfere with interpretation of x-rays or image intensification.

7 After operation on a knee joint, a pressure dressing usually is applied to prevent serum accumulation. This may be a Robert Jones dressing, which includes a soft cotton batting roll, sheet wadding, and cotton elastic bandage. A cotton roll, or other bulky material, may be placed on each side of the knee and held in place with sheet wadding. A four-ply, crinkled-gauze bandage or cotton elastic bandage over this provides even, gentle pressure. Depending on the operation, a plaster splint or other type of knee immobilizer may be preferred.

8 After operation on a shoulder, the arm may be bound against the side of the chest for immobilization. A large piece of cotton or sheet wadding is placed under the arm to keep skin surfaces from touching, as they may macerate. The arm is held in a shoulder immobilizer that supports the humerus and wrist, or it may be bound firmly to the side of the chest with a cotton elastic bandage.

9 An extremity is elevated on a pillow.

Types of Procedures

Preoperative assessment of an acute or chronic disability affecting the musculoskeletal system of an extremity includes evaluation of the extent of bony or soft tissue involvement with or without concomitant neurovascular compromise. Because they are the essence of adult orthopaedic surgery, either due to accidental trauma or a degenerative disease process, procedures on the following major anatomic classifications of structures will be discussed:

1 Fracture of bones
2 Reconstruction of joints
3 Repair of tendons and ligaments

FRACTURES

Intact bones are essential to stability and mobility of the upper and lower extremities. The skeleton functions mechanically. A comminuted (splintered) or fractured (broken) bone can cause malfunction and pain. Fractures vary by etiology, location and type of fracture line, and extent of injury.

1 *Traumatic.* The impact, forced twisting, or bending of an accidental injury can break one or more bones in the body. Traumatic fractures are either simple or compound.
   a *Simple Fracture.* The broken fragments do not protrude through the underlying tissues to skin.
   b *Compound Fracture.* Either the proximal or distal end of the bone, or both, protrudes from the fracture site through the underlying tissues and skin.

2 *Pathologic.* Primary or metastatic malignant bone disease can spontaneously fracture a diseased bone without undue stress. Although technically simple fractures, pathologic fractures require more than simple fixation of the bone fragments. Bone cement may be used as an

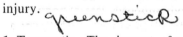

adjunct to fill a bone defect and increase strength of a fixation implant.

When a fracture occurs, mechanical means are used to reduce it and immobilize the parts, maintaining the fragments in proper alignment. Fractures must be handled gently with support above and below the site to prevent further trauma. A physician takes the responsibility for supporting and protecting the fracture site when moving a patient to or from a stretcher, bed, or table. Other personnel should be instructed as to the site of fracture and the special care needed in transferring the patient. The orthopaedist removes or directs the removal of temporary splints or traction. Adequate personnel must be available so the patient can be lifted gently. All lifters should be on the affected side, since this helps support the fracture during transfer.

In treating a fracture, the orthopaedist seeks to accomplish a solid union of the bone in perfect alignment, to return joints and muscles to normal position, to prevent or repair vascular trauma, and to rehabilitate the patient as early as possible. Treatment of fractures usually includes three distinct phases: reduction, immobilization, and rehabilitation. The methods of treating fractures include: (1) closed reduction with immobilization, (2) skeletal traction, and (3) internal fixation.

Closed Reduction

A fracture may be manipulated (set) to replace the bone in its proper alignment without opening the skin. This technique is referred to as a *closed reduction*. Many fractures of the lower leg can be treated by closed reduction. When both bones are fractured, fibula fractures are generally disregarded and the attention is directed to the tibia.

Often performed in the emergency department, the patient may come to the cast room in the OR suite for closed reduction under anesthesia and application of a device for immobilization. A plaster or Fiberglas cast, cast-brace, or molded plastic fracture-brace may be used to hold the reduced fracture site in alignment during union.

Skeletal Traction

Traction is the pulling force exerted to maintain proper alignment or position. In skeletal traction, the force is applied directly on the bone following insertion of pins, wires, or tongs placed through or into the bone. A small sterile setup is required. Traction is applied by means of pulleys and weights. Weights provide a constant force; pulleys help establish and maintain constant direction until the fractured bone reunites.

Forearm or Lower Leg A Kirschner wire, either plain or threaded, or a Steinmann pin is drilled through bone (preferably cortical) distal to the fracture site. For forearm fractures the wire or pin must be strong enough to prevent side-to-side, angular, and rotary motion while the fracture is healing. A traction bow is attached to the protruding ends of the wire or pin. The pulleys are fastened to this bow. Cover the ends of the wire or pin with corks or plaster to protect the patient and personnel from the sharp ends.

Finger A fine Kirschner wire may be drilled through the distal phalanx. The ends may be attached to a banjo splint. Or a cast may be applied to the forearm with a loop of heavy wire incorporated in it that fans out beyond the fingers. The Kirschner wire is fastened to this loop by a rubber band.

Internal Fixation

Open reduction and fixation usually are resorted to for those fractures not amendable to closed reduction or skeletal traction methods of conservative treatment. If vascular structures have been traumatized, internal fixation followed by vascular repair may be necessary to restore arterial tissue perfusion and adequate venous drainage.

Excellent results can be obtained by internal fixation of fractures as soon as possible after they occur. This method gives firm immobilization of the fragments and close approximation of them so that the gap between ends is not too great for the callus to bridge. It reduces to a minimum the space between fragments and movement at the fracture site. Healing seems to take place faster. The patient starts non-weight bearing exercises and progresses to ambulation early, thus reducing joint stiffness and muscle atrophy, and avoids a long period of rehabilitation.

Many types of fixation implants are available. Each type serves its purpose well in the hands of those familiar with its use. Internal fixation implants are made of a metal that is nonmagnetic and electrolytically inert. Only one kind of metal is used in a patient. The implant may be affixed to the cortex of the bone or inserted into the bone through the fracture site.

Screws, Plates, and Nails

Screws Screws alone may be used for fixation of an oblique or spiral fracture of a long bone. Screws must be long enough to penetrate both cortices. Hard cortical bone gives the best fixation and two cortices generally hold better than one. Screws are available in various lengths and diameters. Not all screws have the same type head, e.g., single slot, cross slot, concave cross slot, and Phillips head. The correct screwdriver must be used with each type screw.

Compression Plate and Screws Many fractures requiring open reduction are given rigid fixation through the compression method. Compression plates are heavy and strong. They are held in place by specially designed cortical lag screws. The threads of these screws are deeper than those on other types of screws, and also farther apart, which gives a larger amount of bone between the threads. This construction gives maximum holding power and rigid fixation. A compression instrument may be used. This is connected to the end of the plate and then fastened to the bone with a short screw. By tightening the nut on the compression instrument, the bone fragments are brought tightly together. The rest of the screws are put into the plate and the fracture is fixed. Screws alone are used only in selected situations. A cast may or may not be applied.

Eggers Plate and Screws The plate is slotted, which permits the muscle tone of the extremity to keep the ends of the fragments pressed closely together. The pressure stimulates osteogenesis.

Sherman Plate and Screws The appropriate-size plate is fitted to the contour of the bone, by bending slightly if necessary, before applying the screws. Using a drill guide, holes for the screws are drilled with an electric or air-powered drill in the center of the screw hole and perpendicularly to the plate. The drill bit should be slightly smaller than the screws. The screws should pass through both cortices of the bone.

Nails An intertrochanteric fracture of the neck of the femur may be treated by inserting a nail, compression screw, or multiple pins through the bone of the neck into the head of the femur. Many different types of nails are used. They usually are inserted over or alongside a guidewire. The nail may form a continuous, angulated unit with a plate that fits on the outer lateral cortex of the femur. Or the plate may be attached and the nail, screw, or pins inserted separately. Screws secure the plate to the shaft of the femur before or after the nail is inserted, depending on the design of the implant. Some of the more commonly used implants are:

1 Smith-Petersen cannulated nail with a McLaughlin adjustable plate.
2 Jewett cannulated nail/plate unit. A Jewett overlay plate also may be used with this implant.
3 Neufeld nail/plate unit.
4 Deyerle plate and multiple pins.
5 Lag screw with compression tube and plate.
6 Massie sliding nail and tube assembly.
7 Ken sliding nail.

The patient usually is positioned on the orthopaedic table. The orthopaedist and assistants take the responsibility for moving and positioning the patient (see Fig. 20-1 for position for nailing left hip). If portable x-ray machines are used, one is on the unaffected side for the anterior-posterior view, and one at the foot of the table for lateral view. The film for the AP view is placed on the cassette holder from the unaffected side. All sterile tables are positioned on the affected side. The orthopaedist may sit to operate.

Intramedullary Nailing An intramedullary nail or pin is driven into the medullary canal through the site of the fracture. This brings the ends together for union, splints the fracture, and eases the pain. It permits early return of function so the patient can be ambulatory. Intramedullary implants also provide a method of holding fragments in alignment in comminuted fractures. They usually are used for pathologic fractures or impending fracture of diseased bone.

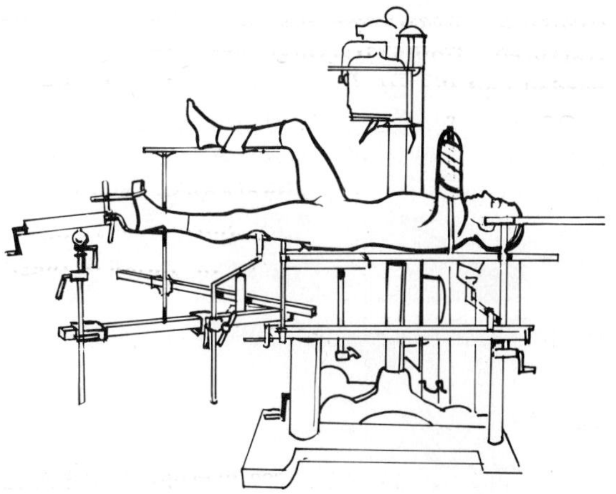

Figure 20-1 Position for nailing left hip. Note arm on affected side suspended from screen to remove it from operative field. Note traction on affected leg and support under knee. Elevated right leg permits x-ray tube to be adjusted under it for lateral view.

Intramedullary nailing may be done with x-ray control following closed reduction when visualization of the fracture site is unnecessary. Or the fracture may be reduced by visual exposure of the site and then the intramedullary implant inserted. In some situations, the medullary canal must be reshaped or enlarged before a nail is inserted. The length, size, and shape of the nail or pin depend on the bone to be splinted. The most commonly used appliances include:

1 Kuntscher nail, for the femur.
2 Hansen-Street pin, for the femur.
3 Zickel intramedullary rod and hip nail, for the femur. This is a particularly strong implant for stabilization of pathologic fractures.
4 Knowles pin, for the femur.
5 Schneider nail, for the femur, tibia, fibula, ulna, or radius.
6 Lottes nail, for the tibia.
7 Rush pin, for all long bones.
8 Steinmann pins, for clavicle, humerus, or ulna.

These implants may be removed after union at the fracture site has taken place.

The patient may be positioned on the orthopaedic table. This permits traction as needed. (See Fig. 20-2 for position of patient for intramedullary nailing of left tibia.)

JOINT RECONSTRUCTION

Joint function depends on the quality of its structures. Articular cartilage covers the two ends of bone where they meet to form the joint. Bones are held securely in place at their articulation by ligaments and the joint capsule attached to both bone shafts. The synovial membrane lining the joint capsule secretes synovial fluid to lubricate the joint. When injured or altered by arthritis or other degenerative disease, normal joint motion is impaired and/or painful.

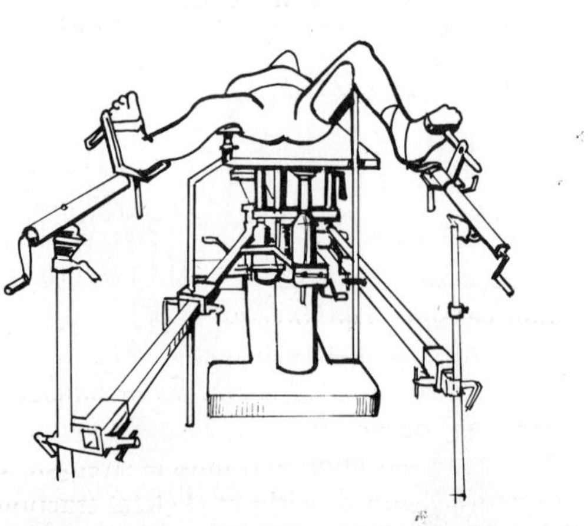

Figure 20-2 Position for intramedullary nailing left tibia. Note left foot anchored to footholder and knee resting on elevated curved kneerest. Right foot is anchored and kneerest adjusted for support of leg.

Arthrodesis

Fusion of a joint may be achieved by removing the articular surfaces and securing bony union, or by inserting a fixation implant that inhibits motion. Arthrodesis may be performed following resection of a recurrent benign, potentially malignant, or malignant lesion that involves the ends of the bones and joint. Following resection of the diseased portion of the bones, the joint may be stabilized with a bone graft or an intramedullary fixation implant. This procedure is performed most frequently for lesions in the distal femur and proximal tibia around or including the knee joint. Arthrodesis also may be performed to relieve osteoarthritic pain or to stabilize a joint that does not respond to other methods of treatment following injury, such as instability of the thumb. Because it limits motion, other joint reconstructive procedures are usually attempted before resorting to arthrodesis.

Triple arthrodesis of the ankle is performed to correct deformity or muscle imbalance of the foot. The subtalar, calcaneocuboid, and talonavicular tarsal joints are fused. Staples sometimes are used to hold bones together.

Arthroplasty

Reconstruction of a joint may be necessary to restore or improve range of motion and stability, or to relieve pain. This may be done by resurfacing, reshaping, or replacing the articular surfaces of the bones.

Cup Arthroplasty of the Hip The hip joint is disarticulated by removing the head of the femur from the acetabulum. The femoral head is smoothed with a bone rasp to a spherical shape and the acetabulum is reamed to the configuration of a perfect hemisphere. A metallic cup is implanted into the acetabulum, to provide a smooth surface for joint movement, before the femoral head is placed back in the socket. Reamers must be correlated to the size of the cup to assure proper articulation.

Femoral and Humeral Head Replacement A metal prosthetic implant can replace the femoral or humeral head and neck. These prostheses have a shaft that is driven into the medullary canal of the bone. The head of the bone is removed. The neck is shaped or removed as necessary for accurate placement of the prosthesis. A reamer may be used to enlarge the canal for insertion of the prosthesis. These prostheses are used:

purpose

1 To replace a comminuted fractured head when soft tissue attachments are destroyed
2 To replace the head if avascular necrosis or nonunion occurs following reduction of fractures
3 To mobilize the joint in arthritic patients

Total Joint Replacement Although prosthetic implants for some joints have not been as well developed as for others, total joint replacement is an accepted therapeutic modality, especially for the hip, knee, and elbow joints. Shoulder and ankle prostheses are available also. A functional design for a prosthesis must consider a combination of load bearing, strain-stress, and kinetics in association with pathologic condition. Positioning of the prosthesis influences distribution of stress and rate of wear.

The bones on both sides of the joints are replaced or resurfaced. Both component parts must be solidly anchored with bone cement to avoid movement of the prosthesis and wear on surrounding tissue. All movement must be between the two parts of the prosthesis. Metal to plastic joints are self-lubricating. Some joint fluids help to lubricate. The rate of wear on these parts is low, so the prosthesis will remain functional in the patient over a period of many years (the exact number not yet determined). Usually performed to improve mobility and relieve pain of severe arthritic joints, total joint replacement may be indicated when other therapeutic measures have failed to correct a congenital defect, traumatic injury, or degenerative disease. The total hip prostheses have greatly reduced the number of arthroplasty procedures previously described.

Silicone rubber prosthetic implants are used to replace metacarpophalangeal joints in the hand. The implant bridges the excised joint and is secured to the adjacent bones by intramedullary stems. This type of prosthesis also may be used to replace small bones of the wrist and great toe.

Arthroscopy

Visualization within the knee joint through the arthroscope not only is used for diagnosis of synovial, chondral, meniscal lesions and gross ligamentous defects, but also is an approach to definitive treatment for some of the simpler chondral and meniscal lesions. Arthroscopy also may be used to obtain a synovial or cartilaginous biopsy in some other rheumatoid arthritic joints.

Arthrotomy

Incision into a joint may be necessary to biopsy synovium or cartilage, to remove bone or cartilage fragments, or to repair a defect in the synovium or joint capsule. Arthrotomy of the knee joint frequently is performed following athletic or motorcycle injuries to excise or repair a torn meniscus, the semilunar intra-articular cartilage. Synovectomy may be the procedure of choice for relief of pain and control of inflammation in a rheumatoid arthritic joint.

Bunionectomy

Hallux valgus, a lateral deviation in the position of the great toe, increases the prominence of the adjoining metatarsal head. Pressure at the metatarsophalangeal joint causes inflammation that creates formation of an exostosis (*bunion*) beneath the bursa and joint capsule. A bunionectomy is done to remove the exostosis. One of several procedures may be selected to correct the deformity.

1 *Metatarsal osteotomy.* Metatarsal alignment is corrected by moving the metatarsal head laterally.
2 *McBride operation.* The abductor tendon is fixed to the metatarsal neck and the sesamoid bone is excised.
3 *Keller arthroplasty.* This includes resection of the proximal third of the phalanx. A silicone implant may be placed in the intramedullary canal to stabilize the metatarsophalangeal joint.

Dislocations

Dislocation of one or more bones at a joint may occur with or without an associated fracture. Tendons, ligaments, and muscles are deranged. The articular surface of the bone is displaced from the joint capsule. The force of displacement damages the capsule, and tears the ligaments and surrounding tissues. Blood vessel and nerve damage, which also can occur, impede circulation and cause changes in sensation and muscle strength. Closed reduction, with or without skeletal traction, may be necessary at the time of acute injury. If closed reduction fails to stabilize the joint and prevent recurrence, internal fixation may be necessary.

Operations to stabilize chronic recurrent dislocations are most frequently performed on the shoulder.

REPAIR OF TENDONS AND LIGAMENTS

Tendons and ligaments may be severed, torn, or ruptured. These injuries are seen frequently in athletes. Total or partial avulsion of major ligaments and tendons torn from their attachments in or around an extremity joint require repair to stabilize the joint.

Tendons can be lengthened, shortened, or transferred. When operation is indicated, tendon repair can be a tedious, meticulous procedure. Close apposition of the cut ends of tendons, particularly extensor tendons, is imperative to successfully restore function. Tendons heal slowly. Stainless steel suture is widely used in tendon repair because of its durability and lack of elasticity. A tendon may be wrapped in a silicone membrane to prevent adhesions after repair. Artificial tendons are made of a polyester center covered with silicone rubber.

Tendon surgery is within the realm of the orthopaedic surgeon; however, many plastic surgeons perform hand reconstruction including tendon repair and transfer. Hand reconstruction has become a subspecialty of both orthopaedics and plastic surgery. The operating microscope frequently is used, especially when vascular and nerve repair also are involved in the reconstruction.

VERTEBRAL COLUMN

Orthopaedic procedures on the back usually are performed to excise vertebral lesions, to relieve pressure on the spinal cord, to stabilize the vertebral column, or to correct gross deformities (refer to Chap. 26, p. 464, for discussion of scoliosis).

Primary neoplasms such as a giant cell bone tumor, bone cyst, hemangioma or osteoid osteoma, and metastatic tumors can occur in the vertebrae. Osteomyelitis, spondylolisthesis, and degenerative diseases also are indications for excision of bone from one or more vertebrae. Fracture, with or without dislocation of one or more vertebra, may be reduced by traction or excision of bony fragments. (Refer to Chap. 24, p. 439, for discussion of cervical traction.)

Laminectomy

Lumbar laminectomy usually is performed by the orthopaedist to remove a lumbar intervertebral disk that is exerting pressure on the spinal cord or nerve roots and causing low back pain. The spinous process and lamina on the affected side are removed. The herniated disk is removed from the intervertebral space (refer to Chap. 24 for details of a laminectomy).

Spinal Fusion

Spinal fusion may be indicated following excision of bone to stabilize the vertebral column. Bone grafts are placed in the intervertebral spaces or along the spinous processes to bridge over or to stabilize the defect. Either a posterior or anterior approach may be used to place the bone grafts. Homogenous cancellous bone from the bone bank may be preferred to provide a larger quantity of bone than can be obtained from an autogenous graft from the crest of the patient's ilium. Cancellous bone usually is preferred for spinal fusion rather than cortical bone.

Internal Fixation

Internal fixation may be preferred to stabilize a fracture or fracture-dislocation of the thoracic or lumbar spine. Harrington instrumentation (refer to Chap. 26, p. 465) may be used to provide decompression of the spinal nerve roots following posterior spinal fusion. An internal spinal splint of stainless steel mesh filled with acrylic bone cement may be preferred to stabilize the spine initially, prior to a second-stage spinal fusion.

CAST APPLICATION

A *cast* is a rigid form of dressing used to encase a part of the body. It supports and immobilizes the part in optimum position until healing takes place. A cast usually includes the joints above and below the affected area. It may suffice as a conservative mode of treatment as for fractures. It can be fitted to any body contour or position, and can be worn for months. Requisites of a cast include:

1. It must fulfill its intended function of maintaining the position of the desired parts.
2. It must not be too tight and must have no pressure areas, to permit adequate circulation. *Postapplication pain is an important symptom and must be promptly investigated.*
3. It must not be too loose. It must be as light as possible, yet strong enough to withstand usage.
4. It must be comfortable, with no binding or chafing.

Padding under Cast

Padding usually is put under casts and serves several functions.

1 It absorbs inevitable ooze from the wound following open operation. Sterile padding is put on over the dressing before applying the cast.
2 It protects the wound and the patient's skin.
3 It protects bony prominences.

Materials Used for Padding

Stockinet A knitted, seamless tubing of cotton 1 to 12 in. (2.5 to 30.4 cm) wide. It stretches to fit any contour snugly.

Sheet Wadding A glazed cotton bandage 2 to 8 in. (5 to 20 cm) wide. It is also available as a sheeting. It is used over stockinet or in place of it.

Soft Roll A thin cotton batting. This has some stretch for smooth contour.

Felt Sheeting made of wool or blends of wool, cotton, or rayon available in thicknesses ranging from $\frac{1}{8}$ to $\frac{1}{2}$ in. (3 to 13 mm). It is cut into desired sizes to fit bony prominences. The felt pads are applied over the sheet wadding. Plaster adheres to them and prevents their slipping.

Foam Rubber Available as a sheeting $\frac{1}{4}$ to 1 in. (6.4 to 25 mm) in thickness. It may be used in place of felt.

Webril A soft, lint-free cotton bandage. The surface is smooth but not glazed, so that each layer clings to the preceding one and the padding lies smoothly in place.

Plaster Casts

Plaster is gypsum or anhydrous calcium sulfate. It is finely ground to break up the crystals, then heated to drive out the water. When water is added again, recrystallization takes place and the plaster sets. It was first used as a method of splinting fractures in the nineteenth century.

Plaster bandages and splints are made of crinoline or other fabric with the plaster powder entrapped in the meshes. These are available in rolls or strips 2 to 8 in. (5 to 20 cm) wide. Plaster splints are either commercially made or made from rolls as the need arises. Usually six or eight thicknesses of the desired length are used. Splints are applied over areas that may weaken from extra strain, to give added strength. Plaster bandages and splints are available with three types of plaster.

1 *Slow setting.* This requires up to 18 minutes to set. It is used in large casts requiring more time to apply and mold. Its use permits blending of the layers.

2 *Medium setting.* This requires up to 8 minutes to set. This type is used in average-size casts.

3 *Fast setting.* This requires 4 to 5 minutes to set. It is advantageous for small casts on children, who are difficult to keep in position. Many orthopaedists prefer the fast-setting type in all kinds of casts; it is the most universally used type of plaster.

Application of Plaster

1 Spread a disposable plastic or nonwoven fabric sheet on the floor around the table to catch the drips.

2 Protect the table. If the orthopaedic table is used, spread a sheet over the table parts, after the patient is suspended.

3 Protect the patient's hair with a cap.

4 Use a disposable plaster pail or a plastic liner bag in a plaster bucket.

5 Fill the bucket with water at room temperature. Water warmer than 70 to 75 °F (21 to 24 °C) will speed setting time and may cause excessive loss of plaster from the fabric. More important, plaster will get even hotter than its normal exothermic reaction if dipped in hot water.

6 Don nonsterile disposable gloves to handle plaster to protect your skin from irritation by lime content.

7 Remove outer wrapping from bandage. Start soaking plaster only when the surgeon is ready to apply it. Keep just ahead in soaking it. Have the next roll ready when needed, but do not prepare several rolls ahead. They may harden and, if used, can produce an ineffective laminated cast. Avoid waste.

8 Hold the bandage under water in the vertical position to allow air bubbles to escape from the rolled end. When air bubbles stop rising, it is soaked through. Compress the ends between fingers and palm of each hand to remove excess water. This procedure prevents telescoping during use.

9 Open the end about 1 in. (2.5 cm) and hand to the surgeon.

10 Fanfold a strip once toward the center, before soaking, leaving the ends free to grasp. When soaking, grasp an end in each hand, press hands together, and submerge the strip in the water a few seconds; remove it and pull the strip taut by the ends. It may seem drippy but the layers blend together well when quite wet.

11 Ask the surgeon if another roll will be needed before soaking it when the cast appears near completion.

12 Handle the cast with care and support the patient in such a way that he or she cannot attempt to bend an incorporated joint. Wet plaster has only one-third to one-half of its ultimate strength when dry. The person who supports an extremity while a cast is being applied takes care not to make finger-pressure areas in plaster that will damage tissue under it.

13 Elevate an extremity on a pillow until the cast hardens. If it is laid on a hard surface, flat pressure areas may be pressed onto it.

14 Clean up as much as possible while the cast is being applied. Wipe plaster off equipment as well as off the patient before it dries. It is easy to remove when still damp; after it dries it must be scraped off. Cast dryer, if used, hastens drying.

15 Avoid splashing plaster on furniture and walls.

16 Clean equipment and table thoroughly. If the sink has a plaster trap, all plaster drip can be washed down the sink and the contents of the bucket can be poured into the sink. If there is no plaster trap, leave the bucket until the plaster in the bottom hardens; then empty the water and throw the plaster pail or plastic liner bag into the trash. Clean a reusable bucket as soon as you have finished with it.

Casts Commonly Used

Cylinder A circular cast, made by wrapping the plaster bandages around an extremity, is used following closed or open reductions of fractures, following some operations for immobilization, or for the purpose of resting a part of an extremity.

Walking Cast A rubber walking heel is applied to the sole of a cylinder cast for ambulation. Use of a lower extremity helps to maintain strength and muscle tone and to prevent atrophy.

Hanging Cast A cylinder is applied to the arm with the elbow flexed. It extends from the shoulder over the hand, leaving the thumb and fingers free. A wire loop is incorporated at the wrist. A strap through this loop and around the neck suspends the arm. The weight of the cast provides needed traction on the humerus.

Shoulder Spica Applied to the trunk, arm, and hand, leaving the fingers and thumb free, a spica cast is used after some operations on the shoulder or humerus, or for fracture of the humerus. The orthopaedic table may be used for its application, or the patient may sit on a stool with the surgeon supporting the arm in the desired position.

Hip Spica This is applied to the trunk and one or both legs, following some hip operations and fractures of the femur. The orthopaedic table is used. The sacrum rests on a sacral rest. The perineal post provides countertraction. Attachments may be used to support the legs of an adult patient.

Minerva Jacket This is applied from the hips to the head. If the head is to be completely immobilized, it is included in the jacket. The plaster is molded to fit around the face and lower jaw. A part of the plaster at the back of the head is cut out. It is used for fractures of the cervical or upper thoracic vertebrae. The orthopaedic table is necessary.

Body Jacket This extends from axillae to hips. It is used to immobilize the vertebrae. The application of this cast usually requires the orthopaedic table with the necessary attachments, although sometimes the patient may stand on the floor; or traction may be applied by an overhead sling. If open operation is to be performed with the patient in a body cast, the cast cutter must be at hand in case of respiratory difficulty. However, a body cast is usually bivalved before a patient is given an anesthetic.

NOTE. An opening is always made over the abdomen of a Minerva or body jacket to allow space for lung expansion and decompresion of abdominal distention that normally occurs with ingestion of food. A folded towel may be placed over the abdomen before the stockinet is pulled over the body. This is removed when the opening is made in the cast to allow more space between the body and cast.

Plaster Shell A body jacket is cut along each side, into anterior and posterior parts. These may be fastened together by heavy straps with buckles, or the patient may rest in one while the other is temporarily removed.

Wedge Cast A wedge-shaped portion is cut from the cast. The edges are brought together and held with plaster reinforcement. It is used to overcome angulation in a fracture.

Plaster Splint Six or more thicknesses of plaster the desired width and length may be applied to the posterior part of an extremity and bandaged with gauze or cotton elastic bandage. The excess water is pressed from the plaster splint after it is immersed in water. A splint may be used for immobilization of a fracture of the ulna or fibula.

Hairpin or Sugar-Tong Splint A splint twice as long as the lower arm and hand is used for fracture of the ulna or radius. After the plaster is soaked, it may be covered with stockinet. Starting with one end of it on the back of the hand, it is placed around the flexed elbow, and the palm of the hand and fingers rest on the other end of it. It is secured with a bandage.

Abduction Hip Splint The splint keeps the hips in constant abduction. If desired for postoperative management, it is applied immediately following hip operation. The patient can be moved safely from the operating table and turned in bed.

Plaster Rope Plaster rope may support the arm in a shoulder spica or join the legs in a bilateral hip spica. It is made by twisting a wet roll of plaster bandage into a rope as it is unwound, fanfolding to the desired length, and drawing it through the cupped hand to blend the strands.

Molds These are made as plaster patterns for removable metal or leather braces for the body, neck, or extremities.

Trimming, Removing, and Changing Casts Rough edges of plaster are trimmed off and the edges of the cast covered with stockinet or adhesive tape to protect the patient's skin. Instruments specifically designed for cutting through plaster must be used for trimming or removing casts. These include:

1 *Plaster knives.* These knives have short, slightly curved blades.
2 *Plaster scissors.* These are heavy bandage scissors.
3 *Electric cast cutter.* This is an oscillating saw. It cuts the cast but not the stockinet or other padding under it, because the padding moves with the oscillations. The patient's skin also moves somewhat and is not injured if touched lightly, although care is always taken not to touch the skin. One model has a vacuum attached to pick up the plaster dust created by the saw.
4 *Cast spreader.* This long-handled instrument has thin, serrated jaws that can be inserted in the cutting line to pry open the cast.
5 *Cast bender.* This is a heavy, forceps-type instrument used to bend a small portion of the edge of a cast away from an area, such as a portion of a jacket away from the mouth and chin, to give freer movement.

Sharp plaster knives or scissors usually are used to trim casts. For large casts the electric cast cutter may be used, for example, to cut an opening over the abdomen of a body jacket. In a hip spica, adequate space is provided for use of the bedpan without soiling. If it is necessary to cut a "window"—a small opening in a cast to remove sutures or to inspect an area—it is put back in place and secured with a few turns of plaster bandage. An opening in a cast encourages swelling of the tissues under it, known as *window edema.*

When edema in a wound under a cast recedes, the cast then does not furnish as much immobilization as may be desired. The cast is usually changed at this stage.

Many times a change of cast also entails removal of skin sutures, if the cast has been applied following operation. A sterile suture removal tray should be ready for use when requested. Sterile sheet wadding may be needed to cover the wound after sutures are removed, before another cast is applied.

If the patient has been in a cast for some time, the skin is apt to be oily, somewhat soiled, and rough. If the surgeon wishes the skin cleansed before applying another cast, only the superficial dirt can be removed. Scrubbing off the oily scales may cause irritation. Usually the skin is not washed but rubbed with cold cream or powdered with talc before applying sheet wadding and a new cast.

Provide a large, empty cardboard carton or plastic-lined trash container in which to put the wrappings, trimming, removed cast, etc., during cast application and removal. (This can be taken directly to the incinerator for disposal with minimal environmental contamination.)

Wash off knives, scissors, cutter, spreader, and bender as soon as finished with them. Apply oil to all instrument joints before putting instruments away to avoid rust and corrosion.

Lightcast II Casting System

An open-weave Fiberglas tape impregnated with a photosensitive resin can be used for casting or bracing. Polypropylene stockinet is applied over the patient's skin. Polypropylene web wrap may be used for extra padding over bony prominences and pressure points. The person applying the cast must coat hands with a silicone hand cream to facilitate smoothing and blending the layers of the Fiberglas tape and to prevent resin pickup on the hands. The tape is applied in the same manner as plaster; however, it does not become rigid until it is cured. Exposure to near ultraviolet light in the 3200 to 4000 angstrom (Å) range, commonly known as *black light,* cures the cast. The lamp generates light energy, not heat, so remains cool during the full 3-minute curing cycle.

When cured, the cast is lighter, thinner, yet stronger and more porous for better ventilation than a plaster cast. It can be immersed in water without deterioration. Because of the advantages it affords, this material is preferred by many orthopaedic surgeons for extremity casts.

ORTHOPAEDIC CART

For closed reduction of fractures, traction, and postoperative applications, many orthopaedic appliances must be available and at hand when needed. An orthopaedic cart can provide the necessary items for these situations. The items may vary somewhat at different hospitals but many will be universally used. The cart can be taken wherever needed in the OR suite. One shelf should be kept for sterile items.

1 Suture removal trays
2 Webril and soft roll
3 Assorted sponges, dressings, bandages
4 Skin antiseptic agents

Another shelf should contain nonsterile items.

1 Pulleys and attachments for beds
2 Ropes, weights, and carriers
3 Felt padding and foam rubber
4 Arm and shoulder immobilizers
5 Pelvic slings and rods
6 Assorted sizes of gauze and muslin bandages, stockinet, sheet wadding, soft rolls, and Webril
7 Stapler
8 Safety pins
9 Cold cream and talcum powder
10 Disposable plaster pail or bucket with plastic liner bag
11 Plastic bag for trash
12 Assorted sizes of plaster rolls and splints
13 Cast cutters, knives, scissors, spreaders, and bender

Splints, overhead traction bars, shock blocks, foot-drop stops, and other bulky items are obtained from the cast room as needed.

Chapter 21

Thoracic and Cardiovascular Surgery

Thoracic and cardiovascular surgery encompass a vast spectrum of clinical pathology. Operative intervention for disease processes, neoplasms, traumatic injuries, and congenital anomalies often involves complex procedures in these highly specialized areas. The inclusion of vital organs of respiration and circulation mandates experienced operating teams with special education and training. Merely a brief overview, with inclusion of a few representative procedures, is given as the extent and complexity of this field preclude detailed discussion beyond the scope of this text.

HISTORICAL DEVELOPMENT OF THORACIC SURGERY

Interest in the thorax and lungs dates back to ancient times. The brutal practice of dissecting live criminals was related by Celsus who noted that when the *diaphragma* or transverse septum was cut, i.e., the thorax was widely opened, the man expired. Vesalius used animals to demonstrate to his students the transparent pleura and motion of the lungs beneath it. As exposure was widened and the pleural cavity entered, the lung was seen to collapse. Experimental animals were revived by tracheotomy with a reed pipe used as a tracheotomy tube. Invention of the stethoscope by René Laennec in the eighteenth century facilitated study of thoracic disease.

Learning safe access to the pleural cavity and lungs was a difficult step in the development of thoracic surgery. Paracentesis with needle and trocar, for open drainage of acute empyema, was performed in the United States in the middle of the nineteenth century, but generally as a last resort since a suppurating cavity often resulted.

Sporadic attempts at thoracic surgery in the nineteenth century, e.g., pulmonary resection, were accompanied by forbidding mortality rates.

In 1913, Torek, a pioneer in chest surgery, successfully removed a carcinoma of the esophagus, resecting ribs but not the scapula as was the mode. Sucking wounds of the chest, created by shell fragments during World War I, drew new interest in thoracic problems. In 1920, Evarts Graham brought attention to the significance of the relaxation of vital capacity to the size of an opening in the thorax and in 1923 presented a staged procedure: cautery pneumonotomy and partial excision of the lung. Cutler, in 1924, utilized a sternum-splitting incision for mitral valvulotomy. The first successful pneumonectomy, using exposure by rib resection, took place in 1931.

Development of thoracic surgery paralleled advances in endoscopy, respiratory tract intubation, mechanical ventilation, closed chest-drainage systems, and respiratory care techniques.

THORACIC SURGERY

Thoracic surgery concerns disorders of the lungs, mediastinum, chest wall, and diaphragm.

Anatomy and Physiology

Thorax The thorax or chest is the part of the trunk between the neck and abdomen. It holds the chief organs of respiration and circulation, the lungs and heart, and the great vessels. These vital organs function under the protection of a bony framework consisting of the sternum, 12 pairs of ribs, and 12 thoracic vertebrae, all encased with soft tissue. The framework is bounded superiorly by structures of the lower part of the neck and inferiorly by the diaphragm. External and internal intercostal muscles, which lie between the ribs, have a corresponding artery, vein, and nerve, which require meticulous dissection to avoid inadvertent injury.

The ribs articulate posteriorly with the thoracic vertebrae. The first seven ribs articulate anteriorly in the midline with the sternum composed of three parts, the manubrium, gladiolus, and xiphoid process. The eighth, ninth, and tenth ribs are joined anteriorly to the cartilage of the rib above each, while the eleventh and twelfth ribs have no anterior fixation. The esophagus, trachea, and great vessels leading to and from the neck and arms pass through the small space between the manubrium and vertebrae. Any structure pushing into this narrow opening, e.g., a mediastinal tumor, may obstruct breathing, venous return from the neck and arms, and possibly swallowing.

The chest cavity is divided into right and left compartments by the *mediastinum,* the space and vertical loose connective tissue wall between the two pleural cavities. The mediastinum has superior, anterior, middle, and posterior sections, each containing structures: the thymus lies within the anterior and superior sections, the thoracic aorta within the posterior, the heart and great vessels in the middle, and esophagus and trachea in the superior section. Organs are surrounded and suspended by the loose tissue diffused throughout the mediastinum. Division of the pleural cavities is flexible and alterations in pressure affecting one cavity are felt in the other.

Lungs The lungs lie in the right and left pleural cavities. The main function of these porous, spongy, conical organs is oxygenation of blood with inspired air. The apex of each extends to the neck; the base rests on the diaphragm. The lungs are enveloped by serous membrane, the visceral or pulmonary pleura. Parietal pleura lines the internal surface of the thoracic cavity. The right lung, with three lobes, is larger than the left lung, which has only two lobes. The left lung is narrower and shares the space in the left chest with the heart.

The ten *bronchopulmonary segments* within each lung are wedges of tissue separated by veins and thin, connective membrane. Although not demarcated by surface fissures like the lobes, these segments represent zones of distribution of the secondary bronchi and may be excised individually, thus preserving the uninvolved portion of a lobe that contains a small lesion. Each segmental bronchus subdivides into numerous increasingly smaller branches that eventually end in terminal bronchioles. These fine tubules invested by smooth muscles can constrict to close off the air passage, as in asthma. The terminal bronchioles give rise to respiratory bronchioles from which arise the alveoli. The approximately 300,000,000 alveoli are the functional units where oxygenation takes place at the capillary level.

The *hilus* of the lung, on the mediastinal surface, is the point of entry for the primary bronchus, nerves, and vessels. The right primary bronchus is longer and a more direct continuation of the trachea. The pulmonary veins and arteries to and from the heart provide pulmonary circulation. Organs of respiration are innervated by the autonomic nervous system.

Size of the thorax varies with the bellows action of the thoracic wall and diaphragm, increasing with inspiration, decreasing with expiration. A partial vacuum exists between the visceral and parietal pleurae, for expansion of the lungs. A negative (subatmospheric) pressure normally exists within the thorax and is essential to life. Alterations of intrapleural pressure are of major concern as an uncontrolled opening in the thoracic wall and pressure change can be fatal. A reduction of negative pressure on one side causes the negative pressure on the normal side to pull on the mediastinum in an effort to equalize pressure. Referred to as *mediastinal shift,* this reaction attends entrance of either air or fluid to the pleural cavity, compressing the opposite lung and causing dyspnea. When the mediastinum has moved its limit, it can no longer accommodate a great pressure change. In such instances, the lung on the affected side collapses. Air in the pleural space between the parietal and visceral pleura constitutes *pneumothorax.* Blood in the pleural space is *hemothorax.*

Mediastinal shift disturbs heart action and circulation. Changes in pressure balance within the thorax reduce *vital capacity,* the greatest amount of air that can be exchanged in one breath. Many diseases and conditions alter vital capacity, for example, anesthesia, thoracic tumors, or injury.

Operative entry into the thoracic cavity can be accompanied by pulmonary distress. However, administration of endotracheal anesthesia under controlled positive pressure prevents physiologic imbalance and prevents lung collapse in the presence of controlled pneumothorax. This is essential for entry into the chest for intrathoracic procedures. An airtight pleural cavity must be restored and negative pressure maintained for maximum pulmonary function postoperatively.

SPECIAL FEATURES OF THORACIC SURGERY

1 Sterile closed water-seal drainage system is essential when the chest has been opened operatively or by trauma, except after a few specific procedures. Chest tube(s) are inserted through a 1- or 2-cm ($\frac{1}{2}$ to 1-in.) incision and are anchored to the chest wall with suture and tape. Sometimes two tubes are inserted into the pleural space and connected to separate drainage systems. The tube at the base of the pleural space is usually inserted at the seventh costal interspace, near the anterior axillary line, to evacuate fluid. An upper tube, if indicated, is inserted at the apex through the anterior chest wall at the second costal interspace to evacuate air leaking from the lung. (Review Chap. 12, p. 247.)
   a Connections must be taped for tight seal. The system must be kept intact.
   b System components must be kept below the level of the patient's body to prevent reentry of air or fluid from the drainage collection system into the pleural cavity.
   c Depending on the surgeon's preference, tubes may be clamped prior to insertion, connection to the system, and during transportation, to avoid introduction of air. *Clamps for the tubing must be with the patient at all times.*
2 Portable chest x-rays are taken immediately and 24 hours after the procedure to assess status of the operative area, pleural cavities, and lung reexpansion.
3 Operating rooms for thoracic or cardiovascular surgery should be provided with electrocardiographic and pressure monitors, cardiac defibrillator, pacemaker, and intra-aortic balloon equipment. Equipment for bronchoscopy, esophagoscopy, and mediastinoscopy must be readily available. Team members especially skilled in meeting emergency situations are essential. These patients require very close observation as changes may occur rapidly. Laboratory facilities must be available on a 24-hour basis.
4 Endotracheal anesthesia permits the unoperated lung to expand and function even when subjected to atmospheric pressure. At conclusion of operation, the operated lung is reexpanded by the anesthesiologist and negative pressure in the chest restored.
5 Properly cross-matched blood for transfusion should be available at all times as hemorrhage is a major threat intra- and postoperatively.
6 Instrumentation includes basic lap setup with addition of thoracic instruments. These include bone instruments and power saws; rib stripper, spreaders, and approximator; large self-retaining chest retractor; bronchus and lung clamps; and long instruments for work in a deep incision.
7 A large variety of sutures may be used for bone, soft tissues, and vessels. The bronchus may be closed with staples.
8 Sponges for hemostasis or blunt dissection are placed on long ring-handled forceps. Periosteal bleeding may be controlled by electrocoagulation. Bone wax may be needed for bone marrow oozing.
9 When a bronchus is opened and sutured, the field is potentially contaminated because of secretions and contact with open air passages. Items and instruments used are isolated in a discard basin. Maintenance of a dry field during bronchial opening and suture is important to prevent aspiration of blood and fluid, predisposing the patient to postoperative pneumonia.
10 Major complications of thoracic surgery are hemorrhage, atelectasis, persistent undrained fluid or air pockets in the pleural space, empyema, bronchopleural fistula, retained tracheobronchial secretions, pulmonary shunting.

THORACIC INCISIONS AND CLOSURES

Factors Influencing Choice of Incision

1 Adequate exposure into thoracic cavity.

2 Physiologic intrapleural pressure changes and constant movement of the chest.

3 Maintenance of integrity of the chest wall and diaphragm. Because of the continuity of the thoracic cavity with the neck and abdominal structures, the cavity may be entered at times for neck

and upper abdominal procedures as well as thoracic procedures.

Access to Thorax

Surgeon preference and the procedure determine method of entrance into the thorax. Access may be gained by various approaches: anterior, lateral, posterior, or a combination of these. Entrance through the rib cage may be intercostal between the ribs, through the periosteal bed of an unresected rib, or by rib resection. By incising near the top of the rib, the surgeon protects nerves and vessels that lie in the intercostal spaces. Intercostal approach may be used to drain an empyema pocket or mediastinal abscess, or to biopsy lymph nodes or the lung. To enter via the periosteal bed, the periosteum of the rib is incised, removed from the unresected rib, and incision made through the bed. For entrance via rib resection, the periosteum is incised and removed superiorly and inferiorly with a periosteal elevator, and the rib divided. Rib spreaders increase exposure but if it is inadequate, the rib above or below the incision may be resected.

Commonly Used Thoracic Incisions

Median Sternotomy (Vertical Sternal Splitting) With the patient supine, incision is carried through the midline from the suprasternal notch to below the xiphoid, which is resected. Retrosternal tissue is dissected and the sternum divided. Caution is used to avoid injury to the underlying mediastinal structures.

At closure, heavy-gauge stainless steel sutures are placed around or through the sternum, tightly pulled together, twisted, and the ends buried in the sternum. Other nonabsorbable sutures may be used to provide firm fixation. The linea alba, subcutaneous tissue, and skin are sutured. Modifications of this incision are used for lesions of the upper mediastinum. Complications are brachial plexus injury, costochondrial separation from too vigorous sternal retraction during operation, and keloid formation. Uses: open-heart procedures, pericardiectomy, mediastinal trauma.

Posterolateral Thoracotomy The classic incision for exploration of the thoracic cavity, this incision permits maximum exposure to the lung, esophagus, diaphragm, and descending aorta. Beginning anteriorly in the submammary fold, about at nipple level, a curved incision is made, extending below the scapular tip, following the course of underlying ribs. Then curving upward and posteriorly, it may be carried as high as the spine of the scapula. The subcutaneous tissue is incised, the latissimus dorsi, lower margin of the trapezius, rhomboideus and serratus muscles are divided and bleeders ligated. In dividing the serratus, special precaution is taken to avoid the neurovascular bundle on the surface.

In closure, the ribs are reapproximated by use of a rib approximator and sutures, the intercostal muscles sutured, and incision in the periosteal bed and pleura closed. Muscles are reapproximated anatomically and sutured, subcutaneous tissue and skin closed. Uses: pulmonary resections, some cardiac operations, repair of hiatus hernia, procedures on the thoracic esophagus or posterior mediastinum.

Anterolateral Thoracotomy With the patient supine, sandbags are placed under the operative side to tilt the shoulder 20 to 45° for extension of the incision posteriorly. A pad behind the buttocks may rotate the hips slightly. Submammary incision, immediately below the breast but above the costal margin, extends from the anterior midline to the mid- or posterior axillary line. To avoid the axillary apex and painful scar, the posterior end of the incision is curved downward. Superiorly, access is desired at about the fourth interspace. Further anterior exposure can be gained if desired by transecting the sternum and continuing the incision to the contralateral interspace. Pectoralis muscles are divided, serratus anterior fibers separated, intercostal muscles divided, and the thorax entered through the intercostal space. When the anterior incision extends to the sternal border, internal mammary arteries and veins are ligated and divided. If the incision is carried far laterally or posteriorly, injury to the long thoracic nerve must be avoided to prevent a "winged" scapula.

In closure, the sternum is reapproximated with heavy suture, ribs are approximated with pericostal sutures, muscles, subcutaneous tissue, and skin closed. Uses: various cardiac operations such as closure of atrial septal defects, or superior vena cava-pulmonary artery shunt, resection of pulmonary cyst or local lesion.

Transsternal Bilateral Thoracotomy With the patient supine, bilateral submammary incision is made. In the midline the incision curves superiorly to cross the sternum at the fourth intercostal space level. Lateral extension is to the midaxillary line. The pleural cavity is entered via the interspace after division of the pectoralis muscles. The internal mammary arteries and veins are ligated and divided, and the sternum divided horizontally.

At closure, the sternum is reapproximated securely, the ribs approximated with pericostal sutures, and the remaining tissue layers closed. Uses: resection of ventricular aneurysm, aortic arch grafts, complicated pericardiectomies. This type of incision is less common and causes more discomfort.

Thoracoabdominal Used also in general surgery procedures, this incision extends from the posterior axillary line to the abdominal midline, paralleling the selected interspace (usually the seventh or eighth). With insertion of a rib spreader, incision in the intercostal muscles and pleura may be extended posteriorly from within for added exposure. The diaphragm may be divided peripherally. This incision exposes the upper abdomen, retroperitoneal area, and lower aspect of the chest.

In closure, the diaphragm is closed with interrupted sutures. Costal margin is secured by approximating the margins of divided costal cartilages with suture. Tissue layers are closed in reverse order of incision. Uses: repair of thoracoabdominal aortic aneurysm, retroperitoneal tumor, cardioesophageal lesions.

Other Less Common Incisions Less common incisions may be used, such as:

1 Cervical mediastinotomy, for drainage high in the mediastinum, e.g., following esophageal perforation

2 Anterior approach, for upper dorsal sympathectomy, exposing upper thoracic ganglia

3 Supraclavicular (scalene approach), for phrenic nerve section, cervicothoracic sympathectomy

4 Axillary approach, for upper mediastinal or lung biopsy, or exposure of second to fifth thoracic ganglia

THORACIC OPERATIVE PROCEDURES

Elective surgery depends on accurate diagnosis by radiologic, endoscopic, physiologic pulmonary-function studies, biochemical, cytological, and histological determinations and evaluations.

Endoscopy

Bronchoscopy In addition to its use in preoperative diagnosis, examination of the bronchi may be performed to ascertain patency of the tracheobronchial tree (refer to Chap. 23, p. 428, for indications).

Mediastinoscopy This procedure may immediately follow bronchoscopy, and also prevent needless thoracotomy. It is performed for assessment of resectability in patients with suspected bronchogenic carcinoma, and for diagnosis of mediastinal lesions. Mediastinoscopy uncovers mediastinal lymph nodes for direct visualization and biopsy. Subaortic nodes draining the left lobe of the lung may be out of reach for biopsy with this technique. With the scope, the mediastinoscopist can see down to the carina and about 4 cm distal to it along each bronchus. If more than one biopsy specimen is obtained, each should be placed in a separate container and identified as to location, to facilitate identification of lesion location. The procedure gives a high percentage of accurate diagnoses and information in staging extent of a lesion and determining operability for curative resection. Sometimes a frozen section is done while the patient is in the OR and resection done immediately following the report.

General endotracheal anesthesia is used. The patient is supine with the neck hyperextended and the head turned slightly to the right. A small transverse incision is made in or about 2 cm above the suprasternal notch between the borders of the sternocleidomastoid muscle. Dissection is carried down to the pretracheal fascia. After blunt dissection, the scope is passed behind the suprasternal notch and advanced behind the arch of the aorta into the superior mediastinum to the level of the carina. Care is exercised because of proximity of great vessels in the region. Bleeding is controlled by coagulation with an insulated electrosurgical suction tip. Usually performed without complication, mediastinoscopy may be accompanied by major bleeding requiring immediate thoractomy. A chest x-ray frequently is obtained after the procedure.

Mediastinotomy

Anterior mediastinotomy may be indicated when x-ray studies show hilar or mediastinal nodal involvement inaccessible to mediastinoscopy. With the patient supine, and under general anesthesia, incision is made over the right or left third costal cartilage. The cartilage bed is incised and extrapleural dissection carried toward the hilus of the lung and biopsy taken. If the desired nodes are deep, the mediastinoscope may be inserted through the incision for a biopsy. Or, the pleural space may be entered for lung biopsy. If the space is entered, closed water-seal chest drainage is required. If not entered, the incision is closed in layers without drainage. Mediastinotomy allows assessment of the extent of lesion involvement.

Thoracotomy

Incision through the thoracic wall is indicated for drainage of pleural spaces, exploration of thoracic cavity, or cardiac and pulmonary operations. Thoracic operations, exclusive of cardiac procedures, include:

Closed Thoracostomy This procedure is performed to establish continuous drainage of fluid from the chest (usually purulent from sepsis), or to aid in restoring negative pressure in the thoracic cavity. It involves insertion of a tube through an intercostal space via trocar and cannula.

Open Thoracotomy This procedure may be employed for spontaneous pneumothorax, for large air leaks that prevent reexpansion of the lung, or for persistent leaks and incomplete lung reexpansion in addition to operative approaches. This type of pneumothorax usually occurs from rupture of a bleb on the lung surface. By posterolateral incision through the fourth interspace, an apical bleb may be ligated or the involved segmental area of lung resected. Abrasion or cauterization of the parietal pleura effects adhesion to the visceral pleura thereby eliminating future rupture of blebs. Open chest drainage also is used to eliminate an empyema cavity, which accompanies chronic disease and lung adherence to the chest wall. With this procedure, portions of one or two ribs are removed to aid establishment of drainage.

Exploratory Thoracotomy This procedure usually is performed to accurately establish diagnosis and extent of involvement of bronchogenic carcinoma or other chest disease, such as mediastinal lesion. Posterolateral intercostal or anterior approach may be used. The lung and hemithorax are exposed after incision, spread of ribs, and opening of the pleura. Biopsy is taken. Etiology of bleeding or detection of injury after trauma are other indications for use. Postoperative pain is due to continuous movement of the chest.

Lung Resection All or part of a diseased or traumatized lung may be resected. Generally, the indications are neoplasms, emphysematous blebs, fungal infection, localized residual lung abscess, tuberculosis, or bronchiectasis stubborn to nonoperative treatment, or continuing bleeding. Neoplasms are the predominant indication. Anterior intercostal incision with division of costal cartilages above and below the incision may be used for excision of pulmonary nodules or lung biopsy, for example. Posterolateral incision commonly is employed for lobectomy and pneumonectomy. Endotracheal anesthesia is used. Special precautions in pulmonary resection include meticulous hemostasis and closure of the bronchus, as well as continual attention to cardiopulmonary function pre-, intra-, and postoperatively. Particular hazards are hemorrhage, which is difficult to control because of size and friability of major pulmonary vessels and proximity to the heart; cardiopulmonary insufficiency; risk of injury to other intrathoracic structures such as the vagus, phrenic, and left recurrent nerves and the esophagus. The following specific operations are included:

Segmental Resection Removal of individual bronchovascular segments of a lobe is conservative and preferred when wide excision is not necessary, as for certain diseases that tend to be distributed segmentally, or for acute hemorrhage. Arteries, veins, and the bronchus to the involved segment are ligated and divided. The segment is separated from surrounding lung tissue and removed. The proximal stump of the bronchus is closed with sutures.

Wedge Resection This also is a conservative procedure performed when a lesion is thought to be benign. With adequate margin of normal lung tissue, the diseased peripheral portion of a lobe is removed and the lung tissue sutured. A lung stapler may expedite removal and closure. Frozen section is done. If benign diagnosis is confirmed, the wound is closed in layers, and water-seal drainage used. If the lesion proves to be malignant, lobectomy or other appropriate procedure may be done. Advantages of wedge resection are its simplicity, little blood loss, and minimum operating time.

Lobectomy This is excision of one or more lobes of a lung where disease or neoplasm is confined to the lobe. The remaining portion of lung expands to fill the space formerly occupied by the removed lobe. Through a posterolateral incision, entrance to the chest may be intercostal or by rib resection. The pulmonary pleura is incised and freed from the hilus of the lobe. Arteries and veins to the pulmonary tissue being resected are ligated and divided. The bronchus of the lobe is identified by lung inflation while the bronchus to be resected is clamped prior to its resection. Suction of blood and secretions from the open bronchus precedes closure of the bronchus by sutures or staples. The suture line of the bronchus is covered with a flap of parietal pleura to prevent leakage. Dissection is completed, the specimen removed, and the chest closed.

Pneumonectomy This is excision of an entire lung. Major indications are malignant neoplasms or extensive unilateral pulmonary disease. The chest wall is opened by posterolateral incision, the pleura incised, the lung exposed, and the pleural cavity examined. Following immobilization of the lung, the hilus is dissected free on all sides; the pulmonary artery and veins are meticulously ligated and divided. The bronchus is clamped, divided, and closed with sutures or staples. The bronchus is checked for air leaks by instillation of saline solution and the bronchial stump covered with surrounding pleura. After closure of the wound, intrathoracic pressure is measured and residual air aspirated from the hemithorax until the desired pressure is reached. Use of chest drainage is governed by surgeon preference, but usually no chest tube is inserted.

Sacrifice of one lung places entire respiratory and circulatory function on the remaining lung. Potential complications are respiratory insufficiency, cardiac arrhythmia, and infection, the latter predisposed by the amount of dead space. The empty hemithorax gradually fills with fluid and eventually consolidates, thus preventing mediastinal shift. Dehiscence of the bronchial closure may produce bronchopleural fistula.

Thoracoplasty This procedure, usually extrapleural, mobilizes the chest wall to obliterate the pleural cavity or reduce thoracic space by resection of one or more ribs. Indications are inadequate expansion of the lung to fill the space after resection, persistent shift of the mediastinum to the empty space after pneumonectomy, or chronic empyema. Tissue fibroses, contracts, and eventually obliterates the space. Thoracoplasty is reserved for patients in whom excessive space in the chest cannot be eliminated satisfactorily by other means to maintain the mediastinum in midline.

Pulmonary Decortication In patients with empyema, a fibrinous thickening or peel on the visceral pleura may restrict pulmonary ventilation. A pleural procedure, removal of the restrictive layer or membrane over the lung, permits the entrapped lung to reexpand and fill the space remaining after drainage of an empyema cavity. Minimum damage to the rib cage by the thoracotomy incision is desired to permit as normal as possible motion of the chest wall. Intercostal incision usually is preferred, but in some patients resection of a rib may facilitate access to the intrapleural space. Adequate postoperative drainage via chest tube(s) is essential.

Repair of Hiatus Hernia

This procedure may be performed by a thoracic or general surgeon (refer to Chap. 17, p. 331).

Correction of Pectus Excavatum (Funnel Chest)

Refer to Chapter 26 for pediatric discussion of this congenital anomaly. Correction sometimes is delayed until adolescence or adult years. A depression deformity of the chest wall, the sternum is pushed back toward the spine. The converse, *pectus carinatum* (pigeon chest), is forward projection or keel of the sternum. *Pectus excavatum* (funnel chest), the more common, is due to elongation of the costal cartilages. Operation is performed for cosmetic improvement or correction of mediastinal compression, to relieve respiratory distress or pressure on the heart.

Various techniques may be employed. Usually, with the patient supine and upper chest slightly hyperextended, the costal cartilages are exposed by muscle splitting and/or division through anterior midline or horizontal inframammary incision. Involved costal cartilages and deformed rib ends are freed from sternal attachments and resected or straightened. The sternum is mobilized and restored to normal position and its corrected position maintained by fixation. An alternate method corrects the contour deformity with a silicone prosthesis introduced through inframammary incision. Dacron patches on the posterior surface stabilize the prosthesis.

CHEST TRAUMA

Trauma to the chest varies in severity and may result in injury to the thoracic wall or intrathoracic organs such as the heart and lungs. If severe, the patient is plunged into critical condition. Rapid initial evaluation of extent of injury is necessary to save life, with priority needs met first. These include resuscitation with relief of airway obstruction, treatment of shock and blood loss, and restoration of as nearly as normal cardiorespiratory dynamics. Impairment of these dynamics may be due to various factors such as disturbance of lung expansion.

Trauma may be categorized as *blunt* or *penetrating.* Blunt trauma usually results from a fall, blow, severe cough, blast, or deceleration injury. The patient may have little overt evidence of chest injury although he or she may be bleeding internally. Penetrating wounds usually are caused by a low- or high-velocity missile, such as knife stab or bullet. Operative exploration usually is required.

Blunt Trauma

Treatment of Fractured Ribs Rib fracture is the most common injury to the chest wall, the fourth to the eighth ribs being the ones mainly involved. Pain may be relieved by intercostal nerve block. Operative treatment usually is not required unless sharp edges or displaced bone fragments puncture the pleura or lung. Extensive pneumothorax requires immediate reexpansion.

Multiple rib or sternal fractures often produce an unstable chest wall resulting in flail chest. Normal respiration changes to paradoxic motion of the chest wall in which the lung fills on expiration and empties on inspiration. As the chest wall expands, the free-floating sternum is sucked inward, compressing the lungs, thus impairing ventilation and producing hypoxia. The following measures are used to stabilize the chest wall:

Internal Stabilization This is achieved by controlled respiration through a tracheotomy tube (refer to Chap. 23). Frequent aspiration maintains a free airway; paradoxical motion and dead air space decrease.

Skeletal Traction Under local anesthesia a wire or pin is inserted through rib or sternal fragments to correct tendency to depression, after open elevation of the bone. Elevation is maintained by traction.

Penetrating Wounds

Anatomical visualization of the path of the projectile or instrument producing injury is important. A knife, for example, should not be removed except under direction of a physician, because it acts as a temporary seal to the pleural cavity and removal may further complicate the injury.

An open chest wound must be converted to a closed chest wound. Air rushes in an open wound building up atmospheric positive pressure inside the pleural space. Pneumothorax followed by mediastinal shift ensues.

Thoracentesis Air or blood in the pleural cavity may be detected and aspirated by needle and syringe. If bleeding persists, the chest is opened and vessels ligated or repaired.

Closure of Sucking Wound Pneumothorax is relieved and further air prevented from entering the chest by suture of the wound and insertion of chest tube(s).

CARDIAC SURGERY

While experiments with transfusion using animal blood flourished during and after the seventeenth century, the most noteworthy disclosure prior to the twentieth century was the discovery of circulation of the blood by William Harvey, an English physician, who published his famous treatise in 1628. Harvey derived much knowledge of comparative anatomy of the heart and blood vessels from lengthy dissections, and conducted experiments on the heart chambers, arteries, and veins.

The evolution of modern cardiovascular surgery began in about 1950 and accelerated rapidly. Early procedures on the heart and vessels included repair of coarctation of the aorta and patent ductus arteriosus. Development of the heart-lung machine, which permits safe direct vision for open-heart operations, is credited to John Gibbon. In 1953, Dr. Gibbon performed intracardiac surgery using the first successful pump oxygenator.

Heart catheterization and angiography, with use of image intensification, provide evaluation of hemodynamics in visualization and recording of intracardiac and intravascular function. Revascularization of ischemic myocardium to increase blood supply has progressed from abrasion of the epicardium with asbestos in the 1950s to the internal mammary artery implantation and the coronary bypass procedures developed in the 1960s. Electronic devices provide cardiac pacing for the irregular heart. Care of cardiac patients immediately following operation has improved markedly, reducing mortality, due in no small measure to increasingly sophisticated monitoring modalities. The greatest challenge to cardiac surgeons remains development of a substitute heart for organs beyond repair.

Anatomy and Physiology

Cardiac operations concern the heart and associated great vessels that enter it. The cardiovascular system is concerned with supplying oxygen and nutrients to body cells and carrying waste away from the cells. The heart, blood, and lymph vessels comprise this system (see Figs. 21-1 and 21-2).

The *heart* is located in the middle mediastinum slightly left of midline. The heart is a muscular "pump" enveloped by a closed, double-walled, fibroserous sac, the *pericardium.* Normally the sac contains a small amount of clear serous fluid that lubricates the heart's moving surfaces. The base of the pericardium is attached to the diaphragm; the apex surrounds the great vessels arising from the base of the heart for a short distance.

The layers of the heart are the *outer epicardium* (visceral pericardium), *myocardium* (muscle fibers), and *endocardium* (inner membrane lining). Divided into right and left halves by an oblique longitudinal septum, each half of the heart has two chambers, a thin-walled upper atrium and a thick-walled lower ventricle. The atria receive blood from veins; the ventricles pump blood into and along the arteries. The heart's rounded apex, formed by the left ventricle, is behind the sixth rib slightly to the left of the sternum. The base is formed by the atria and great vessels. The atria, lying mainly behind the ventricles, continue anteriorly on each side of the aorta to form the auricular appendages. The long axis of the heart extends from base to apex, i.e., from behind forward, downward, and to the left.

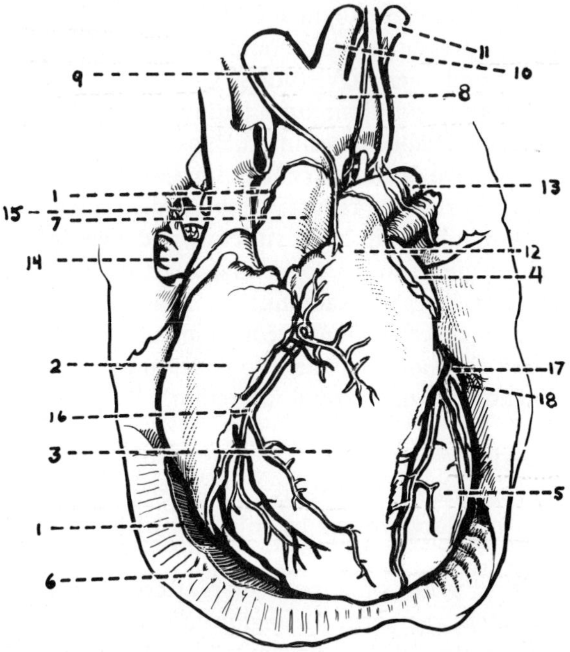

Figure 21-1 Anterior view of the heart and great vessels. (1) pericardium (parietal), (2) right atrium, (3) right ventricle, (4) left atrium, (5) left ventricle, (6) diaphragm, (7) ascending aorta, (8) aortic arch, (9) brachiocephalic artery, (10) left common carotid artery, (11) left subclavian artery, (12) pulmonary trunk, (13) left pulmonary artery, (14) right pulmonary artery, (15) superior vena cava, (16) right coronary artery, (17) left coronary artery, (18) circumflex branch of left coronary artery.

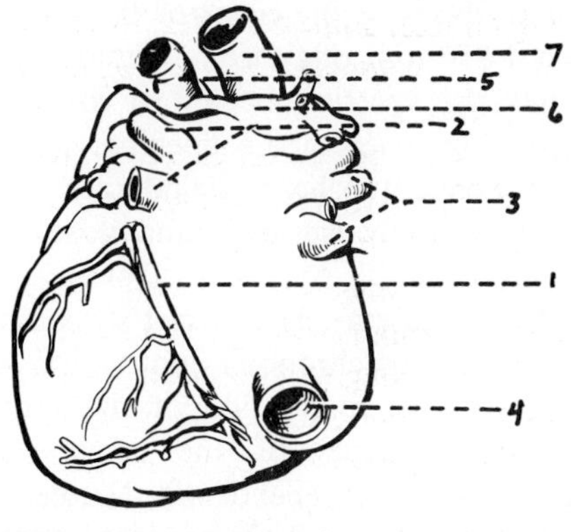

Figure 21-2 Posterior view of heart and great vessels. (1) coronary sinus, (2) left pulmonary veins, (3) right pulmonary veins, (4) inferior vena cava, (5) left pulmonary artery, (6) right pulmonary artery, (7) ascending aorta.

Coronary circulation is alluded to as predominantly right or predominantly left. The coronary arteries arise from the aorta and, with their branches, supply oxygen and nutrients to the heart muscle. The left coronary artery divides shortly after origin into two main trunks:

1. The anterior descending or interventricular branch courses toward the apex of the heart. Its branches distribute over the anterolateral wall of the left ventricle. Septal branches supply the anterior interventricular septum.
2. The circumflex branch passes posteriorly. Following the atrioventricular groove and passing under the left atrial appendage, it meets the right coronary artery at the base of the junction of both ventricles. The right coronary artery is directed to the right, passing to the posterior aspect of the heart and eventually running between the two ventricles. Its branches supply the posterior interventricular septum.

The vagus nerve (parasympathetic) and cardiac branches of the cervical and upper thoracic ganglia (sympathetic) innervate the heart.

Four *heart valves* promote unobstructed unidirectional blood flow. They are the right tricuspid and left mitral atrioventricular (A-V) valves, the pulmonary valve between the right ventricle and pulmonary trunk, and the aortic valve between the left ventricle and aorta. The latter two are referred to as *semilunar valves.* The mitral has two cusps or endocardial leaflets; the other valves have three. Bases of the cusps of the A-V valves attach to the fibrous ring that surrounds the opening. When the ventricle begins to contract, the cusps float up to close the opening, preventing backflow. Sequential heart sounds are heard by stethoscope as the valves open and close.

Conducting System The heart's conducting system permits synchronous contraction of the atria followed by contraction of the ventricles. Right and left sides of the heart function simultaneously but independently. Muscular contractions of the atria and ventricles are controlled by an electrical impulse that originates in the *sinoatrial* (*S-A*) *node*. This "pacemaker" is a dense network of specialized fibers situated at the junction of the right atrium and superior vena cava. These fibers become continuous with muscle fibers of the atrium at the node's periphery. The stimulus is passed to the smaller *atrioventricular (A-V) node* beneath the endocardium in the interatrial septum. A mass of interwoven conductive tissue, this node's specialized fibers are continuous with atrial muscle fibers and the atrioventricular bundle of His. The *bundle of His* provides conduction relay between atria and ventricles. Arising from the atrioventricular node, the band of conducting tissue passes on both sides of the interventricular septum, its branches dividing and subdividing to penetrate every area of ventricular muscle and to transmit contraction impulses to the ventricles. Thus, expansions of conducting tissue, providing coordinated excitation of muscle areas, spread through both atria and ventricles. Each atrial contraction (depolarization) is followed by a period of recharging (repolarization) during which the ventricles contract. Ventricular contraction is followed by a period of recovery while the chambers fill with blood as the atria contract due to higher pressure.

Cardiac Cycle (Circulation) Myocardial contraction is referred to as *systole*, relaxation as *diastole*. Venous blood from the entire body enters the right atrium via the vena cavae and passes through the tricuspid valve to the right ventricle from which it is ejected through the pulmonary valve into the pulmonary arterial trunk. Right and left pulmonary arteries originating from the trunk carry blood to the lungs where it takes up oxygen and gives off carbon dioxide. Oxygenated blood is transported from the lungs to the left atrium by the pulmonary veins and enters the left ventricle through the mitral valve. Contraction of the left ventricle propels blood through the aortic valve into the aorta from which it is carried to all parts of the body by arterial branches. The highest pressure reached during left ventricular systole is the *systolic blood pressure*. Following contraction the ventricle relaxes during which time systemic intra-arterial pressure falls to its lowest level, *diastolic blood pressure*. Each contraction of the right ventricle forces blood through the pulmonary valve into the pulmonary arteries to the lungs. In summary, there are two circulations:

1 *Pulmonary*, from the right ventricle to the lungs and back to the left atrium
2 *Systemic*, from the left ventricle to the aorta, to body tissues and organs and back to the right atrium

Interference in any part of the circulatory system can jeopardize survival.

Diagnostic Methods

Operation is preceded by extensive cardiovascular assessment utilizing noninvasive and invasive studies that dictate subsequent treatment.

Noninvasive Routine examination and electrocardiography are augmented by determination of venous pressure, cardiac output, circulation time, and blood chemistry studies. Chest x-ray reveals heart size, position, and outline. Screening or functional capacity testing such as stress testing is informative. Pulmonary function tests may detect left ventricular failure. Echocardiography by ultrasound reveals heart structure and gives information pertinent to congenital heart disease and valvular disease. Radionuclide imaging may be used to detect regional reductions in myocardial blood flow and thus help to confirm or deny the diagnosis of myocardial infarction.

Invasive

Angiography This is radiographic visualization of blood vessels by injection of a nontoxic radiopaque substance. Selective *arteriography* permits study of a particular artery such as a branch of the aorta. In *angiocardiography*, injection of the substance permits radiographs of the heart chambers and thoracic vessels. Rapid serial radiographs or motion pictures on an enlarged fluoroscopic screen show heart outline and passage of dye in the vessels. *Selective angiocardiography* or *coronary angiography* is done in association with cardiac catheterization to evaluate coronary artery disease and determine extent of obstructive disease in the coronary vessels. Aneurysms also may be diagnosed by angiography (see p. 293).

Cardiac Catheterization Under image intensification fluoroscopy, using aseptic technique, a sterile catheter is introduced through a cutdown into a brachial vein in the arm or femoral vein in the groin and passed into the heart. The procedure permits precise:

1 Evaluation of heart function
2 Measurements of intracardiac pressure
3 Visualization of heart chambers

Catheterization is utilized to diagnose coronary artery disease, valvular heart disease, or congenital anomalies. It is the ultimate tool for diagnosis of ischemic heart disease.

For study of the coronary arteries, a single catheter is passed and the tip inserted into the ostia of the arteries for injection of dye and trace of solution flow. Cinefluorograms record findings. After catheter removal, the incision is closed and pressure dressings applied.

Electrocardiography is monitored continuously by oscilloscope as cardiac arrhythmias may occur.

Special Features of Cardiac Surgery

1 The principles of general and thoracic surgery apply to cardiac surgery but several factors require emphasis:
   a Extra minutes are not available; seconds save lives.
   b The team concept is of utmost importance. An experienced team working together can handle emergencies expeditiously.
   c Comprehensive physical and psychological preparation of the patient precedes operation. Postoperatively the patient is taken to an intensive care unit. The patient is monitored constantly intra- and postoperatively.
2 Basic thoracic setup is used with the addition of cardiovascular instruments, e.g., various noncrushing vascular and anastomosis clamps, cardiotomy suction tips and sump tubes, and cardiovascular sutures.
3 Cardiopulmonary bypass (see below) is used for most intracardiac procedures, e.g., resection of ventricular aneurysm.
4 Local and/or systemic hypothermia may be used intraoperatively to reduce the body's need for oxygen (refer to Chap. 9).
5 Incisional approaches are those used for thoracic procedures, e.g., median sternotomy.
6 Closed water-seal drainage is used postoperatively when the pleura is opened.
7 The operating microscope may be used for anastomosing vessels.

Cardiopulmonary Bypass (Extracorporeal Circulation)

Cardiopulmonary bypass is the technique of oxygenating and perfusing the blood by means of a mechanical pump-oxygenator system. Referred to as the *heart-lung machine,* this apparatus temporarily substitutes for function of the patient's heart and lungs during cardiac surgery, especially open-heart procedures. Venous blood is diverted from the body to the machine for oxygenation, and pumped back to the patient. Bypass permits purposely induced cardiac arrest, thus allowing direct vision of the heart and its interior for repair of intracardiac defects in a dry, motionless field. Deliberate arrest may be effected by:

1 Cross-clamp of the aorta for a limited period
2 Electrical stimulation to produce ventricular fibrillation
3 Local hypothermia, topical application of iced saline slush around the heart or iced Ringer's solution to the heart externally and/or internally
4 Injection of cardioplegic drugs in solution

Bypass time is kept to a minimum as ischemia causes myocardial injury of time-related severity. During bypass the lungs are kept inflated and immobilized. In preparation for bypass, the patient is heparinized to prevent clot formation. Catheters are inserted, for venous diversion, into the inferior and superior vena cavae through small incisions in the right atrium. A catheter for return of oxygenated blood to arterial circulation is placed in the ascending aorta or femoral artery. The catheters are connected appropriately to the machine by sterile tubing before institution of bypass.

Components of the Bypass System

Oxygenator Oxygen is taken up and carbon dioxide removed from the blood. Types of oxygenators include:

1 *Bubble.* Bubbles of oxygen are supplied to the blood by direct blood-gas contact.
2 *Rotating disk.* Blood is directed to an oxygen-saturated atmosphere.
3 *Membrane.* Oxygen and carbon dioxide diffuse through a permeable plastic membrane that contains the blood. This method diminishes blood-gas interface.

Disposable oxygenators are available.

Heat Exchanger Incorporated in the circuit, it regulates blood temperature. Water at thermostatically controlled temperature circulates through the exchanger, which can rapidly produce, control, or correct systemic hypothermia. Hypothermia often is used in conjunction with bypass to reduce oxygen demands of the tissues, and protect the myocardium during arrest.

Pump Rollers turning over the sterile plastic tubing propel the reheated oxygenated blood in a relatively nonpulsatile flow through a blood filter and bubble trap to the arterial cannula for recirculation through the body. Rate of flow can be varied. It is calculated according to patient weight or body surface area. Reduced flow accompanies hypothermia.

Immediately before operation the machine is primed with some type of balanced salt solution, frequently lactated or acetated Ringer's solution. For a hemodilution technique of priming, the system is filled with fluid that will replace blood diverted to the pump-oxygenator system and recirculated through the circuit to remove air bubbles. These solutions are readily available and reduce complications associated with use of transfused blood. Blood is added as needed, however, to maintain adequate oxygen-carrying capacity and perfusion rate.

Bypass may be partial or total. In *partial,* only a portion of venous return is routed to the pump-oxygenator circuitry, the remaining portion following normal systemic circulation. In *total* bypass, all venous return is diverted to the machine for total body perfusion. Cord tapes placed around the caval catheters when inserted are tightened to drain all venous return to the machine, and the heart is arrested.

During perfusion the patient is intensely monitored, i.e., arterial and venous pressures, body and blood temperatures, blood gases and electrolytes, and urinary output. General anesthesia may be maintained by an anesthetic vaporizer that adds vapor to the oxygenating mixture, or by intravenous anesthesia.

At conclusion of defect repair, air is removed from the heart, heartbeat is restored, ventilation reestablished by respirator, the patient is rewarmed, and perfusion gradually decreased to wean the patient from the machine. After discontinuance of bypass, cannulas are removed and the purse-string sutures around the insertion sites are closed. Protamine sulfate is injected to reverse the effect of the heparin previously administered.

Cardiopulmonary bypass also may be employed in conjunction with deep hypothermia during neurosurgical operations, in major organ transplantation, and to perfuse an isolated segment of the body in cancer chemotherapy. (Refer to Chap. 29, p. 496, for complications associated with cardiopulmonary bypass.)

Cardiac Operations

The purposes of heart surgery are to correct anatomical abnormalities, repair or replace defective heart valves, excise ventricular aneurysm, or revascularize ischemic myocardium. The procedures may be performed with or without cardiopulmonary bypass. (Refer to Chap. 26 for pediatric operations.)

Correction of Valvular Disease Valvular disease may arise from a congenital abnormality or be acquired. Abnormal vibrations or heart murmurs may be congenital or the end result of disease such as rheumatic fever or degenerative change. Valves can become thickened and calcified, resulting in loss of valve substance, narrowing of the orifice, and immobility. They then develop *insufficiency,* failure to close completely, and permit blood leakage or regurgitation. Failure to open completely is caused by *stenosis,* which impedes flow. A defective valve is reconstructed if possible. To prevent heart failure, prosthetic valves are inserted in patients who have return of symptoms after reconstruction or have a valve that cannot be reconstructed.

A variety of prosthetic heart valves are available. They may be synthetic or biological. Disc- or ball-type synthetic valves commonly are used. The disc or ball freely opens and closes according to flow of blood. One type consists of a cage in which a spherical ball is enclosed. Other models are constructed with leaflets resembling human valves. The metal ring at the base of the cage may be covered with polyester fabric to facilitate suturing. It also encourages tissue ingrowth, an aid to long-term fixation. Valves also have been developed from homograft or heterograft (porcine or bovine) donor material. An effective prosthesis is nontoxic, nonthrombogenic, and nondeteriorating. The surgeon selects the most suitable type and size for the defect to be repaired.

Closed Mitral Commissurotomy An example of closed-heart surgery, the breaking apart of fused stenosed leaflets of the mitral (left A-V) valve reduces left atrial and right ventricular pressures that decrease lung function. The thorax is entered by left anterolateral incision. To provide hemostasis, purse-string sutures are placed around the left auricular appendage prior to opening it.

The surgeon frees fused leaflets by inserting a finger, valvulotome (knife), or transventricular dilator into the valve. After this is accomplished, purse-string sutures are closed and the auricular appendage is sutured. Lungs are reexpanded, a chest tube is inserted, the incision is closed, and the tube is connected to water-seal drainage.

More commonly, plastic repair, *valvuloplasty,* is done under direct vision of open-heart surgery. A potential hazard of the open method is an air embolism by expulsion of air from the left ventricle into the aorta, but steps are taken to avoid this complication.

Mitral Valve Replacement Cardiopulmonary bypass is used for this open-heart procedure. Through median sternotomy or left thoractomy incision, the pericardium is incised and retracted. When bypass catheters are placed, the left ventricle may be vented with a plastic tube to decompress the heart and prevent overdistention of the ventricle at unclamping of the aorta after anoxic arrest. The left atrium is opened. The mitral valve is exposed, inspected, and removed by circumferential excision and severance of muscular attachments to the ventricular wall. The fibrous ring or annulus surrounding the valvular opening remains intact. The sterile prosthetic valve is inserted, sutured in place, and the atrium sutured. Postoperatively, temporary pacing (see p. 394) may be required; therefore, pacing wires usually are implanted under the wall of the right ventricle during operation. The pericardium is closed. Blood is returned to the heart and air removed from it. Partial cardiopulmonary bypass is resumed as the patient is weaned from the machine. Cannula incisions are closed. Thoracic wound closure is carried out and water-seal chest drainage used.

Excision of Ventricular Aneurysm Atherosclerotic coronary disease predisposes an individual to myocardial infarction. Ventricular aneurysm, a segmental dilatation of predominantly the left ventricular wall, may develop any time from a few weeks but mainly to a few years postinfarction. The thin-walled fibrous aneurysm, result of ventricular force on an area of nonfunctioning scar tissue, often contains clots within it. Left ventricular aneurysm usually produces hemodynamic instability manifested by congestive heart failure, ventricular arrhythmia, or angina. Utilizing cardiopulmonary bypass, it is possible to excise the aneurysm and reconstruct the ventricle.

The chest is opened by median sternotomy and cardiopulmonary bypass established before adhesion between the aneurysm and pericardium is detached. The ascending aorta is cross-clamped to prevent air or blood embolization from manipulation. The aneurysmal sac, entered by stab wound, collapses with suctioning when the heart is empty. Viable myocardium retains shape. The apex is opened with vertical incision and fibrotic myocardium is excised circumferentially with a rim of fibrous tissue left to hold the sutures used to close the left ventricle. Pledgets may be employed to reinforce sutures. All air is removed from the ventricle by suction before completion of closure. Heartbeat is restored, the patient decannulated, and all other incisions closed in the usual manner.

Aneurysmectomy may be done as a single procedure or in conjunction with coronary artery bypass.

Coronary Artery Procedures Coronary arteries supplying the heart may become stenosed or obstructed, referred to as *occlusive coronary artery disease.* Resultant myocardial ischemia may result in angina or myocardial infarction. The number of coronary vessels affected with 50 percent or more occlusion influences survival. Myocardial revascularization to improve blood supply to the affected myocardium is possible by operative intervention in selected patients. The operation relieves anginal pain. Direct coronary revascularization may be accomplished by use of a grafted vein to bypass the occlusion or by direct anastomosis of the internal mammary artery to the affected coronary artery. Results of operation depend on numerous factors such as the patient's preoperative cardiovascular status.

Coronary Artery Bypass Graft Segment(s) of saphenous vein and/or internal mammary artery are used to bypass coronary artery obstruction. The right coronary, left anterior descending, and circumflex arteries most commonly are involved. Single or multiple bypasses are done depending on the number of vessels affected and degree of obstruction present. Use of cardiopulmonary bypass is influenced by the surgeon's preferred technique and extent of grafting.

1 *Saphenous vein bypass graft.* The procedure is expedited by two teams; one harvests the saphenous vein for graft while the other opens the chest and prepares for cardiopulmonary bypass. (A cephalic vein may be used if the saphenous vein is diseased or has been previously stripped.) Adequate vein is removed for sufficient graft material. The distal end of each vein segment removed is identified and the graft placed in heparinized normal saline after harvest. It is handled gently to avoid trauma to the intima.

The chest is opened by median sternotomy and the pericardium incised. Cardiopulmonary bypass is established. After a small opening is created in the aorta, the reversed vein is sutured to the aperture. It is important to position the graft with the distal end of the vein at the aortic anastomosis site to permit normal direction of blood flow through the venous valves. The coronary artery is opened distal to obstruction; the free end of the graft is anastomosed to the artery end-to-side. Cardiopulmonary bypass is discontinued and all incisions closed. Chest drainage is used. After removal from extracorporeal circulation and stabilization of blood pressure, flow is measured in each graft with an electromagnetic flowmeter.

2 *Internal mammary artery anastomosis.* To gain length, the internal mammary artery is dissected up to its origin from the subclavian artery. After mobilization, end-to-side anastomosis is performed between the internal mammary and the diseased coronary artery, distal to the obstruction. The pericardium is not sutured to provide adequate drainage. The wound is closed in the usual manner for sternotomy. Water-seal drainage is employed.

Endarterectomy of Coronary Arteries Removal of an organized thrombus and attached endothelium or atherosclerotic fatty plaques from an arterial wall occasionally is done. Endarterectomy may be combined with venous bypass grafting. Using small endarterectomy spatulas and wire loops, segments of obstructing core are removed to increase blood flow through the graft, especially to the right coronary artery.

Intra-aortic Balloon Pump An intra-aortic balloon pump (IABP) is a supportive device used to assist a patient in left ventricular failure or cardiogenic shock (refer to Chap. 29). It usually is inserted in the OR in conjunction with coronary artery bypass operation. Used prior to or after extracorporeal circulation, IABP reduces left ventricular workload and increases delivery of oxygen to the myocardium, thereby increasing cardiac output and systemic perfusion.

The balloon is inserted into the descending aorta, proximal to the renal arteries, via a prosthetic arterial graft anastomosed end-to-side to the femoral artery. Insertion of the balloon via the graft preserves distal blood flow to the catheterized femoral artery. The IABP utilizes principles of counterpulsation. In contrast to systemic arteries, coronary arteries constrict during systole and fill during diastole. Therefore, inflating the balloon during diastole increases coronary perfusion by counterpulsation for contractility and oxygen transport. When the balloon is inflated, the blood volume displaced increases systemic arterial pressure. When the balloon deflates during systole, resistance that the ventrical must pump against is decreased. Balloons vary in size to provide 20, 30, or 40 ml volume displacement, thus giving maximum assist without total aortic occlusion. When a sterile balloon is placed, the position is verified by x-ray, the complete system is vented of air and filled with either helium or carbon dioxide, for balloon inflation, depending on the type of counterpulsator. The ratio of ventricular assist is determined by the individual patient's hemodynamic status. The pump can be regulated automatically, triggered by an electrocardiogram signal, or operated manually. To prevent potential thrombi, pumping should not be stopped for more than 30 minutes at a time. The IABP is equipped with sensors to minimize danger, e.g., an alarm and an automatic shut-off. Weaning of the patient from IABP is usually gradual in accordance with the patient's tolerance.

Insertion of Cardiac Pacemaker The conducting system of the heart may be altered or interrupted at any point by degenerative disease, drugs, or operative trauma. This may cause diminished cardiac output, arrhythmias, partial or complete heart block. Patients with these conditions may be treated by artificial pacing or delivery of electrical impulse by a pacemaker, a complex electronic battery-driven device. The batteries supply power for years. Nuclear-powered devices also are available.

A pacemaker consists of a pulse generator to produce electrical impulses and electrodes to carry impulses to the heart. An implantable generator is sealed in a plastic or metal container impermeable to body fluids. Electrodes and leads made of plastic-covered metal may be unipolar or bipolar and intended for transvenous, endocardial, or epicardial use. The pacing system includes electrode-myocardial conduction. Radio-frequency pacemakers eliminate need for wire electrodes. A small receiver is implanted beneath the pericardium. A transmitter worn outside the body transmits radio energy that is converted by the electrical stimuli delivered to the ventricles.

Pacemakers are of two types: the synchronous fixed-rate model that delivers impulse for contraction at a regular predetermined rate, and the more commonly used standby demand type. The latter is intermittent and noncompetitive with the patient's own pacing mechanism. The device monitors the heart's normal activity. The impulse to stimulate the heart is not emitted unless the rate of heartbeat falls below a certain preset level.

Effective external pacing for ventricular standstill led to development of partially implanted electrode leads connected to an external stimulator for longer-term pacing. Fully implantable pacemaker systems for long-term use became available in 1960 and rapid development led to a wide variety of systems. Selection of system depends on specific pacing requirements of the individual patient. Pacemakers may be temporary or permanent; temporary pacing may be diagnostic or therapeutic. Transvenous catheter or external electrodes may be used. Temporary pacing is necessary prior to and during permanent-system implantation. Systemic complete heart block is the most frequent indication for permanent implantation. Permanent pacing may be initiated by various methods.

Insertion of Transvenous Permanent Pacemaker This system utilizes transvenous endocardial electrodes. The lead is placed in the endocardium of the apex of the right ventricle and attached to the pulse generator. Incision is made at the base of the neck if the external jugular vein, the more common, is used, or beneath the clavicle if the cephalic vein is desired. Under fluoroscopy an endocardial electrode catheter placed in the selected vein is advanced via the superior vena cava to the apex of the right ventricle where it is wedged into the myocardium and/or sutured to the ventricular wall. Through a separate incision in the anterolateral, prepectoral portion of the chest, a subcutaneous pouch is dissected for placement of the pulse generator. The proximal end of the endocardial electrode, brought to the second incision, is attached to the pulse generator prior to its implantation in the pouch.

Placement of Epicardial Electrodes Permanent pacing also is possible with the use of epicardial electrodes. Several approaches to the heart are possible. For an extrapleural parasternal approach, the pericardium is entered by subperichondrial resection of the fifth costal cartilage. Two epicardial sew-on or screw-on type electrodes are implanted 1 cm apart in the epicardium of the right or the left ventricle. After measuring pacing thresholds from an external generator source, electrode leads are tunneled under the costal margin to the battery case implanted in a subcutaneous pocket in the left upper quadrant of the abdominal wall. Patients with pacemakers require adequate followup and should carry identification containing serial number, model, rate, and manufacturer of the pacemaker. The circulating nurse must record this information in the patient's chart at the time of pacemaker insertion. Also, patients with demand units or radio-frequency pacemakers should be warned to avoid proximity to radar devices since electrical interference may stimulate heart activity.

PERIPHERAL VASCULAR SURGERY

For centuries human beings have been plagued with peripheral vascular disease and its complications such as pain, loss of an extremity or life. Longevity has increased the number of people suffering from diseases of the vascular system. The decades of the 1960s and 1970s have seen marked advancement in this field because of the development of many new operations requiring improved instrumentation, sutures, synthetic grafts, angiography, and microvascular techniques. Circulatory problems may affect any part of the body, but this discussion focuses on the most common pathology amenable to particular vascular operations.

Special Considerations

1 A thorough understanding of principles of general surgery should be combined with special training in vascular operative techniques. An experienced operating team is essential because of the tendency of blood to clot. Speed and accuracy are imperative.

2 Diagnostic procedures include angiography, sonography, and consultation between surgeon and radiologist prior to and often during operation.

3 Local or attended local anesthesia usually is preferred for most angiographic studies. General anesthesia or regional block is used for the operative procedure.

4 Meticulous care must be exercised in anastomosing vessels since any loose adventitia falling into the suture line or being carried into the lumen of the vessel increases the danger of postoperative thrombosis.

5 To prevent undue trauma to vessels an assortment of scissors, noncrushing vascular clamps, and forceps specifically designed for vascular surgery is included in the instrument setup. Umbilical tape or Vesseloops are used for retraction and vascular control.

6 Heparinized solution must be available for local use as an anticoagulant.

7 Certain preferred sutures include several different synthetic materials that pass through vessel walls easily with minimal trauma and tie securely. Swaged needles also minimize trauma. Frequently, double-armed needle sutures are employed for vessel anastomosis.

8 A variety of straight and bifurcated woven or knitted grafts in various lengths and diameters are required in different situations. Pieces of synthetic material may be cut to size for use as patch grafts. Grafts are sterilized in see-through packages to permit the surgeon to select the appropriate size once exposure is completed. Synthetic grafts must be porous enough to allow growth of fibrous tissue. Therefore they must be preclotted before insertion. For the preclotting process, the surgeon withdraws blood from the vessel at the operative site and transfers it to the scrub nurse who may inject it into the lumen of the graft and/or soak the graft in the blood in a sterile basin. The prime goal in preclotting is to make the wall of the graft impervious to blood by filling the interstices with fibrin. The fabric-fibrin conduit later becomes firmly placed in the tissues and provides a hypothrombogenic flow surface.

9 Blood must be available at time of operation, since it is lost by flushing of clots and debris.

10 The most serious immediate postoperative complications are thrombosis and hemorrhage. The patient may need to return to the operating room for *immediate* correction of these problems.

Arterial Bypass

Occlusive vascular disease often involves only a segment of an artery. Arterial injury may occur due to trauma or indirectly occur near the site of fractures. The vessel lumina above and below the lesion usually are normal. Vascular reconstruction is performed in an attempt to restore normal circulation. The surgeon may choose a method to bypass the obstruction.

1 The involved segment may be excised and the ends anastomosed if they can be approximated without tension. If this is not possible, a graft is interposed.

2 The involved segment is excised and an autograft, or synthetic prosthetic graft, is used as replacement.

3 The lesion can be bypassed using the long saphenous vein from one thigh as a vein graft, or a synthetic prosthetic graft may be used. Ends of the graft are anastomosed to the artery proximal and distal to the lesion. The obstructed segment of the artery is not resected.

When a saphenous vein graft is used as the bypass, two surgeons may work simultaneously, one exposing the artery while the other surgeon prepares the vein for grafting. A separate sterile table, supplied with fine vascular instruments and basin of heparinized saline for flushing the vein, is used for vein preparation. The surgeon may use magnification loupes to check for imperfections while preparing the vein.

Femoral Popliteal Artery Bypass In a lower extremity, the femoral artery is most prone to obstruction by occlusive vascular disease. A femoral popliteal bypass may be the procedure of choice, and is the most frequently performed bypass operation in an extremity. The patient is positioned supine on the operating table with the thigh slightly abducted and the knee flexed and supported. The entire extremity is prepped and draped to allow adequate exposure. A longitudinal medial incision extends the entire length of the popliteal artery, or separate incisions can be made to expose the arteries and explore the area before bypassing the obstruction in the femoral artery. During operation the pulsations of the proximal and distal popliteal artery are checked as well as pulsations in the foot. Postoperatively, the distal pulsations may be checked with the Doppler pulse detector, an instrument that detects blood flow through the arteries by means of ultrasound.

Endarterectomy

Atherosclerotic plaques may cause localized stenosis in major arteries such as the femorals and carotids. A loosely attached plaque can be pulled from the vessel wall and removed with vascular wire loops, spatulas, and/or catheters.

Carotid Endarterectomy The operation is done to remove atherosclerotic plaques at the carotid bifurcation that cause localized stenosis or ulceration. Endarterectomy is indicated when arteriography shows narrowing of 50 percent or more. The patient is positioned supine with the head turned away from the operative side. Care must be taken not to place undue extension on the neck as this may occlude the vertebral flow. The incision is carried through the subcutaneous tissue, platysma muscle, and the anterior border of the sternocleidomastoid muscle. Retraction of the sternocleidomastoid muscle and jugular vein allows exposure of the carotid artery and its branches. After systemic heparinization, special vascular instruments are used to clamp above and below the occluded area. In certain instances a shunt will be inserted in the artery to maintain blood flow to the brain while the plaque is removed. Many surgeons use a shunt routinely while others use alternative means of cerebral protection such as deliberately producing mild to moderate hypertension or hypercapnea. In any event, prolonged delay of the procedure at this time may cause serious neurological complications. The carotid is incised and the plaque is removed. Reconstructive procedures may include patch-graft angioplasty or bypass grafting. Bilateral endartectomies may be indicated for severe bilateral occlusion, but the operations are performed at least 1 week apart.

Aneurysmectomy

An *aneurysm* is a localized abnormal dilatation of an artery with formation of a sac due to pressure of blood on the weakened vessel wall. Atherosclerosis is the most common cause but trauma may be an etiologic factor. Cystic medial necrosis causes dissecting aneurysm, usually of the thoracic aorta. Loss of structural integrity is implicit in every aneurysm. The abdominal aorta, femoral and popliteal arteries, and less frequently the thoracic aorta are the vessels usually affected. Diagnostic evaluation combines physical examination, laboratory findings, x-ray studies, and arteriography. Location and extent of lesion determine operability and type of reconstruction. However, a ruptured aneurysm precludes further evaluation and operation must be performed *immediately*.

Resection of Abdominal Aortic Aneurysm Abdominal aneurysmectomy may be a lifesaving operation. It is associated with serious hazards including massive hemorrhage and injury to the ureters and other nearby structures. Renal failure is a potential complication. Modern techniques have greatly reduced the mortality rate and survivors of the operation enjoy the same life expectancy as other patients with comparable arteriosclerotic disease.

A variety of monitoring techniques is essential to avoid prolonged periods of unrecognized hypotension. Blood flow of the extremities must be checked frequently. Urinary output must be carefully calculated and recorded. Blood must be available for transfusion.

The patient is in supine position. The entire abdomen from the nipple line to pubis is prepped and draped. The groin and thighs may be prepared if a bifurcated graft will be used for aortic replacement. A long midline incision usually is used. The abdomen is thoroughly explored, the small intestinal mesentery mobilized, then the posterior peritoneum overlying the aorta incised to expose the aneurysm. The small intestine and ascending colon may be delivered outside the abdomen to increase exposure and to prevent injury. Warm moist tapes, plastic sheeting, or a Lahey bag may be used to protect these structures.

Before occlusion of the aorta, blood is withdrawn to be used for preclotting in the graft. Heparin is injected locally. Appropriate-sized aortic clamps are placed proximal to the aneurysm and the iliac arteries are clamped distally. The aneurysmal wall is opened. The clot and loose intraluminal debris are removed. A graft of appropriate size is sutured into place at the upper limit of the aneurysm and to the common iliac or appropriate arteries distally. Living tissue, for example, the posterior portion of the aneurysm sac or mesentery, must cover the prosthesis to prevent contact of the prosthesis with the intestines. Failure to accomplish this may result in fistula formation. The long abdominal incision usually is closed with nonabsorbable sutures placed in the midline fascia. Retention sutures frequently are used.

Embolectomy

An *embolus* is a mass of undissolved matter carried by the bloodstream until it lodges in a blood vessel and occludes it. Most often part or all of a thrombus, an embolus may be an air bubble, fat globule, clump of bacteria, piece of tissue, or a foreign body. The occlusion of a blood vessel by an embolus causes various syndromes, depending on the size and location of the occluded vessel. Occlusion of a vessel in the brain, lungs, or heart can cause rapid and sudden death. Surgical intervention may be necessary when anticoagulant or other medical therapy fails or is contraindicated. To perform an embolectomy, the affected blood vessel is incised and the embolus removed. If accessibility to the vessel is too hazardous to perform an embolectomy, a sympathectomy may be beneficial (refer to Chap. 24, p. 441).

Pulmonary Embolus An occlusion of the pulmonary artery or one of its branches usually occurs from emboli originating from veins in the lower extremities or the pelvis. Emboli pass up the inferior vena cava to the right side of the heart and are ejected from the right ventricle into the pulmonary artery. Diagnosis of pulmonary embolism has been improved with the use of lung scans, pulmonary angiograms, and phlebograms. Operation may be indicated when anticoagulant therapy fails or is contraindicated, to prevent the passage of emboli to the lungs. Blood flow may be partially interrupted with plastic serrated clips or filter blocks. The inferior vena cava may be ligated to prevent passage of septic emboli arising from infected pelvic veins.

Mobbin-Uddin Filter Procedure This is one effective technique for partial interruption of the inferior vena cava. A long applicator with stylet and loading cone is assembled with the collapsed umbrellalike filter inside. Under fluoroscopy with television amplification, the applicator is inserted through a right internal jugular venotomy. The filter is ejected and fixed in position below the renal veins and above the point of juncture of the iliac veins. This procedure may be performed on poor-risk patients under local anesthesia with an anesthesiologist in attendance.

Vena Cava Ligation/Plication This may be performed by abdominal approach in patients who are reasonable risks for general anesthesia. The surgeon may choose midline transabdominal, retroperitoneal, or subcostal intraperitoneal approach, depending on the exposure needed. After exposing and freeing of the inferior vena cava, a clip is passed around the vein and secured with a suture ligature, or the vein may be ligated. This allows blood to return to the right ventricle of the heart without passage of emboli. Thighs and legs frequently are wrapped with elastic bandages and elevated before the patient leaves the OR to prevent postoperative edema, the main complication.

Vascular Shunts

Normal circulation can be altered to increase or decrease blood flow to a specific organ. A prosthetic vascular shunt may be inserted to establish an external route for diversion of blood flow through a mechanical device.

Arteriovenous Shunts and Fistulas Access to the vascular system through an arteriovenous shunt or fistula can be a lifesaving technique employed for patients suffering from chronic uremia who need renal dialysis, or for patients requiring a series of exchange blood transfusions. The actual insertion of a shunt or creation of an internal or external fistula requires meticulous attention to detail since longevity is an important consideration. The most frequent complications are thrombosis and infection. (Refer to Chap. 19 for renal dialysis procedures.)

Portacaval Shunt This extensive vascular operation is performed in selected patients with gastrointestinal bleeding due to esophageal varices. Portacaval shunting is definitive therapy when bleeding is not controlled by conservative methods. The purpose of the operation is to reduce portal venous hypertension and/or portal venous blood flow. Hypertension, increase in portal pressure, is caused by obstruction to flow of blood from the portal vein to the liver as a result of cirrhosis, hepatitis, or thrombosis. The increased pressure thus produced results in venous dilatation.

Anastomosis of the portal vein to the inferior vena cava relieves hypertension by bypassing obstruction and diverting return flow of blood to the liver from the portal vein. The anastomosis usually is end-to-side. Shunting does not repair the already damaged liver, but, if successful, prevents further hemorrhage.

Subcostal, transabdominal, or thoracoabdominal incision may be used. Abdominal, vascular, and thoracic setups are prepared. Pressure within the portal vein is measured with a manometer, via a cannulated branch of the superior mesenteric vein, at the beginning and conclusion of operation. Because of venous distention and vascularity of the operative area, hemorrhage is a major intraoperative hazard. Care is taken to avoid injury to adjacent structures including the hepatic artery and common duct. Following a thoracoabdominal operation, chest drainage must be established.

Splenorenal Shunt This technique generally is employed when the portal vein is not available for shunting because of obstruction in the hepatic portal venous system. It involves removal of the spleen and anastomosis of the splenic and left renal veins. A splenectomy usually is performed; however, some surgeons advocate a selective splenorenal shunt leaving the spleen *in situ.*

Superior Mesenteric-Inferior Vena Caval Shunt This operation generally is employed when previous shunts have failed, or if a splenic vein is too small for a successful shunt. This procedure is well tolerated by young patients.

Chapter 22

Ophthalmology

HISTORICAL INTRODUCTION

Disorders of the eye have plagued man since time immemorial. None has been as well documented as *cataract,* an opacification of the crystalline lens of the eye. The word *cataract,* originally derived from Greek, was translated in Arabic to mean "mist of a waterfall." Throughout history cataract has been called by various names, such as "pearl of the eye."

Awareness of cataract probably extends back at least 3000 years. The finding of Bronze Age (2000–1000 B.C.) instruments like those used for an ancient couching treatment helps substantiate this belief. Couching consisted of striking a blow to the front of the eye with a sharp instrument to spontaneously dislocate the opacified lens and push it back into the vitreous cavity. Light then entered the pupil. Couching was used by the Hindus, Greeks, Romans, and Arabs.

The rise of Buddhism in the sixth century B.C. forbade dissection and shedding of blood; much knowledge was buried. The Arabians, by translating Greek and Roman writings, kept ophthalmic knowledge alive until it was translated by the monks of the Middle Ages.

A treatise written by a reknowned Hindu surgeon, Súsruta, many years before Christ is believed to be the earliest authentic record. Súsruta taught that cataract was an opacity of the lens due to a disorder of eye fluids. Hippocrates wrote that pupils of the eyes sometimes became distorted, taking on the color of the sea.

In the early Christian era, Celsus differentiated between incipient (beginning) and mature cataracts. Galen thought the white opacity to be partly in the lens, partly in the aqueous humor in the form of a membrane floating between the lens and the iris. That belief was held, and couching practiced sporadically, until the mid-eighteenth century when J. Daviel, a French surgeon, performed the first deliberate lens removal. The intracapsular technique, however, was not accepted and refined until the 1930s and 1940s, when it became a standard procedure of cataract removal.

The first corneal transplant in which a scarred cornea was replaced with a clear cornea was performed around 1817. It failed because heterograft tissue was used instead of homograft tissue. The first reported successful full-thickness graft of full corneal depth, that remained clear, was transplanted in 1905. Although attempted in the interval, corneal transplantation did not become an established technique until after World War II.

The early square grafts were replaced by round ones. Since then technique has been refined to produce a high rate of favorable outcome.

Fruitless attempts were made to implant lenses in the early eighteenth century. The modern era of implantation began, and the concept of plastic intraocular lens evolved from an incidental observation. Surgeons in England noted a lack of reactivity to fragments of plastic from shattered plane canopies that penetrated the eyes in World War II fighter pilots. Posterior chamber fixated lenses in the 1950s produced disappointing long-term results mainly because of dislocation. The first series of anterior chamber lenses were unsuccessful because of delayed corneal damage. Sophisticated support systems reduce damage to corneal epithelium. The iris-supported lenses were designed to avoid this complication. Much of the original research was done in Holland.

THE EYE

The main causes of blindness are retinal disorders, glaucoma, and cataract. A substitute system for vision in the eye, one of the most intricate organs in the body, does not exist, but modern ophthalmology can cure or greatly improve many types of impaired vision.

Anatomy and Physiology

A thorough understanding of the anatomical structure and physiology of the eye is fundamental to comprehension of the operative procedures (see Fig. 22-1). The *globe* or *eyeball* is situated within the bony orbit surrounded by a padding of fatty tissue. Its position is maintained by extraocular muscles and fascial attachments. The outer wall of the globe is called the *sclera,* and is contiguous with the transparent *cornea* anteriorly. The *conjunctiva* is the mucous membrane that lines the inner side of the eyelids and the exposed portion of the sclera except for the cornea.

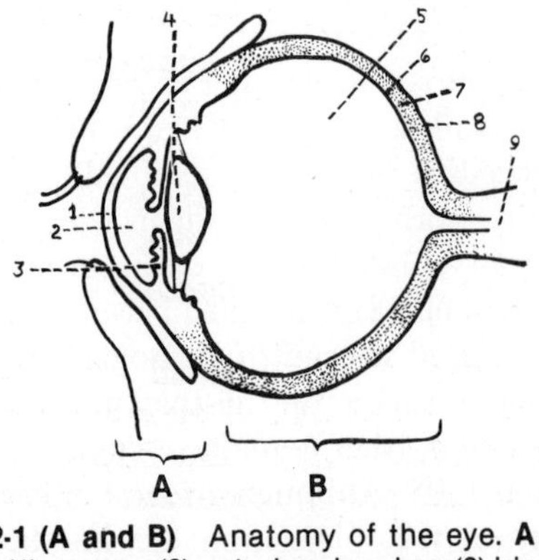

Figure 22-1 (A and B) Anatomy of the eye. **A** anterior segment: (1) cornea, (2) anterior chamber, (3) iris, (4) lens. **B** posterior segment: (5) vitreous body, (6) retina, (7) choroid, (8) sclera, (9) optic nerve.

The *anterior segment* of the eye includes the cornea, the anterior chamber filled with aqueous fluid (humor), the iris, and the lens. The portion of the eye lying behind the lens is known as the *posterior segment.* This part contains the vitreous fluid, which must be clear for vision, the retina, and the choroid linings, which are the vascular nourishing layers.

The function of vision requires:

1 Visual apparatus
2 Source of light
3 Interpretation by the brain of what is seen

Basically the eye resembles a camera with a compound lens system. Light rays emanating from an object in the field of vision are transmitted to the eye, where they traverse the optical system to get to the retina. The retina corresponds to the film of the camera. The optical system is comprised of the transparent cornea or window of the eye, the aqueous fluid behind the cornea, the pupil or opening in the colored iris, and the lens. The lens, by bending the light rays, focuses them to form an image on the retina, the innermost layer of the eye that contains the visual-nerve endings. These sensory cells are connected to nerve fibers, which enter the brain via the optic nerve. The occipital portion of the brain interprets the light-ray images registered on the retina. The intensity of light is automatically determined by the size of the pupil, which is controlled by the iris muscles. The iris action functions like the shutter of a camera.

OPERATIVE OCULAR PROCEDURES

Operative treatment of the eye can be divided for convenience into two main classifications:

1 Extraocular, or conditions affecting the exterior surface of the eye or the orbit
2 Intraocular, or those pertaining to the interior contents of the eye

Extraocular Procedures

Eyelid

Plastic Repair of Lacerations This involves approximation of anatomical layers. If the laceration includes the lacrimal canaliculus or tear duct, special probes are used to identify the proximal portions for rejoining. Penetrating wounds such as animal bites are debrided.

Biopsy or Excision of Neoplasm of Lid This may be performed with a knife, electrodesiccation (high-frequency electric current), or cryosurgery. An extremely common but benign tumor of the lid is the *chalazion,* a cystic alteration of one of the oil-secreting meibomian glands in the lid. The resulting accumulation of oil forms a hard tumor of the lid, requiring excision. This is usually an office or ambulatory operative procedure.

Plastic Repair of Defects Following removal of a lid malignancy, plastic repair employs the usual plastic procedures such as Z-plasty in addition to sliding flaps from adjacent areas and full- or partial-thickness flaps from the opposing lid to close the defect.

Correction of Ptosis (Drooping of the Upper Lid) While more commonly congenital (see Chap. 26), ptosis may be acquired in adults. An incision is made on the front or back surface of the lid to expose the levator muscle. The muscle is then dissected free of its adjacent attachments and a variable amount excised in proportion to the degree of ptosis.

Repair of Acquired Malformation of the Lid Conditions such as senile ectropion or entropion most commonly affect the lower lid. *Ectropion* is a condition in which either lid is *everted* (turned out) so as to expose the conjunctival surface of the lid. *Entropion* is the opposite condition in which the lid margin is *inverted* (turned in). Frequently the lashes then abrade the cornea. Various procedures may be employed with principles common to both conditions. A triangle of lid tissue is excised to erect the lid: in ectropion, the base of the triangle is up; in entropion, the base is down.

Blepharoplasty In this procedure the redundant fold(s) of skin and herniated pockets of fat are removed. Defects in the muscle layer are repaired. Two common results of aging are stretching of the eyelid skin and bulging of orbital fat from between the muscle fibers of the lids. Both cause cosmetic disfigurement or "baggy lids" and in extreme cases may obstruct vision. (Refer to Chap. 25, p. 449.)

Lacrimal Apparatus

Lacrimal-Duct Dilatation This is performed for excessive tearing. A series of probes, graduated in size, are introduced one by one into the duct system to permit freer drainage of tears.

Dacryocystectomy (Extirpation or Removal of the Lacrimal Sac) This is performed for chronic dacryocystitis. It does not reestablish the tear-drainage system.

Dacryocystorhinostomy (DCR) This is the construction of a new opening into the nasal cavity for the tear sac. It is done to correct congenital malformation or trauma to the nasolacrimal duct. A new tear-drainage system is constructed.

Extraocular Muscle Procedures Procedures on oculomotor muscles, those that control eye movement, are performed to correct misalignment that interferes with the ability of the two eyes to remain in simultaneous focus on a viewed object. The operations correct muscle imbalance by strengthening a weak muscle or by weakening an overactive one. While commonly performed on children (see Chap. 26), muscle procedures may be required in adult patients:

1 Those with untreated childhood strabismus (squint)

2 Those who obtained an unsatisfactory result from childhood operation

3 Those who sustained trauma to the brain stem or to the orbit with resultant muscle injury or paralysis

4 Those with systemic disease, such as thyroid exophthalmos, and muscle paralysis

5 Those who suffered a cerebrovascular accident (CVA) and muscle paralysis

Orbital Procedures

Decompression This is the operative treatment for severe exophthalmos that does not respond to medical treatment.

Exploration for Tumors This may be performed as indicated through a suitable approach such as the lateral wall or roof of the orbit, depending on location. The procedure may involve an interdisciplinary team of surgeons.

Reduction of Orbital Fractures This procedure may fall within the province of a multidisciplinary team of surgeons. The injury may involve the rim or the floor of the orbit, or both. Extent of the trauma should dictate the most appropriate operative management.

1 *Fractures of the orbital rim,* frequently associated with fractures of the zygoma, are usually detected by deformity. The fracture is reduced by appropriate means. Fragments are wired into place as necessary.

2 *Blowout fracture of the orbit* may result from a direct blow to the eyeball, which is in turn transmitted to the very thin floor of the orbit. A typical fracture is in the medial third of the floor with dislocation of floor fragments into the maxillary sinus. Occasionally the fracture may extend into the ethmoid plate. Consequently orbital contents, which may include the inferior extraocular muscles, are usually herniated into the antrum. This produces limitation of upward gaze and some degree of enophthalmos or recession of the eyeball into the orbit. The herniated orbital contents must be reduced from the antrum back into the orbit with special attention to freeing the entrapped muscles. A plastic or metal alloy plate may be used to close the defect in the floor. Or, the fragments may be elevated by packing the antrum through a Caldwell-Luc (sinus) approach. Diagnosis of the condition may be overlooked unless a laminogram is taken.

Procedures for Removal of Eye

Enucleation This is the complete removal of the eyeball and severing of its muscular attachments. The muscle stumps are preserved. The space between them forms a pocket into which a spherical implant is usually inserted. The overlying fascia and conjunctiva are closed so as to contain the sphere in the socket. Contraction of the eye muscles cause the sphere to move in the socket. This movement is transmitted to the artificial eye (prosthesis) so as to simulate normal eye movements.

Evisceration In contrast to enucleation, evisceration consists of removal of the contents of the eyeball only, leaving the outer coats (sclera and muscles) intact. This procedure reduces the danger of transmission of intraocular infection to the orbit and brain. It provides points for attachment of a prosthesis. Predisposing factors include destruction of the eyeball by injury or disease, and absolute glaucoma (hard blind eye).

Exenteration This is removal of the entire eye and orbital contents (tendon, fatty and fibrous tissues). It is done for tumors of the lids or the eyeball that have extended into the orbit. Extensive plastic reconstruction is necessary before fitting an artificial eye.

Intraocular Procedures

Corneal Procedures Although resilient tissue, the cornea, continually exposed to the environment, is especially susceptible to injury and infection.

Repair of Laceration This repair is preferably accomplished by direct appositional suturing of the edges. For very irregular tears not suitable for suturing, a conjunctival flap is used to seal off the tear.

Removal of Foreign Body This is done very gently under aseptic technique to avoid secondary infection and further trauma.

Cauterization Cauterization with chemicals or heat is sometimes used for corneal ulceration that does not respond to antibiotics.

Pterygium This is a benign growth of conjunctival tissue over the corneal surface. One of many operative techniques devised for its eradication is the McReynolds transplant, which involves subconjunctival transplanting of the head of the pterygium. Beta radiation may be used as an adjunct to operative treatment.

Corneal Transplant (Keratoplasty) This is indicated when scars or opacities form on the cornea reducing or destroying vision by prevention of transmission of a clear image. It is the most successful transplantation procedure with considerably less rejection phenomenon than accompanies transplantation of other tissues, except bone.

Two types of grafts are used:

1 Full-thickness, the common type, in which the entire thickness of the cornea is replaced, usually 6.5 to 8 mm.

2 Partial-thickness or lamellar, less popular, in which only the top layer of the cornea, not its entire depth, is replaced.

Fresh, healthy tissue, cornea cut from the promptly enucleated eye of a relatively young donor within 4 hours of death, is considered the best for transplantation. It should be inserted in the recipient eye as soon as possible, but within 24 hours, to preserve viability and prevent opacity. Moist chamber storage is used. An opaque cornea is an optically nonfunctioning one. Corneas may be preserved for 3 days if kept in a special (McMurray-Kaufman) solution. Other methods, researched at corneal centers, will, it is hoped, offer preservation of tissue for longer periods.

Corneal tissue is sometimes cryopreserved for use at a later time. The frozen tissue may be stored for about 6 months. The cornea has five layers. Precise freezing and defrosting methods are of crucial importance in preventing injury to the endothelium, the very sensitive inner single layer of corneal cells. This layer must be kept intact for eventual transparency of the graft.

A protective agent, dimethyl sulfoxide (DMSO) replaces water in the corneal cells during cryopreservation. It prevents the formation of ruinous ice crystals. When this solution is thawed, drawn off, and replaced with 25% salt-poor albumin solution to remove the DMSO, the team must work very fast because of the extreme time limitation. The recipient eye must be trephined to receive the donor cornea and the cornea transplanted within 10 minutes of its thawing to reduce the possibility of endothelium damage. Corneal metabolism resumes with defrosting; thus the tissue must be placed immediately within its natural anatomical environment to enhance the option for successful grafting. Between thawing and placement in the recipient eye, the donor cornea is kept in an ice bath. Understandably, adequate preparation, teamwork, and a standardized procedure are imperative.

The greatest advance in modern technique to reduce the rate of rejection and restriction of activity during convalescence has been the use of the operating microscope and microsutures. Continuous 10-0 nylon sutures can be left *in situ* for an extended period, even up to 6 months, with minimal tissue reaction.

NOTE. Available corneal tissue is in limited supply, placing restraints on transplantation. Numerous *eye banks* in the United States comprise the Eye Bank Association of America. The latter is associated with the International Eye Bank. These groups are central clearinghouses for dispersion of accessible tissue. They follow a stringent code of ethics in their function to inform the public of the need for eye donations, procure donated eyes, assist in optimum use of donor corneas locally, or arrange for transportation to an area of greater need.

Iris Procedures

Excision of Prolapse This may follow eye laceration or an operation on the anterior segment. Fresh prolapses may be reduced mechanically at operation or pharmacologically with drugs. Older prolapses should be excised to avoid intraocular infection.

Procedures for Glaucoma Glaucoma is a disease characterized by an abnormally increased intraocular fluid pressure; it often involves the iris. If uncontrolled, glaucoma progresses to atrophy of the optic nerve, hardening of the eyeball, and blindness. The incidence of glaucoma in persons over 40 increases with each decade. There is a familial predisposition to the disease.

One method of estimating intraocular pressure is the use of the mechanical (Schiotz) tonometer. This device records the depth of indentation of the cornea by a plunger of known weight. The degree of indentation is calibrated on the tonometer to correspond to the intraocular pressure. This tonometer can be sterilized for use in the OR for preoperative pressure measurement.

Two basic types of glaucoma are classified anatomically by the size of the angle between the iris and the cornea: narrow-angle or angle-closure glaucoma, and wide-angle or open-angle glaucoma. These two forms may be referred to as *primary glaucoma.* If the angle is narrow, the iris may mechanically obstruct the outflow of aqueous. This will cause the pressure within the eye to rise and precipitate an attack of acute glaucoma, which is very painful. Operative intervention affords relief and is always necessary for this condition to open the angle and reduce pressure.

1 *Iridectomy* is the excision of a sector of iris to deflate the mechanical obstruction, thus increasing drainage by permitting normal outflow of aqueous from the posterior to the anterior chamber.

NOTE. Another use of iridectomy is to create a new pupillary opening to improve visual acuity in patients with corneal or lens opacity from causes other than glaucoma.

Wide-angle glaucoma is a chronic type, often of insidious onset, which may cause permanent vision loss before it is detected. The obstruction is not mechanical but physiological, a lack of ability to filter aqueous. Operations for this type of the disease are performed only if medical therapy is unsuccessful.

2 The operation usually involves a *filtering type of procedure* of which there are many variations, such as *trephining* and *trabeculectomy.* Common to all these procedures is the creation of an artificial fistula between the angle of the anterior chamber and the subconjunctival space. Iridectomy is usually performed as part of the procedure to eliminate blockage of the fistula by the underlying iris.

3 *Iridencleisis* employs a wick of iris in the fistula to help keep the fistula patent.

4 *Cyclodialysis, cyclodiathermy,* and *cyclocryothermy* are performed to diminish aqueous secretion by the ciliary body. Cyclodialysis involves severing the blood supply of the ciliary body. Cyclodiathermy and cyclocryothermy utilize the application of heat or cold respectively for the same purpose.

Secondary glaucoma is a complication of inflammation such as iritis, neoplasm, vascular obstruction, trauma, or hemorrhage. Treatment is directed to the primary etiology. Operative intervention is avoided whenever possible.

Congenital glaucoma is manifested soon after birth (refer to Chap. 26 for discussion).

Cataract Procedures Cataract is an opacification of the crystalline lens, its capsule, or both. The more or less opaque lens does not transmit clear images to the retina. Symptoms are related to the location and configuration of the opacity. Etiology may be a known factor such as metabolic disease, toxic material, radiation, trauma, or an unknown factor. With advancing age, persons are more prone to develop cataracts, so the incidence is increasing. Cataracts may be classified as:

1 Congenital
2 Senile or primary
3 Secondary, resulting from local or systemic disease, or eye injury

Modern therapy is much less disturbing and restrictive to the patient, but operative removal, followed by appropriate optical rehabilitation, is the only treatment. The operative procedure is determined by the patient's age and type of cataract. Time of operation is planned according to visual requirements, general health, and potential for rehabilitation. Microsurgery has revolutionized cataract extraction, one of the most frequently performed operations in the United States.

Intracapsular Extraction In this procedure, the entire lens within its capsule is delivered through a moderately-sized incision made in the region of the *limbus,* the junction of the cornea and the sclera. Prior to delivery, an iridectomy or multiple iridotomies are performed for several reasons. These are chiefly to prevent iris prolapse and to preserve communication between the anterior and posterior chambers. The lens is grasped by the method of surgeon's preference, i.e., mechanical forceps, suction devices, or cryoextractor. A miniaturized cryoprobe freezes onto the surface of the cataract, thus obtaining very secure adherence. This efficient method facilitates removal of fragile or dislocated cataracts (see Figs. 22-2 and 22-3). Also, the freezing technique greatly reduces inadvertent rupture of the capsule during extraction. The scrub nurse should have a balanced salt solution irrigator available for use in case it is necessary to unfreeze unintentional attachment of the cryoextractor to the iris or cornea. The wound is closed watertight with multiple sutures.

Conventional Extracapsular Extraction This involves a similar but much smaller incision than for intracapsular extraction. The anterior capsule is incised and largely removed. The remaining cortex and nucleus are extracted by irrigation and expression. The wound is closed with a few sutures. Occasionally the posterior capsule will remain opaque, in which case discission (needling) is performed at a later date to provide an optically clear opening.

Linear Extraction Linear extraction is performed in young adults. A small incision is made through the limbus. The anterior capsule is incised and the major portion of it excised with a *cystotome,* a miniature hook-shaped knife. The soft cataractous material is irrigated from the anterior chamber.

Phacoemulsification (Phacofragmentation) This is the newest method. Although aspiration technique is commonly used in young persons, it was not successful in adults with senile cataracts

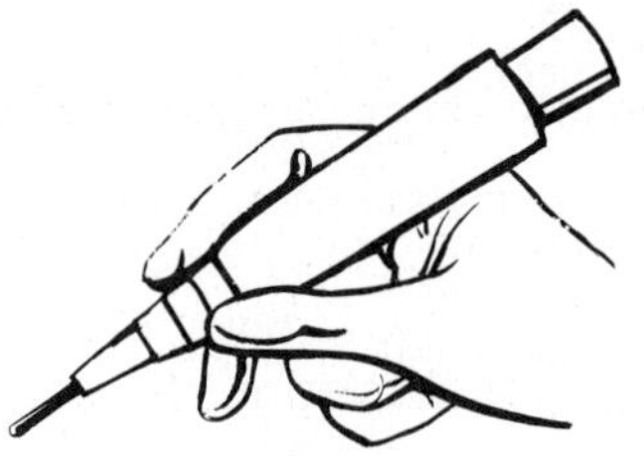

Figure 22-2 One type of sterile disposable cryoextractor used for cataract extraction. (*Cryophake, Alcon Laboratories, Inc., Dallas, Texas.*)

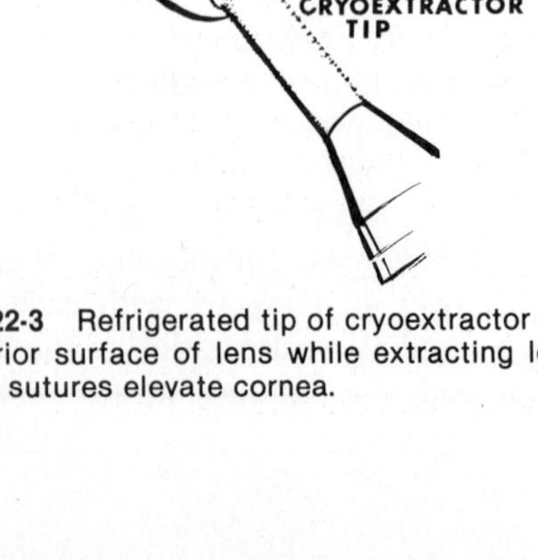

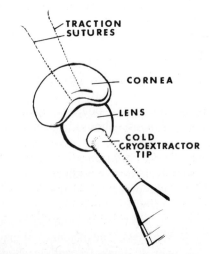

Figure 22-3 Refrigerated tip of cryoextractor adherent to anterior surface of lens while extracting lens. Two traction sutures elevate cornea.

until the late 1960s. At that time a sophisticated machine, the *phacoemulsifier,* was developed to break up and remove hard, insoluble nuclei. This machine, with components for ultrasonic vibration, irrigation, and aspiration, permits extracapsular extraction through a very small incision in the limbus. All functions are controlled by foot pedal.

The handpiece of the phacoemulsifier consists of a 1-mm hollow titanium alloy needle surrounded by a silicone sleeve. The needle is inserted into the anterior chamber following removal of the anterior capsule with a cystotome and prolapse of the lens nucleus into the chamber through a widely dilated pupil. The activated needle breaks up the lens with ultrasonic vibrations. While the lens is thus emulsified, a constant flow of irrigating solution through the sleeve prevents heat buildup and dissolves the soluble lens. The irrigation-aspiration flow is automatically regulated to maintain anterior chamber depth. The aspirator removes the fragments. The posterior capsule is left intact unless an opacity remains, in which case it may be incised during operation or at a future time. The limbal incision is closed with one stitch.

Phacoemulsification has certain *advantages:*

1 It dramatically shortens convalescence. The patient usually returns to full activity in 1 or 2 days.
2 It employs a small incision and minimal suture.
3 It retains the posterior capsule of the lens to preserve a more physiologically normal condition, and to protect the retina from postoperative edema and reduce risk of post-lens-extraction retinal detachment.
4 The posterior capsule supports an implanted intraocular lens.

The procedure also has *disadvantages:*

1 It is not suitable for many patients. Contraindications are corneal disease, dislocated lens, shallow anterior chamber, difficult-to-dilate pupils, completely hard, stonelike cataracts.
2 It requires special techniques which, if not thoroughly mastered, may precipitate operative complications such as temporary or permanent corneal damage (opacification), prolapse of lens into the vitreous, vitreous loss.
3 It may injure the cells because of the necessary substantial amount of anterior chamber irrigation. Corneal cells are very sensitive to manipulation and can respond by loss of function.
4 It requires meticulous technical monitoring of the machine. Usual precautions for use of electrical equipment also are observed.

Rehabilitation Following Cataract Extraction Rehabilitation consists of substitution for the missing part, the lens, so the optical system can function to focus incoming light on the retina. Patients with no optical substitute see only blurred objects of large size with no detail.

Spectacle correction of *aphakia,* absence of the lens, provides focusing of light. However, because the *spectacle lens* is approximately 2 cm in front of the original lens, it magnifies images so that they are approximately 35 percent larger than those the patient saw before the development and extraction of the cataract. This magnification requires considerable readjustment to judge distances. Also, peripheral areas are distorted. Spectacle type of replacement is intolerable in patients who have good vision in the unoperated eye because attempts to fuse the dissimilar images of the two eyes causes double vision.

A *contact lens* rests on the cornea only 2 to 3 mm from the original lens. Consequently it causes only 7 percent magnification and provides a full, undistorted field of vision. The better-tolerated contact lens is often used to replace the optical deficiency caused by cataract extraction, but it is difficult for many elderly persons to handle and care for because of lack of manual dexterity from infirmities or ocular defects in the unoperated eye. For such patients, an *implanted intraocular lens* offers a feasible substitute.

Implantation of Intraocular Lens

An intraocular lens is implanted in almost the identical position of the original lens and therefore does not change the size of the retinal image. Spacial displacement as seen by the aphakic eye, narrowing and distortion of the visual field are eliminated. An intraocular lens is intended to remain *in situ* permanently. The implant usually is inserted through the same incision used to remove the cataractous lens. This is called *primary insertion.* Some surgeons prefer to implant the lens at a later time; this is referred to as *secondary insertion.* Some lenses may be inserted in conjunction with intracapsular cataract extraction. Others require extracapsular extraction.

Prescription of the implanted lens (refractive power) involves complex preoperative calculations based on the patient's corneal curvature, anterior chamber depth, and eyeball axial length.

Ultrasonography is helpful in making these determinations.

The optical portion of the lens is made of an inert plastic, polymethyl methacrylate (PMA), well tolerated by tissues. The fixation portion is made of plastic, synthetic nonabsorbable suture, or less frequently, metal alloys. Some types are fixed in position with polypropylene suture.

Lenses differ in design and method of fixation. Some utilize fixation by suturing. Those not sutured in place require the use of miotic drugs to hold them in position until fixation to adjacent tissues is effected by healing.

Lenses can be classified according to the method of fixation.

Angle Fixation The lens of longest survival is the Choyce lens, which was developed in England. It consists of a band of plastic of length sufficient to traverse the anterior chamber from one angle to the other. The optical portion is centrally located in the anterior chamber, in front of the pupil. The pupil remains mobile because iris adhesions are not required for fixation. Although this lens is commonly inserted primarily, it is the most popular one for secondary insertion.

Iris Fixation Other anterior chamber lenses employ fixation to the iris, anteriorly and posteriorly. Examples are:

1 Worst medallion, developed in 1970. The lens has two posterior loops and a round anterior haptic. A *haptic,* used for fixation, is an extension or appendage of the optical part. The round haptic is sutured to the iris with a single stitch. Primary insertion is used.
2 Binkhorst four-loop. This lens has four vertical loops, two anterior and two posterior, which enclose the iris between them. Further fixation is acquired by suturing the two superior loops together through the iridectomy. This lessens the possibility of lens dislocation.
3 Some lenses include a metal post that may be used instead of suturing for fixation (safety-pin action).

Iris Plane The optic is placed in the pupil in the same plane as the iris. The lens is held in position by the optic and four haptics, in the shape of a Maltese cross. The two posterior ones are inserted behind the iris. The two anterior ones are placed in front of the iris. An example is the all-plastic Copeland lens, noted for its simplicity. The pupil appears square after insertion (primary) because the iris molds to the square base of the implant.

Capsular Fixation This type attaches to the capsule of the crystalline lens. Therefore, it can be inserted only following extracapsular extraction. The lower loop is inserted into a pocket of capsule created before extraction of the cataract. An example is the Binkhorst two-loop lens, held in place by the miotic-constricted pupil until the anterior and posterior capsule portions of the pocket adhere to each other. Additional fixation may be gained by suturing.

Indications for Implantation

1 Elderly patients with disabling bilateral cataracts and others who cannot manage a contact lens
2 Patients with occupations having specific visual requirements (airplane pilots), or difficult working environment (ranchers in a dusty area)
3 Children with traumatic cataract, to prevent amblyopia

Sufficient time has not elapsed for long-term evaluation but apparent *contraindications* are:

1 Impossible patient followup. An experienced implant surgeon should observe the patient for late complications.
2 Ocular conditions such as poorly controlled glaucoma or previous retinal detachment.
3 Diabetes.
4 Poor result in previous implant.
5 Patient anxiety in regard to the procedure.
6 Young patients; congenital cataracts.

Advantages are:

1 Superior spatial orientation
2 Permanent device unless complication develops
3 Additional option for postcataract refractive correction

Complications are:

1 Corneal damage or latent edema
2 Dislocation or malposition of the lens, which can damage the cornea
3 Prolonged inflammation such as iritis or vitreitis
4 Cystoid macular edema
5 Secondary cataract, opacification of the anterior vitreous, from recurrent iritis

Retinal Procedures

Repair of Detached Retina This is indicated when the retina becomes separated from its surrounding nourishing layer, the *choroid.* Serious visual disturbance results. The condition may be due to displacement of the retina by blood, fluid, or tumor. In the last instance, enucleation of the eye is usually indicated. In some cases of accidental or operative trauma or in degenerative diseases, tears or holes may form in the retina. Such defects in continuity can permit seepage of vitreous fluid into the potential space between the retina and the choroid, causing the retina to become detached. Reattachment is effected only by operative intervention, in which the retinal defect is sealed off and, often, the subretinal fluid drained. The type of operation is determined by the type and location of the detachment.

1 The traditional procedure involves the application of *diathermy coagulation* to an area of the sclera overlying the region of the retinal defect. The resultant localized inflammation acts to seal off the break. Coagulation is delivered by a specialized short-wave diathermy unit.

2 Some surgeons prefer *cryosurgery* to diathermy because of the type of adhesion obtained. The therapeutic applications of cryosurgery are basically similar to those of diathermy. Tissue reactions that superficially resemble each other are obtained by both methods.

3 To achieve reattachment of the retina, internal elevation of the sclera may be increased by the *scleral-buckling procedure.* This technique involves the implantation of a wedge of silicone epi- or intrasclerally. On some occasions, an encircling band of silicone is used to keep constant external pressure on the buckle.

4 *Injection into the vitreous cavity* of air or slowly absorbable inert gas is sometimes used to further approximate the retina to the choroid.

Photocoagulation This is used if a retinal hole not surrounded by any detachment is found. The hole may be prophylactically sealed by photocoagulation or by laser burns.

These therapeutic modalities, usually performed in an ophthalmic treatment area rather than the OR, were the outgrowth of a traumatic phenomenon. The idea of using intense heat for a beneficial burning effect to create a scar evolved from observation of numerous retinal burns caused by watching the eclipse of the sun. The origin of the photocoagulator concept was investigated by a physician using a mirror and series of lenses on a hospital roof to reflect the sun's rays.

The photocoagulator utilizes an intense source of multiwavelength light furnished by a xenon tube. This is optically focused and concentrated into a delivering device that is basically a direct ophthalmoscope. The latter also can be used to view the area to be treated as well as to aim the light beam. The light may be directed to any of the various pigmented (light-absorbing) layers of the eye such as the iris or retina. These darker layers of the eye readily absorb the xenon tube's white light. The optical system of the eye is used in the process of focusing the light beam on the desired area.

The xenon arc photocoagulator is a reliable, simple machine without motors or moving parts. No part requires sterilization. The amount of power and exposure time are completely controlled by the operating ophthalmologist. Triggering the xenon flash automatically inserts a protective filter in front of the operator's eye, although the view remains unobstructed. The operator uses the coagulator primarily in multiple sessions of a gauged amount of treatment each time. Vitreous shrinkage possibly leading to an inoperable detachment can be a complication of its use. The pupil of the eye under therapy must be dilated to give maximum visibility to the surgeon. The eye must be immobilized by local anesthesia to prevent undesired movement in order to eliminate the possibility of burning an area other than the one selected for treatment, and to prevent pain caused by the intensity of the heat.

Optical Laser Similar to the photocoagulator in principle and use, this is often preferred because of its advantages. In contrast to the monocular viewing of the photocoagulator, the laser delivery system employs the binocular microscope of the slit lamp, thus giving stereopsis and greater magnification. The nature of the laser beam permits extremely rapid delivery of radiant energy that produces a more sharply defined burn. The smaller lesion it produces can be placed close to the macula. Because of this short exposure time, immobilization of the eye is unnecessary unless the area for treatment is close to the macula, to avoid accidental macular burn. However, pupillary dilation is essential.

The argon laser is effective in treating conditions other than retinal holes or tears. One of its major uses is in treatment of diabetic retinopathy. Diabetes causes many bodily changes, which increase in frequency with duration of the disease. For example, a person who has been a diabetic for over 15 years has very significant likelihood of having some form of retinopathy such as the formation of abnormal blood vessels. These fragile vessels may rupture spontaneously, producing hemorrhage into the retina and/or vitreous humor, with loss of vision. The eventual result may be partial or complete blindness. Pan-retinal photocoagulation (PRP) is one method of eliminating abnormal vascularization. PRP consists of the application of hundreds of laser burns to the peripheral retinal tissue to partially destroy it. The beneficial effect is apparently produced by reducing retinal metabolic need for oxygen.

The laser is also used for other retinopathies such as central serous retinopathy (swelling of the macula), angiomas and hemangiomas, small tumors, bleeding (to seal the vessel), and aneurysms. The red blood cells take up the energy, causing the two sides of the vessels to adhere together, thereby closing the aneurysm.

Vitrectomy This is the deliberate removal of a portion of *vitreous humor,* also called *vitreous body,* that fills the area between the lens and the retina. It is performed for vitreal opacities, vitreal hemorrhage, and certain types of retinal detachment.

Whereas aqueous fluid is clear, the vitreous is normally a transparent, gelatinous, viscid material containing fibrils. The vitreous helps give shape to the eyeball, in addition to serving a refractive function.

Alterations in the vitreous can have serious consequences. Loss of vitreous during operative procedures has always been a dreaded complication, particularly of cataract extraction, because temporary deflation of the globe can lead to collapse. Subsequent to retinal hemorrhage, not uncommon in diabetic patients, bands of scar tissue may opacify the vitreous as well as insert into the retina near the original bleeding vessel. Traction on the retina by these bands or further cicatrization, scarring, can lead to retinal tears or detachment. Persistent hemorrhage, lasting over 1 year, is permanent. It will not absorb spontaneously.

For years the vitreous was considered an inaccessible inoperable area. Research and the advent of microsurgery changed this belief. Loss of vitreous from the posterior segment during operation is rendered relatively innocuous if the anterior segment is cleared of vitreous. Thus, no residual strands are present to block visual function. Also, the eye tolerates subtotal vitreal excision in the posterior segment if the vitreous body is proportionately replaced with balanced salt solution (BSS).

Vitrectomy is performed with the *vitrector* (ocutome or vitreous infusion suction cutter, VISC). This device, incorporating a micromotor, terminates in a needlelike tube that contains a cutting mechanism. In addition, it has auxilliary connections for aspiration of vitreous and replacement with BSS. A fiberoptic light source may be attached to the head of the instrument. Two approaches to the vitreous body are:

1 Through the posterior segment, via the pars plana, the anterior attachment of the retina. Since the pars plana has no visual function, entry there is relatively nontraumatic, with least chance for retinal detachment. The anterior segment remains intact; intraocular pressure is maintained. Used to incise opacified vitreous, old hemorrhage, or bands of scar tissue, thereby giving a clear view of the retina and restoring visual function.

2 Through the anterior segment, via incision at the limbus. A large corneal section is folded back and the vitreous exposed through the pupillary opening. Used for removal of vitreous inadvertently displaced into the anterior chamber during cataract removal, to avoid postoperative complications. The vitreous volume is replaced with BSS.

TRAUMA TO THE EYE

Various forms and degrees of trauma may occur as a result of injury. *All types of injury require immediate appraisal by an ophthalmologist.* Delay of even minor ones may result in temporary or permanent loss of vision. Complications include hemorrhage, infection, iritis or tears of the iris, retinal tears or detachment, macular edema, secondary cataract. Treatment may be immediate, or secondary, if delay is necessary because of life-threatening injuries. Improved operative management, such as vitrectomy, and microsurgery have reduced the loss of severely injured eyes. Optical result is especially crucial in patients with bilateral eye injuries. Patients with eye injuries should be kept supine if possible until seen by the ophthalmologist.

Evaluation of the injury may necessitate sedating or anesthetizing the patient to prevent further damage at examination. Pressure to the eye must be avoided as bone fragments may be displaced, or globe contents emptied.

Injuries may be simple, involving only the external layers, or compound, including inner structures. They may be nonpenetrating, usually caused by a blunt object, or penetrating, more commonly caused by a sharp object. The more structures involved, the more difficult it is to salvage the eye.

Treatment, determined by type or combination of injuries, aims to:

1 Promote healing and prevent anatomical distortion by reparative techniques
2 Preserve maximum vision and/or restore it
3 Control pain, by medication
4 Prevent infection and inflammation, by antibiotic and steroid administration

Nonpenetrating Injuries

Lacerations of the Eyelid These are repaired according to anatomical principles.

Burns These may be caused by ultraviolet radiation such as sunlamps or sunlight, or electrical flash. These burns are basically self-limited but rarely operative. *A chemical burn constitutes an emergency.* Initial treatment consists of flooding the cornea with water. Alkali burns may be further neutralized with a specific substance. Severe burns may be treated with specific amino acids but often progress to corneal opacity and blindness.

Contusions of the Globe These may or may not be operative. If there is hemorrhage, treatment consists of bed rest and antiglaucoma therapy to keep intraocular pressure controlled. It is not unusual for a secondary hemorrhage to occur on the third or fourth day after injury. If the intraocular pressure remains high, blood staining of the cornea and damage to the optic nerve may result. It is then sometimes necessary to perform a *paracentesis,* an incision into the anterior chamber to drain the blood. If an organized clot is found, judicious irrigation may supplement incision.

Penetrating Injuries

Lacerations of the globe may occur with or without retained foreign body and with or without prolapse of ocular contents. In injuries to the globe, an ophthalmic surgeon should repair tissues adjacent to the eye, in addition to the eye wound.

With this type of injury there is the possibility of an eventual *sympathetic ophthalmia,* inflammation of the uninjured eye. Antitetanus therapy should be included in treatment of penetrating injuries.

Without Foreign Body

Conjunctival Laceration This is usually debrided and, unless large, permitted to heal without suturing. If it is large, with loss of conjunctival tissue, sutures or rotating flaps of conjunctiva may be necessary for repair.

Corneal and Scleral Lacerations These are of great concern. Small ones may be covered with a bandage therapeutic soft lens over the eye to seal it and hold the edges together. A larger wound requires accurate appositional sutures best placed under the operating microscope. The microscope is especially useful for irregular complicated or multiple tears. Adequate exploration, particularly of a scleral wound, is necessary to determine extent of injury as well as ensure uncovering of the entire wound for repair. In instances of vitreous fluid presentation or loss, it is preferable to remove the fluid from the wound and the anterior chamber with the vitreotome before proceeding with repair. This is done to avoid undesirable vitreous adhesions postoperatively.

Prolapse of the Iris Prolapse of the iris or other uveal tissue is usually excised, except in very early clean wounds where repositioning it may be attempted.

Posterior Rupture of the Globe This usually involves herniation of retinal and uveal tissue into the orbit. Although such injuries are self-healing, the eye is irreparably damaged. *Avulsion* (tearing) of the optic nerve produces permanent blindness although the rest of the globe may be intact. This injury usually results in enucleation.

With Foreign Body

Extraocular These injuries are usually not extensive. A corneal foreign body is removed with a sharp probe (spud) and the surrounding rust ring taken off with a rotating burr.

Intraocular The type, size, and position of a foreign body should be determined accurately before removal. Localization is accomplished by:

1 Direct vision with the ophthalmoscope
2 X-ray, using a contact lens containing radiopaque landmarks
3 Berman locator, a small but extremely sensitive version of the mine detector, which may indicate the exact location of a metallic foreign body

Fragments of ferrous metals often can be retrieved by utilizing the attraction of a strong electromagnet. In some cases these foreign bodies can be withdrawn along the path of entry.

Nonmagnetic foreign objects present a more serious problem. Frequently they may be secured only by passing a delicate forceps into the globe. Such instrumentation cannot avoid being traumatic to ocular structure. Therefore, end results often are unsatisfactory in comparison to those obtained with the electromagnet.

In summary, traumatic injuries may introduce infection or produce severe inflammatory reaction in greater degree than elective operative procedures. Proper early treatment is indicated to save vision. Early reintervention, before scar formation, may be necessary in some patients.

GENERAL CONSIDERATIONS

The ophthalmic patient faces impaired or loss of vision if the outcome of operative intervention is unfavorable. Special features of ophthalmic surgery aim to prevent such a loss. Operation on the eye is extremely delicate, requiring precision instrumentation, a steady hand, and quiet surroundings.

1 The patient is positioned on the operating table so the head and body are aligned. The top of the head is in line with the edge of the table for accessibility. The head is stabilized. For intraocular procedures, the patient's gown is untied at the neck to prevent pressure. Also, the head must not be turned greatly in either direction. Any obstruction to venous circulation can cause undue pressure in the eye, which can produce loss of vitreous humor when the eye is opened.
2 Refer to Chapter 11 for preparation and draping.
3 Many ophthalmic surgeons use the operating microscope for all operative intervention, especially procedures in the anterior segment.
4 An absolutely quiet eye is mandatory, especially at high magnifications with the microscope. Even when general anesthesia is used, most surgeons administer a retrobulbar block for immobility and lowering of intraocular pressure.
5 Except in children and selected patients, local anesthesia is used. The patient is prepared as ordered. Local anesthesia consists of:
   a Retrobulbar block. The needle is inserted behind the eyeball into the muscular cone, the common origin of the extraocular muscles, to obtain anesthesia of the globe and paralysis of the muscles.
   b Anesthetic drops are instilled topically.
   c Most operations are referred to as *attended local,* i.e., an anesthesiologist is present to monitor the patient, administer oxygen, or supplement the local anesthetic if necessary. Tolerance to procedures is increased because of minimal anesthesia.
6 Frequently, mydriatic or miotic drops are administered to dilate or constrict the pupil. The circulating nurse instills such medications, as well as the anesthetic drops, as ordered, prior to the prep. Common abbreviations are O.D., right eye; O.S., left eye; O.U. both eyes. *To instill eye drops:*
   a Identify the correct medication, eye, and patient.
   b Explain the procedure.
   c Tilt the patient's head back. Tell him or her to look up. While gently pulling down on the lower lid, instill the medication on the inner aspect of the lower lid, in the middle third. Release the lid while the patient slowly closes the eye to retain the drop. Let the patient close the eye between repeated drops. Gently blot excess fluid to prevent drainage into the tear duct, nose, and stomach. Some medications such as atropine may have a systemic effect. In small infants or young children, systemic absorption is avoided by applying finger pressure over the lacrimal sac region (inner canthus) of both eyes simultaneously for 1 minute. In a struggling child, have the patient tilt the head back and close both eyes. Instill the medication at the inner canthus. The drop will roll into the eye as the patient reopens it.
   d Only the specified number of drops, no more, no less, must be given.
   e Read the label on the vial *each* time before instillation.
   f Each patient should receive a fresh, single-use, disposable vial that is discarded after use.
   g Usually one drop of anesthetic is administered to the unoperative eye in case of inadvertent splash during the prep.
7 Medications that may induce vomiting are avoided. Any straining may cause intraocular hemorrhage or expulsion of ocular contents through the wound.
8 Sponges are of precut, compressed cellulose on sticks.
9 A wide variety of fine-sized absorbable and nonabsorbable sutures is used. The scrub nurse follows the manufacturer's recommendations for handling these delicate materials and needles with appropriate needleholders. Special techniques are used in microsurgery (see Figs. 22-4 and 22-5).
10 The surgeon should verify the operative eye with the patient as well as with the office records. To avoid error, after confirmation some surgeons also place an indelible mark on the side of the patient's neck that corresponds to the operative eye.
11 Many of these patients are of age extremes. Reassurance is given as needed. A patient with a drape over the face is often apprehensive and fearful of suffocation. Oxygen or air is deliv-

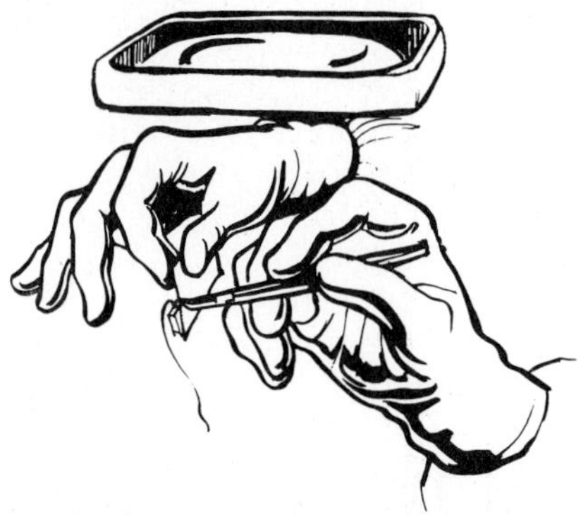

Figure 22-4 Surgeon arming needle on needleholder from primary suture wrap held by scrub nurse under broadfield lens.

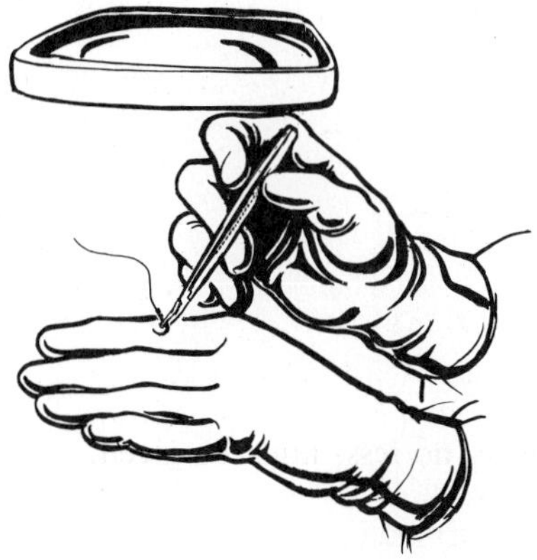

Figure 22-5 Surgeon arming needle on needleholder with suture extended over scrub nurse's hand.

ered to the nostrils beneath the drape for comfort.

12 Emphasis is placed on the need for extreme constant care with *ophthalmic solutions.* Nearly all are colorless and may be in similar receptacles. *Solutions must be immediately and individually labeled* by the scrub nurse. *Identity must not be confused,* as an error could result in total, irrevocable blindness for the patient. If identification is missing, discard the solution. *Solutions for intraocular use must be separated from all others* and ideally should be filtered with micropore filters. Medicine glasses may be properly inscribed or a sterile, metal labeling clip may be attached to the glass as soon as the solution is poured. This clip should hang outside the glass because contact with the solution in some cases inactivates the solution. An example is alpha chymotrypsin. *Sterile solutions commonly used:*

a On the Mayo stand, in medicine glasses in a rack:

(1) Local anesthetic. Hyaluronidase is sometimes added to expedite spread of the anesthetic through the tissue and create more profound anesthesia.

(2) Epinephrine hydrochloride 1:5000 (1 to 2 ml) with an eye dropper, for hemostasis. After a drop is added to the local anesthetic, this glass is removed to the instrument table so the medication is *never* inadvertently injected.

(3) Alpha chymotrypsin (an enzyme solution) to soften the zonules holding the lens, prior to cataract extraction.

(4) Small sterile bottles of balanced salt solution to which a convenient cannula may be attached are commercially available for anterior chamber irrigation and for keeping the cornea moist.

b On the instrument table, in a basin, saline or distilled water for rinsing instruments during operation.

13 No foreign material should be introduced into the operative wound. In intraocular procedures, no portion of any instrument or item intended to enter the eye should be touched by a gloved hand. Sterile plastic drapes are often placed over cloth drapes to prevent lint, especially in lens implantation. Intraocular lenses are soaked and rinsed in BSS before insertion to remove *any* debris or impurity.

14 Inflammation must be kept as minimal as possible since even a slight infection may result in total functional loss. Steroids are often administered locally, subconjunctivally, and sometimes systemically. Antibiotic drops are often instilled topically for 24 hours pre- and postoperatively. The eye may respond violently to the slightest amount of trauma.

15 At the conclusion of operation, a sterile eye pad is applied to the eye. A protective shield is secured over it to guard against mechanical injury.

16 Outcome of ophthalmic procedures includes a cosmetic as well as a functional aspect.

17 Arm restraints are essential for infants and young children (see Chap. 26). Restraints are applied to adults only under extreme circumstances such as disorientation. Use of side rails usually is standard procedure for patients over 65.

18 Ideally, the ophthalmic patient should be physically separated, from admission to discharge, from patients of other services. Not only does segregation minimize cross infection, but also provides for the specialized care required on the unit and in the OR. Ophthalmic surgery has progressed to a highly refined state.

19 The tendency is toward earlier ambulation and shorter hospitalization. A most important aspect of postoperative care is to inform the patient not to get out of bed alone. A fall or jar to the eye can obviate an otherwise successful operation.

Chapter 23

Otorhinolaryngology

Otorhinolaryngology is the surgical specialty that concerns the study and treatment of diseases of the ear (*oto*), nose (*rhino*), and throat (*laryngo*). Specialists commonly called *ENT surgeons* practice within the total field. Some choose to subspecialize as, for example, otologists, who confine their practice to the ear.

HISTORICAL INTRODUCTION

Recognition of abnormal conditions of the ear, nose, and throat began in early times. Some of the first permanent records mentioning them, attributed to the Egyptians, date from 3500 B.C. Breathing was thought to occur through the ears via the eustachian tubes. Therefore, attempts were made to remedy deafness and ear discharges. Study of anatomy antedated the Christian era, leading to the practice of primitive procedures in India. For example, nasal fractures were splinted by insertion of a tube into the nostril.

Hippocrates realized that irregular teeth could cause various mouth and ear disorders. He also recognized otitis media as well as the fact that congenital deafness was incurable. Immediate reduction of nasal fractures was advocated by this reknowned Greek physician.

The early centuries of the Christian era brought attempts to devise mastoid operations. Tracheotomy, thought to have been known 2000 years ago, was described in detail by Antyllas, a surgeon of the second century A.D. In the seventh century, physicians advocated its use to prevent suffocation in persons with laryngeal obstruction. Tracheotomy was performed frequently in 1610 during a diphtheria epidemic in Europe. The lifesaving value of this procedure was further proved in later centuries when used for patients with severe croup or tuberculosis. The seventeenth century also saw removal of the tongue for tumor.

Animal dissection led to a clearer knowledge of anatomy and physiology. Leonardo da Vinci described the nasal sinuses well in the fifteenth century.

In 1855, tuning-fork tests, used in evaluating actual and residual hearing, were described by Rinné. European surgeons in the latter part of the nineteenth century attempted to restore hearing by operative incision of the eardrum and removal of the tympanic membrane and stapes. Eventually, operations such as fenestration and stapes mobilization were developed. Stapedectomy, devised in the 1960s, has largely replaced those procedures.

Research resulting in refined equipment, techniques, and prostheses has brought the specialization of the present. One of the greatest advances in treatment was the development of antibiotics, which often eliminates the need for operation.

Continued research in nerve deafness and in transplantation may well produce a cure for many persons now consigned to a world of silence.

THE EAR

Anatomy and Physiology

The structures of the ear (see Fig. 23-1) are concerned with two functions:

1 Hearing, i.e., receiving sound, amplifying it, and transmitting it to the brain for interpretation
2 Maintaining bodily equilibrium

Anatomically, the ear is divided into three parts: the external, middle, and inner ear.

External Ear The outer ear consists of the *auricle* or *pinna* composed of cartilage and skin except for the lobe, and the *external auditory canal.* The meatus of the auricle leads via the ear canal to the *tympanic membrane* or *eardrum.* This membrane separates the external and middle ear. Color change of the translucent eardrum, visible through a speculum, may be indicative of middle ear disease. The outermost lining of the tympanic membrane is derived from skin of the ear canal while the inner lining is continuous with middle ear mucosa. The eardrum protects the middle ear but may be perforated by injury or pressure built up in the middle ear by infection.

Middle Ear The middle ear consists of the *tympanic cavity,* a closed chamber that lies between the tympanic membrane and the inner ear. Within this cavity are the three smallest bones in the body, an *ossicular chain* comprised of the malleus, incus, and stapes, so named because of their resemblance to a hammer, anvil, and stirrups respectively. The malleus, attached to the eardrum, joins the incus, the extremity of which articulates with the stapes, the innermost bone. The footplate of the stapes fits in the *oval* or *vestibular window,* an opening in the wall of the inner ear. The bones of the ossicular chain must be able to move mechanically in order to conduct sound from the eardrum to the inner ear. The *round* or *cochlear window,* also between the middle and the inner ear, equalizes pressure that enters through the oval window.

The middle ear opens into the nasopharynx by way of the eustachian tube. Normally closed during swallowing or yawning, the eustachian tube aerates the middle ear cavity. This mechanism is essential for adequate hearing.

Posteriorly the middle ear exits to the *mastoid process,* the inferior projection of the temporal bone that is a honeycomb of air cells lined with mucous membrane. Since the antrum of the mastoid process connects with the middle ear, infection in the latter may produce mastoiditis. The middle ear is situated in the tympanic portion of the temporal bone, the inner ear in the petrous portion, which integrates with the base of the skull. The tympanic portion also forms part of the ear canal.

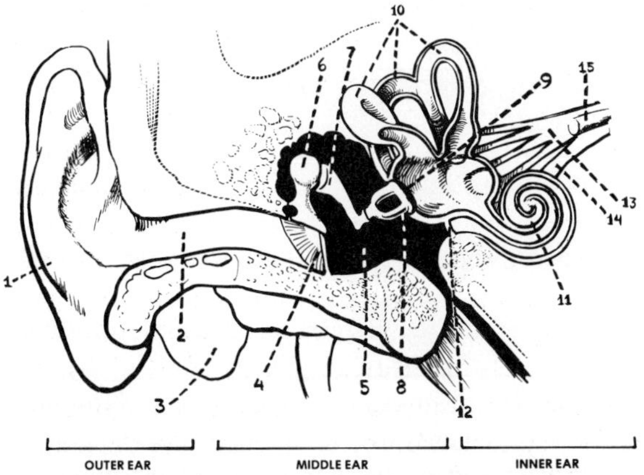

Figure 23-1 Anatomy of the ear. (1) pinna, (2) auditory canal, (3) mastoid process of temporal bone, (4) tympanic membrane, (5) tympanic cavity, (6) malleus, (7) incus, (8) stapes, (9) oval (vestibular) window, (10) semicircular canals, (11) cochlea, (12) round (cochlear) window, (13) vestibular nerve, (14) cochlear nerve, (15) facial nerve.

Inner Ear The end organs of hearing and equilibrium are situated in the inner ear. The two main sections, cochlear and vestibular, have precise functions, although coordinated. The *cochlea,* a bony spiral, relates to hearing. The *vestibular labyrinth,* composed of three semicircular canals, relates to equilibrium. These structures house two separate fluids, *endolymph* and *perilymph,* which nourish and protect the hearing receptors. Neuroepithelium of the *organ of Corti,* the end organ of hearing, holds thousands of minute hair cells, which respond to sound waves that enter the cochlea via the oval window. Neuroepithelium of the vestibular portion also contains hair cells. Rapid head motion produces current in the endolymph that may result in nausea or vertigo. The *vestibular nerve,* a portion of the acoustic nerve, governs reflexes to muscles to maintain equilibrium.

Proximal Structures The middle and the inner ear are adjacent to many important tissues. The seventh cranial or facial nerve is enclosed in a bony canal running through the tympanic cavity and mastoid bone. The meninges of the temporal lobe of the brain are also near the middle ear and the mastoid. Facial paralysis, meningitis, and intracranial infection such as brain abscess are therefore potential complications of ear infection.

Significant blood vessels in the area are the internal carotid artery, internal jugular vein, as well as the lateral sinus. Thrombosis and infection of the lateral sinus of the dura mater is a potentially lethal complication of otitis media, with or without mastoiditis.

Auditory Process Sound or pressure waves enter the auricle. They pass along the ear canal to the tympanic membrane where the vibration of the waves is transmitted across the middle ear sequentially by the ossicles. At the footplate of the stapes, sound pressure is transferred to the inner ear via the oval window. The hair cells of the organ of Corti are set in motion by disturbance of the inner ear fluids as sound pressure moves from the oval to the round window. Mechanical energy is converted to electrical potential, which is delivered to the brain along auditory nerves that enter the inner ear. The brain interprets the sound as hearing.

Amplification of sound is effected to some extent by the mechanical action of the ossicles but mainly by areal ratio, i.e., a large volume of sound-wave pressure from the tympanic membrane is funneled to a small reactive area, the stapedial footplate, thereby resulting in intensification.

Loss of Hearing There are numerous types and causes of deafness. Hearing loss in varying degrees may result from:

1 Disease, such as otosclerosis, in which changes in the bony capsule of the labyrinth occur. Otosclerotic bone invades the footplate of the stapes resulting in its fixation and ultimate inability to vibrate in the oval window. Hearing loss is gradual but progressive. This type of hearing deficiency can be corrected by operation when there is no destruction of auditory nerve endings.

2 Trauma, such as perforated eardrum, requiring repair to restore its function and proper areal ratio.

3 Infection, usually controlled by antibiotics. While more common in children, infection also may occur in adults. It may cause accumulation of fluid in the middle ear. Mastoiditis results from extension of otitis media.

- **a** Serous otitis media may result from obstruction of the pharyngeal orifice of the eustachian tube. If blocked, for example, by hypertrophied adenoid tissue, infection, or allergic swelling, the tube is unable to equalize pressure because air cannot enter the middle ear from the pharynx. The vacuum or negative pressure thus created causes serum to be drawn into the tympanic cavity from blood vessels in the middle ear mucosa. Recurrent otitis media may require drainage of purulent exudate if conservative treatment fails.
- **b** Acute otitis media may require drainage of purulent exudate if conservative treatment fails.
- **c** Chronic otitis media with or without mastoiditis may follow recurrent otitis media with tympanic membrane perforation. It can produce a chronically draining ear.

Auditory acuity is measured by various tests. Measurements that compare bone conduction and air conduction are important in differential diagnosis. The audiogram is one such measurement tool. *Bone conduction* refers to hearing as transmitted through the skull; *air conduction* refers to transmission of sound waves from the tympanic membrane to the inner ear via air. Hearing loss caused by a defect in the external or the middle ear, referred to as *conductive loss,* is a mechanical obstruction of air conduction that usually can be helped by operative intervention. When the decrement is in the inner ear, referred to as *perceptive* or *sensorineural loss,* damage to nerve tissue and/or sensory paths to the brain is not benefited by operation.

OTOLOGIC OPERATIVE PROCEDURES

New concepts, techniques, instrumentation, and the operating microscope have greatly enhanced the ability of otologists to remedy hearing loss. Moreover, the advent of antibiotics has greatly alleviated the necessity for operative intervention which was prevalent in previous decades. Emphasis was formerly on the relief of infection and the conversion of a draining ear to a dry one. Now that infection is generally controlled pharmacologically, attention has turned to operative measures for improvement of hearing following damage from chronic infection, and to restoration of hearing by reconstruction of the ear. These procedures comprise the majority of otologic operations.

External Ear

Removal of a Foreign Body Removing a foreign body from the outer canal is performed most frequently in children. The object is washed out or removed to prevent purulent infection. A plant seed or vegetable foreign body such as a pea is not irrigated as it may swell in the ear and increase the difficulty of removal. General anesthesia sometimes may be required. Trauma must be minimal during removal to prevent stenosis of the canal or perforation of the object through the eardrum.

Drainage of Hematoma Usually the result of injury, a hematoma is drained to avoid infection with subsequent chondritis and deformity of the auricle.

Excision of Tumor This may involve a benign or a malignant lesion. Extent of operation depends on the size and type of tumor. Basal-cell lesions do not metastasize but squamous-cell lesions often do. A malignant lesion usually is excised in a wedge shape, and the incision closed. If the lesion is extensive, the auricle may be completely excised. Radical temporal bone resection is indicated if the bone (canal) is involved.

Otoplasty This is a cosmetic procedure commonly performed to correct congenital deformity such as a protruding external ear.

Middle Ear

Myringotomy This is incision of the eardrum for drainage in acute otitis media associated with pain. By aspiration of fluid and pus, pressure is released, pain relieved, and hearing restored and preserved. Myringotomy is done to prevent perforation of the eardrum and possible erosion of middle ear ossicles. When the exudate is especially viscid, the patient is said to have "glue ear" or mucoid otitis media.

Myringotomy most commonly is performed in association with the insertion of a plastic tube in the incision to facilitate continued aeration of the middle ear space and prevent the reformation of serous otitis media. Premature extrusion of the tube before normal eustachian tube function resumes may necessitate repeated operation.

Tympanoplasty A general term, this refers to any procedure performed to repair defects in the eardrum and/or middle ear structures for the purpose of reconstructing sound conduction paths. The degree of hearing improvement following tympanoplasty is related to the degree of damage.

Preferably the ear is dry and uninfected at the time of operation. If not, infected tissue must be removed to protect the inserted graft. Various autogenous materials such as fascia, fat, or vein graft are utilized to repair perforations in the eardrum. Vein graft is taken from the patient's hand. Fascia, more commonly used as a patch over a perforation, is obtained from the temporalis muscle.

In an effort to conserve the middle ear hearing mechanism, homograft transplantation of ossicles may be used for rebuilding the chain. Or, the tympanic membrane or a graft replacing it may be brought in contact with the stapes directly, permitting transmission of sound.

Mastoidectomy This is eradication of the mastoid air cells.

1 In *simple mastoidectomy* the mastoid region behind the ear is opened and the air cells removed without involving the middle ear or external canal.

2 *Modified radical mastoidectomy* consists of simple mastoidectomy and removal of the posterior wall of the ear canal to provide drainage from the mastoid to the canal. It preserves the tympanic membrane and middle ear ossicles. It may be done in association with tympanoplasty.

3 *Radical mastoidectomy* is performed rarely in patients with chronic mastoiditis. In addition to simple mastoidectomy, the middle ear cavity and mastoid antrum are combined into a single cavity for easy inspection and cleaning. The ossicles and tympanic membrane are partially removed.

Tympanoplasty with Mastoidectomy This allows drainage and cleaning of the mastoid area prior to reconstruction of the eardrum or middle ear ossicles. Following incision behind the auricle, the tympanic membrane and tympanic cavity are inspected. The mastoid antrum is entered by drilling through mastoid bone.

Sometimes in chronic otitis media, the mucous membrane of the tympanic cavity is replaced by epithelium from the ear canal as it grows through a perforation in the eardrum. Desquamated skin cells then cannot escape and form a ball or cyst known as a *cholesteatoma.* If present in the middle ear or mastoid, a cholesteatoma is removed during mastoidectomy and/or tympanoplasty.

Stapedectomy with Insertion of a Prosthesis This gives excellent results in restoring the conductive hearing loss of otosclerosis. The surgeon aims to restore vibration from the incus to the mobile oval window membrane to transmit sound. A partial stapedectomy involves removal of only the fixed footplate. The remaining superstructure is used to reconstruct the sound-conducting mechanism (see Fig. 23-2). More commonly, however, the entire stapes, including the footplate, is removed and replaced by a prosthesis, thus rebuilding the ossicular chain.

Incision is made deep in the canal near but not in the eardrum. The eardrum is folded over, giving access to the middle ear. The stapes is disconnected from the incus, fractured by fine microinstruments, and removed. The oval window is sealed by a graft of vein, perichondrium, fascia, fat, or Gelfoam over the oval window. A prosthesis is inserted and connected to the incus and to the graft, thus restoring sound conduction. Prostheses are made of various inert materials such as polyethylene, stainless steel, or tantalum (see Fig. 23-3).

By performing the microsurgical procedure under local anesthesia, the surgeon can reposition the eardrum and use voice testing to see if hearing is improved. Otosclerosis usually involves both ears but stapedectomy is performed on only one ear at a time.

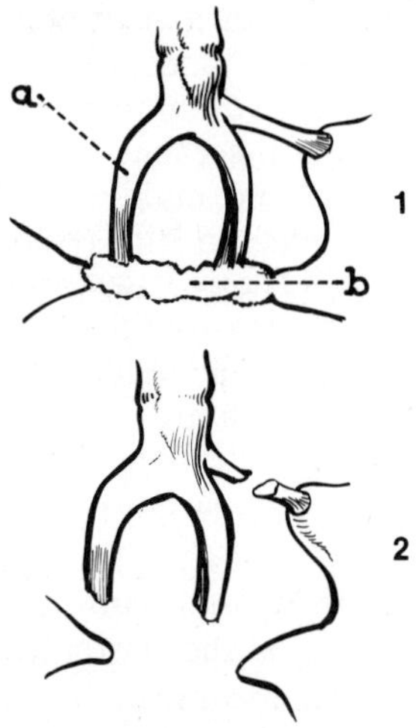

Figure 23-2 Partial stapedectomy. (1) stapes superstructure (a) attached to fixed otosclerotic footplate (b), (2) footplate removed; superstructure remains.

Stapes Mobilization This may be performed instead of stapedectomy. The stapes is manipulated at the footplate with the aim to restore normal function. A break through an otosclerotic lesion is achieved by means of transcrural pressure or direct application of chisels and picks to the footplate. A mobile, noninvolved portion of a functioning stapes remains. Various techniques are used, some with and some without use of prosthetic devices. The advantage of the procedure is that the preserved stapedial footplate provides natural protection for the inner ear. The disadvantage is that frequently a continuing otosclerotic process causes the footplate to become refixed. Therefore, stapedectomy is more popular because it produces more long-lasting results.

Stapes procedures are performed under direct vision with the operating microscope. The procedures do not disturb the integrity or position of the eardrum.

Inner Ear

Removal of Acoustic Neuroma This may be performed by an otologic surgeon and/or a neurosurgeon, depending on its location and extent of neurological involvement. An *acoustic neuroma* is a slow-growing, encapsulated, benign tumor of the eighth cranial, the acoustic, nerve. It originates in the neural sheath, but grows to involve nerve fibers. Initially the patient experiences unilateral hearing loss and disturbances, especially tinnitus, and equilibrium problems such as mild vertigo. The syndrome may resemble Ménière's disease or an expanding intracranial tumor. Early differential diagnosis is enhanced by audiometric

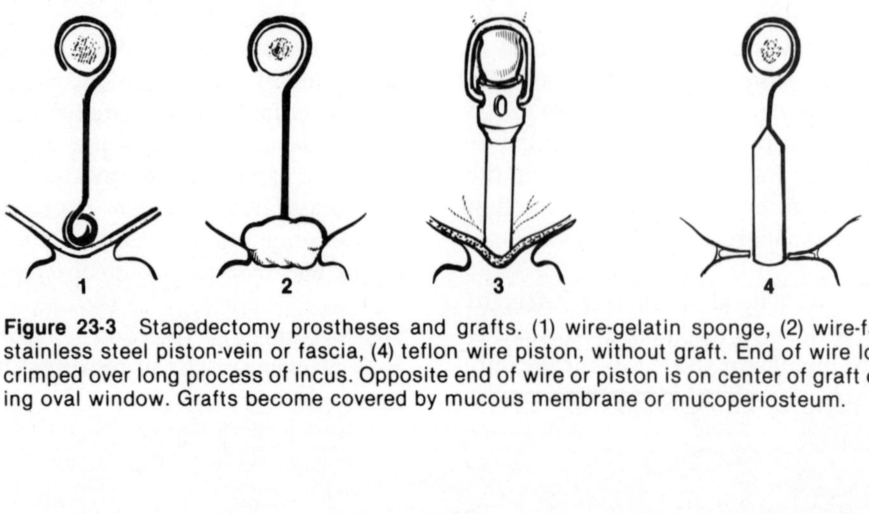

Figure 23-3 Stapedectomy prostheses and grafts. (1) wire-gelatin sponge, (2) wire-fat, (3) stainless steel piston-vein or fascia, (4) teflon wire piston, without graft. End of wire loop is crimped over long process of incus. Opposite end of wire or piston is on center of graft covering oval window. Grafts become covered by mucous membrane or mucoperiosteum.

evaluation, posterior fossa myelography, and vertebral angiography.

A small neuroma, confined to the internal auditory canal, may be resected by the otologist using microsurgical technique. A translabyrinthine approach is used to gain access to the internal auditory canal posterior to the inner ear structures. The patient has no practical hearing remaining at the time of the operation. Acoustic neuromas extending into the cranial cavity usually are resected by the neurosurgeon (refer to Chap. 24, p. 435).

THE NOSE

Anatomy and Physiology

The supporting structures of the nose consist of two nasal bones and the nasal processes of the maxillary bones superiorly, lateral cartilages and connective tissue inferiorly, and the septum. The *septum,* composed of bone posteriorly and cartilage anteriorly, divides the nose into two chambers lined by mucous membrane. The *anterior portion* or *vestibule* holds the nasal hairs. The external anterior orifices are called *nares.*

The internal portion of the nose, the *nasal cavity,* extends back to the *nasopharynx,* the space behind the *choanae* or funnellike posterior nasal orifices. The nose communicates with the ear via the eustachian tube. The hard and soft palates divide the nasal and oral cavities. Separation of the nasal and cranial cavities is achieved by the ethmoid bone.

The *paranasal sinuses* are the frontal, maxillary, ethmoid, and sphenoid. *Ostia* (openings from the sinuses and nasolacrimal ducts) are located in the nasal lateral walls. The ostia provide a drainage system for the sinuses as well as aerate them. Three turbinate bones (superior, middle, and inferior) also are situated in the lateral walls. These bones are covered with a vascular mucosa. Beneath each turbinate is a corresponding meatus. Tears drain into the nose through the nasolacrimal duct that enters the inferior meatus. Drainage from the paranasal sinuses is passed to the nose through the middle and superior meatuses.

External and internal carotid arteries and their branches supply blood to the nasal region. Because of the extensive vascularity, lymphatic supply, and proximity to the brain, infections on or about the face are potentially very dangerous. Microorganisms readily may be carried to or thrombi form in the cavernous sinus. The sensory nerve supply of the nasal area is associated with the trigeminal or fifth cranial nerve.

The *function of the nose* is twofold:

1 It provides filtered air to the respiratory system. Fine cilia in the mucous membrane propel mucus toward the nasopharynx. Air is warmed and moistened as it passes to the trachea and lower respiratory tract.

2 It contains the end organs for smell in the olfactory epithelium, which differs from other nasal epithelium. When nasal obstruction blocks off the olfactory epithelium, loss of smell (*anosmia*) results. The senses of smell and taste are closely related.

NASAL OPERATIVE PROCEDURES

Nasal operations are concerned with two factors: adequate ventilation to accessory spaces and adequate drainage from them. Abnormalities in structure, congenital or traumatic, and disease processes hinder function. Corrective procedures are done for several purposes as described below.

To Relieve Obstruction

Nasal obstruction may be due to allergies or nonoperative conditions. Operative intervention, however, can provide relief in certain instances.

Foreign Body or Abnormal Growth

Removal of Foreign Body This is more frequent in children. Often it is not suspect until discharge develops. After shrinkage of the mucosa with a vasoconstrictor and suctioning of secretions, the object is removed with a forceps. Usually local anesthesia suffices but general anesthesia may be necessary if the child is uncooperative or the removal difficult.

Incision and Drainage of Nasal Abscess or Hematoma This is indicated to drain infection and relieve pressure. Accumulation of blood or pus separates the *perichondrium,* connective tissue covering, from the underlying cartilage. This may cause necrosis of cartilage with resultant deformity. Infection must be removed to avoid extension to the brain.

Adenoidectomy This is the removal of adenoid tissue at the roof of the nasopharynx and behind the posterior choanae to facilitate breathing and prevent recurrent otitis media. Adenoid tissue atrophies after adolescence so the procedure is most often performed in children (refer to Chap. 26).

Polypectomy This is indicated when the posterior choanae are obstructed by *polyps,* soft edematous masses projecting from the nasal or sinus mucosa. Polyps may be unilateral, bilateral, single, or multiple. In addition to impeding ventilation, they may obstruct the sense of smell if the olfactory epithelium is blocked off. Multiple or large polyps are excised with a snare-type instrument. Packing, to control bleeding, is usually left in place 2 to 3 days. Since polyps frequently recur, persistent regrowth can be deterred by more extensive removal, i.e., by external or intranasal *ethmoidectomy,* removal of ethmoid sinuses, where most polyps originate.

Removal of Tumors Benign or malignant tumors should be removed as early as possible. Basal-cell carcinoma is a common type. Operation alone may be used, or combined therapy. Immediate repair by skin graft or pedicle flap accompanies excision of well-defined lesions (see Chap. 25). Reconstruction is postponed in multicentric (many-centered) cancer or doubtful extension of the tumor. More advanced lesions require replacement of the nose by prosthesis.

Erosion of a growth in one of the sinuses into an adjacent nasal wall can occlude the air passage.

Nasal Deformity

Reduction of Nasal Fracture This should be performed as soon as possible to bring the parts in apposition, but 7 to 10 days may be allowed to pass without affecting outcome to permit edema to subside. Frequent fracture of the septum or nasal bones accompanies other trauma to the head. Intranasal manipulation in the OR under anesthesia is required to elevate depressed bone or cartilage that may be pushed into the paranasal sinuses. Bleeding from laceration must be controlled and drained. Intranasal structure compatible with air passage must be preserved.

If the zygoma or maxilla is involved, reduction may be done through a small incision anterior to the ear and superior to the zygomatic arch. Periosteal elevators are used to raise depressed bone and fragments.

Blowout fracture of the orbit was discussed in Chapter 22. In these patients, orbital contents may be depressed into the maxillary sinus. Operative exploration through an orbital or a transsinal approach is indicated.

Septoplasty, Septal Reconstruction, Submucous Resection These terms are used interchangeably to describe correction of a deviated nasal septum. Often the result of injury, the condition interferes with breathing and drainage. Under local anesthesia one side of the septum is incised its entire length. Membranous coverings are detached from cartilage and bone. The deformed part of the septum is removed, or it may be straightened and replaced. Bilateral nasal packing is inserted to hold the tissues in place and to prevent bleeding. The procedure creates a patent airway and straight septal line, thereby reducing sinus disease and polyp formation.

Rhinoplasty This is a plastic procedure to correct deformity of the nose. It may be performed by a rhinologist or a plastic surgeon (refer to Chap. 25). An aesthetic operation to improve appearance, rhinoplasty is a major procedure involving reconstruction and molding of the bones and cartilages. Septoplasty and rhinoplasty may be performed together; *septorhinoplasty* restores both function and cosmetic appearance. Local anesthesia usually is used. The skin is taped postoperatively to maintain nasal structures in alignment. A rigid shield is applied for protection. This dressing must not be disturbed without specific order from the surgeon. Temporary ecchymosis from operative trauma surrounds the eyes postoperatively.

Repair of Perforated Septum This is performed most often for perforations in the anterior cartilage. If bleeding and crusting are severe, the perforation may be covered by rotated mucoperichondrial flaps. Or, the mucosa of adjacent intact septum may be denuded and a skin graft applied to cover the perforation (refer to Chap. 25). Nasal packing is inserted.

To Ensure Drainage

The paranasal sinuses are air-filled spaces in the skull. Since the sinus mucous membrane lining is continuous with the mucous membrane lining of the nose, nasal infection readily may spread to the sinuses. Various procedures provide drainage in patients with chronic sinusitis that may result from repeated nasopharyngeal infection. Swelling of nasal mucosa can trap microorganisms and infection within a sinus cavity. Abnormalities in the walls of the nasal cavity also interfere with breathing and drainage. Sinus procedures are executed through an external or an intranasal approach.

Maxillary Sinus Operation The *maxillary sinuses* are located bilaterally between the upper teeth and the eyes.

Caldwell-Luc (Antrostomy) This involves an approach to the maxillary sinus contents through incision of the oral mucous membrane above the canine teeth. The flap is retracted. A section of maxillary bone is cut out to create a large nasoantral window for aeration and permanent drainage by gravity into the nasal fossa under the inferior turbinate. Any polyps and diseased tissue also are removed. At completion of operation, the sinus is packed with gauze impregnated with antibiotic ointment. One end of gauze is brought through the window and into the nose. The incision under the upper lip is sutured. The packing eventually is removed through the nose. Antrostomy usually is limited to adults because of unerupted teeth in children. Caldwell-Luc incision also is used for removal of a tumor in the maxillary sinus.

Ethmoid Sinus Operations The *ethmoid sinus* cells lie bilaterally between the nose and the orbits. The maxillary sinuses are below the ethmoid bones, the frontal sinuses above them.

Ethmoidectomy This is performed to remove diseased tissue from the ethmoid labyrinth, middle turbinate, and meatus. A large cavity is formed to facilitate aeration and drainage. Severe ethmoiditis can cause orbital abscess requiring drainage through intranasal, or external (Lynch) incision that extends from the inner half of the eyebrow downward along the side of the nose.

Turbinectomy This includes removal of portions of the inferior and middle turbinates to increase aeration and drainage. The cavity is packed at completion of operation.

Frontal Sinus Operations The *frontal sinuses* are situated above the eyes. Usually approached through the external incision described for ethmoidectomy, a coronal incision may be made for exposure. This entails incision across the scalp from ear to ear.

Osteoplastic Flap Procedure This is performed to remove diseased tissue and ensure drainage. The bone covering the frontal sinus is exposed and incised. Contents of the interior of the sinus, such as a *mucocele,* a cyst lined with mucous-secreting glands, are extracted. The lining of the mucocele sac is then removed and the cavity packed with fat, from the abdominal wall, to obliterate the sinus with fibrous tissue that fills in the cavity. The incised bone flap then is repositioned and the incision sutured.

Killian Operation This is used to eliminate diseased tissue from the frontal sinuses. The cavity is reached by removal of the floor or anterior wall of the sinus through external incision above the eye. A large communication and drainage channel into the nose is formed.

Sphenoid Sinus Operation The *sphenoid sinus* is deep, almost in the center of the skull. It may be approached intranasally or via the external ethmoidectomy incision through the eyebrow.

Sphenoidotomy This involves the creation of an opening into the sphenoid sinus for drainage.

To Resect Tumors

Procedures for Carcinoma of Paranasal Sinuses Although rare, carcinoma does occur in the ethmoid sinuses and the maxillary antrum. The incidence increases with age. The sinuses are proximal to the orbits, oral cavity, and base of the skull. Tumor in the maxillary sinus may be associated with oral or nasal symptoms such as loosening of the upper teeth, bleeding from the nose, or asymmetry of the face. Malignancy in the ethmoid sinus may be accompanied by displacement of the eye, disturbance of smell, and nasal obstruction.

Chronic sinusitis is thought to play a role in etiology because of an associated replacement of respiratory epithelium by stratified squamous cells. Most sinus tumors are squamous-cell carcinoma. Often the bony walls are invaded and destroyed by the time symptoms appear since the tumor tends to extend in all directions. *Exploratory operation* by Caldwell-Luc incision provides the best chance of early diagnosis.

Radical craniofacial resection may be indicated. Resection may include *partial or total maxillectomy* and removal of surrounding tissues. The cavity usually is covered by skin graft. Unilateral enucleation of the eye may be necessary. Radical operation for ethmoid tumor also may involve removal of part of the base of the skull, excision of the maxillary antrum and the palate on the affected side.

In providing maxillofacial prostheses to replace facial structure following various procedures, the prosthodontist works closely with the surgeon and radiation therapist. Splints or stents hold tissue grafts in place, seal cavities from each other, or unite bony segments. A dental prosthesis to close the defect in the upper jaw and eye prosthesis following enucleation contribute to the patient's rehabilitation following extensive operation.

To Control Epistaxis

Nasal bleeding may be spontaneous, as in patients with arteriosclerosis, hypertension, or blood dyscrasia, or may result from trauma. Bleeding is unilateral except in persons with systemic disease such as leukemia, or severe fracture. Dehumidified air also may cause changes in the mucosa and splitting of tiny vessels. Management consists of locating the precise bleeding site and promptly instituting appropriate therapy. Hypovolemia should be corrected preoperatively. A bleeding patient is in a precarious condition.

Placing an Anterior Pack This will control the majority of nosebleeds. The vascular anterior portion of the nasal septum is a frequent site of bleeding (anterior epistaxis). Local vasoconstriction and pressure to the side of the nose are employed, and the bleeding point cauterized if necessary. When bleeding is from the anterior ethmoid artery, inaccessible to cautery, packing is applied to the area of depression between the septum and the middle turbinate.

Placing a Posterior Pack This may be necessary for constant pressure when bleeding in the posterior part of the nose is severe. Or, operative intervention may be indicated. The pack consists of rolled gauze securely tied to the middle of a length of narrow tape or strong string. Commercial packs are available. The gauze is lubricated with antibiotic ointment before insertion to control infection and odor. After passing a catheter into the mouth via the nose, one end of tape is tied to the oral end of the catheter. The catheter and attached tape then are drawn back through the mouth and out one nostril, thereby pulling the pack up into the nasopharynx. Thus one end of tape comes out the nose, the other end out of the mouth. These ends are secured to the patient's cheek with adhesive tape. The nasal end is taped to prevent the pack from slipping into the throat; the oral end facilitates removal of the pack. Some oozing may persist in spite of packing. The pack is left in place until bleeding is arrested, usually for at least 48 hours, but prolonged use can lead to otitis media or paranasal sinusitis.

Patients with postnasal packs often are apprehensive and uncomfortable. They must breathe through the mouth. Posterior packs tend to reduce arterial oxygen tension. All patients, especially the elderly or those with marginal pulmonary function, should be observed carefully for respiratory problems that may result from the pack dropping into the hypopharynx. Severe bleeding additionally may require anterior packing of the nose and correction of hypovolemia.

Artery Ligation A microsurgical technique, this is increasingly performed to control persistent nasal hemorrhage by reducing the blood supply to the posterior portion of the nose. Some surgeons prefer this modality to packing. Or, it may be performed with a pack in place.

A Caldwell-Luc incision, with removal of the posterior wall of the maxillary sinus for exposure, is used for the transantral ligation. Terminal branches of the internal maxillary artery, a branch of the external carotid artery, are exposed, identified, and ligated with metallic clips. Electrocoagulation is employed to control intraoperative bleeding but if it is excessive during operation, creation of a nasoantral window establishes drainage. The replaced posterior mucosal flap is covered with absorbable gelatin sponge, and the Calwell-Luc incision closed.

Incision along the left side of the nose and ligation of the anterior and posterior ethmoidal arteries is helpful in controlling bleeding in the superior aspect of the nose.

THE ORAL CAVITY AND THROAT

Anatomy and Physiology

Structures in the oral cavity are associated with both respiration and *deglutition* (the act of swallowing). Pathology may affect any of the structures: the lip, tongue, floor of the mouth, palates, salivary glands, or pharynx. Abnormalities result from infection, trauma, congenital malformation, improper occlusion or jaggedness of teeth, or tumors.

The tongue, occupying much of the oral cavity, is joined posteriorly to the soft palate and pharynx by folds of mucous membrane. The *hard palate* forms the floor of the nasal cavity as well as the anterior part of the roof of the mouth. Normality of tongue, lips, and palate is essential for proper speech. The *soft palate,* a musculomembranous structure posterior to the hard palate, occludes the nasal cavity during swallowing. The *oropharynx* includes the tonsillar fossae, base of the tongue, and oropharyngeal walls.

There are six major salivary glands, in addition to lesser glands, whose ducts secrete saliva into the mouth. These are the paired submandibular, sublingual, and parotid glands, the latter being the largest.

The funnel-shaped pharynx, which leads to the esophagus below, consists of three sections: nasopharynx (above), oropharynx (middle), and hypopharynx (below). The nasopharynx closes during swallowing but the other two parts communicate. The *pharynx,* posterior to the larynx and to the nasal and oral cavities, consists of constrictor muscles essential to swallowing. The proximity of food and air passages and the joint function of the pharynx in air and food passage, contribute to the hazard of aspiration. The pharynx contains masses of lymphoid tissue consisting of the adenoids or pharyngeal tonsils, hanging from the nasopharyngeal roof, the lingual tonsils, tissue in mucosal crypts, and the palatine tonsils, which lie in fossae on either side of the oropharynx. The palatines are referred to as the *tonsils*; a fibrous capsule adheres to each laterally. The tonsils are supported in the fossae by anterior and posterior pillars.

The *larynx,* situated anteriorly between the hypopharynx superiorly and trachea inferiorly, consists of three major cartilages supported by ligaments and muscles: the thyroid cartilage, which protects the soft inner structures, the cricoid cartilage directly beneath it, and the paired arytenoid cartilages posterior to the thyroid and joined to the cricoid. The thyroid cartilage is incomplete posteriorly but the cricoid is a complete ring. The cricothyroid space lies between the thyroid and cricoid cartilages. In this area the airway is readily accessible and therefore the site for emergency tracheotomy (see p. 426).

The main functions of the larynx are as an organ for speech and for closure of the glottis during swallowing to protect the respiratory passage and prevent aspiration. Extrinsic muscles open and close the *glottis,* the space between the true vocal cords. Intrinsic muscles regulate vocal cord tension. Movement of the paired arytenoid cartilages opens and closes the glottis. Folds of membrane covering muscle, the *true vocal cords* are attached to the arytenoid cartilages posteriorly and to the thyroid cartilage anteriorly. The cords are an integral part of phonation as they vibrate to produce sounds by rhythmically moving air particles. Production of vocal sound involves coordination of musculature of the lips, tongue, soft palate, pharynx, and larynx. The mouth and pharynx are the resonating cavities.

The tenth cranial or vagus nerve innervates the larynx. Its major branch to the larynx is the recurrent laryngeal nerve. Trauma to the nerve can result in laryngeal paralysis, devastating if both nerves are paralyzed.

The *trachea* is a tube composed of rings of cartilage anteriorly and membrane posteriorly. This membrane also forms the anterior wall of the *esophagus,* the musculomembranous canal between the pharynx and stomach. The trachea extends from the lower larynx to the carina in the chest, the point at which the trachea bifurcates to form the right and left main bronchi leading to the lungs.

OPERATIVE PROCEDURES OF THE ORAL CAVITY AND THROAT

The comon procedures in these anatomic areas fall within two major classifications: those for trauma and those for neoplasms.

Repair of Lacerations of the Lip or Mouth This is necessitated by injury. Edges are carefully sutured together.

Excision of Leukoplakia This is performed to resect a precancerous lesion. Chronic irritation can result in an abnormal whitening of the mucous membrane of the lip and tongue, a lesion primarily seen in heavy smokers.

Excision of Oral Carcinoma Lesions of the lower lip, tongue, floor of the mouth, as well as tonsillar pillars are included. Because of the proximity of cervical lymph nodes, metastasis occurs early. A painful bleeding ulcer should be suspect. However, oral cancer in its earliest stages may be asymptomatic and painless. Small tumors require only irradiation or local excision with primary closure. Larger lesions compel more extensive procedures.

1 *Partial or hemiglossectomy* is removal of part or half of the tongue.

2 *Total glossectomy* is removal of all of the tongue and often of the floor of the mouth. Cervical flaps or pectoral or forehead pedicle flap are used often to restore intraoral lining in reconstruction (refer to Chap. 25). Cervical metastases are indications for uni- or bilateral neck dissection.

3 *Mandibulectomy,* partial or total removal of the lower jaw, is performed for extension of tumor into the bone of the floor of the mouth. It may be performed with glossectomy and radical neck dissection (see p. 425) for wide excision. Mandibular replacement combines bone graft and synthetic materials for restoration of speech and appearance. If the patient is dentulous, relationship of the opposing teeth is maintained; if edentulous, the patient wears a denture. Whenever possible during operation, mandibular tissue is preserved.

Reduction of Fracture of the Mandible This requires interdental wiring if the patient has upper and lower teeth. If he or she is without teeth, open reduction and internal fixation with wire may be necessary. A wire scissors must be kept at the patient's bedside.

Excision of Tumor of Lip The procedure may be minor, with V-wedge excision, or extensive, depending on the stage of malignancy. Extensive lesions require a flap procedure for reconstruction.

Excision of Tumor of Salivary Gland This involves a subtotal or total parotidectomy (see Chap. 25, p. 451). If the neoplasm involves the mandible, the procedure is more complex including mandibulectomy requiring reconstruction. Radical neck dissection also may be indicated. Incision must be adequate to expose the entire gland and the facial nerve. A nerve stimulator is used to identify the nerve and its branches. Sometimes the nerve also must be resected in order to remove the entire tumor. In these patients nerve grafting may be done, as permanent paralysis causes disfigurement.

Incision and Drainage of Peritonsillar Abscess While less common since the discovery of antibiotics, this may follow acute tonsillitis. It is done to drain purulent material posterior to the tonsillar capsule. The anterior tonsillar pillar is the site of incision.

Tonsillectomy This is the removal of hypertrophied or chronically infected tonsils (refer to Chap. 26 for tonsillectomy in children). The adult patient may be positioned in semi-Fowler's or sitting position on the operating table or may sit in a specifically designed chair, with the surgeon sitting in front of him or her. Local anesthesia frequently is used. The throat is anesthetized with a topical agent and local infiltration.

With sharp or blunt dissection, the tonsil is separated from the pillars and capsule and removed from the fossa with a tonsil snare. Special attention is given to hemostasis so the operative area is clearly visible and aspiration prevented.

The scrub nurse assists by retracting the tongue, identifying the various colorless solutions used, and preparing sutures. Sponges are placed in forceps. The circulating nurse, in addition to monitoring the patient, should observe how much blood is being drawn into the suction bottle and report an abnormal amount.

Removal of Tumor of the Tonsillar Area This usually involves resection of a malignant neoplasm. Superior progression of the tumor may reach the supratonsillar fossa, soft and hard palates, and uvula. Inferiorly, tumor may spread to the posterior and lateral walls of the larynx, base of the tongue, and pyriform sinus. Metastatic nodes are common. Smoking has been implicated in the etiology. Diagnosis is made by biopsy and histopathological examination. Symptoms include dysphagia, sore throat, ear pain, or lesion in the throat.

OPERATIVE PROCEDURES OF THE ESOPHAGUS

Esophageal disorders may be congenital or acquired (refer to Chap. 26 for congenital). Abnormalities result from trauma, inflammation, or neoplasm. Esophageal problems may include study by a gastroenterologist and/or otorhinolaryngologist.

Esophagoscopy This is the endoscopic or direct visualization of the interior of the esophagus. It is performed to remove foreign bodies, obtain biopsy, brush cytologic or secretion specimens for diagnosis, and examine the esophagus and esophageal orifice of the stomach for organic disease. Inspection is made for diverticula, varices, strictures, lesions, or hiatus hernia, which may be manifested by symptoms of obstruction, regurgitation, or bleeding. (Refer to Chap. 15 for discussion of endoscopes, endoscopy, and care of endoscopic equipment.)

Esophagoscopes are rigid hollow metal tubes or the flexible fiberoptic type of scope that reduces discomfort and trauma. Accessory instruments, such as aspiration tubes and biopsy forceps, are similar for all endoscopes. Removal of an obstructing mass such as a steak bolus in the esophagus is better accomplished with the rigid metal scope. Various sizes of scopes are available to suit the individual patient.

Preoperative preparation and endoscopic technique are similar for esophagoscopy, laryngoscopy, and bronchoscopy. General anesthesia usually is used, but local topical anesthesia may be employed in some patients. For the procedure the patient is supine with the neck hyperextended and the head supported by a team member. The esophagoscope is passed through the mouth and cricopharyngeal lumen to the cardiac sphincter at the esophagogastric junction. The entire area is carefully scrutinized. The esophagus may be distended by insufflation of air to assist in viewing in the presence of stenosis.

A laryngoscope may be self-retaining by suspension in a special appliance placed over the patient's chest, thus giving the surgeon bimanual freedom in use of the operating microscope.

As following any anesthetization of the throat, postoperative orders include nothing by mouth for a specific number of hours until throat reflexes have returned, to prevent aspiration.

Removal of Foreign Bodies Removal of foreign bodies from the pharynx and/or esophagus is relatively common. Persons who wear upper dentures are especially prone to swallowing sharp bones that cannot be felt against the covered palate. Pieces of meat or dental bridgework may lodge or impact in the food passage, occluding the airway by pressure. This is an emergency situation necessitating provision of a patent airway by endotracheal intubation or tracheotomy and endoscopic removal of the bolus or foreign object. Acute esophageal obstruction increases salivation creating danger of tracheopulmonary aspiration.

Children frequently swallow objects such as coins, buttons, parts of toys, or safety pins that may remain in the throat. Metallic objects are visible on roentgenograms but many others are not.

It is dangerous to attempt to push an object toward the stomach as esophageal perforation can result. Esophagoscopy is the method of choice for removal, although the procedure is often difficult and painstaking. All effort is made to prevent trauma, with resultant mediastinitis.

Dilation of Stricture This may be indicated when the esophageal lumen has narrowed because of formation of scar tissue resulting from inflammation or burn at any level. Treatment consists of regular dilation with mercury-filled bougies of graduated sizes. Steroid administration is adjunctive therapy.

When an individual suffers a severe burn as from swallowing a caustic material, gastrostomy may be indicated in order to bypass the esophagus until it heals. Dilation of such strictures utilizes retrograde fusiform bougies with spindle-shaped shafts that are linked together. They are carried through the gastrostomy, up the esophagus, and out the mouth. The treatment must be continued for an extended period of time.

Dilation of stricture at the cardioesophageal junction may be necessary in patients with cardiospasm (*achalasia*). Gross dilatation above the stricture, often the result of muscular atrophy, leads to regurgitation. Diagnosis is made by roentgenography, esophagoscopy, or gastroscopy. If dilation is unsuccessful, a myotomy at the esophagogastric junction (Heller procedure) is performed to enlarge the opening into the stomach. Severe unyielding strictures may necessitate resection or esophageal replacement.

Diverticulectomy Diverticulectomy, or removal of sacs or outpocketings of lower pharyngeal mucous membrane in which food collects, may be performed in extreme cases where regurgitation presents hazard of aspiration. The neck of the sac is dissected from the posterior pharyngeal wall and ligated. The stump of the excised sac is inverted into the pharyngeal wall. Diverticuli may be removed endoscopically, especially in high-risk patients.

Neoplasms of the Esophagus Most often malignant, these are treated by resection or irradiation. Dysphagia or obstruction demands immediate investigation. Operative procedures fall under the classification of gastrointestinal surgery.

OPERATIVE PROCEDURES OF THE LARYNX

Trauma or disease of this cartilaginous tube, which joins the pharynx and the trachea, invariably causes respiratory obstruction. Operation is directed toward eliminating etiology of the obstruction and maintaining the larynx's dual function in respiration and phonation or production of speech.

Examination of the Larynx

Indirect Laryngoscopy This is use of a laryngeal mirror inserted through the mouth to the base of the tongue, with the patient in sitting position. Light is reflected to the area by the surgeon's headlamp. This is a simple ambulatory procedure.

Direct Laryngoscopy This is the insertion of a hollow tubular laryngoscope into the larynx for direct visualization of the interior. Direct laryngoscopy and endolaryngeal microsurgery are performed for diagnosis, such as biopsy, often an ambulatory procedure, and/or for treatment. Suspension laryngoscopy is used for most intralaryngeal operations. Some treatment procedures may require general anesthesia. Endoscopic principles are applicable. Laryngoscopy is employed for *removal of*:

1 *Foreign body,* such as a coin or small toy.
2 *Papilloma of the vocal cords,* which prevent accurate cord approximation and normal voice.
3 *Laryngeal polyps,* with stripping of polypoid mucosa to alleviate recurrence.
4 *Juvenile papilloma,* multiple growths on the larynx, epiglottis, vocal cords, and trachea. These may be treated by cryosurgery or laser beam in lieu of excision.
5 *Leukoplakia,* a white thickening on the vocal cords, causing hoarseness. The lesion must be examined histologically for differentiation from carcinoma.
6 *Laryngeal web,* adherence of the anterior aspects of the vocal cords as a result of removal of mucous membrane, or following inflammation. After excision, a metal or plastic plate may be put between the cords until normal mucous membrane regenerates. The plate is then removed.

Care of Laryngeal Injuries

Treatment is concerned primarily with maintenance of the airway, which may be occluded by edema, hematoma, torn mucosa, or cartilagenous fragments. Preservation of voice is of major concern also. The anterior, unprotected location of the larynx predisposes it to trauma, such as crushing injury.

Tracheotomy may be necessary to prevent asphyxia. An intraluminal stent inserted into the larynx superiorly to the tracheotomy tube, and fixed to it for stabilization, may be worn for several months until the laryngeal laceration heals and an intralaryngeal airway reforms. The stent is used to mold the tissues.

Patients with any laryngeal condition bear close watching for respiratory distress.

Severe laryngeal injury may result in permanent voice impairment.

In unilateral vocal cord paralysis, because of muscle atrophy and muscle imbalance, a weak, hoarse ("air-spilling") voice is present. Inadequate glottic closure can be treated by injection of polytef paste into the affected cord, to augment its size and thus help to bring the two cords into apposition. The injected material becomes firm and retains shape. A functioning cord and markedly improved voice quality result. This modality is used commonly when the recurrent laryngeal nerve is affected.

Procedures for Carcinoma of the Larynx

Procedures vary depending on the size and location of the lesion, extent of invasion, presence of regional or distant metastasis, age, general condition, and rehabilitative capacity of the patient. Radiological examination of the lesion by various methods such as contrast laryngography is a valuable adjunct in selecting an appropriate therapeutic modality. Laryngograms can identify mucosal irregularity, vocal cord thickening or tumor, and outline the lesion, as well as portray functional alteration of laryngeal structures.

Classification of malignancy by location includes *glottic* (true cords), *supraglottic* (above true cords), and *infraglottic* (below true cords).

Symptoms vary as well. Hoarseness of over 2 weeks duration often signals origin of malignancy of the glottis, as a result of cord fixation by the lesion. Dysphagia is suggestive of tumor at the esophageal opening. Dyspnea from airway obstruction is a late manifestation.

Total Laryngectomy with/without Neck Dissection This is performed for advanced lesions of the true vocal cords or hypopharyngeal area. The entire larynx (epiglottis, false and true cords) and upper tracheal rings are removed, destroying connection between the pharynx and trachea. Pharyngeal walls and lower trachea are preserved. Thereafter the patient breathes and expels bronchial secretions through a permanent stoma in the neck created by suturing the tracheal stump to the skin (*tracheostomy*). Size of the stoma should be recorded on the patient's record in case of emergency need for a tube at a later time. Air no longer is humidified by the nose. Sense of smell also is lost because the nasal olfactory epithelium is not stimulated by inhalation. Acclimatization to air intake through the neck constitutes a major adjustment for the patient.

A nasogastric tube may be inserted at operation for temporary feeding. Although the laryngectomee no longer has normal voice, normal eating is resumed after healing takes place.

Formation of a salivary fistula is one complication of laryngectomy. Swallowed saliva leaks out through a weakness in the pharyngeal suture line and through the skin. Rupture of the carotid artery, especially in preirradiated patients, is another complication. This may occur if radical neck dissection was performed also, which places the artery in the operative area. (Further discussions of neck dissection follow in this chapter and in Chap. 25.)

Rehabilitation of the laryngectomee should begin preoperatively with diagnosis and include the family. It incorporates input from many professional disciplines since major disability results from the operation. In working with the speech pathologist, the patient learns to develop esophageal speech. By intake of a bolus of air into the esophagus and vibration by cricopharyngeal muscles, sound is produced to articulate speech. Persons unable to perfect the technique can use an artificial larynx, an electronic device that includes pitch and volume. Practical help and moral support are offered the newly laryngectomized patient by others who are members of numerous groups such as the International Association of Laryngectomees and the Lost Chord Club. The American Cancer Society also is a notable resource for assistance.

Total laryngectomy is a radical procedure. Whenever possible and for smaller lesions the surgeon instead will perform *conservation surgery of the larynx or partial laryngectomy.* These procedures yield the same rate of cure of selected malignancies as the radical procedure, without sacrificing phonation, deglutition, and respiratory function. Some natural voice is retained and a neck stoma may not be necessary for breathing.

Supraglottic Laryngectomy A conservation technique, this is performed for carcinoma of the epiglottis and/or false cords, which are removed in addition to the hyoid bone. Horizontal incision is made above the true vocal cords, thus preserving the voice and normal airway. Neck dissection may be done simultaneously. A prophylactic tracheotomy is always part of the procedure because of the danger of aspiration. With the epiglottis removed, liquids in particular can easily spill into the trachea. Use of a cuffed tracheotomy tube (see p. 427) is a necessary precaution.

Vertical Hemilaryngectomy Also a conservation method, this may be performed by several techniques. In hemilaryngectomy, through a vertical incision, one true cord, false cord, arytenoid, and half the thyroid cartilage are removed. The epiglottis, cricoid, and opposite cord are preserved. Following healing, scar tissue that fills in the operative defect almost approximates the remaining vocal cord. Thus the patient has a usable although hoarse voice, satisfactory airway, and normal eating. Sometimes a muscle flap is used for glottic reconstruction to improve voice quality. A prophylactic tracheotomy may be done.

Subcutaneous emphysema, infiltration of air under the skin, is a potential complication.

NOTE. 1. In the early stages, cancer of the larynx is one of the most curable of all malignancies because of the sparse lymphatic supply in the region of the vocal cords.

2. In patients with a permanent stoma, resuscitation always must be via stoma.

Radical Neck Dissection

This procedure gives the patient with cancer of the cervical lymphatic chain a chance for cure and arrest of spread. It involves removal of all cervical lymphatics on one or both sides of the neck when metastasis there is known to be present or is highly suspect because of location or stage of the malignancy. The operation is predicated on the assumption that metastases if present are regional and not distant.

In an attempt to eradicate all cancer foci, neck dissection may be performed at a time later than removal of a primary lesion of, for example, the larynx or tongue, or simultaneously with it as a one-stage procedure. This composite resection removes primary tumor and metastatic lesions at the same time en masse. Sometimes, however, metastasis occurs before a primary lesion is discovered.

The operation includes massive tissue resection, removal en bloc of all nonvital structures of the neck on the side of the tumor. More specifically, these structures are the jugular vein, eleventh cranial (spinal accessory) nerve, sternocleidomastoid muscle, and submaxillary salivary gland. Elimination of the motor nerve to the trapezius muscle contributes to muscular atrophy, subsequent shoulder drop on the affected side, and possibly decreased strength in raising the arm. If possible, all vital structures such as the carotid artery system, facial, vagus, phrenic, and hypoglossal nerves as well as the brachial plexus are preserved.

A prophylactic tracheotomy may be performed to protect the patient from respiratory distress in neck dissection alone. It is always done in a composite resection.

A nasogastric tube or cervical pharyngostomy tube, for anticipated extended extraoral feeding, permits suction to avoid aspiration and gastric distention in addition to providing a feeding route. The tube usually is inserted in the OR.

Effective drainage of the wound is important to healing. This is accomplished by application of continuous negative pressure to catheters inserted through stab wounds below the clavicle. Drainage protects viability of the thin skin flaps and facilitates approximation of wound surfaces.

There are numerous potential complications of neck dissection, depending on the tumor itself, irradiation therapy, or necessary sacrifice of vital structures. Intraoperatively, hemorrhage may occur from injury to a major vessel or the thoracic duct. Postoperatively, invasion of overlying skin necrosis into a major vessel wall, such as the carotid artery, can cause an often fatal blowout of the vessel. Slight previous bleeding may be forewarning.

Various techniques are used to close a large defect in the anterior neck caused by resection of involved skin when malignancy penetrates anteriorly, or to rebuild a removed part (refer to Chap. 25).

OPERATIVE PROCEDURES OF THE TRACHEA

Upper respiratory tract obstruction and ventilatory failure may require operative intervention when the need for intubation or positive-pressure ventilation would be long-term or of indefinite duration, or when severe laryngeal obstruction is present. The obstruction is bypassed.

Tracheotomy

Tracheotomy is the formation of an opening into the trachea into which a tube is inserted, through which the patient breathes. It is performed in any age group to improve or maintain patency of the airway or relieve obstruction. The opening in the trachea provides easy accessibility for suctioning secretions from the tracheobronchial tree or administering anesthesia to patients with facial trauma or burns.

Airway crisis may result from mechanical obstruction due to a tumor, foreign body, infection, or secretions. It also results from congenital, neurologic, or traumatic conditions. Some of the many indications for the procedure are foreign body in the hypopharynx or larynx, acute laryngotracheal bronchitis or epiglottitis in infants and children, laryngeal edema, or any other condition that obstructs respiration.

Tracheotomy is commonly a controlled procedure, such as a prophylactic procedure in conjunction with glossectomy, but can be an acute emergency. An endotracheal tube may give temporary relief prior to and during tracheotomy.

Tracheotomy is often done under local anesthesia. The patient is supine with support under the shoulders to hyperextend the neck. A transverse incision is made, producing better cosmetic result, or a midline vertical incision is made between the cricoid cartilage and the suprasternal notch. The overlying isthmus of the thyroid gland is retracted or divided and the exposed third or fourth tracheal ring is incised. After tracheal aspiration to remove blood and secretions, a previously selected and prepared tube is inserted with the obturator in place. Immediately after insertion the obturator is removed to open the airway. However, it remains with the patient constantly in case of future need. The outer cannula is suctioned, the inner cannula fixed in place. The wound is closed with a few sutures, or superficial edges of the area above the tube may be sutured and the area below left with natural tissue approximation, for drainage. A smooth-edged dressing split around the tube protects the skin. Commercial tracheotomy dressings are available. Tapes that are tied to the ends of the outer cannula are secured around the neck. Proper tension allows insertion of one finger between the tape and skin. If tied too tightly, the tapes may compress the jugular vein; if too loosely, the tube can obtrude with coughing. The tube should not be removed in the first 24 to 48 hours by any person unable to perform tracheotomy, as the tract to the trachea may occlude and not be immediately located.

A sterile tube identical to the one inserted and a tracheotomy set must accompany the patient from the OR and constantly remain with him or her. The set is eventually released by surgeon's order.

A tracheotomy is an open wound. While rigid asepsis is not possible, every effort is made to keep contamination to a minimum. Only sterile equipment, with minimal handling, is used to prevent infection. Suctioning through a tracheotomy tube is done as a sterile procedure, with sterile catheter and gloves. Careful suctioning prevents trauma. Insert the catheter without application of suction, to protect tracheal walls and prevent suctioning out oxygen in the borderline patient. Apply suction as you withdraw the catheter. Run sterile solution through the catheter after use to clean it and maintain patency. Disposable catheters are recommended.

Some tracheotomized patients come to the OR for change of tube or other procedure. These patients may require suctioning while waiting in the holding area. Knowledge of and preparation for each patient is a prime responsibility of the circulating nurse.

Tracheotomized patients require humidified air, deliverable by various devices, to keep secretions liquefied and to prevent drying of tissues. Other needs are constant observation and special communication.

Tracheotomy Tubes While an endotracheal tube may provide ventilation for short-term therapy, a tracheotomy tube is easier to suction and immobilize for extended use. It also reduces possibility of laryngeal injury.

Various materials such as plastic, nylon, and silicone largely have replaced silver tubes. The plastic tubes have certain advantages:

1 They can be left *in situ* during radiation therapy.
2 They are lighter in weight, softer, more pliable, less traumatic.
3 They can be cut to length.
4 They are bonded to the inflatable cuff.

The inside and outside diameters of some tubes are labeled in millimeters. French or Jackson scale is stated on others. All hospitals keep a variety of sizes and types of sterile tracheotomy tubes available in the OR suite, in the emergency department, and on emergency carts.

Most tubes consist of three parts—the outer cannula, inner cannula, and obturator. The inner cannula is periodically removed and cleaned to prevent blockage by crusting of secretions. *It always must be replaced immediately within the outer cannula* so that the latter remains free of crusting. The obturator provides a smooth tip during tube insertion to prevent trauma to the tracheal wall. Some plastic tubes do not require an inner cannula because they are relatively crust-free. However, if crusts do form, the tube must be changed.

Some tubes have a built-in soft cuff that is inflated to eliminate any free space between the tube and the tracheal wall, thus preventing aspiration of drainage down the trachea. Cuffed tubes also facilitate function of any ventilatory apparatus. A pilot balloon in the inflation line, attached to the outer cannula, indicates cuff inflation or deflation. *Proper cuff inflation-deflation is highly important.* Irritation and pressure of the cuff against the tracheal wall can cause damage such as ulceration and necrosis of the mucosa, which can lead to infection, tracheobronchial fistula, erosion into the innominate artery, or stenosis from scarring. Precautionary measures include deflation at regular intervals, by written order, to increase blood flow to the cuff site, use of low-pressure or controlled-pressure cuff, constant monitoring of intracuff pressure, and minimum inflation to ensure a leak-free system. Overinflation can reduce tube diameter as well as cause the cuff to extend over the tip of the tube, thus obstructing ventilation. Or, the tracheal wall may herniate over the tube end. Underinflation may cause subcutaneous emphysema. Cuffs also should inflate symmetrically. The amount of air needed for inflation varies with the size of the trachea and the tube. Understandably, less air is needed for larger tubes. Usually 2 to 5 cm of air provide a closed system.

Specific tubes have special variations, such as an opening in the wall opposite the bevel to permit ventilation in case of bevel occlusion. Others have a radiopaque tip that allows radiologic visualization of tube position. Many have connectors, some of which are a built-in swivel type permitting lightweight, flexible, easy connection to a ventilating system. These connectors reduce hazard of accidental disconnection. Still others have a fenestration in the outer cannula permitting air to flow through the larynx. These tubes are used in patients no longer requiring mechanical ventilation to allow assessment of spontaneous breathing and coughing in preparation for decannulation. With air passing through the larynx, the patient can speak with the proximal end of the cannula plugged. A so-called speaking tube permits introduction of humidified air and oxygen through a special line and with upward flow of the gas through the larynx, the patient can speak.

Tracheotomy Set A tracheotomy set, with all essential equipment for performance of tracheotomy, should be in the operating room during any extensive operation on the face or neck, such as drainage of Ludwig's angina, thyroidectomy, or radical neck dissection. If a tracheotomy tube is inserted during operation, the obturator must accompany the patient at all times. If a tube is not needed, the tracheotomy set accompanies the patient and remains at the bedside for a few days postoperatively, in case of development of respiratory obstruction due to edema. A set is kept at the bedside of a patient on a respirator. The number of sets in the inventory is governed by individual hospital need. Sterile sets *always* must be available. Tubes are wrapped and sterilized individually to permit free selection.

OPERATIVE PROCEDURES OF THE BRONCHUS

Disorders of the trachea and bronchus often overlap and most commonly are infection, foreign body, trauma, or neoplasms. Diagnosis is made by radiologic study and endoscopy.

Bronchography

This is the radiologic study of the tracheobronchial tree. It is frequently done in conjunction with bronchoscopy.

Bronchoscopy

This is direct visualization of the tracheobronchial tree through a bronchoscope for:

1 Diagnosis: securing uncontaminated secretion for culture, taking a biopsy, or finding the cause of cough or hemoptysis
2 Treatment: removing a foreign body, excising a small tumor, applying a medication, aspirating the bronchi, or providing an airway during performance of tracheotomy

Foreign bodies in the trachea and bronchi are very serious, requiring careful history and immediate bronchoscopy with preparation for potential tracheotomy. Maintaining a safe airway during extraction is a major risk. If the airway is not seriously obstructed, the aspirated foreign body may remain in the bronchus for months without producing symptoms until suppuration develops. Coughing and hemoptysis bring the patient to the physician.

GENERAL CONSIDERATIONS IN ENT PROCEDURES

1 Illumination is provided by the overhead spotlight, the operating microscope, or by the surgeon's reflective headlamp that enables him or her to see up and under surfaces. Some surgeons prefer a fiberoptic headlamp.

2 Anesthesia is mainly local. It minimizes bleeding and postoperative discomfort in addition to affording the surgeon observation of patient response. It utilizes patient cooperation. Also, presence of an endotracheal tube, routine with general anesthesia, can distort features during operation.

- **a** The circulating nurse observes the usual precautions for local anesthesia, i.e., monitoring the patient (and ECG) in the absence of a standby anesthesiologist. She must record the amount of local anesthesia used on the anesthesia record and write intraoperative nursing notes. A patient may be conscious of nausea, vertigo, or a sense of falling, from stimulation of the vestibular labyrinth in otologic operations.
- **b** If the patient experiences syncope, it must be differentiated rapidly from reaction to the local anesthetic (refer to Chap. 9). The patient may be in a fairly erect position, for example, local tonsillectomy, which may contribute to postural hypotension.
- **c** Patients for local anesthesia are permitted to wear pajama bottoms to the OR in some hospitals.

Microsurgical laryngeal operations and endoscopies usually require general anesthesia.

3 Although the operative area is often contaminated, such as the oral cavity, only sterile equipment and sterile technique are used to avoid introducing exogenous microorganisms.

4 Instrumentation is quite varied but suited to the area. It includes very delicate, small microsurgical implements in addition to bone instruments, because of the extensive involvement of cartilage and bone in facial structures and skull. These areas have relatively little soft tissue. Many instruments are angulated to permit insertion into areas of difficult access and curving passages. Various endoscopes are used.

5 Sponges used in ENT procedures are relatively small and a distinct hazard when blood-soaked, as they can occlude an airway. Sponges placed in the postnasal area are easily controlled if a 10- to 12-in. (25 to 30cm) suture is attached to them.

6 Various colorless solutions are on the table. Each container must be accurately and clearly labeled for foolproof distinction between, for example, cocaine, lidocaine, and epinephrine. Preferably the surgeon draws the solution into the syringe to avoid potentially fatal error.

7 Suction must be available at all times including several patent cannulae. The degree of suction should be variable. A foot pedal may be used to interrupt wall suction so the surgeon has control of it for grasping and releasing an object, e.g., in handling a prosthetic graft.

8 Cryosurgery is used to destroy tumorous tissue in accessible areas, especially those that bleed profoundly if incised.

9 Microsurgical techniques are used for many ENT procedures because they facilitate distinction between normal and diseased tissue and allow more accurate dissection. e.g., in infinitely small areas such as the middle ear.

10 One or two drops of blood can obscure a microsurgical field. The nurse must have hemostatic aids ready at all times. Gelfoam pledgets soaked in 1:1000 epinephrine are used frequently.

11 Care with prep solutions is necessary as they are very painful and irritating if allowed to touch a perforated eardum. Disposable, lint-free drapes are often preferred for otologic operations. A patient may experience anxiety with drapes over the head. Air and oxygen administered during the procedure afford relief.

12 Special care with electrical appliances is indicated. Electrocoagulation is employed to control oozing. Compressed air or compressed nitrogen drills with foot-pedal control are used on bone, such as the mastoid area. There are a number of drills for the smaller extremely fine work, such as stapes sculpturing, which are powered by small electric motors fitted into the handpiece.

13 Irrigation equipment and solution at body temperature must be available to remove bone dust, clean burrs, and rinse suction apparatus. The very fine suction needles used in stapedectomy must be irrigated constantly to avoid blockage.

14 It is mandatory in otologic surgery that gloves be powder- and lint-free. Formation of granuloma in the oval window can cause sensorineural (irreversible) hearing loss. Handle tissue grafts and gelatin sponges with forceps, not the hands. Gelfilm, which is brittle, may be cut while in the primary wrap.

15 Tissue grafts must be kept from drying out prior to use. A convenient method is to place the graft on a moist cellulose sponge in a sterile, covered Petri dish. Some surgeons intentionally dry a temporalis fascia graft to facilitate handling.

16 Preoperative explanations and postoperative instructions are vital to outcome. For example, following ear or nasal procedures the patient must avoid blowing the nose, which would force air up the eustachian tube to cause infection, force air through the incision, or dislodge a graft. In sneezing he or she should keep both nose and mouth open.

Chapter 24

Neurosurgery

Neurosurgeons specialize in surgery of the central and peripheral nervous systems. More than 200 clinical disabilities are associated with dysfunction, disease, or injury of the nervous system. The nervous system includes the brain and spinal cord (the *central nervous system,* CNS) and the cranial, spinal, and autonomic peripheral nerves (the *peripheral nervous system,* PNS). The neural tissues control motor and sensory functions throughout the body. Generalized cerebral function is manifested in overall behavior, level of consciousness, orientation, and intellectual performance. These functions may be altered by a metabolic disorder, a chromosomal defect, a disease process, or a traumatic injury. Assessment of neurological deficits or changes in functional activity establishes the indications for neurosurgical intervention. The scope of neurosurgery is broad to include: removal of pathological lesions; relief of pain, spasm, or other neurophysiological conditions; and repair of nerve injuries and tissue defects.

HISTORICAL DEVELOPMENT

The earliest time in which operative procedures were done is not known. The evidence of it is shown in trephined skulls from prehistoric burial sites. It is possible that these trephines were done to let out evil spirits. This may be considered the forerunner of psychosurgery to treat mental illness by frontal leukotomy or topectomy, procedures rarely performed since the advent of the tranquilizing drugs.

The Smith Papyrus from Egypt is the first authentic recorded documentation of wound care. From the seventeenth century B.C., it describes treatment of head and vertebral column injuries as well as methods of holding wound edges together.

Ancient Greeks and Romans used cranial instruments. Hippocrates described the use of a trephine to treat headache. He also treated skull fractures, epilepsy, and blindness.

Surgery of the nervous system advanced slowly through the centuries. Cranial surgery, for example, was limited until the 1880s to treating trauma or trephining to evacuate pus or blood. The first brain tumor was removed in England in 1884 by Sir Rickman Goodlee. In 1887, W.W. Keen of Philadelphia was the first surgeon in the United States to excise a tumor from the brain.

Sir Charles Sherrington (1857–1952) was a pioneer in the study of the physiology of the spinal cord. In 1887, Sir Victor Horsley removed a spinal cord tumor. Subsequently Horsley (1869–1939) attempted operations on the brain. He was the first to approach the pituitary gland. He may be considered the first neurosurgeon.

The recognized father of modern neurosurgery, however, is Harvey W. Cushing (1869–1939). Among his many accomplishments, Cushing described the relationship of intracranial pressure to blood pressure in 1900 and, in 1932, pituitary basophilism, commonly known as *Cushing's disease.* He established at Harvard the first school of neurosurgery, which resulted in the development of a discipline recognized throughout the world.

The application of increasing knowledge of neurophysiology and the advances in diagnostic methods, such as those of Dandy and Moniz prior to the impact of computerized axial tomography, led to the success of intracranial and intraspinal operations. Stereotaxis led to the development of less destructive techniques to replace some extensive invasive procedures and of treatments for otherwise inoperable lesions.

The operating microscope opened up a new field of microneurosurgery that has created interest in cerebral revascularization techniques previously unattempted, and offers advantages in operative management of many other pathological lesions.

SPECIAL CONSIDERATIONS IN NEUROSURGERY

Neurosurgical procedures may be classified, as will be discussed in this chapter, according to the anatomic location of the nervous system involved, i.e., the brain and cranial nerves, the spinal cord and nerve roots, the autonomic and somatic peripheral nerves. Regardless of the location of the operative site, neural tissue must be handled gently to minimize functional disability of surgical trauma. Hemostasis is a critical factor to sustain vital functions of circulation and respiration. Visibility of structures in the operative site also must be assured.

Hemostatic Agents

Refer to Chapter 12 for a complete description of the methods of hemostasis. The hemostatic agents commonly used by the neurosurgeon for most procedures include:

Bone Wax Victor Horsley discovered the value of beeswax to seal bleeders in bone during his animal experiments in 1885. Now supplied as a refined blend of beeswax and a synthetic ester, bone wax is used by neurosurgeons on cranial and vertebral bones.

Compressed Absorbent Patties Made of rayon or cotton, patties are used on fragile, delicate neural tissues to absorb blood and fluids, rather than mesh gauze sponges. They also are used to protect wound edges and for hemostasis. An assortment of sizes are moistened with saline and pressed out flat on a metal surface easily accessible to the neurosurgeon. Although they have no loose fibers, they could pick up lint if placed on a towel. Moisture must not soak through drapes.

Policy for sponge counts may include counting these patties. They must be retrieved before the operative site is closed. Some neurosurgeons use only patties with a thread securely attached to each one. This reminds the surgeon that they are in the wound and facilitates their removal.

Electrosurgery Small vessels are coagulated. Current frequently is conducted through hemostatic forceps, fine smooth-tipped tissue forceps, or metal suction tip to the bleeding vessels. A combination of suction-fulgeration tip may be used.

Gelatin Sponge or Microcrystalline Collagen These agents may be used following resection to control bleeding from large vessels, sinuses, or the surface of a tumor bed. The scrub nurse must moisten gelatin sponge with normal saline or thrombin before handing it to the neurosurgeon. Microcrystalline collagen is applied dry. The tips of tissue forceps should be dry to prevent this substance from adhering to them.

Ligating Clips Clips are applied on larger vessels where electrocoagulation would be insufficient or its thermal effect would be hazardous. Some clips, such as intracranial aneurysm clips, are specifically designed only for neurosurgical use. Each type and size clip requires a specific applier.

Adjuncts to Visibility

Neural tissues must be as clean, dry, and visible as possible without damaging them. Visibility is enhanced by:

Irrigation Most wounds are irrigated frequently with normal saline or lactated Ringer's solution. The scrub nurse should keep a bulb syringe filled ready for use. The solution must be maintained at room to body temperature. A thermometer in the basin of solution helps provide a safety check.

Suction Suction is necessary to evacuate blood, cerebrospinal fluid, and irrigating fluid from the operative site so the neurosurgeon can identify structures. Necrotic tissue, pus, or cystic matter also may be aspirated. Usually a Ferguson-Frazier tip is used. Caution is taken to avoid applying vacuum directly on normal neural tissue, especially brain tissue. This tissue is protected by compressed absorbent patties. Suction must be available for all neurosurgical operations.

Lighted Retractors Because visibility of structures is critical, retractors with a lighting system incorporated into them may be used, especially for intracranial operations. A fiberoptic headlamp also is used by some neurosurgeons for supplemental lighting in the operative site.

Endoscope An endoscope with a fiberoptic side-viewing telescope may be used to enhance visibility at obscure angles in otherwise visually inaccessible areas. This endoscope is particularly useful to identify lesions in the sella turcica, cerebral aneurysms, and intervertebral disks, for example. An endoscope may be used for placement of electrodes for stimulators. (These procedures will be further discussed later in this chapter.)

CRANIAL SURGERY

Anatomic Approaches

An understanding of basic anatomy and physiology is essential to preparing for the approach the neurosurgeon will use to reach the desired section of the brain or a cranial nerve. The brain must be approached through the skull. Although several bones are fused together to protect and support the brain, the skull is described as divided into three areas: the anterior, middle, and posterior fossae. The brain has three distinct anatomical units that consist of several subdivisions as shown in Figure 24-1.

Cerebrum Consisting of two hemispheres, right and left, the cerebrum occupies most of the area within the skull. Each hemisphere is divided into four lobes.

1 The *frontal lobe* lies within the anterior fossa.
2 The *parietal lobe* lies in the superior and anterior portion of the middle fossa.
3 The *temporal lobe* lies inferior to the frontal and parietal lobes within the middle fossa.
4 The *occipital lobe* lies posteriorly within the middle fossa.

The *hypothalmus* and *thalmus* also lie within the cerebrum. Although it lies in the sella turcica outside the cerebrum, the pituitary body attaches to the hypothalmus.

Cerebellum Also consisting of two hemispheres, the cerebellum lies below the occipital lobes, posterior to the brainstem, within the posterior fossa. It is about one-fifth the size of the cerebrum.

Brainstem Including the midbrain, pons, and medulla oblongata, the brainstem lies anteriorly within the posterior fossa. It extends from the cerebral hemisphere to the base of the skull, where it merges with the spinal cord. It also contains the nuclei of 10 of the 12 pairs of cranial nerves, all except the olfactory (I) and optic (II) nerves.

Ventricles The lateral ventricles, one lying in each hemisphere, are within the cerebrum. These open into a central cavity, the third ventricle, which is connected by the aqueduct of Sylvius with the fourth ventricle lying anterior to the cerebellum and posterior to the brainstem. Cerebrospinal fluid produced in the choroid plexuses lining the ventricles circulates, through the subarachnoid space, around the meninges covering the brain and spinal cord to cushion these structures. An obstruction to the flow of cerebrospinal fluid causes intracranial pressure.

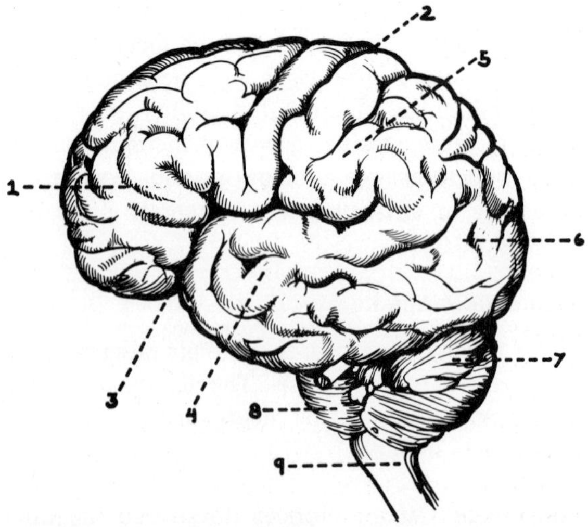

Figure 24-1 Left lateral view of cerebral hemisphere. (1) frontal lobe, (2) central fissue of Rolando, (3) lateral fissure of Sylvius, (4) temporal lobe, (5) parietal lobe, (6) occipital lobe, (7) cerebellum, (8) pons, (9) medulla oblongata.

General Considerations

1 Preparation of the patient in the OR usually begins with clipping hair. Hair on the head is considered the patient's personal property. When all of it must be removed, it is saved unless permission is granted by the patient to destroy it.

Hair usually can be removed from a male patient with electric clippers. A female head is shaved after initial hair removal with clippers. The neurosurgeon or assistant usually removes the hair.

2 Location of the intended line of incision determines the headrest that will be needed to position the patient. The basic unit of the neurosurgical headrest attaches in place of the head piece on the standard operating table. The headrest stabilizes and supports the head. If the patient will be in supine position, the configuration of the headrest contours to the back of the head. For prone position, the padded headrest equalizes weight distribution around the face.

Fowler's or sitting position may be desired. The headrest is attached at the head end of the operating table to support the back of the head for a unilateral or nasal approach. For a posterior fossa approach, the headrest is attached to a crossbar attachment placed in the stirrup holders on the table. The forehead is supported. A special neurosurgical chair may be used.

The circulating nurse must be familiar with the neurosurgical headrest attachments for each desired position. The supine position is used most commonly for approaches to the frontal, parietal, and temporal lobes within the anterior and middle fossae. Lateral position may be preferred for some operations. Prone position is used to reach the occipital lobe. It also may be used for a suboccipital approach, but most neurosurgeons prefer the sitting position to approach the posterior fossa.

3 Infiltration of a local anesthetic agent beneath the scalp is desirable for many intracranial procedures. The scalp, extracranial arteries, and portions of the dura mater are the only structures covering the brain that are sensitive to pain. Epinephrine may be added to the agent to prolong its effectiveness and to constrict superficial blood vessels. The anesthetic may be injected before the patient is prepped and draped.

4 Administration of general anesthetic agents via endotracheal tube may be preferred for extensive intracranial operations, although the skull and brain are insensitive to pain. The patient is positioned after he or she is anesthetized, before prepping and draping.

5 Anticipation of difficulty in achieving hemostasis by the methods previously discussed is not unusual for some operations to remove vascular intracranial lesions. Controlled hypotension may be initiated by the anesthesiologist, with the concurrence of the neurosurgeon, to lower blood pressure (refer to Chap. 9).

6 Prevention of cerebral edema during repair of cranial injuries may be accomplished with hypothermia. Hypothermia also may be used to decrease cerebral blood flow and venous pressure, and to decrease brain volume and intracranial pressure (refer to Chap. 9).

7 Prevention of potential air embolism in patients in Fowler's or sitting position must be considered. The brain is higher than the heart in these positions. Venous pressure may be lower than atmospheric and can allow for entry of air into the heart via an open venous channel. An antigravity suit may be used (refer to Chap. 12, p. 249). This extends from the patient's rib margin to the ankles, and is inflated if the patient becomes hypotensive.

8 Function or organic activity of the brain may be monitored by electroencephalogram periodically throughout the operation. Sterile subdermal needle electrodes may be used, if surface scalp electrodes cannot be used.

9 Reduction of intracranial pressure and brain volume may be accomplished by withdrawing spinal fluid. An intrathecal catheter or Tuohy needle is inserted, before prepping and draping, for the anesthesiologist to remove cerebrospinal fluid during operation as desired by the neurosurgeon.

10 Demarcation of the desired outline for the incision may be made on the scalp after the skin prep, prior to draping. A sterile disposable skin marker is available.

11 Instrumentation usually is arranged on a large table over the patient in supine or prone position. The scrub nurse must stand on a tiered platform to easily set up and reach the instruments for the neurosurgeon. The drapes over the head are attached to the table drapes (refer to Chap. 11, p. 233 for procedure).

A double Mayo stand setup usually is preferred if the patient will be in Fowler's or sitting position. These Mayo stands are placed above and lateral to drapes over the patient. Mayo stands are also used for microneurosurgical procedures.

12 Armamentarium may include air-powered instruments for cutting through the skull. For cranial surgery, a dura guard attachment must be used to protect the dura mater.

Craniectomy

Craniectomy is removal (*-ectomy*) of a portion of the bones of the skull (*cranium*). Bone must be perforated or removed to approach the brain. This may be accomplished through one or more burr holes or twist drill holes. Each hole is drilled manually with a Hudson brace and burr or with an electric or air-powered instrument. ***Burr holes*** are approximately $\frac{1}{2}$ in. (13 mm) in diameter. Some diagnostic and therapeutic procedures are performed through them. Additional bone may be removed with a rongeur to increase exposure of the brain for more extensive procedures, such as an approach to the cranial nerves or tumors in the posterior fossa or suboccipital region.

Bone may be cut between the burr holes with a flexible multifilament wire (Gigli saw) or air-powered craniotome. This is performed to raise a large area of bone for temporary or permanent removal. Attached to the muscle, which acts as a hinge, the bone may be turned back to expose the underlying dura. This is referred to as raising a *bone flap.*

Burr holes may be plugged with a soft, pliable silicone, disc-shaped cover, with or without a channel for introduction of a hypodermic needle. The cover may be used to eliminate a cosmetically undesirable indentation of scalp into the surgically created bone defect. Postoperative access to the cranial cavity through the hole or channel in the burr hole cover can be used for drainage of fluid or installation of chemotherapeutic drugs. Intracranial pressure monitoring devices also can be attached.

A hollow subarachnoid screw, introduced into the subarachnoid space through a twist drill hole in the skull, may be preferred for continuous or intermittent intracranial pressure monitoring. An intraventricular catheter, inserted through a burr hole, may be preferred for installation of antibiotics directly into the ventricular system or for intracranial pressure monitoring.

Electrode plates of a brain pacemaker are implanted through small occipital and suboccipital craniectomies. Silicone-coated polyester fiber mesh plates, each with four pairs of platinum-disc electrodes, are applied to the anterior and posterior surfaces of the cerebellum. One or two receivers, implanted just below the clavicle prior to the craniectomies, are attached to the electrodes on the cerebellum by subcutaneously placed leads. Stimulation of the pacemaker electrodes is controlled by an external transmitter through an antenna placed on the skin over the subdermal receiver. This device is used to control muscular hypertonia and seizures related to cerebral palsy, epilepsy, stroke, or brain injury.

Craniotomy

Scalp, bone, and dural flaps are raised to expose a large area of the cerebrum for exploration, definitive treatment, or excision of lesions within the brain. The three semicircular or U-shaped flaps are turned in opposite directions. Hemostatic forceps or compression clips designed to control bleeding from the scalp are applied to the galea and over the edge of the skin flap. The bone flap is turned as described for craniectomy. Moistened sponges protect both the scalp and bone flaps. The dural flap is protected with large compressed patties. For wound closure, the thin but tough fibrous dural flap is laid over the brain. Usually it is sutured with many interrupted stitches to provide a tight seal that prevents leakage of cerebrospinal fluid. The bone flap may be anchored with stainless steel suture or silicone burr hole buttons. The galea is closed with interrupted sutures before the scalp is sutured or approximated with staples.

A silicone rubber suction drain may be placed in the subdural space to drain residual fluid from a subdural hematoma or the bed of a brain tumor, or to remove red blood cells in cerebrospinal fluid after craniotomy.

Intracranial tumors can originate from the neural tissues of the brain itself, the meninges, glandular tissue, choroid plexuses, cranial nerves, blood vessels, embryonal defects, or metastatic lesions. A craniotomy may be performed to remove a circumscribed, encapsulated, slow-growing, benign brain tumor. Some of these tumors, such as a meningioma, are highly vascular. Primary or metastatic malignant tumors are broadly classified as *gliomas.* These have an unregulated cellular proliferation of rapidly growing cells, which invade surrounding brain tissue. *Glioblastoma multiforme* is the most common and most malignant type of brain tumor. Anatomical location makes many tumors impossible to remove. Due to the hemorrhagic and edematous effects of a rapidly growing tumor, a lobectomy may be performed to give the brain area for expansion and to impede mortality. The rigid characteristics of the skull prevent its expansion or contraction; however, the brain can expand or contract. Subdural decompression by craniectomy to reduce intracranial pressure and papilledema may be the palliative procedure of choice. By anatomic location, some benign tumors are considered malignant because they cannot be safely removed without severe neurological deficits or threat to life-sustaining functions.

Cranioplasty

Traumatic or surgically created skull defects are corrected with autogenous bone grafts or a synthetic or metallic prosthesis. Large defects in the anterior or middle fossae are covered to protect the brain and for cosmetic effect. The bone flap may be removed following intracranial operation to allow cerebral decompression postoperatively. It is stored under sterile conditions in the bone bank until it can be positioned in the skull.

Bone removed because of an extensively comminuted fracture or bone disease may be replaced with methyl methacrylate. This material contours better than preformed metal plates. The resin powder is mixed with the liquid polymer to form a doughy mass. This is placed in a sterile plastic bag and rolled to the thickness of the skull with a roller. It is then, while still pliable, molded to the contour of the head and the size of the defect. When hardened, it can be trimmed with a rongeur and the edges smoothed with a special small emery wheel mounted on the electric bone saw. The prosthesis is wired to the skull in several places. The brain expands to meet it and leaves no dead space between it and the dura.

> NOTE. The outside of the ampuls of resin powder and liquid polymer and the mixing bag must be sterile. They can be sterilized in ethylene oxide gas or immersed for 10 hours in glutaraldehyde solution. The roller and emery wheel can be steam-sterilized.

Dural defects can be closed with freeze-dried human cadaver dura mater grafts. A trimmed and measured piece of dura mater is freeze-dried, sterilized by exposure to ethylene oxide, and stored in a vacuum container. This may be stored at room temperature indefinitely provided the vacuum is present. The graft is reconstituted by the addition of saline to the container for a minimum of 30 minutes. The majority of these grafts are used for closure of dural defects, but also may be used to repair abdominal and thoracic wall defects.

Intracranial Microneurosurgery

The magnification and lighting afforded by the operating microscope has refined techniques and made possible approaches to many neurosurgical problems. Refer to Chapter 16 for discussion of the operating microscope. Intracranial microneurosurgical procedures include the following.

Excision of Acoustic Neuroma A translabyrinthine approach may be used by the otologist for removal of an acoustic neuroma near the auditory canal (refer to Chap. 23, p. 416). A neurosurgeon resects an acoustic neuroma that more commonly extends into the cranial cavity. An acoustic neuroma progressively can grow into the trigeminal, facial, and abducens nerves, and into the cerebellopontine angle (the area between the pons, medulla oblongata, and cerebellum). Potentially life-threatening, symptoms of these involvements are manifested by facial weakness, paresthesia, and dysphagia.

The suboccipital retrolabyrinthine approach of the neurosurgeon, utilizing the operating microscope, offers the advantage of resecting neuromas with potential for preservation of functional hearing. Particular caution must be taken to obtain meticulous hemostasis, avoid trauma to or resection of the facial nerve, and spare the auditory artery if hearing is to be preserved. It is impossible, however, to salvage facial nerve function in a percentage of patients.

Decompression of Cranial Nerves Microsurgical exploration of cranial nerves with definitive decompression relieves the severe and disabling symptoms of some cranial nerve disorders such as trigeminal or glossopharyngeal neuralgia, acoustic nerve dysfunction, and hemifacial spasm. Initial symptoms of hyperactivity in a cranial nerve can progress to loss of function. Some of these disorders are due to mechanical cross-compression, usually vascular, of the nerve root at the brainstem. Symptoms are dependent upon the sensory and/or motor functions of the nerve.

With the patient in sitting position, a retromastoid craniectomy is performed to explore the cerebellopontine angle. A supracerebellar exposure is used for the trigeminal nerve, and an infracerebellar exposure for the remainder of the cranial nerves. An artery or vein compressing the nerve root may be mobilized away from the nerve. Preoperatively undiagnosed tumors are excised.

Cerebral Revascularization Anastomosis of an extracranial artery to an intracranial artery for bypass of stenotic or occlusive vascular disease distal to the bifurcation of the common carotids provides an additional and significant source of blood to the cerebral circulation. An artery in the scalp such as the superficial temporal, occipital, or another branch of the external carotid artery is anastomosed to a branch of the middle cerebral artery or a cortical branch of the cerebral. The vessels must be 1 mm in diameter or larger. The procedure is primarily prophylactic to prevent the development of a major ischemic stroke in patients who have had transient ischemic attacks or minor strokes with temporary disruption of brain function due to blockage of the cerebral vascular system.

The patient is positioned laterally with the head stabilized flat on the operating table for an approach through a temporal craniectomy. The anastomosis is made on the surface of the brain. Because this operation may take 7 to 10 hours to complete, the circulating nurse must check pressure points on the patient's body to prevent peripheral nerve and circulatory damage.

Occlusion of Aneurysms Aneurysms of the cerebral and vertebral arteries vary from the size of a pea to the size of an orange. Most intracranial aneurysms are located near the basilar surface of the skull and arise from the internal carotid or middle cerebral arteries. Cerebral artery (berry) aneurysms usually are located on the circle of Willis at the base of the brain between the hemispheres of the cerebrum. Most aneurysms are associated with a congenital defect of the media of the intracranial vessel wall. Hemodynamic forces of pulsatile pressure cause enlargement, outpouching and thinning of the arterial wall, which eventually ruptures. This is the most common source of subarachnoid hemorrhage. The majority of aneurysms seal spontaneously, but operation may be indicated to prevent rebleed. If diagnosed, an unruptured asymptomatic aneurysm may be operated prior to rupture.

With the patient in sitting position for suboccipital or subfrontal craniectomy, the aneurysm is exposed for occlusion. The neck (base) is clipped or ligated if it can be isolated. If it cannot be isolated, the aneurysm and parent vessel may be wrapped in fine mesh gauze and coated with methyl methacrylate, ethyl 2-cyanoacrylate, or other epoxy resin to reinforce the wall. Induced hypotension may be used to decrease blood flow in the artery feeding the aneurysm. This aids in dissection and occlusion. The operating microscope is used for delicate dissection of the arteries at the base of the brain.

Extracranial Operations

The cranial procedures previously discussed include access to the operative site through the skull. A few cranial neurosurgical procedures do not require craniectomy or intracranial incision.

External Occlusion of the Carotid Artery When an internal carotid or middle cerebral artery aneurysm cannot be reached or controlled by other operative techniques, a carotid clamp can be applied extracranially. Progressive turns of the clamp in the neck, over several days, cause it to occlude the carotid artery gradually until complete occlusion of blood supply to the aneurysm is accomplished.

Transsphenoidal Operations As a palliative operation, *hypophysectomy,* the enucleation of the pituitary gland, may be performed for pain relief and endocrine ablation in patients with disseminated metastatic carcinoma of the breast or prostate gland, or to relieve intractable pain from other types of disseminated carcinoma. The microsurgical transsphenoidal approach also is used for removal of intrapituitary tumors or other lesions within the region of the sella turcica. Visual loss and endocrinopathy are the main symptoms of pituitary tumor. Tumor tissue in the sella turcica is distinguished both by color and texture from the normal firm, yellowish anterior and red-gray posterior lobes of the pituitary.

The patient is placed in semi-Fowler's position with one anterior thigh exposed. A fascia, muscle, or fat graft may be needed to pack the sella turcica, so this area is prepped and draped also. The head is slightly flexed and tilted so the patient's body is out of the way when the neurosurgeon sits in front of the face to work in the median sagittal plane. The image intensifier is positioned lateral to the patient's head with the horizontal beam centered on the sella turcica. The television monitor is placed behind and just above the patient's head, so the surgeon can look at the screen in line with the binocular of the microscope. Televised radiofluoroscopy is used as an aid in placing instruments and resecting tissue. The image intensifier is switched on and off, as needed, to minimize exposure to radiation.

The floor of the sella turcica is exposed through the sphenoid sinus. A horizontal incision is made under the upper lip, at the junction of gingiva, and carried deep to the bone of the maxilla. Soft tissues are elevated; bone and nasal cartilage are resected. The resected nasal cartilage is preserved on the instrument table for possible replacement. A specially designed nasal speculum is inserted in the oral incision to visualize the sphenoid sinus. This is opened widely until the floor of the sella turcica can be identified. The floor is opened with an air-powered drill. The microscope is brought into position for visualization of the pituitary, other structures and lesions inside and around the sella turcica.

Stereotaxis

Stereotaxis is the accurate location of a definite circumscribed area within the brain from external points or landmarks of the skull. The technique is used to create a lesion in otherwise inaccessible parts of the brain. Operations usually are performed under local or neuroleptic anesthesia because patient cooperation to test motor or sensory function may be needed during the operation.

A *stereoencephalotome,* a specially designed mechanical apparatus, is attached to the skull. With the patient in sitting position, steel screws are tapped through each of four burr holes for fixation of the apparatus and the head. A fifth burr hole is made for positioning the instrument that will make the lesion, and a sixth for introduction of a Scott ventricular cannula for ventriculogram. By determining specific reference points on x-ray, the exact area of the brain for creation of the lesion can be calculated. The lesion may be made by electrocoagulation, freezing (cryosurgery), ultrasound, injection of a chemical or radioactive agent, or mechanical curettage.

Thalmotomy The procedure most frequently performed using stereotaxis, thalmotomy may be done to relieve involuntary tremor or rigidity of muscles, to reduce intractable pain, or to control functional psychotic behavior.

Cingulotomy Cingulotomies are appropriate treatment for relief of pain of benign etiology that has not responded to other methods of treatment. The *cingulum* is a bundle of connecting fibers in the medial aspect of each cerebral hemisphere, between the frontal and temporal lobes. Bilaterally symmetrical radio-frequency lesions are placed with the aid of a stereoencephalotome and x-ray control.

Electrical Stimulation Intermittent electrical stimulation of the brain by stereotaxically implanted electrodes can control a variety of intractable pain problems. One electrode is placed in the somatosensory system to evaluate pain of central origin, and another in the paraventricular gray matter for pain of peripheral origin. Following postoperative evaluation of the effectiveness of electrical stimulation of each electrode, the patient returns to the OR to have a receiver placed under the skin on the anterior chest wall. A connecting wire is tunneled from the receiver to the electrode. An external transmitter and antenna placed over the receiver stimulate the electrode as desired by the patient.

Radio-Frequency Retrogasserian Rhizotomy This procedure relieves the pain of trigeminal neuralgia, also known as *tic douloureux.* The fifth cranial nerve, the trigeminal, carries sensory impulses for touch, pain, and external temperature from the face, scalp, and mucous membranes in the head. Trigeminal neuralgia is an intense paroxysmal pain in one side of the face. It can be controlled by damaging the gasserian (trigeminal) ganglion.

The patient lies in supine position. Using x-rays for control, an insulated cannula with an uninsulated tip is placed through the cheek and foramen ovale, and is advanced to the gasserian ganglion. The ganglion is coagulated when a radio-frequency generator activates the tip of the cannula. Several lesions can be made to achieve the desired extent of paresthesia.

Cryohypophysectomy The cryosurgical probe is introduced into the sella turcica through a frontal burr hole. Cryogenic lesions may be the procedure of choice for treating growth-hormone-producing pituitary adenomas with no suprasellar extension. During creation of the lesion, ocular movements and visual acuity are carefully monitored.

Radioactive seeds also may be stereotaxically implanted into the pituitary for interstitial irradiation (refer to Chap. 27).

Intracranial Aneurysm Thrombosis Thrombosis of a cerebral aneurysm can be accomplished by a stereotaxic magnetic-metallic technique. Tiny particles of iron are injected through a magnetic field into the aneurysm. The purpose is to reinforce the wall of the aneurysm by forming a firm scar that will not grow.

Embolization of arteriovenous malformations also are performed for large dural and many otherwise inoperable cerebral arteriovenous malformations. Some aneurysms or arteriovenous malformations can be electrocoagulated or clipped through stereotaxic instruments.

Head Injuries

When injuries occur in other parts of the body, the head is often injured also. A patient with severe head injury requires *first* a patent airway. Relaxed jaw and tongue should be raised; if necessary, suction through the mouth. An endotracheal tube may be inserted. Ultimately a tracheotomy may be necessary.

Vital signs, blood pressure, dilatation of pupils, and level of consciousness are checked frequently. Osmotic dehydrating IV solution, such as mannitol, may be ordered to reduce cerebral edema if there is no evidence of intracranial hemorrhage. After these supportive measures have been carried out, definitive treatments are initiated.

1 Scalp lacerations are thoroughly cleansed, debrided, and sutured. The scalp is very vascular, so lacerations bleed profusely. Hypovolemic shock is rare, but possible.
2 Simple linear or comminuted fractures usually require no treatment. A depressed skull fracture must be elevated when bone is pressed 5 mm or more into any part of the brain.
3 A compound fracture requires debridement. The extent of operation will depend upon the specific extent of injury. Dura may need to be sutured. Some macerated brain tissue may have to be excised.
4 Intracranial hematoma may be present. Depending on location, intracranial hemorrhage may require immediate, emergency operation.
  a *Epidural hematoma.* Bleeding due to rupture or tear of the middle meningeal artery, or its branches, forms a hematoma between the skull and dura. Usually associated with a skull fracture, symptoms of increased intracranial pressure due to rapid compression of the brain may occur immediately or within a few hours. When hemorrhage is arterial, the patient presents an extreme surgical emergency to evacuate the clot and clip or electrocoagulate the bleeding vessel through a burr hole or small craniectomy.
  b *Subdural hematoma.* Bleeding between the dura mater and arachnoid usually is caused by laceration of the veins that cross the subdural space. A large, encapsulated collection of blood over one or both cerebral hemispheres produces increased intracranial pressure and other neurologic changes. Onset and extent of these changes depends on the cause, size, and rapidity of growth of the hematoma. Treatment may necessitate a burr hole. A bone flap may be raised if more extensive exploration is indicated. Subdural hematoma may be:
    (1) Acute. Usually due to arterial bleeding, symptoms occur rapidly. The vessel must be ligated with clips or electrocoagulated.
    (2) Subacute. Usually due to venous bleeding, symptoms appear within 24 to 48 hours to 5 days after injury.
    (3) Chronic. Symptoms do not appear until 6 or more months postinjury.
  c *Intracerebral hematoma.* Tears in the substance of the brain at the point of greatest impact most commonly occur in the anterior temporal and frontal lobes. Although usually absorbed, hematoma may require evacuation and debridement of necrotic tissue.

SPINAL SURGERY

The bony structure of the vertebral column extends from the foramen magnum at the base of the skull to the coccyx. The 33 vertebrae, which provide support for the body, vary in size and are classified according to location: the 7 cervical vertebrae are in the neck; the 12 thoracic vertebrae articulate with the ribs; the 5 lumbar vertebrae are posterior to the retroperitoneal cavity; the 5 sacral vertebrae are fused to form the sacrum; and the 4 fused coccygeal vertebrae form the coccyx. The spinal cord passes through a canal in the cervical and thoracic vertebrae to a level of the second or third lumbar vertebra. It terminates in a fibrous band that extends through the lumbar vertebrae and sacrum and attaches to the coccyx. Pairs of spinal nerve roots branch off to each side of the body from 31 segments of the spinal cord as it passes through the vertebrae. They carry sensory and motor impulses between the central nervous system and the peripheral nervous system.

Because of the proximity of the vertebral column to the spinal cord, both neurosurgeons and orthopaedic surgeons perform operations in this area. They may work together as a multidisciplinary team. For example, the neurosurgeon may remove a herniated lumbar intervertebral disk and the orthopaedist will do the spinal fusion (refer to Chap. 20). Only the most common operations for spinal lesions performed by the neurosurgeon will be described.

Laminectomy

Removal of the spinous process(es) and lamina from one of more vertebra is performed to expose an intervertebral or spinal cord lesion. A laminectomy usually is carried out through a vertical midline skin incision with the patient in prone or lateral position. However, some neurosurgeons prefer a transverse skin incision with patient in modified prone position. The extent of the incision will depend on the number of laminae to be removed. The fascia and muscles are retracted to expose the spinous processes and laminae. These are cut off with a rongeur, as necessary for exposure of the spinal cord dura, the spinal nerve roots, or an interlaminar lesion. An intervertebral disk, spinal cord tumor, bone fragments, and extradural or intradural foreign bodies may be removed after the laminectomy is completed.

Diskectomy Herniated or ruptured intervertebral disks are the most common spinal problems seen by neurosurgeons. Most of these occur in the lower lumbar and lumbosacral regions and are traumatic in origin. Displaced intervertebral disks are rare in the thoracic area, but do occur in the cervical spine. Normally intervertebral disks are held between each vertebral body by the annulus fibrosis and posterior longitudinal ligament. The disk itself is a fibrocartilaginous substance known as the *nucleus pulposus.* Under stress of lifting or twisting, the nucleus pulposus can protrude through a tear in the annulus fibrosis and posterior ligament. The protrusion compresses the spinal nerve roots within the spinal canal against the vertebrae. This causes pain from the lumbar or sacral region to the lower back and radiating down the sciatic nerve pathway to one leg, or from the cervical region of the neck to an arm. At operation, the herniated nucleus pulposus or ruptured portion of the annulus fibrosis is excised.

Excision of Spinal Cord Tumor Primary tumors of the spinal cord include ependymoma, lipoma, meningioma, and neurofibroma. The posterior segment of the vertebral arch must be removed to expose the dura over the involved section of the spinal cord. The dura is incised and retracted with sutures. The tumor is excised and the dura closed tightly to prevent leakage of cerebrospinal fluid.

Rhizotomy Anterior motor roots of spinal nerves can be divided to control the involuntary muscle contractions associated with torticollis and spastic paralysis. Cutting the roots of the cervical spinal nerves controlling the neck muscles, for example, relieves the muscular imbalance that causes the head to rotate intermittently and tilt significantly in patients with torticollis.

Treatment of Spinal Injuries Vertebral fractures, with or without dislocation, can cause spinal cord compression that denervates the nerve tracts below the injury. The resultant paralysis may be relieved if operation is done within a very short time after injury. Results are frequently discouraging. Damage to the cord may be too extensive for return of function or, at best, only an incomplete return. Care must be taken in moving a patient with a spinal injury to avoid further paralysis.

A lumbar puncture with pressure readings may be done. If a block in flow of spinal fluid is present, a laminectomy is done to decompress the spinal cord in a patient with complete paralysis or partial paralysis that is becoming progressively worse. Laminectomy also may be done to remove bone fragments.

Anterior Cervical Operations

The anterior cervical spine can be exposed through a transverse skin incision in the neck and dissection through the cleavage plane between the carotid artery and esophagus. The spinous processes and laminae remain intact. A ruptured intervertebral disk and/or a fracture-dislocation with bone fragments compressing the cervical spinal cord or nerve roots can be completely explored. Removal of the posterior margins of the vertebral bodies may be indicated to decompress the nerve root. A bone graft may be placed between the vertebral bodies for interbody fusion, usually by an orthopaedic surgeon.

The operating microscope is a valuable adjunct to anterior cervical intervertebral diskectomy and for an anterior approach to other cervical spinal lesions.

Cervical Traction

To stabilize the head and neck of a patient with cervical spine injury, traction is applied by means of a Sayre sling as an emergency measure. A Sayre sling is a canvas or leather halter that buckles around the neck and chin. The patient lies with head at the foot of the bed, to permit traction appliances to be attached to the footboard. Countertraction is accomplished by the weight of the patient, who rests in bed in semi-Fowler's position.

If the patient has a cervical fracture and/or dislocation, the Sayre sling may be replaced, in the OR, by Vinke or Crutchfield tongs for skeletal traction. A sterile table setup with a dissecting set of instruments and a drill is necessary. Through a small incision over the lateral parietal bones on each side of the head, holes are drilled in the skull for positioning the mechanical apparatus. The pins of Crutchfield tongs, when tightened, are controlled by a locking and positioning mechanism that forces the points of the pins medially and upward away from the inner table of the skull. Traction is then transferred from the Sayre sling to the tongs giving the patient free movement of the jaw. The amount of weight applied to the tongs will depend on the extent of injury and weight of the patient.

Relief of Intractable Pain

Many patients suffer intractable pain in advanced stages of some illnesses such as cancer, occlusive arterial disease, myelinating or degenerative diseases, or from some benign lesions. Intractable pain cannot be relieved satisfactorily by drugs without the hazard of narcotic addiction or incapacitating sedation. Operative techniques may be indicated to interrupt the sensory fibers carrying pain sensations through the spinal cord to the brain.

Anterior Cervical Chordotomy Exposure of the cervical spinal cord, through an anterior approach, can be used to sever sensory fibers at the base of the brainstem. A microsurgical technique may be used for this procedure. Good relief from severe pain of advanced carcinoma may be achieved.

Commissural Myelotomy Commissural or sagittal midline myelotomy may be preferred to relieve intractable midline or bilateral pain in the lower half of the body. The sensory nerve fibers of the cervical or thoracic spinal cord are exposed and severed. The operating microscope is a valuable aid to the neurosurgeon in identifying the nerve tracts to be cut or resected.

Percutaneous Cervical Chordotomy To avoid an open operation, a percutaneous approach may be used to destroy sensory fibers. Under local anesthesia, a spinal needle is introduced just below the ear into a cervical interspace. The neurosurgeon avoids the pyramidal tract that carries motor impulses. The position of the needle is checked on x-ray or image intensifier. An electrode wire, inserted through the needle, is connected to a radiofrequency lesion generator. The fibers are destroyed when the positive charge is activated through the electrode. The patient retains sense of touch but not pain.

Electrical Stimulation Chronic intractable pain of organic origin may be relieved by electrical stimulation in some selected patients. Fibers of the peripheral nerves conduct pain impulses to the spinal cord. These pain impulses can be blocked by induced electrical stimulation that modifies the impulses transmitted from peripheral nerve receptors through the spinal cord to the brain. Electrodes to transmit an electric current to the spinal cord or peripheral nerve are placed transcutaneously, percutaneously, or implanted.

Transcutaneous Neural Stimulation (TNS) This is applied to the surface of the skin over the spinal cord or a peripheral nerve. These devices are used for many types of chronic pain problems.

Percutaneous Stimulation This is achieved by inserting an electrode into the spinal canal or subcutaneous tissue adjacent to the peripheral nerve. This is performed in the OR or radiology department under local anesthesia, fluoroscopic control, and sterile conditions. The patient is prepped and draped as for an invasive procedure. For spinal cord stimulation, two platinum-tipped electrodes are threaded cephalad through needles placed in the epidural space. After the electrodes are connected to a percutaneous transmitter, they are manipulated until the patient feels paresthesia in the desired area. When in the correct position, the electrodes are secured to the lumbodorsal fascia by Silastic patches. The distal ends are attached to a lead wire brought through the skin. This connects to an external transmitter for temporary stimulation. When conversion is to be made from temporary to permanent stimulation, the electrodes are attached to a receiver implanted in the lateral chest wall, usually on the left side midway between the axilla and waistline. An antenna, placed on the skin over the implanted receiver, connects to the external transmitter.

Dorsal Column Stimulator (DCS) This operates on the same principle as the percutaneous stimulator. However, a laminectomy must be performed to suture the electrode over the dorsal column of the spinal cord. For permanent peripheral nerve stimulation, the electrode is attached to a major sensory nerve. The receivers for these stimulators are implanted in subcutaneous tissues.

PERIPHERAL NERVE SURGERY

The peripheral nervous system includes the cranial nerves, spinal nerves, and the autonomic nervous system located outside the central nervous system. *Ganglions,* a group of nerve cell bodies also located outside the CNS, can transmit either *autonomic* (involuntary) or *somatic* (both reflex and voluntary) impulses. *Somatic nerves* supply voluntary muscles, skin, tendons, joints, and other structures controlling the musculoskeletal system. *Afferent nerve fibers* carry sensory impulses from the organs and muscles to the CNS. *Efferent fibers* transmit motor impulses from the CNS back to them. Peripheral nerve operations are performed on both the autonomic and somatic nervous systems. The neurosurgeon may identify nerves and test function with a nerve stimulator before or after dissection or repair.

Autonomic Nervous System

The autonomic nervous system is an aggregation of ganglions, nerves, and plexuses through which the viscera, heart, blood vessels, smooth muscles, and glands receive motor innervation to function involuntarily. This system is divided into:

1 *Sympathetic nervous system.* This thoracolumbar division arising from the thoracic and first three lumbar segments of the spinal cord includes the ganglionated trunk near the spinal cord, plexuses, and the associated preganglionic and postganglionic nerve fibers. The efferent fibers transmit impulses that stimulate involuntary activity in the heart, blood vessels, smooth muscle of the viscera, and all glands in the body.

2 *Parasympathetic nervous system.* This craniosacral division includes the preganglionic fibers that leave the CNS with cranial nerves III, VII, IX, and X and the first three sacral nerves, outlying ganglions near the viscera, and postganglionic fibers. In general, this system innervates the same structures, but has a regulatory function opposite to that of the sympathetic nervous system. These efferent fibers act to restore stability for quieter activity.

Operations most frequently performed on the autonomic nervous system are discussed.

Sympathectomy Resection or division of the sympathetic ganglions and nerve fibers of the autonomic nervous system is performed in an attempt to increase peripheral circulation or to decrease pain of peripheral vascular disease or intractable pain of other organic origin. It may be an emergency procedure to relieve severe vasospasm following arterial embolism or freezing of an extremity. The paravertebral ganglionic chains and/or nerve fibers that innervate the affected area are resected or divided. The procedure may be termed a *sympathetic ganglionectomy* or *splanchniectomy,* but usually the operation is specified by the location of the ganglions and nerves. (General surgeons also perform some of the following operations.)

Upper Cervical Sympathectomy This is done to increase blood supply in the internal carotid arteries. Through an anterior cervical approach in the neck, the superior cervical ganglion is resected. Ptosis of the eyelid may occur postoperatively because this ganglion innervates eyelid retraction.

Cervicothoracic Sympathectomy This may aid the patient with Raynaud's disease of the upper extremities by relieving the chronic vasoconstrictive process. It also may be done to relieve angina pectoris or causalgia. Through a transaxillary-transpleural incision, the stellate ganglion of the middle cervical ganglionic chain is hemisected and the lower half resected along with the second through fifth thoracic nerve ganglions.

Thoracic Sympathectomy This is usually done for the relief of chronic intractable pain of biliary and pancreatic diseases. Through a posterior paravertebral incision over the transverse processes of the thoracic vertebrae, the ganglions of the sixth through twelfth thoracic nerves are resected and the splanchnic nerves divided.

Thoracolumbar Sympathectomy This procedure is performed for the treatment of essential hypertension. Usually done in two stages, bilateral resection is necessary to reduce blood pressure by altering vascular tone and denervating the viscera. With the patient in prone or lateral position, a paravertebral incision parallel to the vertebral column extends from the ninth rib downward and then curves anteriorly toward the iliac crest. The lower half of the thoracic and the first through third lumbar chains with the ganglions and splanchnic nerves are resected.

Lumbar Sympathectomy This may be of some value in the treatment of vasospastic disease such as Buerger's disease, ischemic ulcers of the lower extremities due to vasospasm of the peripheral vessels, and some types of causalgia. Usually through a flank incision, the lumbar chain and ganglions located in the retroperitoneal space between the vertebral column and the psoas muscle are resected from above the second to below the third ganglions.

Presacral Neurectomy The hypogastric nerve plexus may be resected for relief of idiopathic intractable dysmenorrhea.

Somatic Nervous System

As the cranial and spinal nerves extend out from the CNS into plexuses and peripheral nerve branches through the body, the somatic nervous system provides involuntary control over sensations and both voluntary and involuntary control over muscles. Loss of sensation and muscular control occurs distal to the site of severed or compressed nerve fibers. Sensation and function will be restored only if regeneration of the nerve axons takes place distally from an unobstructed axis cylinder proximal to the site of disruption.

Most peripheral nerve surgery is performed to repair traumatic nerve injury in an extremity. However, dissection also is done to remove tumors or relieve pain. Etiology determines the location and length of the skin incision.

Neurorrhaphy The suturing of a divided nerve must provide precise approximation of the nerve ends if function is to be restored. Primary repair may be accomplished by suturing the *epineurium,* the outer sheath. Under magnification of the operating microscope, accurate fascicular alignment and perineural suturing of larger nerve bundles are the desired technique to enhance regeneration of function. For a successful result, however, nerves must not be repaired under tension. Primary repair soon after injury may be advantageous to align the fascicles.

A tumor, such as a neurofibroma or posttraumatic neuroma, is excised. If the nerve ends can be brought together without tension, they are anastomosed. Silastic membrane may be wrapped around the anastomosis to prevent adhesions with the surrounding tissue.

Neurolysis Freeing of a nerve from adhesions relieves pain and restores function. Carpal tunnel syndrome, for example, a neuropathy caused by entrapment of the median nerve, produces tingling and numbness over all or part of the hand and compromises hand functions. Release of the transverse carpal ligament overriding the nerve affords relief of this syndrome.

Neurotomy, Neurectomy, and Neurexeresis These procedures may be performed to relieve localized peripheral pain.

Chapter 25

Plastic and Reconstructive Surgery

"Plastic surgery is surgery dealing with restoration of wounded, disfigured, or unsightly parts of the body. It includes cosmetic surgery or cosmetic corrections not necessarily related to the physical health or safety of the patient. The word 'plastic' in its classic sense means 'giving form or fashion to matter.' As used in plastic surgery, the word bears no relationship to the current concept of plastic materials and products."*

However, autografts, allografts, or prosthetic implants may be used to improve or restore contour defects or functional malformations due to congenital, developmental, or traumatic disfigurements. Elective operations desired by an individual in an attempt to improve appearance for psychological well-being are classified as aesthetic or cosmetic surgery. Thus the plastic surgeon's hand extends to alteration of cosmetically unacceptable body contours, as well as to repair and reconstruction of tissue injuries. Plastic surgeons have a philosophy about how tissues can be handled, and a technique for handling them that heals the patient's body and mind, limited only by the surgeon's ingenuity.

*The American Society of Plastic and Reconstructive Surgeons, Inc.

DEVELOPMENT OF PLASTIC SURGERY

Plastic surgery was probably the first form of surgery. Egyptian papyrus scrolls tell of skin grafts and pedicle flaps to replace deficiencies in tissue as early as 3500 years ago. Egyptian mummies have been found with artificial ears and noses. In India over 2000 years ago, the Hindus became skilled in transferring tissue to form noses for those who had lost them as a punishment. These ancient records verify attempts to improve people's appearance.

Two centuries ago, some plastic surgery was done in Europe. The beginning of the present interest and the great strides that have been made in plastic surgery began when Reverdin used pinch grafts. He reported his work with them in 1869. But the transplantation of skin met with mediocre success until World War I.

In the twilight of the nineteenth and the dawn of the twentieth centuries, descriptions of "featural surgery" performed by "cosmetic surgeons" were brazenly advertised, often with unwarranted claims of success. Charles Conrad Miller (1880–1950) has been called both "the father of modern cosmetic surgery" and "an unabashed quack." Practicing in Chicago, Miller began around 1904 to improvise surgical procedures to alter facial features. He did them in his office under local anesthesia, employing a gentle technique of lifting structures by lenticular or crescent excisions and lowering tissues by excisions and vertical closures. He preferred to sew with fine needles and cautioned not to tie sutures tightly as this might cause suture marks. His text, first published in 1907 and expanded in 1925, described cosmetic procedures for upper and lower lid blepharoplasty, subcutaneous sectioning of facial muscles, incisions to change lip posture, and a variety of rhinoplastic techniques.

Vilray Papin Blair became a prominent plastic surgeon when, in 1906, he published the results of closed ramisection of the mandible for micrognathia and prognathism. Within a short time, physicians from all over the United States and Europe sent patients to see Blair in St. Louis, Missouri, for jaw reconstruction and other facial surgery.

Sir Arbuthnot Lane, a contemporary of Miller and Blair, was doing cleft lip, cleft palate, and some mandibular surgery in England. When Blair arrived in England in 1918 as Chief of Plastic and Oral Surgery for the American armed forces, he visited the center Lane had established for treatment of soldiers with facial injuries arriving from the battlefront. The work being done there by Harold Gillies impressed Blair. The high quality of work done at this and other centers during World War I on facial injuries, burns, and reconstruction of other injured parts of the body did much to establish plastic surgery as a surgical specialty.

Upon his return to St. Louis after the war, Blair established the first plastic surgery service in the United States at Barnes Hospital and Washington University.

During World War II, the development of military plastic surgery centers led to rapid progress in the rehabilitation of casualties with maxillofacial and hand injuries. Plastic surgeons worked closely with other specialists in treating many types of war injuries. They found that by replacing lost skin with grafts, fractures under these areas healed better and more quickly and parts returned to normal function sooner.

Today's plastic surgery is largely the refinement of techniques developed during World Wars I and II to restore men disfigured by the ravages of war. These techniques are not only imaginative but precise. They are imaginative because plastic surgeons reshape and replant living tissue and augment tissue with prosthetic implants.

One of the most imaginative surgeons of modern times is Paul L. Tessier of Paris. In 1967, he reported his work to surgically correct gross facial and skull deformities of children with Crouzon's and Apert's syndromes. Tessier's results have had a monumental impact on the development of craniofacial surgery as a new surgical subspecialty. Surgeons are able to systematically dismantle, rearrange, and reconstruct the entire musculoskeletal system between the top of the head and the oral cavity. This requires a multidisciplinary team with a plastic surgeon, neurosurgeon, anesthesiologist, ophthalmologist, oral surgeon, and otorhinolaryngologist. Special craniofacial centers have been established for these complex procedures.

Plastic surgery has been called the "surgery of millimeters" because of the critical margin between good and poor cosmetic results. Each millimeter lack or excess of tissue can have an extreme psychological impact on the patient. If the patient thinks his or her appearance has improved, personality and self-image improve and others respond more positively to him or her.

Plastic surgery has been extended by increased knowledge of the principles and techniques of microvascular anastomosis for replantation and transplantation of tissue.

SPECIAL FEATURES OF PLASTIC SURGERY

Scars are inevitable whenever skin is incised or excised, either intentionally by the surgeon's scalpel or accidentally by trauma. The plastic surgeon attempts to minimize scar formation by meticulous realignment and approximation of underlying tissues and wound edges. The plastic surgeon makes the incision along natural skin lines whenever possible. Many plastic procedures involve only the subcuticular tissues and skin. Reconstructive procedures, however, may include manipulation of underying cartilage, bone, tendons, nerves, and blood vessels.

General Considerations

1 Colorless prep solution may be preferred so the plastic surgeon can observe the true skin color.

2 Sterile dye, such as methylene blue or brilliant green, is often used to outline areas for incision. This can be done with a sterile marking pen after the skin is prepped.

3 Exposure of both sides for comparison usually is required for operations on the face, ears, and neck.

4 Draping often exposes much skin surface, which is unavoidable. A fenestrated sheet frequently cannot be used. The opening does not give adequate exposure, especially for skin grafting procedures. Use towels, towel clips, minor and medium sheets under and around the areas, according to needs, to drape as much of the patient as possible.

5 Local anesthesia is used for many operations on adults. Ephinephrine may be added to help localize the agent, prolong the anesthetic action, and provide hemostasis. Short 26- or 30-gauge needles are used for injection.

6 Number 15 and 11 scalpel blades are routinely used to cut small structures.

7 Instruments must be small for handling delicate tissues. Iris scissors, mosquito hemostats, fine-tipped tissue forceps, and other small-scale cutting, holding, clamping, and exposing instruments are part of the routine plastic surgery setup.

8 Nerve stimulator may be used to help identify nerves, especially in craniofacial, neck, and hand reconstruction procedures.

9 Bone, cartilage, or skin grafts may be needed. Homografts may be obtained from the tissue bank rather than the patient's own tissues.

10 Silicone or other prosthetic implants are used in plastic surgery to reconstruct soft tissue and cartilage defects. They cannot be used unless there is adequate soft tissue coverage. They cannot be used in an infected area (refer to Chap. 13, p. 269, for discussion of handling silicone implants).

11 Small sponges, 2 by 2 or 3 by 3, are used in small areas. Compressed absorbent patties and peanut dissector sponges also may be used.

12 Suture must be of small diameter. Sizes 5-0, 6-0, and 7-0 usually are preferred for peripheral and small structures. The material varies by the personal preference of the plastic surgeon. However, synthetic nonabsorbable materials are more commonly used than natural nonabsorbable fibers and absorbable sutures.

13 Needles of small wire diameter with sharp cutting edges minimize trauma to superficial tissues. An appropriately fine-tipped needleholder must be used with these delicate, curved surgical needles.

14 Skin closure tapes may be used instead of skin sutures, especially to supplement a subcuticular closure if very close approximation of skin is required for good cosmetic results.

15 Fine mesh gauze usually is preferred as the initial dressing. This may be impregnated with petrolatum or an oil emulsion, with or without medication, to cover denuded areas. Several types of sterile nonadhering dressings are commercially available. Dry gauze is not used on a denuded area because it adheres, it acts as a foreign body, and granulations grow through it.

16 Pressure dressings frequently are used following extensive operations to splint soft tissues and prevent contractures. The mild pressure keeps fluid formation in tissues or under a skin graft to a minimum. Commercial dressings for various areas of the body are preferred by some plastic surgeons. (Refer to Chap. 8 for types of pressure dressings.)

17 Stent fixation is a method of obtaining pressure when it is impossible to bandage an area snugly, as the face or neck. A form-fitting mold may be taped over the nose. Long suture ends can be tied crisscrossed over a dressing to immobilize it and exert gentle pressure.

Categories of Plastic Surgery

Four main categories of problems are treated by plastic surgeons.

1 Congenital anomalies, especially in structure of the face and hands. The most commonly corrected anomalies are discussed in Chapter 26.

2 Cosmetic appearance, especially of the face and breasts.

3 Benign and malignant neoplasms, especially those leaving large soft tissue defects. Resection of extensive tumors other than those involving the skin or head and neck are not usually within the province of the plastic surgeon initially, but the patient may be referred for reconstructive surgery and rehabilitation.

4 Traumatically acquired disfigurements, especially facial lacerations, hand injuries, and burns. The objective of the plastic surgeon is to restore function as well as body image.

Tissue may be approximated, supplemented, excised, transferred, or transplanted. Many procedures are done in stages before complete reconstruction and restoration of function are achieved. Tissue flaps and grafts, prosthetic implants, and external prosthetic appliances may be required for functional and cosmetic restoration as a result of ablative surgery or trauma.

GRAFTING TECHNIQUES

Denuded areas of the body are resurfaced by transplanting or transferring segments of skin and other tissues from an uninjured area to the injured area. The plastic surgeon prefers to transfer tissues of compatible color and texture. Soft tissue autografts are used whenever possible. They are classified by the source of their vascular supply, essential for viability, as:

1 *Free graft.* Tissue is detached from the donor site and transplanted into the recipient site. It derives its vascular supply from the capillary ingrowth from the recipient site.

2 *Pedicle flap.* Tissue remains attached at one or both ends of the donor site during transfer to the recipient site. The vascular supply is maintained from the vessels preserved in the pedicle of the donor site.

Deformities caused by loss of soft tissue substance such as trauma of accidental injury, tumor resection, or radiation therapy may require a graft to fill in deficiencies in order to restore contours or to cover tendons and bones. Free grafts and pedicle flaps may be taken from various areas of the body to reconstruct soft tissue defects.

Free Skin Grafts

The epidermis including *corium,* the basal layer of the dermis that generates new skin, is transplanted from the donor site to a recipient site in which it becomes a part of the living tissue in that area. The depth of the graft will vary according to its purpose:

1 *Split-thickness graft.* The epidermis and half of the corium to a depth of .010 to .035 in. (.3 to 1 mm) is removed. The donor site heals uneventfully unless it becomes infected. Split-thickness grafts are widely used to cover large denuded areas on body surfaces as the back, trunk, and legs.

2 *Full-thickness graft.* The epidermis, corium, and subcutaneous fat at a depth greater than .035 in. (1 mm) is removed or elevated. Full-thickness grafts inhibit wound contraction better than split-thickness grafts and, therefore, may be preferred on the face, neck, hands, elbows, axillae, knees, and feet.

The desired thickness of a free skin graft is predetermined by the plastic surgeon before the skin is incised. The appropriate cutting instrument is selected to obtain the graft.

Dermatomes A dermatome is a cutting instrument designed to excise split-thickness skin grafts. The thickness of the graft can be calibrated by adjusting the depth gauge. The width of the graft is determined by the width of the cutting blade. Blades are detachable and many are disposable, which always ensures a sharp new blade for every patient. The length of the graft may be limited by the type of dermatome used.

Oscillating-Blade Type Brown and Hall dermatomes may be electrical or air-powered with compressed nitrogen. The length of the graft is limited only by the donor site. The surgeon checks the adjustable depth gauge before cutting the graft. The oscillating-blade dermatome usually is not used on the abdominal wall where underlying support is not firm. The oscillating blade, free of vibrations, takes an accurate graft from other donor sites.

NOTE. Extreme care should be used in handling these precision dermatomes. If electric, the circulating nurse should remove the foot pedal as soon as the graft is taken. If air-powered, the scrub nurse and surgeon should place a thumb under the lever on the handle while preparing the instrument for use. These dermatomes *cannot be immersed in water* nor put in a washer-sterilizer or ultrasonic cleaner. Follow manufacturer's instructions for use, care, and sterilization.

Drum Type Padgett and Reese dermatomes consist of one-half of a metal drum, which is one-half of a circle. A metal handle through the center of the drum has an arm on each end. These arms hold the bar that carries the blade. The bar swings around the drum to cut the graft. The size of the graft is limited by the width and length of the drum. An adhesive must be placed on both the skin surface and the drum to keep the skin in contact with the surface. The knife blade is moved from side to side as slight tension is exerted on the skin by rotating the drum. The drum-type dermatome is used on flat, open areas, as it is bulky. Its use is limited by body contour and amount of skin on the donor site.

Dermatome tape must be used with the Reese dermatome. Packaged sterile, the tape has an adhesive coating on each side covered with a paper backing. Remove the backing on one side and apply to the drum with care to line up the edges of the tape and the drum. After the backing paper is removed from the other side of the tape, the drum is placed on the skin, which adheres to it.

NOTE. When handling a drum-type dermatome, *always* grasp the blade carrier to prevent its swinging around the drum and seriously injuring your hands. Leave the dermatome in the rack when not in use or until the blade is removed.

Kinds of Free Skin Grafts

Split-Thickness Thiersch Graft Removed with a skin-graft knife or dermatome, Thiersch grafts are used to cover superficial defects. The surgeon may use sutures or skin staples along the edges of the graft to hold it to underlying subcutaneous tissue. This prevents movement and helps obliterate dead space in the recipient site. The skin of the donor site regenerates rapidly and the same area can be used again in 2 or 3 weeks if necessary, or sooner if a thin graft is taken, from an infection-free donor site.

Split-Thickness Meshgraft This graft makes it possible to obtain a greater area of coverage from a split-thickness skin graft. After removal with a dermatome, the graft is placed on a plastic dermacarrier, cut side down. This is a rigid base to keep the graft spread out flat while it is put through a mesh dermatome. This instrument cuts small parallel slits in the graft. When expanded, the slits become diamond-shaped openings. This permits expansion of the graft to cover three times as large an area as the original graft obtained from the donor site. The meshgraft can be placed over the recipient site with slight tension. The increased edge exposures are conducive to rapid epithelialization. The mesh minimizes serum accumulation. A piece of sterile nylon net may be applied over the grafted area to hold the graft in place.

Full-Thickness Wolfe Graft The graft is cut exactly to size and shape of the recipient site with a skin-graft knife, and sutured into place under normal skin tension. It is used on face, neck, or hands to fill in superficial denuded areas and over joints to prevent contractures. This graft does not become viable readily on granulated surfaces, and the amount that can be transferred is much more limited than in a Thiersch graft.

Full-Thickness Pinch Graft Small, full-thickness pieces of skin a few millimeters in diameter may be cut from the donor site with a razor. A fine-tissue forceps or a sharp straight needle is used to pick up and hold the skin taut while it is cut. These bits of skin form islands that grow outward from the edges to cover the denuded area. Pinch grafts do not result in a smooth surface, either on the donor or recipient sites. Their removal destroys the donor site as a future source of split-thickness graft and, therefore, they are seldom used by most plastic surgeons.

Free Myocutaneous Grafts

Free island grafts of skin, subcutaneous fat, and muscle can be resected and transplanted from one area of the body to another to cover a denuded area. In this procedure, also known as the *microvascular free flap,* the main artery and vein supplying the tissues of a graft must be anastomosed to vessels in the recipient site under the operating microscope.

The iliofemoral area is the most common donor site, using the superficial circumflex iliac artery and vein or the superficial epigastrics to maintain the vascular supply. After resection, the defect in the groin is partially closed primarily, and the rest of the area is covered with a split-thickness skin graft. The gluteal region also may be a donor site.

The recipient site may be the cheek, scalp, neck, leg, foot, or arm.

Free Composite Grafts

A composite graft may include, along with myocutaneous tissue and its blood vessels, nerves, bone, and other tissues. Fascicles of nerves must be anastomosed to restore sensation, as well as microvascular anastomoses of arteries and veins to maintain viability of the graft.

Free Omental Grafts

Omentum, grafted to provide vascularity, can be resected from the peritoneal cavity and transplanted to an avascular area if sufficient recipient blood vessels are available for anastomoses to the right or left gastroepiploic artery and vein. An omental graft can be used, for example, to resurface the scalp. The gastroepiploic vessels can be anastomosed to the temporalis artery and vein. Split-thickness skin grafts are placed over the omental graft.

Pedicle Flaps

Creation of a pedicle flap may be the procedure of choice to reconstruct deformities of soft tissue loss that will create, or have created, an obvious aesthetic or functional disability for the patient. The *pedicle,* which is the attachment of elevated tissue to the donor site, must contain a vascular bundle to maintain blood supply to the tissue. Pedicle flaps are constructed from several types of tissues and sources of the vascular bundles.

Arterialized Skin Flap A full-thickness skin graft contains a vascular bundle within the subcutaneous tissue and skin. Arterialized flaps may be:

1 Those with axial vasculature from axial vessels that supply a fairly definite area of skin and subcutaneous tissue. A direct cutaneous artery flows through the length of the flap.

2 Those with random or local vasculature from the subdermal plexus of musculocutaneous arteries.

3 Those with both axial and random vasculature. A deltopectoral flap, for example, has axial vessels from the pectoral region and random vessels from the deltoid.

Myocutaneous Flap This incorporates the muscle, overlying fascia, subcutaneous tissue, and skin. It receives a vigorous blood supply from the vascular pedicle that supplies the underlying muscle. It may include a neurovascular bundle with nerve fibers to innervate the muscle in the flap. Usually done as a one-stage procedure, myocutaneous flaps can be created from the following and other muscles:

1 Trapezius
2 Sternocleidomastoid
3 Lattisimus
4 Rectus abdominis
5 Gracilis
6 Gluteus maximus
7 Biceps femoris

Muscle Flap Divided section of a muscle with its proximal blood supply intact can be rotated over a soft tissue defect, such as an ulcer on the leg or buttock. The muscle flap may be covered with a split-thickness skin graft.

Omental Flap Omentum is mobilized from the peritoneal cavity, without compromise of the vascular pedicle, to cover the defect in the chest wall following resection for irradiation necrosis or neoplasm. The vascularity of the donor omentum revascularizes the reconstructed chest-wall recipient site. Split-thickness skin grafts, which may be meshgrafts, cover the omental flap. If additional rigidity is needed to restore the chest wall, polypropylene mesh may be sutured inside the rib cage to supplement the strength of the omental flap.

Types of Pedicle Flaps

Rotational Flap One end of the flap is rotated and sutured to the recipient site to cover a denuded area. The flap tissue is obtained from an area near the recipient site. Myocutaneous, muscle, omental, and arterialized skin pedicle flaps with axial vasculature are rotated in a one-stage procedure.

Cross-Finger, -Thigh, or -Calf Flap Tissue at the donor site is undermined and rotated to cover the defect in an adjacent extremity site. For example, a flap can be sutured between two adjacent digits. Or an ankle can be covered by a flap from the thigh or calf of the opposite leg.

Pocket Flap A full-thickness skin flap is elevated on the abdomen or anterior surface of the thigh. Both ends are left attached. A denuded hand or wrist is placed under the flap and sutured along the edges of the flap. It remains under the flap until the blood supply becomes established. The flap is then divided along each side of the resurfaced extremity, and the donor area is covered with a split-thickness skin graft.

Distant Tubular Flap Both ends of an elevated full-thickness skin flap are attached to the donor site. The skin edges are approximated and sutured together into the form of a cylinder. A Thiersch graft covers the tissue under the tube. After vascularity is well established, one end of the flap is freed and transferred to an intermediate site. Again after vascularity is established, the other end is freed from the original donor site and transferred to the intended recipient site. For example, the tubular flap may be elevated on the abdomen: one end transferred to an arm; the other end attached to the face. In this way, a pedicle flap may be migrated from the abdomen to arm to face, and it is kept viable by its vascular attachment at each stage of the procedure.

Delayed Skin Flap In this procedure, which is done in several stages, the blood supply in the flap is permitted to become established between stages. A tubular flap is one process of delay. Sometimes, preliminary to making a tube, the plastic surgeon elevates the tissue for the flap, leaving the ends attached, then sutures it back to its original site. This stimulates the random vasculature in the tissue to increase size of blood vessels, and thus increases the viability of the flap when it is rotated or migrated to the recipient site.

General Considerations for All Tissue Autografts

1 Skin is prepped with a colorless antiseptic agent so the plastic surgeon can see true skin color and assess vascularity of the donor graft.

2 Donor and recipient sites are prepped and draped separately, but concurrently, care being taken that cross contamination does not occur from the one site to the other.

3 Recipient site is covered with a sterile towel or sheet until ready to apply free graft or pedicle flap, if preparation of this will be the first procedure. If the recipient site must be prepared to receive the donor graft or flap, the donor site is covered.

4 Separate sterile instrument table is prepared for the donor site. This includes appropriate instruments for obtaining the graft or flap and dressings for the donor site.

NOTE. *Always* put a dermatome on a separate, small sterile table, never on the recipient instrument table. Handle dermatomes carefully so the depth gauge is not disturbed.

5 Graft must be kept moist by covering with a sponge wet with warm normal saline. A free skin graft is gently spread out on a flat surface covered with a moistened sponge, with the cut surface down. The edges of skin tend to curl.

6 Hemostasis is obtained during operation by warm saline packs, pressure, or thrombin.

7 Dressings over grafts vary by surgeon preference. Stent fixation to obtain pressure on the grafted area may be preferred. Some plastic surgeons omit pressure dressings and use the exposure technique on grafts for selected areas. The surgeon can keep a close watch on the graft and incise a hematoma if necessary. The graft is kept covered with sterile, moist saline sponges to keep the skin moist until revascularization occurs. A plaster cast frequently is applied to immobilize extremities during migration or transfer of pedicle flaps.

HEAD AND NECK RECONSTRUCTION

Craniofacial Operations

Craniofacial refers to the cranium and face. Craniofacial surgery of increasing complexity has been performed since World War II. However, the approach developed by Tessier has led to previously inaccessible anatomical areas. Exposure for dissection of soft tissues and bone to restore contour and symmetry in practically every type of facial deformity, whether congenital, neoplastic, or traumatic in origin, can be accomplished by a multidisciplinary team of surgeons. Some operations require over 100 separate maneuvers and may take as long as 14 to 16 hours to complete. Many of the concepts developed for these very complex procedures are applied in the more common and less complicated operations to reshape sections of the skull or reconstruct soft tissues. Craniofacial reconstruction should be performed as soon as indicated by the physiological and psychological impacts of the deformity upon the patient, regardless of age. Early operation not only decreases psychological trauma, but may prevent craniofacial distortion due to brain and nerve damage of a disease process or traumatic injury.

Aesthetic Procedures

Blepharoplasty Redundant skin and/or protruding orbital fat is excised to correct deformities of the upper or lower eyelids of one or both eyes. *Blepharochalasis,* loss of elasticity of the skin of the eyelids, can occur at any age and usually is of unknown etiology. *Dermatochalasis* primarily involves hypertrophy of the skin of the upper lids. Resection of the excessive redundant skin removes the mechanical visual obstruction caused by these two conditions. *Protrusion of intraorbital fat* into the lids is the most common eyelid deformity. This fat must be removed from the compartments in the upper and/or lower lids to correct the deformity. This may be associated with dermatochalasis. A free graft of cartilage and mucosa from the nasal septum may be necessary to reconstruct lower eyelid defects. *Hypertrophy of the orbicularis muscle* appears as a horizontal bulge below the lower lid margin. A skin-muscle flap resection may be performed. An operation for lifting the eyebrows will secondarily correct a hooding deformity of the upper lids caused by ptosis of the eyebrows.

These procedures usually are performed under local anesthesia. The patient should wear dentures to the OR, because facial contour is distorted without them and the surgeon could remove too much or too little redundant skin. Because of proximity to the eye, these oculoplastic procedures may be performed by an ophthalmologist, as mentioned in Chapter 22.

Otoplasty Deformities of one or both external ears of an adult usually are the result of traumatic avulsion. A segment of the external ear that is partially or completely amputated often can be reattached to the remaining segment and buried beneath a flap of postauricular skin. The area over a completely severed auricular cartilage, which cannot be sutured back in place, is covered with a split-thickness skin graft initially. Later reconstruction may include insertion of cartilage taken from the rib cage or a silicone prosthetic implant.

Rhinoplasty An operation for reshaping the nose, although usually performed for cosmetic appearance desired by the patient, may be necessary to correct defects caused by trauma or surgical resection of neoplasms. Subtle changes with limited nasal reduction, preservation of the normal physiology and anatomy, and augmentation of the nasal tip with the patient's own nasal cartilage can result in aesthetically attractive and physiologically normal noses in most patients. A pedicle flap may be necessary to close a large tissue defect. Bone or cartilage grafts may be needed for septal reconstruction. Prosthetic reconstruction for partial or total loss of the nose may be the procedure of choice.

Rhytidoplasty Commonly referred to as a "face lift," rhytidoplasty involves extensive dissection from above the ear downward along the jaw line and upper neck. The skin is freed from underlying fascia. Wrinkles and folds of the normal aging process smooth out as the skin is lifted up and sutured in place. Redundant skin is trimmed away. Frequently other procedures, such as blepharoplasty or rhinoplasty, accompany this operation. Meticulous hemostasis is essential to prevent hematoma formation, the foremost complication of rhytidoplasty. Hypotensive anesthesia may be used to help reduce this incidence. Closed-wound suction drainage frequently is used with or without a pressure dressing applied after operation.

Maxillofacial Operations

Maxillofacial pertains to the part of face formed by the upper and lower jaws. Most maxillofacial operations are designed to reconstruct defects in the lips, the buccal sulcus, maxilla, alveolar ridge, floor of the mouth, mandible, and/or chin. These defects may be the result of trauma or resection of tumor. Congenital deformities are discussed in Chapter 26.

Transfacial Nerve Grafting Restoration of the quality of facial expressions in a patient with severe facial nerve paralysis can be accomplished by transfacial nerve grafting. A segment of nerve is brought through a tunnel across the upper lip from the normal side of the face to the paralyzed side. The overpull of the mouth and lower face toward the normal side is balanced when the nerve graft is anastomosed between fascicles of the intact facial nerve innervating the zygomaticus muscle to the same fascicles on the denervated side.

Lip Reconstruction Lips can be adequately reconstructed by a variety of techniques to restore sensation and motor function following trauma or surgical resection. Lip cancer is the most common type of cancer in the upper respiratory and digestive tracts. Operations to reconstruct lips may be classified as:

1 Those amendable to repair by primary closure of the remaining lip segments.
2 Those that can be closed with a full-thickness cross-lip flap from the opposite lip.
3 Those that utilize arterialized or myocutaneous flaps from adjacent cheek or nasolabial tissue.
4 Those that employ distant flaps. Arterialized and innervated myocutaneous flaps from the forehead or deltopectoral region may be used. These require staged procedures.

The ideal repair yields a lip that is not tight, has a good vermilion border, an adequate sulcus, good sensation, and good muscle tone.

Erich or Jelenko Splint A pair of metal splints are used as a method of fixation in fractures of the mandible and maxilla. Wires are passed between the teeth to anchor the splints on the upper and lower jaws. Each splint contains a series of small lugs. Tiny rubber bands, placed around opposing lugs, hold the teeth in occlusion. Frequently splints are not used for fixation of these fractures. The teeth may be held in occlusion by wires passed around opposing teeth.

NOTE. Following fixation of the mandible or maxilla, a pair of wire scissors must accompany the patient from the OR and remain at the bedside as long as wires or rubber bands are in place. If the patient experiences respiratory difficulty, the wires may need to be cut to prevent aspiration. Fluids may be difficult to swallow.

Mentoplasty The chin can be reshaped by removing sections from or adding to the mandible. *Prognathism,* the forward jutting of the jaw, is corrected by removing bone. *Micrognathia,* abnormally small jaws (usually the mandible), is augmented with bone or cartilage grafts or silicone implants. These operations usually are performed in combination with orthodontic treatment. Bands on the teeth may be applied when the upper or lower jaws are moved for correction of malocclusion.

Neck Dissections

Tumors, benign and malignant, occur in the head and neck regions. Although the origin of many of these neoplasms is technically in the head, the cervical lymph nodes frequently are involved secondarily by metastases from a primary head or neck malignant tumor. Treatment is directed toward definitive management for eradication of the tumor, and metastases, with consideration for rehabilitation. Various reconstructive techniques provide immediate restoration to improve speech, reestablish oral function, or prevent airway obstruction. Others involve delayed reconstruction. The method of repair depends on the type of defect resulting from excision of the lesion. Preoperatively, the patient's emotional stability is analyzed if the operation will result in cosmetic deformity. Reconstruction is planned prior to or at the time of the operation so local tissue can be used whenever feasible, and normal function preserved whenever possible. The aim of reconstruction is to restore function and appearance. Some plastic surgeons subspecialize in resection of tumors or lesions approached through the oral cavity or neck.

Parotidectomy Parotidectomy is performed through an incision in the neck below the angle of the mandible and extending upward to one or both sides of the ear. Swelling beneath the skin in the area in front of or below the ear is almost invariably within the substance of the parotid gland. This may be a benign, mixed, or malignant tumor. Benign lesions localized superficially may be excised by superficial subtotal parotidectomy. Lesions deep within the gland, extending under the mandible, frequently present in the oral cavity by displacing the soft palate. Radical neck dissection or hemimandibulectomy may be indicated to remove a highly invasive malignant tumor. For most parotid tumors, the facial nerve can be isolated and preserved during total parotidectomy, unless the nerve is inextricably involved in the tumor. If the facial nerve must be sacrificed, the nerve may be primarily grafted to prevent total facial nerve paralysis.

Radical Neck Dissection Malignant tumors of the oral or pharyngeal cavities, cutaneous malignant melanoma, and skin cancer in the head and neck region often require wide resection of the primary lesion and excision of all the cervical lymph nodes on one or both sides of the neck. The head and neck surgeon must plan the operation with reconstruction in mind, so that the incisions will allow good exposure, but provide as much local flap tissue as possible for reconstruction. Incisions used for the tumor resection will necessarily vary according to the type of reconstruction planned. Thus, no single operative procedure can be used to treat all lesions. However, certain basic features remain common to all neck dissections.

All lymph-bearing tissue from the midline anteriorly to the trapezius muscle posteriorly and from the mandible superiorly to the clavicle inferiorly is removed. All tissue between the deep cervical fascia and the platysma muscle externally is removed except the carotid artery system, the vagus, phrenic and hypoglossal nerves, and the brachial plexus.

Attention is given to preservation of the occipital, posterior auricular, facial, and superior thyroid arteries. When these can be preserved, arterialized skin flaps designed to incorporate branches from these vessels can be constructed with length up to three or four times the width. Otherwise the length of a flap should not exceed twice the width. A deltopectoral pedical flap or a myocutaneous graft may be needed. An exposed carotid artery must be covered. Cervical flaps carrying their own blood supply may be used for this, and to restore the oral pharyngeal lining intraorally.

The mandible is preserved, unless involved by direct extension of tumor into the bone. Access through a mandibular osteotomy or partial mandibulectomy is usually required for effective resection in the posterior oral cavity. Solid bony continuity and realignment of the dental arches must be established for functional restoration of speech and chewing. A bone graft from the rib or iliac crest, or cancellous bone chips, may be used to stabilize the mandible.

A tracheostomy tube and feeding esophagostomy tube are inserted. Although reconstruction begins at the time of primary neck dissection, the patient usually requires considerable postoperative rehabilitation, psychologically, and staged operations before cosmetic and functional reconstruction is complete.

RECONSTRUCTION OF OTHER BODY AREAS

Adipose Tissue

Lipectomy is an excision of excessive fat and redundant skin from the upper arms, abdomen, buttocks, or thighs.

Breast

Augmentation Mammoplasty This procedure is often performed for aesthetic effect on women who desire larger breasts; however, unilateral augmentation is sometimes performed following mastectomy to reconstruct breast contour. A silicone prosthesis may be inserted at the time of simple mastectomy. Following modified radical or radical mastectomy, the wound should be well healed, the scar mature, and the skin well vascularized prior to breast reconstruction. Technical maneuvers of the general surgeon at the time of mastectomy will influence the possibility of an aesthetically acceptable result following breast reconstruction by the plastic surgeon. A prosthesis can be implanted only when reliable skin is available to cover it. Skin flaps should be cut as thickly as consistent with a curative mastectomy. If sufficient skin flaps are not available to insert a prosthesis, the plastic surgeon may transfer a pedicle flap from the abdomen to the chest wall. Aesthetically the end result is a semblance of a breast.

An inflatable breast prosthesis may be inserted. Made of polyurethane-covered silicone gel, this implant has a self-sealing valve that can be filled by percutaneous injections of dextran or saline. The prosthesis is gradually inflated over a period of several weeks while the skin flaps are healing without tension. An areola and nipple complex may be constructed in a second-stage operation.

A prefabricated or vulcanizing silicone prosthesis for soft tissue defects incorporated with the prosthetic breast may be implanted for chest wall reconstruction following radical mastectomy.

Hematoma, infection, and skin necrosis are potential complications following prosthetic implantation for breast augmentation performed either unilaterally or bilaterally.

Reduction Mammoplasty This is usually performed for comfort as well as aesthetic improvement in body image. Hyperplasia of the breasts is reduced by resection of skin and glandular tissue. The nipple-areola complexes may be placed slightly inferiorly to prevent high-riding nipples postoperatively. If this cannot be done initially, several other procedures have been developed, which allow the nipple-areola complexes to be transferred intact with the underlying breast tissue, maintaining the blood and nerve supply. In younger patients, these are preferred to procedures involving amputation of the breast tissue with a free nipple graft.

Hand

The plastic surgeon is dedicated to salvaging injured tissues whenever possible. Therefore, it is not surprising that those who subspecialize in hand reconstruction have turned to the operating microscope. Microsurgical revascularization and primary nerve repair salvage many traumatized hands that have lost their blood supply and sensation. Neurovascular island flaps also reinnervate and revascularize digits. Other traumatic hand injuries can be repaired by resurfacing with free skin grafts or pedicle flaps. Lacerated tendons are sutured or grafted. Hand reconstruction also is performed to correct joint deformities of degenerative diseases or for secondary release of contractures. (Refer to Chap. 20, p. 371, for general considerations pertaining to operations on an extremity.)

Scars

Dermabrasion Dirt and cinders can become embedded in the dermis from a brush-burn injury. The plastic surgeon sandpapers out this dirt and irrigates it from the area with warm saline solution. Sandpapering also is done to improve acne scars. However, this procedure is not always satisfactory if many pitted scars are too deep to reach or there are changes in pigment of scars. Some plastic surgeons prefer chemical dermabrasion in selected patients for face peeling.

Sandpaper, in the form of narrow abrasive bands, is mounted on a hollow core attachment to an electric drill. This is used for small areas of deeply embedded dirt and cinders or acne scars. For more superficial areas, sandpaper may be cut into 1-, 2-, or 3-in. (2.5, 5, or 7.5 cm) widths and wrapped around a gauze bandage. Waterproof sandpaper can be steam-sterilized.

Scar Revision The plastic surgeon attempts to make a scar as fine a line, as level, and as smooth as possible at the time of primary wound closure or as a secondary scar revision. Scar formation, the body's mechanism for healing wounds, is inevitable whenever skin is incised. The plastic surgeon can excise an aesthetically displeasing scar, realign wound edges, and resuture or close them with anticipation of a better cosmetic result. The direction of a scar can be changed to be less conspicuous in the natural skin lines. Scars are frequently revised following extensive reconstructive procedures or following a laceration with or without other soft tissue trauma, particularly a facial scar. Z-plasty, W-plasty, Lazy-S, Y-V-plasty, and many other techniques are used to improve the appearance of a hypertrophied or prominent scar.

BURNS

Skin and underlying tissues can be destroyed by thermal, chemical, or electrical injury. Burns are open wounds. As in other injuries, initial treatment is aimed at saving the patient's life. Then the treatment is directed toward preserving or restoring to normal, or as near normal as possible, the patient's bodily functions and appearance as rapidly as possible. Depending on the depth, extent, and location of the burn, reconstruction may extend over long periods of time: months to years. The patient must be helped to accept the disfigurement; thus rehabilitation from a psychological standpoint is important. Psychotherapy as well as surgery and physiotherapy may be necessary to promote as early a return to normalcy and usefulness as possible.

Classification of Burn

The severity of injury is determined by individual factors such as age, pretrauma medical history, other injuries sustained, location and etiology of the burn. Burns are classified by depth and extent as soon after injury as possible. The depth of a burn may be:

First-Degree Burn The outer layer of the epidermis only is involved. Superficial erythema, redness of the skin, and tissue destruction occur, but healing takes place rapidly.

Second-Degree Burn This is a partial-thickness burn in which all epidermis and varying depths of the corium are destroyed. This is usually characterized by blister formation, pain, and a moist, mottled red or pink appearance. Hair follicles and sebaceous glands may be destroyed. Reepithelialization can occur provided the deepest layer of the epithelium is viable. However, superimposed infection can interfere with healing.

Third-Degree Burn In this full-thickness injury, the skin with all its epithelial structures and subcutaneous tissue is destroyed. This is characterized by a dry, pearly-white, or charred-appearing surface void of sensation. The destroyed skin forms a parchmentlike *eschar* over the burned area. If removed or left to slough off, eschar leaves a denuded surface that can extend to the fascia. Third-degree burns require skin grafts for healing to occur unless the area is small enough for closure by reepithelialization.

Fourth-Degree Burn Sometimes referred to as *char burns,* fourth-degree burns may damage bones, tendons, muscles, blood vessels, and peripheral nerves. An electrical burn, for example, causes damage much deeper than is apparent on the skin surface. Often muscle and bone necrosis must be excised.

Estimation of Burn Damage

Two methods are used to estimate the total percentage of body surface burned and the percentage of each degree of burn.

Lund and Brower Chart The percentage sizes of the head and lower extremities differ between infancy, childhood, and adulthood. Per guidelines of this chart, percent of burn is estimated on the basis of age in addition to anatomic location of the burn.

Rule of Nines The body surface of an adult can be divided into areas equal to multiples of 9 percent of the total body surface.

1 Head and neck—9 percent
2 Anterior and posterior trunk—18 percent each
3 Upper extremities—9 percent each
4 Lower extremities—18 percent each
5 Perineum—1 percent

Initial Care of Burn Patient

1 *Stop the burning process.* All clothing, jewelry, metal, and synthetic objects in contact with patient's skin are removed.
2 *Ensure a patent airway.* The respiratory system may be damaged from inhalation of superheated air or toxic gases. Endotracheal intubation is attempted initially. Tracheotomy may be required several days later for prolonged respiratory assistance if burn includes head and neck or respiratory tract injury.
3 *Establish intravenous fluid therapy.* Blood samples are drawn for laboratory analysis, type, and cross match when a venipuncture or cutdown is performed to establish an intravenous route for fluid and nutritional administration. Fluid and electrolyte balance must be restored as quickly as possible. An electrolyte, such as lactated Ringer's

solution, is infused initially. Plasma or other nutrients may be infused later.

4 *Insert a retention catheter.* Urine specimens are sent for analysis and then checked for pH and specific gravity at frequent intervals. Hourly output is recorded.

5 *Cleanse the wound.* All burns are treated aseptically. A mild cleansing agent, such as povidone-iodine, and *warm* saline or water are used to gently remove debris and loose devitalized tissue. Areas surrounding the burn should be shaved. Copious amounts of water, along with appropriate neutralizing agents, are used to cleanse and irrigate chemical burns. After cleansing, wet sheets under and around the patient must be removed and dry, sterile ones applied. Nonwoven sheets specifically designed for burn care are commercially available.

6 *Estimate percent and depth of burn.* Definitive treatment may be completed in the emergency department, or the patient may be transported to an immersion tank for further cleansing and debridement, or to the operating room for initiation of further therapy as indicated by assessment of the burn. The burned area is covered with sterile or clean linen for transfer of the patient from the emergency department.

Methods of Operative Treatment

Prevention of infection and promotion of healing are of utmost concern in the treatment of burned patients. The probability of infection developing increases in greater proportion to the percentage of body surface burned. Colonization may begin as early as 24 hours postburn.

Excisional Therapy Primary excision of necrotic tissue from deep second-degree and all full-thickness third-degree burned areas, followed immediately by skin grafting, is performed beginning as soon as possible after injury. Debridement can be accomplished with a scalpel, free-hand skin-graft knife, dermatome, electrosurgical knife, or laser beam. The surgeon selects the most appropriate instrument for the particular burned area to be excised. Hypotensive anesthesia may be used to help control massive blood loss during extensive excisions.

Tangential Excision Burned tissue is excised until normal dermal tissue is reached below the depth of the wound. The wound base, containing some viable dermal structures necessary for regeneration, is covered with a split-thickness autograft or homograft. A homograft may be used when sufficient autografts cannot be harvested from the patient, or to cover the area temporarily as regeneration proceeds. If neither an autograft or homograft is available, a heterograft may be applied.

Massive Degloving Excision Eschar is removed. The burned area is excised down to the fascia when viable tissue in more superficial layers is not evident, except on the hands, neck, or face. All denuded areas created by excision are covered with split-thickness autografts, if sufficient skin is available, or temporary skin transplants.

NOTE. Temporary skin transplantation refers to the use of homografts or heterografts as biological dressings for a *prolonged* period of time. Immunosuppression may be used to delay rejection of the skin transplant, which usually occurs within 12 to 20 days without immunosuppression.

Other Operative Procedures During the course of hospitalization a burned patient may come to the operating room for one or many procedures.

Escharotomy Shrinkage of eschar may occur and cause a tourniquet effect in circumferential burns of the extremities or thorax. Bilateral incisions through the eschar, not including the fascia, are made to improve circulation to an extremity. Multiple incisions on the chest wall relieve respiratory distress. Site of incisions avoid major peripheral nerves to prevent irreversible neurological complications.

Fasciotomy If adequate decompression does not occur following escharotomy, incision may be extended into underlying fascia.

Amputation of Digits Amputation may be necessary to control infection in the extremity and septicemia.

Debridement Debridement of underlying tissues helps prevent extension of tissue loss. Nonviable tendons, cartilage, or bone may be excised, as from the hand, ear, or skull.

Full-Thickness Skin Grafts With or without tarsorrhaphy, full-thickness skin grafts are used to prevent contracture of the eyelids. The cornea must be protected from exposure.

Split-Thickness Skin Grafts Autografts are applied to debrided areas as rapidly as possible. Hands and face are first priority to restore function; joints and flexion creases are second to prevent contractures; extremities and trunk are lowest priority. Skin from donor sites is cut thin if the site will be used again. Meshgrafts frequently are used to cover very large surfaces or irregular areas such as the perineum.

Biological Dressing Changes Instead of leaving a biological dressing in place until rejection, with attendant inflammatory reaction, a biological dressing may be replaced every few days until the area is ready for autograft or skin for autograft is available. Biological dressings may be homografts of human skin from a living or cadaver donor, or amniotic membranes, or a heterograft of porcine skin. Porcine dressings frequently are applied initially on second-degree burns as a temporary dressing, or used in conjunction with extensive excisional therapy. A biological dressing is used for several reasons.

1 It helps to control infection by covering denuded areas.
2 It prevents loss of serum.
3 It decreases pain.
4 It seems to stimulate formation of epithelium in dermis under it.
5 It promotes growth of granulation tissue.

Dressing Changes Occlusive dressings must be changed frequently if infection develops under them. An antimicrobial or chemotherapeutic agent may be applied as an integral part of the dressing.

1 Silver and/or zinc sulfadiazine or cerium nitrate cream may be applied directly onto the burned area. This makes removal of a dressing less painful and does not disturb the healing process as it is removed. Fresh cream is applied after cleansing and debridement. A layer of fine mesh gauze is laid over it (unless the open-exposure method will be used for further healing). Then soft, absorbent material, such as fluffed gauze, and a preformed splint may be used. These are held in place by a cotton elastic bandage. An occlusive dressing may be used to hold a hand, foot, or joint in functional position.

2 Silver nitrate solution may be preferred. After cleansing and debridement, multiple-thickness dressings are applied to the area. These are kept saturated with 0.5% silver nitrate solution and changed every 12 hours. When doing a debridement, sterile distilled water is used for irrigation as saline may cause the precipitation of silver salts.

NOTE. Care is taken to avoid splashing silver nitrate solution on walls and floors as staining can occur. If disposable drapes and gowns are not used, stained linen must be laundered separately from other linen.

Serial Biopsy Cultures Through two linear incisions, a biopsy of tissue including subcutaneous fat is excised for culturing. This is done every 2 or 3 days, until the eschar begins to separate, to monitor the colonization of microorganisms in the wound. The results of serial biopsy culture enable the surgeon to make decisions specific to the therapeutic needs of the patient. An antimicrobial or chemotherapeutic topical agent is selected or changed according to these results.

Curling's Ulcer Gastrointestinal complications may occur anytime from the early postinjury period through rehabilitation. Complaints must be carefully evaluated. The patient who develops massive bleeding from a Curling's or stress ulcer in the stomach and duodenum must be operated on. Vagotomy with antrectomy is most frequently performed by a general surgeon.

Environmental Considerations for Burn Patients

1 Environmental control is perhaps the essence of burn therapy. The environment must protect the wound from further injury and microbial invasion. A burn wound is always potentially contaminated until epithelialization occurs. Open exposure of the wound to room air may be the choice of the plastic surgeon for selected patients. Regardless of method of treatment, the following adjuncts are used, if the equipment is available, in the care of burned patients in addition to strict adherence to all the principles of aseptic technique.

- **a** *Reverse isolation technique.* This can be practiced in every hospital by all personnel. The goal is to protect the patient, whose resistance is low, from cross infection from personnel. Caps, masks, shoe covers, sterile gowns and gloves are worn by all personnel attending the patient. This may be referred to as *protective isolation.*
- **b** *Hyperbaric oxygen.* Hyperbaric oxygenation causes an intense vasoconstriction without creating a hypoxic state. Intermittent exposures in the immediate postinjury period reduce plasma loss. Healing is accelerated and tissue loss diminished.
- **c** *Laminar airflow.* Downward unidirectional airflow away from the wound helps minimize airborne contamination.
- **d** *Plastic isolator.* The patient is protected by clear plastic access walls through which nursing and medical care is given. Personnel do not directly enter this isolation unit. The environment around the patient inside the isolator is controlled at 90°F (32°C) and 94 per-

cent relative humidity to conserve heat loss by evaporation.

2 Patients with extensive burns may be placed on a Stryker frame or a circle electric bed specially designed to facilitate handling and turning. They are transported to the OR on these frames or beds. Patients must be turned slowly and gently, because they are often hypovolemic postinjury.

3 Hypothermia must be prevented. The patient's thermoregulatory mechanism is altered by the destruction of skin that normally acts as an insulator. Heat loss is the greatest single problem the burn patient poses in the OR. Room temperature should be increased to between 80 and 90°F (27 and 32°C) with low relative humidity of about 30 percent. Warm hyperthermia blankets can cover the operating table. Solutions should be warmed prior to irrigation or infusion.

4 Operating during nighttime hours is advantageous for the patient:

a Normal schedule for oral intake is not interrupted.

b The OR can be preheated to above-normal temperature.

Chapter 26

Pediatric Surgery

The surgical problems peculiar to children from birth to maturity are not limited to any one area of the body nor to any one surgical specialty. Malformations and diseases affect all body parts and therefore may require the skills of any of the surgical specialties. However, pediatric surgery is a specialty in itself and is not adult surgery scaled down to infant or child size. Skill is required in performing pediatric operations, and specialists in all fields must develop it as a refinement of their specialties. Surgeons who perform pediatric surgery must have knowledge of the physiological, embryological, and pathological problems peculiar to the newborn, infant, and child.

PEDIATRIC STAGES OF DEVELOPMENT

1 Newborn infant, sometimes referred to as a neonate:
  a True premature. Gestational age is less than 37 weeks; birth weight is 2500 g or less.
  b Large premature. Gestational age is less than 37 weeks; birth weight is more than 2500 g.
  c Term neonate. Gestational age is 37 weeks or more; birth weight is appropriate for gestational age, usually over 2500 g. If less than 2500 g, the neonate is considered dysmaturely small-for-date.

2 Infant: birth to 18 months.
3 Toddler: 18 to 30 months.
4 Preschool: $2\frac{1}{2}$ to 5 years.
5 School age: 6 to 12 years.
6 Adolescent: 12 through 16 years.

CLASSIFICATIONS OF PEDIATRIC SURGERY

Pediatric surgery in all specialties can be divided into three classifications:

Congential Anomalies

A congenital anomaly is a deviation from normal structure or location in any organ or part of the body. It can alter function or appearance. Multiple anomalies often are present at birth. If the anomaly does not involve sustaining life functions, surgical intervention may be postponed until the results can be maximized and the risks of operation are minimized by growth and development of body systems. If the newborn has a poor chance of survival without operation, the risk is taken within hours or days after birth. Defects in the alimentary tract are the most common indication for emergency operation during the newborn period, followed in frequency by cardiac and respiratory system defects. Mortality rates in the newborn are influenced by three uncontrollable factors: the multiplicity of anomalies, prematurity, and birth weight.

Acquired Disease Processes

Appendicitis is the most common surgically corrected childhood disease process. Malignant tumors do occur in infants and children but the frequency in comparison to adults is minimal. Benign lesions, such as hypertrophied tonsils, are surgically excised usually without further difficulty to the child.

Trauma

Accidental injury is the leading cause of death in children. Injury can occur during the birth process and anytime thereafter to any part of the body. Trauma can be the cause of major physical deformity, prolonged hospitalization with multiple operations, and emotional problems. In the emergency department it is very important that the difference in response to injury between a child and an adult is observed and quick action taken. The margin for error in diagnosis and treatment of a child is less than that of an adult with a similar injury. A child's blood volume is small and even a small loss of blood can be critical, and the comparatively large skin area causes rapid heat loss. The child's chest capacity is small so abdominal or chest injury can be critical. Fatal collapse can result rapidly. It is imperative that diagnosis be made quickly, the patient be sent to the operating room if indicated and lifesaving measures be taken immediately.

GENERAL CONSIDERATIONS

Knowledge has advanced pediatric surgery so that many anomalies, diseases, and traumatic injuries formerly considered fatal or inoperable now yield to successful surgical intervention. This is due to:

1 Recognition of differences between newborns, infants, and children from adults.
2 Accurate diagnosis, especially in the premature and term neonate. Many defects can be repaired if diagnosis is made early.
3 Understanding of preoperative preparation of the total patient.
4 Advances in anesthesiology: new agents, perfection of techniques of administration, and understanding of responses of infants and children to anesthetic agents.
5 Refinements in operative procedures and instrumentation.
6 Understanding of postoperative care.

Differences by Age Factor

Newborns, infants, and children through adolescence differ from each other according to age. All differ from adults. Infants, for example, have great vitality beyond that indicated by their size, but their reactions are different than those of adults.

Metabolism Infants have relatively greater nutritional requirements than adults to minimize loss of body protein; thus they develop disturbances more rapidly than adults. Complications increase proportionately with increase in time of fluid restriction. Procedures on infants and small children should have priority on the operative schedule so as to deprive them of food and fluid for as short a time as possible, and to return them to normal routine as quickly as possible.

1 Infants are given regular formula or a varied diet up to 4 hours before anesthesia and clear liquids, usually dextrose in water, up to 2 hours prior to operation. The number of missed feedings is thereby reduced and curds are absent from the stomach. Infants should not miss more than one or two feedings. Oral intake is resumed promptly after the infant recovers from anesthesia except following an abdominal operation.
2 Toddlers and preschool children usually are permitted clear liquids up to 4 hours preoperatively.
3 Children under 8 years of age should not be without supplemental glucose and clear liquids for more than 6 hours preoperatively.
4 Older children may require slower progression of oral dietary intake postoperatively, and are maintained with supplemental intravenous therapy that includes protein and vitamins. Vitamins K and C may be given to any age group.

Fluid and Electrolyte Balance The newborn is not dehydrated and withstands major operative procedures within the first 4 days of life without extensive fluid and electrolyte replacement. The renal system can be easily overloaded with the administration of intravenous fluids. The newborn has a lower glomerular filtration rate and less efficient renal tubular function than an adult. (Renal function improves during the first 2 months of life and approaches adult levels by 2 years.) Ten to thirty milliliters of fluid may be administered during the time of an average operation on a newborn. Blood loss, in most cases, is small, but must be measured. Blood volume of the average newborn is 250 ml, approximately 75 to 80 ml per kilogram of body weight. Significant blood loss requires replacement. Blood is typed and cross-matched in readiness.

Infants become dehydrated rapidly as they have a relatively larger body-surface area to body-mass ratio than adults. When the body becomes dehydrated, body functions are disturbed, as is the acid-base balance. Plasma proteins differ in concentration from an adult's. Fluid and electrolyte replacement are necessary, as is significant blood loss. Hemoglobin level is lowest at 2 to 3 months of age. A loss of 30 ml may represent 10 to 20 percent of circulating blood volume in an infant. The small margin of safety demands replacement of losses exceeding 10 percent of circulating blood volume. When replacement exceeds 50 percent of the estimated blood volume, sodium bicarbonate is infused to minimize acidosis.

1 Dehydration is avoided and therapy for metabolic acidosis, should it develop, is guided by measurement of pH, blood gases, and serum electrolytes. Blood-volume loss is measured and promptly replaced.

2 Rapid transfusion of blood may produce transient but severe metabolic acidosis in an infant.

3 Intravenous fluids and blood are infused through pediatric-size cannulated needles or catheters connected to drip-chamber adaptors and small solution containers. A cannula is placed in a vein before an extensive operation starts. Scalp veins are used frequently on infants; a cutdown on an extremity vein, usually the saphenous, is necessary for toddlers and older children. An extremity should be splinted to immobilize it. An extra length of tubing may be needed between the cannula and the solution container, so the tubing will reach under the drapes and the container can be elevated high enough for the solution to drip. Remember that the tubing lies on the operating table under the drapes. Take care that instruments are not placed on it to obstruct the flow. A cardboard box, with ends cut out, can be placed over the tubing as a protection. A 250-ml solution container is used to help avoid the danger of overhydration. Adaptors are set for accurate control of the desired flow rate.

Body Temperature Newborns, especially prematures, infants, and children have wider average body temperature variations than adults. This can vary with environmental changes. Body temperature in the newborn tends to range from as low as 97 to 100 °F (36 to 37.7 °C). Temperature begins to stabilize within this range 12 to 24 hours after birth if the environment is controlled. The relatively high rate of heat loss in proportion to heat production in the infant results from an incompletely developed thermoregulatory mechanism and from body-mass ratio with a thin layer of subcutaneous fat for insulation. Extensive superficial circulation also causes rapid dissipation of heat from the body. Oxygen consumption is at a minimum when abdominal skin temperature is 97 °F (36 °C). A room temperature 5 ° cooler than that of abdominal skin produces a 50 percent increase in oxygen consumption creating hazard of acidosis. These factors account for the infant's susceptibility to environmental changes. Heat loss can occur in infants by:

1 *Evaporation.* When the skin becomes wet, evaporative heat loss can occur.

2 *Radiation.* When heat transfers from the body surface to surfaces such as walls of the room that are not in direct contact with the body, radiation heat loss can result.

3 *Conduction.* When air currents pass over the skin, heat loss by convection results; cold diapers and blankets can cause heat loss by conduction.

Newborns, infants, and children must be kept warm during the operation to minimize heat loss and to prevent undesired hypothermia. Body temperature tends to fall in the operating room because of air conditioning, open body cavities, etc. Precautions to be taken include:

1 Hyperthermia blanket or a water mattress is placed on the operating table and warmed before the infant or child is laid on it. Covered with double thickness of linen, temperature of an electrically controlled blanket or water in a mattress is maintained at 100 °F (37.7 °C) to avoid skin burns and elevation of temperature above normal range. Excessive hyperthermia can cause dehydration and convulsions under anesthesia.

2 Telethermometer monitors the body temperature throughout the operation. A *telethermometer* is an electronic instrument that when connected to a probe provides direct temperature readouts on the dial. Rectal, esophageal, or tympanic probes are used. A probe placed into the rectum must not be inserted more than 2 or 3 cm (an inch) because severe trauma to an infant through perforation of the rectum or colon can occur.

3 Solutions should be warm when applied to tissues to minimize heat loss by evaporation and conduction. The circulating nurse should pour warm skin preparation solutions immediately prior to use. The scrub nurse dampens sponges in warm saline before handing them to the surgeon.

4 Blood can be warmed prior to transfusion by running the tubing through a blood warmer or basin of warm water. Intravenous solutions also should be warmed.

5 Drapes must permit some evaporative heat loss to maintain equalization of body temperature. Studies indicate that even though slight temperature rises can occur during prolonged operations, these cannot be attributed to any specific draping techniques as discussed in Chapter 11.

6 Blankets should be warmed to place over infant or child immediately after dressings are applied and drapes are removed. Keep infant covered whenever possible before and after operation to prevent chilling from the air conditioning.

Hyperthermia, core temperature of the body over 104 °F (40 °C), during operation presents a hazard. Causes are fever, dehydration, decrease in sweating from atropine administration, excessive drapes, drugs that disturb temperature regulation such as general anesthetics and barbiturates. Dire consequences ensue. Operation should be delayed if the patient is febrile preoperatively to allow reduction in temperature and to permit fluid administration. If immediate operation is necessary and fever persists, anesthesia is induced and external cooling employed.

Cardiopulmonary Response The heart rate is unstable and fluctuates widely in infants, toddlers, and preschool children. After age 5, cardiopulmonary response to stress resembles that of a young adult. Cardiac and respiratory sounds are continuously monitored by precordial or esophageal stethoscope. Blood pressure, vital signs, and other parameters as indicated also are monitored throughout the operation.

Infants and toddlers are particularly susceptible to respiratory obstruction because of anatomic structure. They have small nares, relatively large tongue, presence of lymphoid tissue, small diameter of trachea causing disproportionate narrowing of airway. Cylindrical thorax, poorly developed accessory respiratory muscles, and increased volume of abdominal contents limit diaphragmatic movement.

Infection Newborns and infants are susceptible to nosocomial infection and show less resistance to overcoming it than adults. Many premature infants suffering from respiratory distress and circulatory problems survive due to advances in perinatal medicine. This has increased the population of high-risk and debilitated infants with reduced humoral and cellular defenses to infection. Aseptic technique is essential in handling these and all other pediatric patients.

Elective operation should be delayed in the presence of respiratory infection because of the risk of airway obstruction. Intubation of inflamed tissues may cause laryngeal edema. *Coryza,* inflammation of mucous membranes of the nose, is often a premonitory sign of an infectious respiratory disease.

Pain Infants and children differ greatly from adults in their sensitivity to pain. Pain may be intense, but infants, toddlers, and preschool children are unable to describe its location and nature. School-age children may refer pain to a part of the body not involved in the disease process. Insecurity and fear in an older child may be more traumatic than pain itself. Children must be observed for signs of pain. Children also differ from adults in their response to pharmacological agents; their tolerance to analgesic drugs is altered.

Preparation of the Total Patient

Preoperative visits are made by an OR nurse to see and talk to the infant or child and/or parents. The pediatric surgical patient must be considered as a whole person with individual physical and psychosocial needs assessed in relationship to natural stages of development. Equally important to the patient are the adjustment and attitude of the parents toward the child, the illness, and the hospital experience. Parents' anxiety about the impending operation may be transferred to the child. Emotional support of both patient and parents as well as parent/child teaching are important aspects of preoperative preparation. Most adults face stress with more control when fear of the unknown is eliminated; children do not differ in this respect. Understanding does, however, vary with age.

1 Psychologically it is better for the infant as well as the parents if a congenital anomaly is repaired as soon after birth as possible. The infant under 1 year of age will not remember the experience. Parents will gain confidence in learning to cope with a residual deformity as the infant learns to compensate for it.

2 Separation from the mother or mother-equivalent is traumatic for the infant over 1 year, the toddler, and the preschool child. Such young children may fear strangers. The mother's presence is mandatory for the toddler and she should be encouraged to stay with the hospitalized child as much as possible. The child should be permitted to bring a toy or other security object to the OR suite, where mother cannot be present. In some hospitals a parent is permitted to rejoin the child in the recovery room, if condition permits.

NOTE. If feasible, arrangements can be made for the child to enter the hospital an hour or two before the operation and return home following recovery from anesthesia. This minimizes the trauma of separation. Physical examination and laboratory tests are completed upon admission for ambulatory surgery before the child enters the OR.

3 Fear of body mutilation or punishment may be of paramount importance to a preschool or young school-age child. This child needs reassurances and explanations in vocabulary compatible with developmental level.

4 Anxiety in the school-age child may be stimulated by remembrance of a previous experience. Many children undergo two or more staged operations before the deformity of a congenital anomaly or traumatic injury is cosmetically reconstructed or functionally restored. Familiarity with the nursing staff reassures the child. Ideally, the OR nurse who circulated for the first operation should visit preoperatively and be with the child during subsequent operations.

5 Fear of the unknown about being put to sleep may become exaggerated into extreme anxiety with fantasies of death. The school-age child and adolescent need facts and reassurances. Parents must be honest with their child and transmit confidence by maintaining a confident manner. The OR nurse must do the same. However, do not give a school-age child information not asked for; answer only questions and correct misunderstandings.

NOTE. Some hospitals hold "parties" for children and their parents prior to hospital admission or after admission prior to operation to explain hospital routines and procedures. Others take children to the OR suite so they can see the different attire, lights, tables, anesthesia machine, and other equipment that might interest them. A child-size anesthesia mask becomes a play toy and not something to be feared. A plastic mask, like those pilots wear in an airplane, is less psychologically traumatic to a child than an opaque black rubber mask. An effective method of explaining to children is to use a doll and dress it as the child will look postoperatively. For example, show a plaster hip spica cast on the doll to explain the cast if the child will have one postoperatively.

OR Nursing Procedures

The basic principles of the nursing care and operating room techniques discussed in preceding chapters appy to pediatric surgery. A few points specific to pediatric surgery are mentioned to differentiate this specialty from care of adult patients.

1 Hair is not removed with a depilatory or shaved, except for cranial operations and as ordered by the surgeon for an adolescent.

2 Diagnostic studies may be done in the OR under local anesthesia prior to induction of general anesthesia for an open operative procedure. An infant may be swaddled on a padded board to restrain him or her from moving while x-rays are taken and to permit easy change of position. A sugar nipple will help comfort and keep the infant quiet.

3 Care must be taken to protect the patient from injury:
   - a Guard against fall from a crib or stretcher. Siderails must be up at all times. An overbed cage on a crib helps confine a toddler without restraint. Children must be restrained on a stretcher or in a specially designed pediatric cart.
   - b Do not leave a crib where the patient can reach an electrical outlet or any article that can be picked up and cause injury.
   - c Pad the wrists and ankles after an infant is asleep with several turns of sheet wadding. Restrain with muslin or roller gauze and pin the straps to the sheet on the operating table. The sheet wadding prevents possible abrasion of delicate skin by the restraint straps. Care must be taken not to restrict circulation.
   - d Safety pins, open or closed, must not be left within reach of an infant or child.

4 Catheters as small as size 8 French are available for use as needed in newborns and infants. A plain tip or whistle-tip catheter is used for a stomach tube. If a urinary retention catheter is needed, a Foley with a 3-cc bag is used. Small, calibrated drainage containers are connected to permit accurate determination of output.

5 Positioning principles are essentially the same as described in Chapter 10. Correspondingly smaller towel rolls, pillows, and sandbags are used to protect pressure points and to stabilize

anesthetized infants and children. Size of the child or adolescent determines appropriate supports to maintain desired position. A small towel roll at each side of the body takes the weight of drapes off the small body of an infant or keeps the patient in lateral position.

6 Disposable drape sheet without a fenestration often is advantageous; the surgeon can cut an opening of the desired size to expose the site of intended incision. Small towels and towel clips are used with a laparotomy sheet if self-adhering and disposable drapes are not used. A standard opening 3 by 5 in. (7.6 by 12.7 cm) in a pediatric lap sheet frequently is too large for a newborn or infant. Part of the fenestration must be covered with a towel.

7 Sponges are weighed while still wet; blood loss through suction is measured and in drapes is estimated. The surgeon and anesthesiologist will determine if blood replacement is necessary, volume for volume, as it is lost.

8 Adhesive tape is abrasive to tender skin and should be avoided when possible. An adhesive spray or collodion is adequate over a small incision with a subcuticular closure, and is especially desirable under diapers, unless dressings are needed to absorb drainage. Care must be taken that the clothing or blanket does not touch this substance until dry. Skin closure strips may be used instead of a liquid adhesive substance.

9 Dressings on the face or neck must be protected from vomitus and food soil as well as from an infant's or toddler's hands. The elbows must be splinted when the patient potentially may disturb the incision, dressings, or a tube. This is particularly important following eye surgery, cleft lip or palate surgery, and when a tracheotomy tube is inserted.

10 Stockinet pulled over dressings on an extremity protects them from soil and helps keep them in place. This can be changed easily if soiled, leaving the dressings in place.

Instrumentation

Gentleness and precision in handling small structures and fragile tissues are essential. Thus basic or standard instrument sets, sutures, needles, and other items used for operations on adults must be duplicated in miniature to take care of infants and children in each surgical specialty. The OR nurse and technician must be informed about their patient and then use good judgment in preparing supplies for pediatric surgery.

1 Size and weight are more critical factors than age in the selection of instruments, sutures, needles, and equipment.

2 Small instruments must be used on small, delicate tissues of a newborn, infant, or small child.

3 Hemostats should have fine points. A mosquito hemostat will clamp a superficial vessel, but not a major artery.

4 Noncrushing vascular clamps permit occlusion of major blood vessels and can be placed across the intestine of a newborn or infant rather than using a large, heavy intestinal clamp.

5 Light-weight instruments will not inhibit respiration. Instruments not in use on tissues must *never* be laid on the patient, especially not on the chest. The weight of them could restrict respiration or circulation, or cause bruises. Return instruments to the Mayo stand or instrument table immediately after use.

6 Umbilical tape is used frequently to retract blood vessels and small structures. This gives the surgeon greater visibility in a small operative site and eliminates the weight of retractors.

7 Needleholders must have fine-pointed jaws to hold small, delicate needles.

8 Operation on an adolescent will require adult-size instruments.

9 An efficient scrub nurse will watch the tissue being dissected closely and select the instruments to hand the surgeon accordingly.

COMMON OPERATIONS

General Surgery

Anastomosis within the Alimentary Tract Alimentary tract obstruction is the most frequent cause for emergency operation of the newborn or young infant. The common sites of obstruction are in the esophagus, duodenum, ileum, colon, and anus. *Atresia,* an imperforation or closure of a normal opening, and *stenosis,* a constriction or narrowing, are the common causes of obstruction. The obstructive lesion usually is resected and the viable segments of the viscera anastomosed. A temporary gastrostomy, ileostomy, or colostomy may be necessary. Intestinal obstruction can develop in infants and children months to years after the newborn period from a predisposing or associated congenital anomaly or acquired disease process.

Appendectomy *Appendicitis,* an acute inflammation of the appendix requiring removal of the organ, is the most common cause for abdominal operation in the school-age child.

Herniorrhaphy Hernia repair is the most frequently performed elective operation in infants and children by general surgeons. Of the four types of hernias seen in pediatrics, indirect inguinal hernia is the most common; it occurs much more frequently in males than females and appears during the first 10 years of life. Although frequently seen, most umbilical hernias do not require surgical intervention. Hiatus (diaphragmatic) hernia and femoral hernias require surgical correction, but are rarely acute problems in childhood. A hiatus hernia is a surgical emergency in the newborn if abdominal contents are in the chest causing acute respiratory distress. Hernias seen in infants and children are caused by congenital weakness in the fascia, abdominal wall, or diaphragm.

Omphalocele Failure of the intestines to become encapsulated within the peritoneal cavity during fetal development results in herniation through a midline defect in the abdominal wall at the umbilicus. The intestinal contents of the omphalocele are reduced back into the peritoneal cavity and primary closure of fascia and skin is attempted. For large defects, synthetic mesh or sheeting may be used with primary skin closure. Delayed secondary fascia closure may be necessary.

Pyloromyotomy *Pyloric stenosis,* a congenital obstructive lesion in the area of the pylorus of the stomach, is relieved by cutting through the serosa and dividing the muscle layers of the pylorus. Onset of symptoms usually occurs between the third and eighth weeks of life.

Splenectomy Removal of the spleen may be indicated to correct hypersplenic disease, either congenital or acquired. Emergency splenectomy is necessary following rupture of the spleen, usually from blunt trauma.

Tracheoesophageal Fistula Esophageal atresia, with or without tracheoesophageal fistula, is an acute congenital problem in the newborn. Primary repair is performed by division of the fistula and anastomosis of the trachea and esophagus.

Urology

Pediatric urology concerns itself basically with the diagnosis and treatment of infections and congenital anomalies within the genitourinary tract. Some type of anomaly of the genitourinary system may be found in 10 to 15 percent of newborns. Secondary infections frequently are associated with congenital anomalies; chronic diseases frequently are associated with infections. The following operative procedures include those most commonly performed by pediatric urologists.

Circumcision Excision of the foreskin of the penis may be done to prevent *phimosis,* in which the foreskin becomes tightly wrapped around the tip of the glans penis, or to remove redundant foreskin. Circumcision is the most commonly performed pediatric operation.

Cystoscopy Diagnostic evaluation and therapeutic removal of obstructions within the structures of the genitourinary tract may be performed through an infant- or child-size cystoscope. Cystoscopes from $9\frac{1}{2}$ through 16 French are used for infants and children. A size 3 ureteral catheter can be introduced through the smallest-size cystoscope.

Exstrophy of the Bladder A congenital anomaly, the bladder herniates through the lower abdominal wall in the suprapubic region. Repair requires reconstruction of the lower abdominal wall and external genitalia as well as provision for the passage of urine. This usually can be accomplished in one operation on the female infant, but requires two or more staged operations in the male infant. If urinary continence cannot be established, urinary diversion through ureteral reimplantation may become necessary.

Nephrectomy, Nephrostomy, or Pyeloureteroplasty Hydronephrosis, congenital or acquired, may necessitate one of these operations. Nephrectomy is indicated only if severe disease is unilateral with the contralateral kidney capable of life-sustaining function. More conservative operations are indicated for bilateral or moderate to mild kidney disease. Nephrectomy is necessary to resect a *Wilms's tumor,* a sarcoma of the kidney that develops rapidly in a child usually under 5 years of age.

Orchiopexy One or both testicles that failed to descend during fetal development can be brought into the scrotum and stabilized with a traction suture until healing takes place. Frequently done as a two-stage Torek orchiopexy, the testicle and supporting structures are dissected free from the inguinal region. Adequate length of the spermatic vessels must be obtained to permit the testicle to reach the scrotal sac. After it is pulled down through the scrotum, the testicle is sutured to the fascia of the thigh. Two to three months later at the second-stage operation, the testicle is freed from the fascia and embedded into the scrotum.

If one or both testicles are absent, silicone prostheses may be inserted into the scrotum for cosmetic appearance. Psychologically for the child and parents, undescended (*cryptorchism*) or absence (*agenesis*) of the testicles usually are repaired at age 5 or 6, before the boy begins school.

Ureteral Reimplantation Repositioning of the ureters may be performed to correct either congenital or acquired total urinary incontinence or vesicoureteral reflux.

Incontinence, involuntary leakage of urine from the bladder, causes parents to seek help for the infant or child. Incontinence usually is not due to a single factor, so the urologist must plan the operation on the basis of an accurate assessment of the anatomic and physiologic etiology. Creation of a tubularized trigonal muscle, when reconstructed into a new bladder neck, acts as a sphincter to maintain continence. With the ureters in the normal position, this muscular tube in the bladder wall cannot be constructed. Therefore, the ureters must be reimplanted superiorly into the bladder using a tunnel technique. Care must be taken so the ureters are not hooked or angled, but follow a smooth curve into the bladder.

Vesicoureteral reflux is the most common reason for reimplanting ureters in pediatric patients. Chronic reflux, regurgitation of urine from the bladder into the ureters, can lead to pyelonephritis and hydronephrosis. Ureteral reimplantation may be required to prevent kidney damage. The objective of the operation is to position a segment of the ureters at a higher level within the bladder wall so that the urine lies below the orifices and intravesical pressure prevents reflux.

Urethral Repair The external opening of the urethra may be displaced at birth. *Hypospadias* is an anomaly in the male in which the urethra terminates on the underside of the penis or on the perineum; in the female, the urethra opens into the vagina. *Epispadias* in the male, the urethra terminates on the dorsum of the penis; in the female, it terminates above the clitoris. Multistage procedures are necessary to correct these anomalies.

Orthopaedic Surgery

Pediatric orthopaedic surgery is principally elective and reconstructive in nature to correct deformities of the musculoskeletal system. These may be congenital, idiopathic, pathologic, or traumatic in origin. The extensiveness of the anomalies and functional disorders often involve prolonged immobilization and hospitalization. Many patients require a series of corrective procedures. Some of the conditions most commonly seen in the operating room include the following:

Congenital Dislocated Hip Displacement of the femoral head from its normal position in the acetabulum can be present at birth, either unilaterally or bilaterally. If diagnosed early in infancy, closed reduction with immobilization usually corrects the dislocation without residual deformity. The thighs are hyperextended and the knees flexed. The position is known as "frog" position. Splints or a cast hold the hip in abduction and flexion. The infant cast table is used to apply a hip spica cast.

If the deformity is not found until after the child has begun to walk, an open reduction of the hip with an osteotomy to stabilize the joint may be necessary.

Fractures Fractures occur in infants and children and are treated generally as in adults as described in Chapter 20. However, fixation devices are not well tolerated by children and often prevent uniting of fracture. Closed reduction of long bone fractures is preferable.

Leg-Length Discrepancies The epiphyseal cartilaginous growth lines progressively close as the child matures. Bones lengthen from the activity of the epiphysis. The absolute physiologic criterion for the completion of childhood is when this cartilage becomes a part of the bone. A discrepancy in the activity of an epiphyseal line may retard or overstimulate growth of a bone in one extremity and not its contralateral counterpart. When this occurs in one femur, the legs become unequal in length. The orthopaedic surgeon corrects leg-length discrepancies, usually in excess of 1 in. (2.5 cm), by epiphyseal arrest—stopping the growth of the bone. This may be done in the contralateral leg to let the shorter extremity catch up.

Slipping of the upper femoral epiphysis causes displacement of the femoral head. This can occur as a result of traumatic injury or as a chronic disability usually seen in obese adolescents. Fusion of the epiphysis to the femoral neck may be necessary to prevent slipping and leg shortening.

Scoliosis Scoliosis is a lateral curvature and rotation of the spine, most frequently seen in rapidly growing school-age children or adolescents. Treatment depends on the degree and flexibility of the curvature, the chronological and skeletal age of the child, and the preference of the surgeon. The child may be fitted with a Milwaukee brace, immobilized in a cast, or stretched by traction. If untreated at an early stage, scoliosis produces secondary changes in vertebral bodies and in the rib cage. Spinal fusion must ultimately be performed if the curvature has become severe or must be stabilized following corrections.

1 A wedge body jacket or Minerva jacket (see Chap. 20, p. 378) may be applied. Turnbuckles may be incorporated. These are adjustable metal rods placed along the edges of the wedge of the cast. Gradual opening of the turnbuckles by the surgeon as tolerated by the patient corrects the lateral curvature of the spine.

A Sayre sling, an appliance used for head traction (see Chap. 24), is used sometimes when applying a body jacket to correct slight scoliosis. Traction is obtained by means of pulleys and a rope suspended from the ceiling or an arm of the fracture table.

2 Halo traction is used to stretch the spine in some patients in whom the spine is too rigid to be straightened in a cast. A metal band is applied to the skull by means of four pins inserted into the cortex of the skull. A Steinmann pin is inserted into the distal end of each femur. A traction bow is put on each one. Weights, usually equal, are put on the Halo and Steinmann pins and gradually increased as tolerated. When x-rays show maximum correction, a spinal fusion is done. The traction may be continued until healing has taken place to the degree that there will be no loss of correction; then a plaster jacket is applied.

3 Risser jacket is applied a few days preceding posterior spinal fusion to gain as much correction as possible. The orthopaedic table is used. Traction is applied by a chin strap, similar to a Sayre sling, and countertraction by a pelvic girdle. The spine is straightened as much as possible and the body and head encased in plaster.

4 Posterior spinal fusion may be performed as a two-stage procedure: vertebral body wedge resection at the first stage, and insertion of Harrington rods with fusion at the second stage. Bone fragments removed during the first stage may be saved for the second-stage fusion or sent to the bone bank. Harrington rods are stainless steel. Harrington instruments are required to insert them. Two rods are inserted, one on either side of the curvature. These are secured to the spine and force it into a more nearly normal position. The spine is then fused.

The operation may be done through a window in the Risser jacket, but usually the cast is bivalved and the patient lies in the anterior section during the operation. If the operation is done through a window, an electric cast cutter should be at hand to bivalve the cast if the patient has any respiratory difficulties. After operation the bivalved posterior part is put in place and the jacket is fastened together by several rounds of plaster or by webbing straps with buckles. The patient is in the Risser jacket for a year. Progress is checked by x-ray.

5 Anterior spinal fusion through a transthoracic approach is performed as a one-stage operation to correct severe curvatures in patients who have malformed vertebral bodies. Using Dwyer instruments, titanium staples are fitted over the vertebral bodies on the convex side of the curve. Each staple is held in place by two titanium screws. A multistrand titanium cable, threaded through the heads of the screws, is tightened to compress the vertebrae and straighten the curve. A series of staples and screws are secured the full extent of the curvature. A plaster body jacket may be applied after operation to immobilize the back until the fusion is healed. The patient then is ambulatory.

Talipes Deformities Combinations of various types of deformities of the foot, especially those of congenital origin, are referred to as *talipes* plus the medical term to describe whether the forefoot is inverted (*varus*) or everted (*valgus*) and whether the calcaneal tendon is shortened or lengthened.

Talipes varus, the condition known as *clubfoot*, is the most common of these deformities. Either unilateral or bilateral, the forefoot is inverted and rotated, accompanied by shortening of the calcaneal tendon and contracture of the plantar fascia. Conservative treatment by casting during infancy usually corrects the deformity before the infant bears weight on the foot. A wedge cast with turnbuckles may be applied to an older child to allow gradual manipulation. If conservative treatment is unsuccessful, arthrodesis or other open operative procedure may be necessary to correct the deformity.

Tendon Repair Tendons may be lengthened, shortened, or transferred to correct congenital deformities of the hand or foot. Lacerated tendons must be repaired to restore function. A tourniquet is always used to control bleeding. Tourniquet cuff size must be appropriate for the size of the infant or child. Padding under the cuff must be applied smoothly. Sheet wadding may be used under an infant cuff to protect delicate skin. The cuff must be tight but without restricting circulation before inflation. Time of inflation must be closely watched to prevent ischemia. The surgeon may ask the circulating nurse to release the pressure every 30 minutes on an infant; up to 1 to 2 hours depending on age of older child. Tendon procedures are often lengthy.

Cardiovascular Surgery

Congenital heart defects are the result of abnormal embryological development of the heart or major vessels. Most are diagnosed in infancy, often when the symptoms of congestive heart failure develop within the first few days or months after birth. Palliative or corrective operations are necessary to sustain or prolong life of these infants. Many of these operations are enhanced by or possible only with cardiopulmonary bypass and profound hypothermia (refer to Chap. 21). Congenital heart defects in infants or children amendable to surgical intervention include the following:

Anomalous Venous Return Failure of any one or combination of the pulmonary veins to return blood to the left atrium precludes the full complement of oxygenated blood from entering the systemic circulation. The anomalous pulmonary vein(s) must be transferred and anastomosed to the left atrium.

Coarctation of the Aorta A *coarctation* is a narrowing or stricture in a vessel. This is one of the more common congenital heart defects, usually occurring in the aortic arch. It may cause hypertension in the upper extremities above the obstruction and hypotension in the lower extremities from slowed circulation below the coarctation. If the infant develops severe heart failure, operation must be performed in infancy. Usually it can be deferred until the child is older and operation less risky. To correct the defect, the coarctation is resected and the aorta anastomosed. An aortic graft may be necessary when the length of the coarctation prevents anastomosis.

Patent Ductus Arteriosus During fetal life the ductus arteriosus carries blood from the pulmonary artery to the aorta to bypass the lungs. Normally this vessel closes in the first hours after birth to prevent recirculation of arterial blood through the body. If closure does not occur, blood flow may be reversed by aortic pressure causing respiratory distress. Closure often is delayed in premature infants. Surgical intervention is indicated in true premature and term neonates, in lieu of prolonged ventilatory support, to prevent development of chronic pulmonary changes. The patent ductus arteriosus is clamped and ligated.

Septal Defects Open-heart operation with cardiopulmonary bypass is necessary to close abnormal openings in the walls separating the chambers within the heart.

Atrial Septal Defect An opening in the wall between the right and left atrium may be sufficiently large to allow oxygenated blood to shunt from left to right and return to the lungs. This can increase pulmonary blood flow with eventual pulmonary hypertension if the defect is not closed. If the defect cannot be closed with sutures, a patch graft is inserted.

Ventricular Septal Defect The defect usually is located in the membranous portion of the septum between the right and left ventricles. The most common of the congenital heart anomalies, patients with small defects are relatively asymptomatic and repair may be unnecessary. Large defects with left-to-right shunting of oxygenated blood back to the lungs, thus increasing pulmonary hypertension, are closed. A patch graft may be required to close the defect.

Tetralogy of Fallot Tetralogy of Fallot is a combination of four defects:

1. Ventricular septal defect
2. Stenosis of the pulmonary valve and/or outflow tract into the pulmonary artery
3. Hypertrophy of the right ventricle
4. Displacement of the aorta to the right so it receives blood from both ventricles

Often referred to as "blue babies," the infants are cyanotic because insufficient oxygen circulates to body tissues. Total correction of the multiple anomalies is difficult in these infants. Generally assessment of the technical ease of correction is the dominant consideration. If cyanosis is severe, a palliative shunt operation may be performed during infancy to increase pulmonary blood flow.

1. *Blalock-Taussig operation*: end-to-side anastomosis of the right subclavian artery to the corresponding pulmonary artery. Mixed arterial-venous blood from the aorta flows through the shunt to the pulmonary artery and into the lungs for oxygenation.
2. *Potts-Smith-Gibson operation*: side-to-side anastomosis of the aorta and left pulmonary artery. The shunt enlarges as the child grows, but is more difficult to reconstruct than a Blalock

shunt at a later time when corrective operation is performed.

3 *Waterston operation*: anastomosis of the aorta and right pulmonary artery. The anastomosis is placed on the posterior aspect of the aorta to provide perfusion to both pulmonary arteries.

Total correction usually is delayed until the child is 4 years or older. With cardiopulmonary bypass and hypothermia, the ventricular septal defect is closed with a patch graft that also corrects the abnormal communication between the right ventricle and the aorta. Then the obstruction to pulmonary blood flow is relieved. This may include enlarging the pulmonary valve and/or widening the outflow tract. Resection of obstructing cardiac muscle may be necessary with insertion of prosthetic outflow patch. An aortic allograft containing the aortic valve with the septal leaflet of the mitral valve and the ascending aorta attached may be inserted. The septal leaflet of the mitral valve is used as a portion of the right ventricular outflow patch. All or part of the aortic valve and ascending aorta is used as a new conduit with the pulmonary artery or as a patch graft.

Transposition of the Great Vessels The aorta rises from the right ventricle and the pulmonary artery from the left ventricle. This essentially creates two separate circulatory systems: one systemic and the other pulmonary. Life depends upon the presence or creation of associated defects to permit exchange of blood between the two systems. These defects may include a patent foramen ovale, patent ductus arteriosus, atrial septal defect, or ventricular septal defect. Palliative operations are performed in the newborn, usually to enlarge the atrial septal defect, to sustain life until the infant grows enough to tolerate a corrective procedure that may include partial transposition of the pulmonary veins.

Tricuspid Atresia Absence of the tricuspid valve between the right atrium and ventricle prevents normal blood flow through the chambers of the heart. Blood flows through an atrial septal defect, into an enlarged left ventricle, through a small right ventricle to the pulmonary artery. The Glenn procedure, anastomosis of the superior vena cava to the right pulmonary artery, or other type of aorta-pulmonary artery shunt is created as a palliative procedure to increase pulmonary blood flow.

Truncus Arteriosus A single artery carries blood directly from the heart with a large associated ventricular septal defect, to the coronary, pulmonary, and systemic circulatory systems. An initial palliative banding of the pulmonary arteries, as close to their origins off the truncus as possible, decreases pulmonary blood flow in the infant in congestive heart failure. At a later stage a corrective procedure can be performed to close the ventricular septal defect and insert a conduit with an ascending aortic graft and aortic valve. Correction in infancy requires replacement of the conduit as the child grows.

Valvular Obstructive Lesions Congenital aortic and pulmonary valve stenosis require valvulotomy.

Thoracic Surgery

Pectus Excavatum A congenital malformation of the chest wall, pectus excavatum is characterized by a pronounced funnel-shaped depression over the lower end of the sternum. The deformity is corrected by resecting the lower intercostal cartilages and substernal ligaments to free up the sternum. The sternum is elevated and the cartilages fitted to the sides of it. The operation is done primarily for cosmetic purposes, but occasionally it is necessary to establish normal respiratory and circulatory function.

Ophthalmology

Oculoplastic Procedures on Eyelids Congenital malformations such as *ptosis* (drooping of an upper or lower eyelid) are corrected by extraocular procedures.

Extraocular Muscle Operations Operations on muscles to correct strabismus or squint are the third most commonly performed pediatric operations between ages 6 months and 6 years. The trend is to correct the congenital type during infancy, and the acquired type in the preschool years. The patterns of using the two eyes together are more flexible and adaptable in the younger child. These operations on extraocular muscles are done to correct muscle imbalance, either by strengthening the weak muscle or by weakening an overactive one. The mechanical advantage of a weak muscle can be increased by:

1 *Tucking.* A tuck is sutured in the muscle to shorten it, thereby increasing its effective power.

2 *Advancement.* The attachment point of the muscle is freed, and it is reattached closer to the cornea, thereby increasing its leverage.

3 *Resection.* Part of the muscle is removed to shorten it, and the cut ends are sutured together.

An overactive muscle can be weakened by:

1 *Tenotomy.* The point of attachment of the muscle is severed, and the muscle is dropped back, held by ligaments only.
2 *Recession.* The muscle is detached from the eyeball and reattached farther back to decrease its action.
3 *Myotomy.* The fibers of a section of muscle are divided in order to diminish muscle action.
4 *Myectomy.* A section of the muscle belly is excised.

Intraocular Procedures

Cataract Operations Discission or needling procedures are performed for congenital cataract or cataract in young children. The capsule is incised, and the lens substance is broken up. The aqueous humor has a solvent action on the exposed lens material so that a clear opening for the passage of light is obtained.

Goniotomy Performed for congenital glaucoma, this microsurgical procedure involves dividing a congenital layer of abnormal tissue covering the drainage angle of the anterior chamber. This is performed under direct observation by use of a contact lens that permits visualization of the angle. Incision is made through an opening in the contact lens.

NOTE. Since the majority of surgical eye patients are children and aged persons, detainers are used as needed postoperatively. Elbows of infants and toddlers must be prevented from bending by use of arm splints so they cannot disturb dressings (refer to Chap. 22).

Otorhinolaryngology

Middle Ear Tympanoplasty Congenital deafness may occur in varying degrees, and as yet no cure has been found for the nerve type. Congenital or acquired conductive deafness may be helped by tympanoplastic operative techniques (refer to Chap. 23, p. 415).

Correction of Choanal Atresia When bone or fibrous tissue blocks the posterior choanae, operative excision of the obstructive tissue corrects the problem. Newborns are obligate nose breathers and may die at birth if choanal atresia is undiagnosed. They are unable to breathe and feed properly without adequate nasal airway.

Adenoidectomy Preferably a patient should be at least 2 years old before having adenoid tissue in the nasopharynx removed, but it may be done earlier. This procedure is usually done in conjunction with a tonsillectomy.

Tonsillectomy Excision of hypertrophied or chronically infected tonsils is the second most commonly performed pediatric operation. The operation is not generally advised before 3 years of age. General anesthesia is used for patients up to about 14 years of age. Frequently tonsillectomy and adenoidectomy are performed together, appearing on the operating schedule as "T&A." Sterile technique is carried out throughout the operation. Precautions during operation include control of bleeding and prevention of aspiration of blood or tissue.

Esophageal Dilation Children, usually of preschool age, may ingest caustic agents that cause chemical burns of the mouth, lips, pharynx, and corrosive esophagitis. Long-term, gradual esophageal dilation with bougies may be necessary to restore an adequate oral intake of food after the acute phase of traumatic injury. When all attempts at dilation fail, the esophagus must be replaced. The most satisfactory source of esophageal replacement is the colon.

Tracheal or Laryngeal Stenosis Some accidental injuries result in a narrowing of the trachea or larynx. Of greater concern are the injuries that result from therapy for respiratory problems, especially in newborns. Prolonged endotracheal intubation can lead to injury from tubes that are too large for the available lumen, are too long, or move too much. These injuries may require dilation and/or endoscopic resection of the stenotic area. Most infants then require an intraluminal stent to maintain patency of their airways.

Tracheotomy Tracheotomy is advisable in situations of severe inflammatory glottic diseases, when endotracheal intubation would be required longer than 72 hours, and when respiratory support is necessary for longer than 24 to 48 hours to treat respiratory problems. The appropriate sizes and types of tracheotomy tubes for infants and children must be available. Tubes that are too large, too rigid, too long, or have an improper curve can produce ulceration and scarring at pressure points. Strictures that develop at the site of tracheotomy may require resection to relieve airway obstruction after decannulation.

Neurosurgery

Children of all ages sustain head injuries with hematomas that must be evacuated (refer to Chap. 24, p. 438). Brain tumors do occur in children; however, the more frequently performed pediatric neurosurgical procedures are related to correction of congenital anomalies.

Craniosynostosis If one or more of the suture lines in the skull, normally open in infancy, fuses prematurely, the skull cannot expand during normal brain growth. The surgeon removes the fused bone, a *craniectomy,* to reopen the suture line. A strip of polyethylene or Silastic film may be inserted to cover the bone edges on each side, or the newly formed suture lines may be cauterized with Zinker's solution, to prevent refusion. More extensive freeing of other bones may be necessary to achieve decompression of the frontal lobes and orbital contents.

Encephalocele Brain and neural tissue can herniate through a defect in the skull. This is present at birth as a sac of tissue on the head. Usually these lesions can be removed 6 to 12 weeks after birth, unless complicated by hydrocephalus.

Hydrocephalus Usually congenital, dilatation of the ventricles by obstruction, excessive formation of cerebrospinal fluid, or failure of the absorptive mechanisms produces impairment in the normal circulation of cerebrospinal fluid. Fluid accumulates in the ventricles. Pressure thus created causes enlargement of the infant's head, if it develops prior to fusion of the cranial bones, and often causes brain damage. Operative treatment involves establishment of a mechanism for transporting the excess fluid from the ventricles to maintain a close-to-normal ventricular pressure. This may be done by implantation of a shunt, which carries the fluid from the lateral ventricle to the peritoneal cavity (*ventriculoperitoneal shunt*) or to the right atrium of the heart (*ventriculoatrial shunt*). Other types of shunts are used, but less commonly, to bypass localized obstructions.

One end of the shunt catheter is put into the ventricle; the other end may connect to a one-way valve, which in turn is connected to the catheter that drains fluid distally from the head. Most of the catheters are silicone rubber. An antithrombotic coating may be incorporated into the distal end. Some valves are regulated to open for drainage when predetermined pressure in the ventricle is reached. Other valves are designed as flushing devices to keep the distal catheter patent; the skin over the device is manually depressed to flush the system. The surgeon chooses the shunt mechanism for each patient that will be safest for the particular type of hydrocephalus being treated. Follow-up minor revisions are sometimes necessary, generally due to growth of the child.

Myelomeningocele A saclike protrusion bulges through a defect in a portion of the vertebral column that failed to fuse in fetal development. If the nerves of the spinal cord remain within the vertebral column and only the meninges protrude into the sac, the congenital anomaly is a *meningocele.* However, if the sac contains nerves, it is a *myelomeningocele* with associated permanent nerve damage. The degree of impairment depends on the level and extent of the defect. Clubfeet, dislocated hips, hydrocephalus, neurogenic bladder, paralysis, and other congenital disorders often accompany myelomeningocele. Each patient must be evaluated and treated individually according to priorities of needs. In general, it is best to delay operating to repair the myelomeningocele until danger of hydrocephalus developing is passed or the cerebrospinal fluid has been shunted. If the sac is covered with a thin membrane, *meningitis* (infection of the meninges) is an imminent danger unless the defect is repaired soon after birth, usually within the first 48 hours, to close the cutaneous, muscular, and dural defects.

Spina Bifida Incomplete closure of the paired vertebral arches in the midline of the vertebral column may occur without herniation of the meninges. A spina bifida may be covered by intact skin. Laminectomy may be indicated to repair the underlying defect.

Plastic and Reconstructive Surgery

With the exception of burns and other traumatic tissue injuries, most plastic and reconstructive surgery performed on infants and children is done to correct congenital anomalies. The most common of these include the following:

Cleft Lip Lack of fusion of the soft tissues of the upper lip creates a cleft or fissure. Cleft lips vary in degree from simple notching of the lip to extension into the floor of the nose. They may be unilateral or bilateral. The number of operations required for correction depends on the severity of the deformity. Some plastic surgeons do a primary *cheiloplasty,* closure of cleft lip, within the first few days after birth to facilitate feeding and to minimize psychological trauma of the parents. Those surgeons who prefer to wait until the infant is older follow the "rule of 10": 10 weeks, 10 g of hemoglobin, 10 lb of body weight. Regardless of preferred timing, infiltration of local anesthetic agent with epinephrine usually is the anesthesia of choice.

To relieve tension on the incision postoperatively, a Logan bow (a small curved metal frame) may be applied over the area of incision and held in place by narrow adhesive strips, to splint the lip. Skin closure strips may be used. Arm or elbow restraints are imperative to prevent the infant from removing the bow or strips and injuring the lip. These restraints are applied in the OR.

Cleft Palate Failure of the tissues of the palate to fuse creates a fissure through the roof of the mouth. Palatal clefts may be only a defect in the soft palate or may extend through both hard and soft palates into the nose and include the alveolar ridge of the maxilla. Cleft palate often is associated with cleft lip; however, the two deformities are closed separately. *Palatoplasty,* closure of the palate, usually is done between 18 and 24 months of age. Before this time, the oral cavity is too small for adequate exposure of tissues. But more importantly, the soft palate is closed before speech begins to avoid speech defects. A mouth gag must be used during operation to permit access to the palate without obstructing the airway. General anesthesia is administered via endotracheal tube. This may be supplemented by infiltration of local anesthetic agent. When epinephrine is used by the surgeon to minimize bleeding, the anesthesiologist must be informed. Elbow restraints are always applied before the toddler leaves the OR.

In patients with bilateral and frequently unilateral clefts, an additional operation to the nose will be performed before the age of 4 years to elevate the tip of the nose and correct the asymmetry.

Hemangioma Hemangiomas are the most common of all human congenital anomalies. An angioma that is made up of blood vessels is a hemangioma that may pigment or appear as a growth on the skin. All hemangiomas have abnormal patterns of hemodynamics, which is the effect of blood flow through tissues, but variations in vessel size distinguish the different types of these tumors. Surgical excision in combination with skin graft or pedicle flap repair is the treatment of choice primarily for intradermal capillary hemangiomas (port-wine stain). Cryosurgery, surgical excision, or steroid therapy may be used for some other cavernous-type tumors.

Microtia Abnormally small or absent external ears can be reconstructed in several operative stages. Autogenous rib cartilage graft or silicone prosthesis is used for the supporting framework to produce the anatomic contour. Usually necessitated by microtia, a congenital anomaly, reconstruction of the external ear can follow traumatic injury with loss of all or part of the pinna.

Otoplasty procedures to correct protruding or excessively large ears are performed more frequently than procedures for microtia. These often are done on preschool-age children, usually boys, to prevent psychological harm from teasing.

Syndactylism Webbing between the fingers is the most common congenital deformity of the hand. The tissue holding the digits together must be cut to separate the fingers. Separation of webbed digits almost always requires skin grafts to achieve good functional results. Syndactyly may occur in the foot also.

PEDIATRIC ANESTHESIA

Pediatric anesthesia has become increasingly specialized as the many variables in the management of infants and children have become better understood.

Premedication

Premedication varies considerably by age and weight of the patient and routine of the anesthesiologist. Some anesthesiologists prefer children to be well medicated; others favor minimal sedation. Crying greatly increases mucus in the respiratory tract. Atropine sulfate frequently is used for premedication to inhibit secretions. In some instances meperidine hydrochloride (Demerol) is given to infants and children over 20 lb in body weight. Dosage is approximately one-half mg per pound (1.1 mg per kg) of body weight given IM. Barbiturates or diazepam also are used sometimes for relaxation so anesthesia can be more easily induced. Whether asleep or awake upon arrival in the OR suite, the patient should not be disturbed so the premedication can be effective.

Induction

1 Restrain the patient during induction. If the patient is a newborn, infant, or toddler, restraint straps are omitted while the circulating nurse holds the patient during induction. A toddler or preschool-age child is less frightened holding onto someone's hands. Restraints can be applied after the patient is asleep.

2 If the child is awake, crying, or struggling, apprehension during induction can be avoided by distraction and rapport. It is not easy to establish rapport with young children. Their cooperation may be solicited by counting out loud, singing the alphabet song, blowing up a balloon, taking a "space trip," or discussing a favorite plaything or television character. The face mask can be held slightly above the face, permitting anesthetic gas to flow by gravity, and lowered gently as the child becomes drowsy.

3 Induction may be accompanied by regurgitation and aspiration of gastric contents in infants with pyloric stenosis, tracheoesophageal fistula, intestinal obstruction, or food in the stomach. The hazard is minimized by aspirating gastric contents by sterile catheter prior to induction, and leaving the tube in place for drainage during operation. Or, if solid food is present or suspected, the stomach may be emptied completely before induction by induced vomiting. A stomach tube may be passed and gentle suction applied after intubation to relieve gastric distention.

Intubation

1 Endotracheal intubation is used by some anesthesiologists for all procedures in infants under 1 year of age. It is mandatory for intra-abdominal, intrathoracic, neurosurgical procedures, and those about the head or neck areas.

2 Airway obstruction in infants and children usually occurs early during anesthesia administration. When anesthesia deepens, airway insertion is essential after prior assisted ventilation. Assisted or controlled ventilation reduces the labor of breathing and, therefore, metabolism. Intubation and suctioning are preceded and followed by oxygen administration.

3 Sterile equipment and gentle manipulation to avoid soft tissue injury are essential for intubation and suctioning. Nasotracheal tubes are avoided as they may inadvertently dislodge adenoid tissue and carry it into the trachea.

4 A newborn's head must be maintained in a neutral position midway between full extension and full flexion, while an endotracheal tube is in place. The tip of the tube should be placed at the mid-trachea position. The average distance between the vocal cords and the carina, where the trachea separates into two branches, is only 4 or 5 cm (about 2 in.) in a term neonate and much less in a premature. If the head shifts, the tube can slip up or down and cause disastrous consequences.

Anesthetic Agents

1 Topical agents are generally avoided because of the hazard of overdose.

2 Any general anesthetic agent may be used. Halothane is popular and few cases of hepatotoxicity in children have been reported. Depth of anesthesia is judged by muscle tone, respiratory rate, color of blood, circulatory changes, and chest compliance. Simple, lightweight, sterile equipment, offering low resistance to breathing, is used. Disposable equipment is popular.

3 Neuromuscular blockers are used judiciously. Infants under 1 year exhibit a greater degree of blockade from succinylcholine than older children. Also, bradycardia and intraocular tension rise are more conspicuous in infants. Response decreases with age. Dosage varies.

Extubation

Extubation of an infant or child is a treacherous time. It is preceded and followed by oxygen administration and performed either under deep anesthesia or on return of spontaneous respiration since laryngospasm is possible between these periods. Heart and breath sounds are monitored following extubation. If spasm occurs, oxygen is given by positive pressure.

Postoperative Care

The patient should not be taken from the OR if body temperature is below 95 °F (35 °C), a crucial level below which there is high incidence of bradycardia, hypotension, and apnea. Dehydration and low humidity increase viscosity of secretions. Pediatric patients require *close* watching for development of laryngeal edema noted by croupy cough, sobbing inspiration, intercostal retraction, tachypnea, or tachycardia. Laryngeal edema greatly reduces the small diameter of the airway of an infant or toddler. Controlled humidity and oxygen are vital.

Chapter 27

Oncology

Oncology is the study of scientific control over neoplastic growth. It concerns the etiology, diagnosis, treatment, and rehabilitation of patients with known or potential neoplasms. Clarification of terminology is essential to an understanding of oncology.

DEFINITIONS

Neoplasm An atypical new growth of abnormal cells or tissues.

Tumor Any neoplasm in which cells are permanently altered but have the capability of growth and reproduction. A tumor consists of two elements: the tumor cells themselves, and a supporting framework of connective tissue and vascular supply.

Benign Tumor An aggregation of cells closely resembling those of the parent tissue of origin. The tumor usually grows slowly by expansion, is localized, and is surrounded by a capsule of fibrous tissue.

Malignant Tumor A progressively growing tumor originating from a specialized organ such as the lung, breast, or brain, or localized to a specific body system such as bone, skin, lymph nodes, or blood vessels. Four characteristics differentiate malignant from benign tumors. A malignant tumor:

1 Is anaplastic. Cells, resembling embryonic cell forms, are morphologically and functionally differentiated from the normal tissue of their origin. They vary in size, shape, and texture.
2 Infiltrates and destroys adjacent normal tissue.
3 Grows in a disorganized, uncontrolled, irregular manner, usually rapidly increasing in size perceptibly within weeks or months.
4 Has power to metastasize. The tumor cells migrate from a primary focus to another single focus or to multiple foci in distant tissues or organs via lymphatic or vascular channels.

Cancer A broad term describing any malignant tumor within a large class of diseases. More than 100 different forms of cancer are known, with many histologic variations within each. Cancerous tumors are divided into two broad groups:

1 *Carcinoma.* A malignant tumor of epithelial origin affecting glandular organs, viscera, and skin.
2 *Sarcoma.* A malignant tumor of mesenchymal origin affecting bones and muscles.

-oma A suffix denoting a tumor or neoplasm.

Oncologist A specialist in the study and treatment of neoplastic growths.

TREATMENT AND PROGNOSIS OF CANCER

The treatment and prognosis of cancer are based on the extent of the disease. Each type of cancer differs in its symptoms, behavior, and response to treatment. Cancer is a potentially curable disease, but it is the second leading cause of disease-related death in the United States.

Clinical Signs and Symptoms

1 Palpable tumor
2 Abnormal bleeding
3 Steady decrease in weight, appetite, and energy
4 Chronic cough or change in bowel habits

High-Risk-Related Factors

1 Exposure to *carcinogens,* cancer-producing agents such as coal tar, chemicals, radiation
2 Age, sex, or racial predisposition
3 Predisposition to cancer due to specific environmental conditions, genetics, hereditary or acquired conditions, or diseases

Extent of Disease

Carcinoma *in situ* Normal cells are replaced by anaplastic cells but the growth disturbance of epithelial surfaces shows no behavioral evidence of invasion and metastasis.

Localized Cancer The malignant tumor is contained within the organ of its origin.

Regional Cancer The invaded area extends from the periphery of the organ or tissue of origin to include tumor cells in adjacent organs or tissues, e.g., the regional lymph nodes.

Metastatic Cancer The tumor has extended by way of lymphatic or vascular channels to tissues or organs beyond the regional area.

Disseminated Cancer Multiple foci of tumor cells are dispersed throughout the body.

Curative versus Palliative Therapy

Cancer is basically a systemic disease. Therapy is *curative* if the disease process can be totally eradicated, but success largely depends on early diagnosis. When a cure is not possible, *palliative* therapy relieves the symptoms, but does not cure the disease. Tumors are classified to determine the most effective therapy.

Tumor Identification System

A standardized tumor identification system, which includes classification and staging, is essential to establish treatment protocols and to evaluate the end result of therapy. Hospitals maintain a tumor registry of patients to evaluate therapeutic approaches to specific types of tumors.

Classification includes the anatomical and histological description of a tumor. *Staging* refers to the extent of the tumor. The three basic categories of the system are:

T: primary tumor
N: regional nodes
M: distant metastases

The TNM categories are identified by pretherapy clinical diagnosis, tissue biopsy, and/or histopathological examination following operative resection of tumor. Subscripts are used to describe the findings, e.g., bronchogenic carcinoma$_T$ meaning primary tumor in the lung without regional nodes or distant metastases. Older staging systems are referred to in the literature as stages I, II, III, and IV.

Adjunctive Therapy

Operative resection, endocrine therapy, radiation therapy, chemotherapy, immunotherapy, hyperthermia, or combinations of these procedures are used in the treatment of cancer. The surgeon or oncologist must determine the most appropriate therapy for each patient. Consideration is given to:

1 The type and site of the tumor, its extent, and whether lymph nodes are involved
2 The type of surrounding normal tissue
3 The age and general condition of the patient, including nutritional status, and whether other diseases are present
4 Whether curative or palliative therapy is possible

OPERATIVE RESECTION

In the past, operative resection was the modality of choice to remove tumors. Resection of a malignant tumor is, however, localized therapy for what usually is a systemic disease. Each patient must be evaluated and treated individually, and the extent of the operative procedure must be planned appropriately for the identified stage of disease. The surgeon selects either a radical curative operation or a salvage palliative operation, depending on localization, regionalization, and dissemination of the tumor. In planning the operation, the surgeon considers the length of expected survival, prognosis of surgical intervention, and the effect of concurrent diseases on the postoperative result.

Accessible, well-differentiated primary tumors are frequently treated by excision. Extremely wide resection may be necessary to avoid recurrence of the tumor. The pathologist is able to make judgments about questionable margins by making rapid frozen sections while the operation is in progress. The pathologist's findings guide the surgeon as to the extent of resection needed so residual tumor is not left in the patient.

Many of the operations described in previous chapters are performed for the ablation of tumors by primary resection. In addition, *lymphadenectomy* may be performed as a prophylactic measure to inhibit metastatic spread of tumor cells via lymphatic channels. Other modalities of therapy may be administered pre- and/or postoperatively to reduce or prevent recurrence.

Specific Considerations

Malignant tumor cells can be disseminated by manipulation of tissue. Because of their altered nutritional and physiological status, patients with cancer may be highly susceptible to the complications of postoperative infection. To minimize these risks, specific precautions are taken in the operative management of these patients.

1 Skin over the site of a soft tissue tumor should be handled gently during hair removal and antisepsis. Vigorous scrubbing could dislodge underlying tumor cells.

2 Gowns, gloves, drapes, and instruments are changed following a biopsy, e.g., a breast biopsy, before incision for a radical resection, e.g., a mastectomy. The tumor is deliberately incised to obtain a biopsy for diagnosis. However, margins of healthy tissue surrounding a radical resection must not be inoculated with tumor cells.

3 Instruments placed in direct contact with tumor cells are discarded immediately after use. Even when the tumor appears to be localized, most cancers have disseminated to some degree. Therefore, some surgeons prefer to use each instrument once and then discard it.

4 Antibiotics are administered pre-, intra-, and postoperatively as a prophylactic measure to provide an adequate antibacterial level to prevent wound infection.

5 Time-honored precautions such as gentle tissue handling, keeping blood loss to a minimum, and avoiding an unduly prolonged operation influence the outcome for the patient.

6 Messages should be conveyed periodically during a long radical operation to the patient's anxiously awaiting family, to reassure them that their loved one is receiving care from a concerned OR team.

ENDOCRINE THERAPY

Tumors arising in organs that are usually under hormonal influence, such as the breast and uterus in the female and the prostate in the male, may be stimulated by hormones produced in the endocrine glands. Cellular metabolism is affected by the presence of specific hormone receptors in the tumor cells: estrogen and/or progesterone in the female, androgens in the male. Some breast, endometrial, and prostatic cancers depend on these hormones for growth and maintenance. Recurrence or spread of disease may be retarded by therapeutic hormonal manipulation. Endocrine manipulation does not cure, but it can control the dissemination of disease if the tumor progresses beyond the limits of effective operative resection or radiation therapy. Cancer of the breast or prostate may metastasize to soft tissues, or to the brain, lung, liver, and bone.

Hormonal Receptor Site Studies

Identifying hormonal dependence of the primary tumor by receptor site studies is a fairly reliable way of selecting patients who will benefit postoperatively from endocrine manipulation. Following a positive diagnosis of cancer, either by a frozen section biopsy or by pathologic permanent sections, the surgeon probably will request receptor site evaluation of a primary breast, uterine, or prostatic tumor. The tissue specimen removed by operative resection should *not* be placed in Formalin preservative solution, since this will alter the receptor cells enough to negate hormonal study.

Endocrine Ablation

Since 1896, surgeons have described positive clinical responses in patients with metastatic breast cancer treated by *endocrine ablation,* the surgical removal of endocrine glands. If the surgeon plans to eliminate endocrine stimulation surgically in a patient with a known hormone-dependent tumor, all sources of the hormone should be ablated.

Bilateral Adrenaloophorectomy Both adrenal glands and ovaries may be resected to prevent recurrence, control soft tissue metastases, or relieve bone pain from metastatic breast cancer. These may be removed as a one-stage operation. If two separate operations are preferred, bilateral oophorectomy precedes bilateral adrenalectomy except in menopausal women in whom only the latter operation may be indicated (see Chap. 18, p. 349 for discussion of oophorectomy and Chap. 19, p. 358 for discussion of adrenalectomy).

Bilateral Orchiectomy and Adrenalectomy Both testes may be removed following radical prostatectomy for advanced carcinoma of the prostate to eliminate androgens of testicular origin. Bilateral adrenalectomy also may be indicated. (See Chap. 19 for discussion of these operations.)

Hypophysectomy Enucleation of the pituitary gland may be indicated in patients with recurrent or progressive breast or prostatic cancer to eliminate stimulating hormones produced by the pituitary (see transsphenoidal operations in Chap. 24, p. 436).

Hormonal Therapy

Hormones administered orally or intramuscularly can alter cell metabolism by changing the systemic hormonal environment of the body. To be effective, tumor cells must contain receptors. Hormones must bind to these receptors before they can exert an effect on the cells.

Androgens A male sex hormone is given to women with cancer of the breast to inhibit estrogen action following oophorectomy or during the normal postmenopausal life cycle. Preparations of testosterone are most commonly used.

Corticosteroids When bilateral adrenalectomy or hypophysectomy is contraindicated, corticosteroids may be administered to suppress estrogen production. Prednisone, cortisone, hydrocortisone, or some other preparation of corticosteroids may be administered as an anti-inflammatory agent along with chemotherapeutic agents given for control of disseminated disease.

Estrogens A female sex hormone is given both to men with prostatic carcinoma and to women with breast cancer. Diethylstilbestrol is one of the most common estrogens for both sexes.

Progesterones Progesterone inhibits proliferation of endometrium and will retard the growth of some endometrial carcinomas. It also is given to retard renal cell and breast cancers.

Antiestrogen Therapy

Patients with medical contraindications to an endocrine ablation may receive antiestrogen therapy. An estrogen antagonist deprives an estrogen-dependent tumor of the estrogen necessary for its growth. Nafoxidine hydrochloride, a synthetic nonsteroidal drug, inhibits the normal intake of estrogen at the estrogen receptor sites. It is given orally.

RADIATION THERAPY

Treatment of disease with any type of radiation (referred to as *radiation therapy* or *radiotherapy*) includes the use of high-voltage irradiation, radium, or other radioactive elements to injure or destroy cells. Like operative resection, radiation is localized therapy applicable in only a limited number of specific tumors. Radiation is the emission of electromagnetic waves or atomic particles from the disintegration of the nuclei of unstable or radioactive elements. Ionizing radiation is used for therapy.

Ionizing Radiation

Ionization is a physical production of positive and negative ions capable of conducting electricity. Radiation of sufficient energy to disrupt the electronic balance of the atom is called *ionizing radiation.* When this takes place in tissue cells or extracellular fluids, the effect can range from minor changes to profound disturbances. Radiation may come from particles of the nuclei of disintegrating atoms or from electromagnetic waves that have no mass. Types of ionizing radiation include:

Alpha Particles These relatively large particles have a very slight penetrating power. They are stopped by a thin sheet of paper. They have dense ionization, but can produce tremendous tissue destruction within a short distance.

Beta Particles These relatively small particles are electrical and travel with the speed of light. They have greater penetrating properties than alpha particles. Their emissions cause tissue necrosis. They produce ionization, which has destructive properties.

Gamma Rays and X-Rays Electromagnetic radiation of short wavelength but high energy, gamma rays and x-rays are capable of completely penetrating the body. They affect tumor tissue more rapidly than normal tissue. Rays are stopped by a *thick* lead shield. Protons ranging in energy from 30 kilovolts to 35 million electron volts are available for treatment of various cancers. Gamma rays are emitted spontaneously from the nucleus of the atom of a radioactive element.

Effects of Radiation on Cells

Cancer cells multiply out of normal body control. They are in a state of active, uncontrolled mitosis, the nuclear division of the cytoplasm and nucleus. Radiation affects the metabolic activity of cells. Cells in an active state of mitosis are most susceptible. Thus radiation has the ability to destroy malignant tumors without permanently injuring normal tissue in therapeutic dosages. Gamma rays and x-rays, acting over a period of time, cause a cessation of cell growth and a regression of the tumor mass. The cells die and are replaced by fibrous tissue.

Sensitivity to radiation varies. Some tumors can be destroyed by a small amount of radiation; others require a large amount. The sensitivity of the normal cells from which the tumor cells are derived determines the sensitivity of the tumor cells. Cells originating from bone marrow and lymphoid tissue are especially susceptible to radiation. Tumors in bone are resistant.

Dosage of radiation cannot be limited solely to the area to be treated. The danger of injuring normal surrounding tissue is a limiting factor in the dosage and selection of the most appropriate type of radiation therapy. The factor in dosage is the ratio of tumor tissue to the surrounding normal tissue. Dosage is computed in rads. A *rad* (roentgen absorbed dose) is the unit used to measure the absorbed dose of radiation. One rad is the amount of radiation required to deposit 100 ergs of energy per gram of tissue. The dosage of irradiation delivered to a specific tissue site is measured by the distance from source and duration of exposure by radiophysics or by instruments such as Geiger counters or scintillation probes. The doses are measured in rads to determine if dosage is adequate for therapy and not so excessive that it would cause damage to normal tissues.

Radiation energy penetration is calculated from the rate of decay or disintegration, known as half-life. *Half-life* is the time required for half the radioactive element to disintegrate and to lose one-half of its activity by decay.

Sources of Radiation

Although the effects of radiation are similar, its sources and their application for therapy differ. Some sources are implanted into the body in direct contact with tumor tissue; others are passed through the body to the tumor from an external beam.

Radium Radium is a radioactive metal. Mme. Curie, a research chemist, and her husband, a physicist, discovered and named it in 1898. Several years earlier, Mme. Curie had been given the task of finding out why pitchblende would record its image on a photographic plate. She and her husband knew that pitchblende emitted more radiation than the known minerals in it justified. It took 6 years of painstaking, difficult work for the Curies to isolate radium as a pure element and learn of its radioactive properties.

Metallic radium is unstable in air. Radium chloride or bromide salts emit fluorescence and heat. One gram gives off 134 calories per hour. Alpha and beta particles and gamma rays are products of its disintegration. The half-life of radium is about 1620 years; half the remaining life is lost in another 1620 years, and so on. The final product is lead.

A close associate of the Curies carried a tube of radium salts in his vest pocket and subsequently developed a skin ulceration under it. This led to animal experimentation and research in the treatment of skin lesions, and thus began the use of radium in medicine. Radium is used in the treatment of many malignant tumors.

Radon Radon is a dense radioactive gas liberated as the first byproduct from the disintegration of radium. Mme. Curie discovered this gas and first named it "emanation." Radon is collected by an intricate process in gold capillary tubing. Seeds for implantation are then cut and sealed. Dosage is computed for the hour of insertion into tissue. It is measured in millicurie-hours. The half-life of radon is 4 days; its total life is about 30 days.

Radionuclides A radionuclide is an element that has been bombarded in a nuclear reactor with radioactive particles. It shows radioactive disintegration and emits either alpha and beta particles or gamma rays. Those emitting alpha and beta particles are used primarily for treating malignant tumors (see Chap. 15 for use of radionuclides in diagnostic procedures). Therapeutic radionuclides may also be referred to as *radiopharmaceuticals.* Historically they were known as *radioactive isotopes* or *radioisotopes,* and these terms are still found in the literature. Cesium, cobalt, iodine, and iridium are the most commonly used elements for therapy.

Radionuclides are controlled by the Atomic Energy Commission and are released only to individuals trained and licensed to use them. Available in liquid or solid forms, they may be ingested orally, infused intravenously, instilled into a body cavity, injected or implanted into tumor, or applied to skin externally. The ionizing radiation emitted has an action on tissue similar to that of radium, but radionuclides differ from radium in the following ways:

1 Half-life is short. Radionuclides disintegrate at varying rates depending upon their type. Each element has a specific half-life, but each one is different. They vary from a few hours, such as the 6 hours of technetium 99, to the 8 days of iodine 131 or the 5.3 years of cobalt 60.

2 Irradiation does not spread so much into adjoining tissue; thus a stronger dose can be used in a malignant tumor. Radiation is not absorbed by bone and other normal body tissues.

3 Irradiation can be more easily shielded. The surgeon and other personnel do not get as much radiation exposure in placing or removing radionuclides.

4 Precautions in handling patients who are receiving treatment may be less stringent. However, exposure to radionuclides, like exposure to radium and radon, is always potentially dangerous. Radiation may treat cancer, but it can also cause a malignancy.

Implantation of Radiation Sources

All radiation sources for implantation are prepared in the desired therapeutic dosages by the nuclear medicine department. Many types of sources are used to deliver maximum radiation to the primary tumor. No single type is ideal for every tumor or anatomic site.

Interstitial Needles Interstitial needles are hollow sheaths, usually made of platinum or Monel metal. Radium salts or radionuclides are encased in platinum or platinum-iridium short units or cells, which in turn are sealed in the metal sheath of the needle for implantation into tumor tissue. Radium needles are used occasionally in treatment of tumors in the vagina, cervix, tongue, mouth, or neck. Radionuclide needles, usually containing cesium 137, are also implanted in tumors that are near the body surface or accessible enough to permit their use. In the OR, these needles are inserted at the periphery of and within the tumor. They are usually left in place for 4 to 7 days depending on the planned dosage to the tumor bed.

A needle may contain one or several short units or cells of the radiation source depending on the length of the needle to be used. The dosage is measured in milligram-hours, which can be converted to rads. The needles vary in length from 10 to 60 mm, with a diameter of 1 to 2 mm. The choice of length depends upon the area involved as well as the dosage.

One end of the needle is pointed and the other has an eye for a heavy (size 2) suture. A square knot is tied about $\frac{1}{8}$ in. (3 mm) from the eye of the needle. Needles are threaded to prevent their loss while in use and to aid in removing them. After the surgeon inserts the needles, the ends of the sutures are tied or taped together and taped to the skin in an adjoining area.

Interstitial Seeds Sealed seeds containing radon, cesium 137, iridium 192, or iodine 125 may be implanted or injected directly into tumor tissue. Radon seeds are permanently implanted; the radionuclide seeds are removed after the desired exposure. Seeds are particularly useful in body-cavity tumors, localized areas, and tumors that are not resectable because they are located near major vessels or the spinal cord. Seeds can be inserted with or without an invasive operation. Because they are small, seeds can be placed to fit a curved area well without immobilization of the tongue or lips, for example, as do needles. However, they may move about if there is much motion. A seed that is inadvertently implanted in a blood vessel may migrate from the site and present a slight danger.

Seeds are 7 mm or less in length, 0.75 mm in diameter, with a wall 0.3 mm thick. The length depends on the desired dosage. Seeds may be strung 1 cm apart on a strand of suture material or placed in a hollow plastic tube. With a needle attached, the strand or tube is woven or pulled through the tumor. Seeds in a hollow plastic tube may be inserted like a catheter through a trocar.

More commonly, seeds are implanted individually. If seeds are to be placed through the skin or in the mouth, the surgeon usually marks the location for insertion of each seed with a sterile dye such as alcoholic gentian violet before beginning to insert them. The seeds are then inserted by means of long, rigid or flexible-shaft needles. These needles have stylets which should extend about $\frac{1}{16}$ in. (1.5 mm) beyond the tips so the seeds can be pushed into the tissue. When the seeds are received from the nuclear medicine department, two persons should count them and record the number received. As many needles as there are seeds must be sterilized. Check each needle before sterilization to be sure each stylet extends beyond the needle point; discard the needle for repair if it does not. For insertion of seeds:

1 Drape a small table for the seeds, needles, and seed forceps. Also place a sponge with a small amount of petroleum jelly on this sterile table. Do not put seeds on a gauze sponge, as they slip through the meshes.

2 Withdraw the stylet about $\frac{1}{2}$ in. (13 mm).

3 Hold the bevel of a needle against the table at the end of a seed and, with a slow forward and rotating motion, push the needle lumen over the seed. A seed forceps may be used to stabilize the seed while doing this. However, there is danger of the forceps slipping off the seed and flicking it onto the floor. *Be careful.*

4 When the seed is in the end of the needle, run the needle *forward and upward* through the edge of the petroleum jelly, which entraps the seed in the needle. Never pull the needle backward through the petroleum jelly, as this will pull the seed out of the needle.

5 When handing the needles to the surgeon, keep the tips high. Count the number quietly as each one is passed. Handle carefully, keeping eyes on the needle tip.

6 As the surgeon hands back a needle, check it to see whether the seed has been expressed. Keep empty needles on the opposite side of the table from the loaded ones.

Intracavitary Capsules A sealed capsule of radium, cesium 137, or cobalt 60 may be placed into a body cavity or orifice. Usually used to treat tumors in the cervix or endometrium of the uterus, a capsule is inserted via the vagina. The capsule may be a single tube of radium pins fixed in a tandem loading or a group of individual capsules each containing one radium pin. These methods are used for treating cancer of the uterine corpus.

In a patient with cervical cancer, an instrument such as an Ernst applicator is employed. A metal tube with radium pins is inserted in the uterus. This tube is attached to two vaginal ovoids, each of which contains a radium pin, that are grouped around the cervix. This type of application delivers the desired dosage in a pear-shaped volume of tissue, which includes the cervix, corpus, and tissue around the cervix, but spares the bladder and rectum from high doses of irradiation.

A blunt intracavitary applicator is utilized to position the parts. The applicator must be held securely and remain fixed to assure proper dosage to the tumor without injury to normal surrounding structures. The surgeon may suture the radium applicator to the cervix for stabilization. Vaginal packing is used. Two different methods of application are employed to insert the radiation source.

Afterloading Techniques These techniques afford the greatest safety for OR personnel. A "cold," unloaded, hollow plastic or metal applicator, such as the Fletcher afterloader, is inserted into or adjacent to tissues to receive radiation. This is done in the OR. After verification by x-ray of correct placement, the radiation source is loaded into the applicator at the patient's bedside.

Preloading Techniques These techniques require insertion of the "hot" radiation capsule in the OR. Nurses and technicians should not be permitted in the room during this procedure. To deliver a uniform dose to the desired area, the surgeon inserts an adjustable device, such as the Ernst applicator, designed to hold the radiation source in proper relationship to the tissues. The bladder and rectum are held away from the area with packs to avoid undesired radiation. The surgeon checks the position of the radiation source on x-ray films of the pelvis to measure distances from critical sites to calculate dosage.

> NOTE. *All* preparations for insertion are made by the nursing team members before leaving the room. (They wait in substerile room during radium insertion.) Preparations include: setting sterile table with vaginal packing, antibiotic cream for packing, radiopaque solutions for x-ray studies, basin of sterile water, etc.; placing x-ray cassette on operating table and notifying x-ray technician; obtaining radiation source; positioning patient; and putting radiation sheet on patient's chart and card on stretcher; etc.

Intracavitary Colloidal Suspensions Sterile radioactive colloidal suspensions of gold or phosphorus are used as palliative therapy to limit growth of metastatic tumors in the pleural or peritoneal cavities. The effect is due to the emission of beta particles, which penetrate tissue so slightly that radioactivity is limited to the immediate area in which the colloidal suspension is placed. A trocar and cannula are introduced into the pleural or peritoneal cavity. The colloidal suspension is injected through the cannula from a lead-shielded syringe. These instruments must be stored in a remote area until decay of radioactivity is complete. Radioactive colloidal gold 198 is most commonly used; it has a half-life of 2.7 days. It also may be instilled within the bladder.

Safety Rules for Handling Radiation Sources

The principles of radiation safety for both personnel and patients listed below apply to the handling of all types of radioactive materials. The cardinal factors of protection are *distance, time, and shielding.*

1. Radiation intensity varies inversely with the square of the distance from it; double distance equals one-quarter intensity, etc. Personnel must stay as far from the source as practically feasible.
2. Radiation sources, i.e., needles, seeds, capsules, and suspensions, are prepared by personnel in the nuclear medicine department from behind a lead screen with hands protected by lead-lined gloves, if possible, or special forceps during handling.
3. Radiation sources are transported in a long-handled lead carrier so that they are as close to the floor and as far away from the body of the transporter as possible. The lead carrier should be stored away from personnel and patient traffic areas while it is in the OR suite.
4. Each needle, seed, or capsule is counted by the surgeon with the radiation therapist when radiation sources are delivered to the OR. The number is recorded.
5. Glutaraldehyde solution is poured into the lead carrier to completely submerge the radiation sources. When ready to use, the lead carrier is transported into the OR, the needles, seeds, or capsules are removed from the lead container with sterile long-handled instruments, and *rinsed thoroughly* with sterile water.
6. All radiation sources are handled with special, long, ring-handled forceps from behind a lead protection shield. *Never touch radiation sources with bare hands or gloves.* Radiation sources are never handled with a crushing forceps since the seal of hollow containers can be broken. A groove-tipped forceps, designed for this purpose, is used.
7. Radiation sources are handled as quickly as possible to limit the time that personnel are exposed to radiation.
8. Monitoring devices should be worn by all personnel who remain in the room during radiation exposure from whatever source (see Chap. 15 for discussion of sources of radiation used for diagnosis).
   a. Badge dosimeters should be distributed to the entire OR team before a procedure involving radiation therapy. These badges are worn on the torso of each person exposed. The reading is recorded for each individual at weekly intervals to monitor accumulated exposure to radiation.
   b. Personal radiation monitors are pocket dosimeters with an additional device that produces audible sounds when exposed to ionizing radiation. The surgeon may wish to wear this during radiation therapy procedures.
   c. Film badges are worn by personnel in the radiology and nuclear medicine departments, and may be used by individual OR personnel. The maximum tolerance dose for a week or month is known. The film badge is worn for a proscribed period and is then developed with a film exposed to the tolerance dose, and the two compared. The exposure on the film badge is measured and recorded for each individual on a monthly basis.
9. To avoid overexposure of any one person, especially a woman of childbearing age, personnel should rotate assignments on procedures that involve radiation. Sterility is a potential hazard. Exposure should not exceed 100 milliroentgen (mR) per week, and staff members may request relief from exposure during pregnancy. The maximum permissible dose to the fetus is 0.4 REM (roentgen equivalent man). All personnel who handle radioactive elements should have a complete blood count every 30 days. Anemia can result from exposure.
10. Account for all radiation sources before and after use. Report any loss at once to the supervisor. Do not remove anything from the room. Call a radiation therapist or nuclear medicine department technician to bring a Geiger counter. This instrument, which is used to locate a lost radiation source, is constructed so that an indicator moves when near radioactive substances.
11. A *radiation sheet* is completed and put in the patient's chart. The surgeon fills in the amount and exact time of insertion and the time the source is to be removed. Each nurse who cares

for the patient on the unit signs this sheet in turn just before going off duty, thus passing the responsibility for checking the patient and the radiation source to the nurse who relieves. To check needles, the sutures attached to each needle are counted.

12 The patient's bed and door of the room are conspicuously labeled with a "radiation in use" card.

13 The radiation source is removed by the surgeon at the exact time indicated so the patient will not be overexposed.

14 Be careful—observe rules. Radiation is not seen or felt. Potential dangers from excessive exposure to personnel are anemia, sterility, and burns.

External Beam Radiation Therapy

Ionizing radiations of gamma or x-rays generated from machines are used externally to alter tumor cells within the body. This type of radiation therapy is noninvasive and is not performed in the OR. A maximum dose of radiation is concentrated on the malignant tumor, and a minimum dose to the surrounding tissue. The angle of approach is changed a number of times during the treatment to spread the amount of radiation to normal tissue over as wide an area as possible. *Orthovoltage,* low-voltage equipment of less than a million volts, and *megavoltage* equipment, such as the cobalt 60 beams and linear accelerators or betatrons, are in use for external beam radiation therapy.

External radiation may be the only therapeutic modality used to cure some cancers. The dosage of radiation that will provide the optimal cure with an acceptable balance of complications is difficult to determine. However, the cure rate has greatly increased with the advent of the megavoltage equipment. These rays can deliver cancercidal doses without permanently injuring normal tissue and causing skin irritation. Even so, most oncologists recommend a combination of radiation therapy and operative resection for many tumors. Radiation therapy may be administered preoperatively, postoperatively, or both. External radiation therapy also may be combined with internal sources such as intracavitary radiation capsules to build up the dosage to the large tumor areas.

CHEMOTHERAPY

In 1854, the first drug used for cancer chemotherapy was synthesized. However, this type of therapy did not attract much attention until after World War II when reports were published purporting that tumor cells circulate in the venous blood of patients undergoing operation. Administration of chemotherapeutic agents during and shortly after operation, in the hope of destroying those cells, seemed justified in selected patients. Nitrogen mustard was first used in 1942. A cooperative clinical study involving 23 medical centers was begun in 1958 to evaluate the efficacy of triethylenephosphoramide following radical mastectomy. Since then, many researchers have investigated over a quarter of a million compounds in search of systemic antineoplastic substances that would kill tumor cells without excessive toxicity or damage to normal cells.

Extensive experience has been gained with the use of chemotherapeutic agents for the systemic treatment of primary and metastatic cancer. A variety of agents are capable, either alone or in combination, of providing measurable palliative remission or regression of disease with decrease in the size of the tumor and no new metastases. In some instances, a complete response with disappearance of all clinical evidence of tumor is achieved. The trend is toward earlier and greater use of adjuvant chemotherapy. More than one agent may be administered to enhance the action of another cytotoxic or antigenic substance. Adjuvant therapy is designed to maximize the benefits of each agent in the combination, while avoiding overlapping toxicities. The following factors are important in determining the ability of tumor cells to respond to chemotherapy:

1 Size and location of tumor. The smaller the tumor, the easier it will be to reach cells. The mechanism for passage of drugs into the brain differs from that to reach other body organs.

2 Type of tumor. Cells of solid tumors in the lung, stomach, colon, and breast may be more resistant than cells in the lymphatic system, for example.

3 Combinations of adjunctive and adjuvant therapy. Chemotherapy may be used as an adjunct to all other types of therapy in selected patients. Precise scheduling of dosages is necessary to attain effective results.

4 Specific biochemical requirements of the tumor. Agents are selected according to the appropriateness of their structure and function. More than one agent usually is given.

5 State of cancer cell life cycle. An understanding of this phenomenon is necessary to understand chemotherapy. Cancer cells go through the same life-cycle phases as normal cells.

Cell Life Cycle

Deoxyribonucleic acid (DNA) is a double molecule in the nucleus of the cell that contains its genetic code. DNA is capable of reproducing itself and also of producing ribonucleic acid (RNA), which in turn synthesizes protein. Protein is essential for cellular function. Therefore, DNA is vital to cell viability. It regulates the processes of growth, rate of mitosis, differentiation, specialization, and death of cells. Cell division requires the assimilation of nutrients in the cell, their incorporation into DNA, the synthesis of new DNA, and the splitting of DNA to form two new cells. RNA is synthesized in the rest intervals between the phases of DNA replication. The duration of the rest interval is related to the proliferative activity of the tissue cells. Malignant tumor cells may proliferate more rapidly than normal cells.

Action of Chemotherapeutic Agents

Antineoplastic cytotoxic agents are destructive to rapidly dividing cells. However, each dose will kill only a fractional portion of the tumor cells present. The action of these agents takes place within the cell, but each agent acts differently to interrupt the cell life cycle. Antineoplastic agents are classified according to their structure and function. Only a few of the many agents in use are mentioned as examples of each classification. Cytotoxic action may be:

1 *Cell-cycle specific.* Some agents affect the cell during one or more phases and have no adverse effect during other phases. Some interfere with DNA synthesis; others inhibit mitosis when the cell is most susceptible; still others prolong the rest intervals.
   - **a** *Antimetabolites* affect most of the cells as they enter the DNA synthesis phase, thus interfering with RNA synthesis. This causes death of the cell by inhibiting the DNA cycle. These agents include fluoruridine (FUDR), fluorouracil (5-FU), and methotrexate.
   - **b** *Mitotic inhibitors* prevent cell division in a subphase of mitosis. They may be plant alkaloids such as vinblastine sulfate (Velban) and vincristine sulfate (Oncovin) or enzymes such as L-asparaginase.

2 *Cell-cycle nonspecific.* These agents affect the cell throughout the entire life cycle. They have a more prolonged action that is independent of the phases of the life cycle.
   - **a** *Alkylating agents* denature or inhibit the DNA to interfere with mitosis and synthesis, thereby preventing rapid cell growth. Their action is similar to that of radiation therapy. These agents include cyclophosphamide (Cytoxan), melphalan (L-phenylalanine mustard, L-PAM), and mechlorethamine nitrogen mustard (Mustargen).
   - **b** *Antibiotics* bind with DNA to block RNA production, thus disrupting cellular metabolism. Those used as antineoplasic agents include dactinomycin (actinomycin-D), bleomycin sulfate (Blenoxane), and dororubicin hydrochloride (Adriamycin).

Indications for Chemotherapy

Patients with systemic signs of advanced or disseminated disease, generally indicated by extranodal involvement, may be candidates for chemotherapy pre- or postoperatively.

Preoperative Therapy The objective may be to shrink the tumor sufficiently to permit radical operative resection. Tumor regression with tumor necrosis may occur with or without adjunctive radiation therapy. Agents may eliminate subclinical microscopic metastatic disease.

Postoperative Therapy Operative resection followed by regional chemotherapy often can control local disease to keep a tumor in remission. Residual metastatic disease may be treated with systemic chemotherapy to cure the patient or prolong life. Multiple doses may be given over a long period of time (several months to a year or more) to delay recurrence of the tumor.

Administration of Agents

The method of administration depends on how disseminated or localized the tumor cells are and on the agent, or combination of agents, selected. Agents can be instilled locally into a body cavity, injected intramuscularly or intrathecally, infused by intravenous push or drip, or ingested orally. A patient with widely disseminated metastatic cells usually receives systemic therapy via the IV, IM, or oral route.

Regional intra-arterial or intravenous infusion may be used for patients whose tumor cannot be removed because of its location, e.g., a primary or metastatic tumor in the liver. An infusion catheter may be placed percutaneously or directly into an artery leading to the tumor site, into a vein, or both. Continuous or intermittent infusion of the chemotherapeutic agent is maintained by means of a pump attached to the catheter. A portable infusion unit is available. Selected patients may receive treatment at home if the intra-arterial catheter is secure, and come to the hospital on an outpatient basis for weekly blood studies.

An extremity, in which the blood supply can be isolated and can form a closed circuit, may be perfused for a short time with one or more agents. Extracorporeal circulation is established for this type of regional perfusion. It is used most frequently to reduce the size of an otherwise inoperable sarcoma or melanoma to an operable tumor mass, or for palliation of incurable disease.

Toxic Side Effects

Cytotoxic agents are destructive to rapidly dividing cancer cells, but they also affect rapidly dividing normal cells such as hematopoietic cells of bone marrow, epithelial cells of the oral cavity and gastrointestinal tract, and hair follicles. Patients must be informed of the toxic side effects to be expected from the specific agents they are receiving. These can include:

1 *Alopecia.* Loss of hair can occur suddenly or gradually. This can be devastating to the patient's self-image. It is most often caused by the alkylating and plant alkaloid agents, and by some antibiotics. Hair grows back after therapy is discontinued.
2 *Bone marrow suppression.* Suppression of bone marrow function is the most hazardous toxic effect from cytotoxic agents. The therapy may have to be discontinued to allow for bone marrow recovery. Suppression increases the patient's susceptibility to:
   a Leukopenia. The white blood cell count is lowered below the normal number of leukocytes in the peripheral blood. Leukocytes protect the body against invasion of microorganisms. The patient with leukopenia is therefore highly vulnerable to the spread of infection from one part of the body to another, or to acquiring a nosocomial infection from the environment.
   b Thrombocytopenia. The number of platelets in the blood decreases below normal with variable consequences. Spontaneous hemorrhage into the skin, sclera, joints, or brain may occur. Normal blood clotting time can be prolonged. The patient may require platelet transfusion.
3 *Gastrointestinal disturbances.* Anorexia, nausea, vomiting, and/or diarrhea are common complaints. Usually these subside within a few hours or days after each dose is administered.
4 *Neurotoxicity.* Symptoms of neurotoxicity to the plant alkaloids usually begin with constipation. Toxicity can progress to impaired sensation, ataxia, and an unsteady gait. The effects are cumulative during the course of therapy, but are reversible when therapy is discontinued.
5 *Stomatitis.* Ulcerative lesions in the mouth and oropharynx are often early signs of severe toxicity from the antimetabolite and antibiotic agents. These can be very painful and may lead to secondary infection.
6 *Vein hyperpigmentation.* A dark discoloration of a vein may occur over the length of the arm during prolonged infusion of some agents. A vesicular rash around the injection site may develop from the use of some other agents. Although unsightly, these effects are not uncomfortable for the patient.

IMMUNOTHERAPY

Immunization against disease is a well-established concept. Ancient Chinese and Arabic writings describe the stimulation of the body's immune system to combat infectious diseases. Immunization against smallpox was practiced in Turkey long before Edward Jenner developed a vaccine in England in the late sixteenth century. The concept developed by Jenner, Pasteur, Salk, and Sabin, to mention a few historic names, of using vaccinations and immunizations to prevent or treat infectious diseases forms the basis of modern immunotherapy.

Immunotherapy utilizes agents that stimulate or activate the body's own host defense immune system to combat disease. This is the same immune system that normally wards off microorganisms which cause infection. Cancer may become clinically apparent only when the immune system ceases to function properly. The immune response may be defective, or become compromised, as the disease progresses. Immunosuppression can stimulate tumor growth and prolong wound healing. If the patient can be helped to regain partial or complete immunocompetence, the immune system can be utilized against the "foreignness" of tumor cells.

Attempts to treat cancer by immunization date back to 1895. However, it was not until 1957 that antigens specific for tumors were conclusively demonstrated in animals by Prehn and Main. Although intensive experimental research was conducted during the 1960s to investigate the applications of immunotherapy as a therapeutic modality, its use in selective types of cancer was not validated by clinical research until the 1970s.

Types and Agents

Tumor antigen evokes an immune response in the patient either by an antibody (*humoral response*) or a specifically reactive lymphocyte (*cell-mediated immunity*). Patients are initially tested for a delayed cutaneous hypersensitivity response to establish an index of immune function. The type of immunotherapy is selected that will most effectively strengthen the immune response.

Active Immunotherapy Antigens are injected to stimulate the development of antibodies against the tumor cells by the patient's own humoral immune response.

1 *Active specific immunotherapy.* A vaccine of specific tumor antigen stimulates the immune response. A series of small doses are administered intradermally.
   a *Autologous vaccine* is prepared from the patient's own tumor cells and reinoculated.
   b *Allogenic vaccine* is prepared from tumor cells of the same type obtained from a donor. This introduces antigens new to the patient's immune system.
   c *Modified tumor cell vaccine* is treated to increase antigenicity.
2 *Active nonspecific immunotherapy.* The vaccine containing antigens other than tumor cells causes increased antibody and lymphocyte production.
   a *BCG* (bacillus Calmette-Guerin) is accentuated bovine tubercle bacillus. The most widely used, it is a potent stimulant of the defensive mechanism of the reticuloendothelial system. It is usually administered intradermally by scarification, the tine grid technique, or injection gun. It may also be injected intralesionally or intrapleurally.
   b *MER* is the methanol extractable residue of BCG.
   c *Corynebacterium parvum* is a gram-positive anaerobic bacillus.
   d *Levamisol* is an antihelminthic given to stimulate host defense.

Passive Immunotherapy Antitumor antibodies can be transferred from one person to another to establish transient, acquired, cell-mediated immunity. Antisera from a cured patient with the same type of tumor or from a family member with natural or acquired immunity may be injected subcutaneously or infused intravenously. The patient's own lymphocytes may be sensitized in the laboratory and reinfused to increase lymphocyte-to-tumor cell ratio. Passive immunotherapy is transient because lymphocytes in antisera are continually made and destroyed by the body.

Adoptive Immunotherapy The patient accepts passive immunity from systemic transfer of immunocompetent cells and then actively maintains cell-mediated immunity. This is maintained by administration of immunostimulant extracts from human white cells called *transfer factor* or of lymphoid extracts from animals called *immune RNA.* These extracts are highly specific, rapid in action, and long-lasting in effect. The transfer of this delayed-type hypersensitivity depends upon the dosage used and the duration of therapy necessary to develop sufficient lymphocytes to inhibit tumor growth.

Advantages of Immunotherapy

1 It attacks only cancer cells.
2 It does not damage normal cells.
3 It can be continued for long periods with fewer hazardous side effects to the patient than chemotherapy.
4 It can be injected subcutaneously, infused intravenously, or applied topically or intradermally as for skin cancer and melanomas.
5 It may significantly increase cure and survival rates.

Immunotherapeutic agents have a relatively weak killing capacity, but no limitation on the kinds of cells they can destroy. Although highly specific, they can destroy small numbers of tumor cells, but are not effective against large numbers. They can regress or eradicate a small tumor mass, or eliminate cells resistant to chemotherapy. Combining these agents may accomplish what neither can do alone, either with or without operative resection—delay recurrence and prolong survival.

HYPERTHERMIA

Hyperthermia has a regressive tumoricidal effect. Total body hyperthermia may be applied externally during operative resections by placing the patient on a hyperthermia blanket or mattress. Radio-frequency hyperthermia may be applied to regional or local tumor sites. Since drug action is greater at higher temperatures, the perfusate is warmed before regional infusion of cytotoxic agents. An extremity is warmed externally during regional perfusion also.

HYPERALIMENTATION

Untreated cancer produces weight loss and can lead to malnutrition, probably because the tumor cells extract nutrients from the patient at a more rapid rate than they are ingested. Malnutrition depresses established cell-mediated immunity to infection and immunologic reactivity to the tumor. The only hope of cure or palliation of cancer in a malnourished patient may be a treatment that itself produces malnutrition. Healing may be delayed following operative resection in poorly nourished tissues of patients who have some degree of malabsorption of nutrients. This can deter resumption of oral intake after head and neck or gastrointestinal operations. Radiation therapy, chemotherapy, and immunotherapy can cause loss of appetite due to nausea, and often produce vomiting or diarrhea that may necessitate delay in therapy. Adequate nutrition can be maintained before and during treatment with intravenous hyperalimentation (see Chap. 3, pp. 59–61). Patients are usually started on IV hyperalimentation prior to oncologic therapy and supported postoperatively or throughout other therapy. A minimum of 10 days is required to derive any benefit from hyperalimentation. If the tumor responds to therapy, appetite returns, weight gain is maintained, and immunocompetent cells return as a defense mechanism against the tumor cells.

FUTURE OF ONCOLOGY

As described above, many therapeutic modalities are used, and researchers are constantly seeking others, to improve survival chances and quality of life for patients with neoplasms. Early diagnosis of the extent of the disease is crucial for the selection of appropriate curative therapy. In poor-risk patients with extensive tumors and advanced disease, only palliative therapy may be possible.

The day when oncologists and surgeons looked only at survival statistics is now past. The National Cancer Act, which Congress adopted in 1971, calls for study of the cause of cancer, as well as the diagnosis, treatment, and rehabilitation of cancer patients. Moreover, patients are demanding that their surgeons give attention to reconstruction of body image and rehabilitation to a useful life. Management of cancer patients must, therefore, be through the efforts of a multidisciplinary team of surgeons in conjunction with pathologists, radiation therapists, pharmacists, immunologists, oncologists, and others. Nurses in all patient care settings must provide, in addition to physical care, psychological support for cancer patients and their families.

Chapter 28

Transplantation and Replantation

TRANSPLANTATION

Transplantation biology is the science of transplantation of living tissues. Concentrated efforts continue in search of compensation for or suitable replacement of deficient tissues and organs. One modality is transplantation or graft, the application to or insertion into the body of tissues or organs taken from another part of the same body or from another body. Indication for transplant is irreversible functional failure of the organ.

Types of Transplants

Allografts (Homografts) Tissue grafted between different or genetically dissimilar individuals of the same species.

Autografts Tissues grafted in the same person from one part of the body to another. The donor is also the recipient.

Isografts Tissues grafted between genetically identical donor and recipient, as between identical twins.

Xenografts (Heterografts) Tissues grafted between two dissimilar species. Experiments in heterografts are done because of unavailability of allograft material.

Orthotopic Transplant Transplant to an anatomically natural or normal recipient site.

Heterotopic Transplant Transplant to an anatomically abnormal location in the host. Heterotopic grafts may function normally in the unnatural site.

Development of Transplantation

Interest in this field is many centuries old. Celsus wrote that tissues could survive after grafting from one part of the body to another. Galen attempted reconstruction of facial defects. Centuries later it was observed that full-thickness autografts survived whereas allografts failed although the reason was not understood.

Darwin's theory of evolution and Mendel's laws of heredity shed new light in the nineteenth century spurring researchers to pursue the study of regenerative capacity in animals. In the early twentieth century, Carrel and Guthrie performed blood vessel anastomoses, an essential component of organ transplantation. Performing heterotopic heart transplants in animals, they demonstrated that a heart could be removed, transplanted, and resume beating.

In the 1930s, the maintenance of organs *in vitro* opened the way to organ preservation. Information concerning patient response to operation was expanded during the decade of the 1940s, a marked advance in operative therapy. Open-heart surgery evolved in the 1950s as well as the acquisition of basic knowledge required for clinical transplantation. Pioneers in transplantation biology, Medawar and Burnet, received the Nobel prize in 1960 for their work on immunologic tolerance in tissue transplantation in animals.

Many scientific disciplines contribute to and fuse information to aid progress in clinical transplantation. Foremost among these are physiology, genetics, immunology, and pathology. Practical application of clinical transplantation became possible in the 1960s after investigative efforts led to the development of supportive techniques such as cardiopulmonary bypass and immunosuppressive drug therapy.

Although kidney transplantation preceded it by more than a decade, the first successful heart transplant, performed by Dr. Christian Barnard in 1967 in South Africa, expanded the era of clinical organ transplantation.

Tissue Transplantation

Some tissues such as skin can function normally even though moved to a different area of the body.

1 Skin grafts provide a protective surface covering, initially acquiring then eventually losing vascular connection with the host. Use of skin grafts offered the first extensive study of rejection reaction (see below).

2 Corneal grafts replace nonfunctioning corneal tissue.

3 Bone grafts afford temporary structural supports and a pattern for regrowth of the host's bone, the graft then being resorbed.

4 Blood vessel grafts are used to bypass or replace diseased or obstructed segments of vessels.

While all these grafts are commonplace and successful in many patients, transplantation of whole vital organs designed to remain as permanent functional units, such as the kidney or heart, presents ethical and philosophical dilemmas in addition to technical factors. A supply of donor tissue from the living involves a real sacrifice. Therefore, primarily cadaver sources are used.

Organ Transplantation

Clinical transplantation of organs in human beings is the result of extensive worldwide research. A large body of pertinent knowledge has been gathered and impressive progress made, although many unsolved problems remain. Transplantation potentially can restore an individual to normal or near-normal physiological status.

Transplant of kidneys has been the most successful and principal clinical application of organ transplantation. If the graft fails, the patient may survive by returning to hemodialysis and receiving another transplant. Transplantation of the heart and liver, although showing increasing success, has not been equal to that of kidneys. In addition, no practical prolonged artificial support exists in the event of allotransplant failure. Transplantation of the pancreas, lung, and intestines are far less successful. Prolonged extracorporeal respiratory support under investigation may provide a more hopeful outlook for lung grafting.

Transplantation of each organ involves unique technical and physiologic problems but the major barriers and causes of failure of all transplants are infection and immunologic rejection, treated by appropriate use of antibiotics and manipulation of immunologic agents. Transplant patients are similar to other critical patients. They are prone to sepsis because of combined lowered host-resistance factors. In addition to severe chronic illness, defense mechanisms are further depressed by immunosuppressive agents. Reverse isolation may be used to protect the patient although endogenous infection may occur.

Immunologic Rejection Many technical aspects of transplantation have been largely solved. However, the body possesses an innate tendency to reject and destroy any foreign material introduced into it except tissue from an identical twin. Transplanted cells from donors even slightly dissimilar to the recipient may be rejected.

Organ rejection, the focus of intense investigation, involves the patient's immunologic system. Both cellular and humoral immune systems seem to be involved in responses to transplanted cells. Activation of the immune response by foreign cells is not clearly understood.

The immunologic reaction usually is accompanied by a febrile systemic reaction, local inflammation, and deteriorating function of the graft. A knowledge of antigens, individual-specific and species-specific, and their genetic transmission is important for avoidance of violent reactions. Many factors influence the strength and rate of a rejection reaction. Some of these are acquired immunologic tolerance, lymphatic depression, or previous sensitization by blood transfusions, pregnancies, or transplants. Rejection may be reversible with intensive therapy, or progressive with cessation of transplant function.

Combating Rejection Attempts must be made to find compatible donors and to minimize rejection.

Preoperative Matching of Donor to Recipient Although time-consuming, this is an essential prerequisite to transplantation. It is accomplished by use of multiple serologic reagents. Histocompatibility implies acceptability by an individual of tissue from another. Histocompatibility tests, while not infallible, result in improved organ survival both from related and cadaver sources. They assist in donor-recipient selection. The better the histocompatibility match and degree of genetic similarity between donor and recipient, the less serious is the rejection. Histocompatibility testing, *tissue typing,* is based on detection of histocompatibility antigens, such as by mixed lymphocyte culture (MLC) or interaction test. Favorable results are expected when fewer antigens are detected by careful typing. Preformed antibodies appear to have a harmful effect on graft survival. Testing employs serological techniques, methods for *in vitro* analysis for study of cell-to-cell interaction and identification of the mediator of the interaction, as well as cell-culture techniques. Complex assay techniques measure effects of antibodies and lymphocytes against donor tissue in a culture setup.

Immunosuppressive Therapy in the Recipient Specific alterations in immune responses are produced by inactivating or destroying lymphoid cells potentially capable of responding to the antigens. The goal is to selectively suppress antigenic reactions to the transplant without impairing the body's defense against pathogenic organisms. An attempt is made to neutralize or modify the body's protective antigenic mechanisms by the use of various immunosuppressive agents to allow the transplant to remain and function. This barrier can be pierced at least temporarily by creating an increase in transplant tolerance or paralyzing the recipient's immunologic system. Since lymphocytes and globulins seem to be mainly responsible for rejection, an attempt is made to vary their synthesis. Antibody formation and immune reaction can be suppressed by certain factors. Protocol is fairly standard in all transplant centers.

1 Use of agents cytostatic or cytotoxic to lymphatic tissue such as the drugs azathioprine and cyclophosphamide. Extracorporeal perfusion with drugs and localized radiation to the transplant may be used but irradiation may incur many new problems. Radiation and drugs can be used separately or concurrently but drug usage alone is more common.

2 Use of corticosteroids such as prednisone for anti-inflammatory effect, useful in reversing early rejection reaction. There is an inverse relationship between steroids and lymphocytes.

3 Use of heterologous (horse) antihuman thymocyte globulin or serum (ATG), the action of which is directed primarily against circulating lymphocyte T cells.

4 Drainage of the thoracic duct or common lymph trunk, splenectomy, and thymectomy, used occasionally.

Employment of immunosuppressive measures is not without complication. Leukopenia and susceptibility to infection are common sequelae. Therapy may not totally abolish rejection by the host but may delay onset and decrease incidence of rejection episodes during the crucial first month or two following transplantation.

Availability of Organ Allografts The goal is selection of a donor-recipient pair with adequate histocompatibility to permit a functioning graft without complications and using the lowest possible safe doses of immunologic drugs.

Cadaver Sources Cadaver sources are used except for some kidney and all bone marrow transplants. Most transplanted kidneys are harvested from nonliving individuals because of the critically inadequate supply of organs. Since written informed consent is required to obtain donor organs, many persons carry a signed identification card stating that in case of death certain organs or any organs may be removed for transplant.

Ideal cadaver donors are young persons with confirmed brain death, often the result of automobile accident, where the organ can be preserved *in vivo.* All donors should be without sepsis or malignancy, preferably under 50 years of age, and with previous good function of the donor organ. *Organ banks* exchange organs, collect organs from donors, and register patients in need of a transplant as well as information about their blood grouping and tissue typing. Less is known concerning potential transmissible disease when cadaver organs are used.

Organs from cadaver sources will be more valuable when improved methods of storage are found. A drawback, in addition to medicolegal issues, is the delay incurred in procurement. Time is paramount when critical organs are involved, for their value depends on preserving maximum functional viability. The time factor is less urgent with less critical tissue.

Living Sources In patients for kidney or marrow transplantation, the use of an organ or marrow from a biologically related living donor has distinct advantages: results are better than with cadaver organs because donor-recipient matches usually are good (identical twin sources are ideal for compatibility), waiting time is reduced, lengthy dialysis avoided, and the procedure planned. Many patients die while awaiting a compatible cadaver organ. Use of living donors involves special protocol.

1 Adults, preferred over adolescents or children, must be able to give informed consent voluntarily without coercion. Children are used as donors only for a twin or for a patient with predictable results. If the donor is a minor, court (legal) consent is required as well as parental or guardian consent, to avoid bias. The donor must fully comprehend the sacrifice; if the physician deems advisable, psychiatric examination is included as well as intelligence testing.

2 The donor must be in excellent health. The *donor's* physician confers with him or her and performs the preoperative physical examination to permit a rational decision. Renal arteriograms are done to confirm bilateral kidneys and identify renal vasculature prior to a nephrectomy.

3 The donor should have no psychiatric complications. Donor reactive depression may follow removal of the organ if adequate gratitude on the part of all, especially the recipient, is not shown promptly.

Preservation of Organ Allografts Successful use of donor tissue depends on rapid organ resection and cooling, since the period of ischemia must be kept to a minimum. Long-term preservation of tissue remains a problem; the search for new techniques utilizes a wide variety of cryoprotective agents. Controlled freezing may produce lethal cell injury. This technique is used for skin, and sperm or blood suspensions, but not for whole organs. Hypothermia above freezing with or without perfusion with cold solutions reduces general metabolic demands thereby providing a safety margin. Methods of hypothermia include:

1 Simple flush techniques with use of special solutions and hypothermic storage by immersion in electrolyte or flush-out solution in a plastic container kept at a specific hypothermic temperature

2 Hypothermic continuous pulsatile perfusion with oxygenated plasma

Human Kidney Allotransplantation

Begun in 1951, kidney transplantation is an acceptable clinical entity and an everyday reality. Combined hemodialysis and transplantation have significantly changed the outlook and notably improved the quality of life of many patients with terminal renal disease. Patients must choose whether to accept transplantation or undergo frequent dialysis for the rest of their lives. Indication for transplantation is end-stage or near-terminal renal disease, most often glomerulonephritis, pyelonephritis, polycystic disease, or nephrosclerosis. Ideal recipients are 5 to 40 years of age without severe extrarenal disease, malignancy, or active sepsis. Pretransplant bilateral nephrectomy may be performed in patients with uncontrollable hypertension. Patients with detected presensitization states have to wait longer for a suitably matched donor and statistically have a lower 1-year graft survival rate than unsensitized patients.

Recipients are carefully prepared preoperatively with kidney dialysis, fluid and electrolyte intake regulation, and control of hypertension. Proper donor-recipient matching is performed. Written informed consent is necessary.

Donor preparation is equally important. Removal of a kidney is associated with low morbidity although the donor must guard against bruising or rupturing the remaining kidney for the rest of his or her life. The donor therefore is advised to avoid body-contact sports.

Transplantation Unless a transported cadaver donor organ is used, two adjoining operating rooms and teams are employed. One team harvests and preserves the donor kidney while the other prepares the recipient site and transplants the kidney. Operative technique has been standardized.

Donor Nephrectomy In a living donor the kidney is removed through a flank incision. Adequate renal perfusion and urinary output, maintenance of adequate blood pressure and ureteral blood supply, as well as gentleness in manipulation, are extremely important intraoperatively. As soon as excised, the kidney is flushed with cold heparinized solution to remove red blood cells. Total ischemia time usually is less than an hour. The donor's incision is closed per routine technique.

Recipient Procedure The iliac fossa is the standard site for transplantation in the adult patient. The hypogastric artery is anastomosed to the renal artery and the common iliac vein to the renal vein. Reconstruction of the urinary tract is the main technical problem. Implantation of the donor ureter into the bladder, *ureteroneocystostomy,* is the preferred technique for urinary drainage. Alternate methods include uretero-ureterostomy and ureteropyelostomy. Postoperative management is similar to that of other surgical patients with emphasis on initial adequacy of renal function, prevention of hazardous effects of immunosuppressive therapy, and observation for allograft rejection. Possible *types of rejection* are:

1 *Hyperacute,* due to presensitization. This is an immediate, acute rejection that occurs immediately after anastomosis of blood vessels or within 24 hours. It includes thrombosis and extensive destruction of allograft vasculature.
2 *Accelerated,* due to presensitization. The graft may function for up to 5 days, followed by rapid loss of renal function. Treatment for both hyperacute and accelerated rejection is immediate removal of the transplant.
3 *Acute.* This usually occurs 1 week to 4 months following transplantation and often is reversible unless the immune response is severe. Systemic and local symptoms are present as well as reduced urinary output and abnormal laboratory findings.
4 *Chronic.* Antibodies developing long after transplantation produce insidious onset with mild hypertension and diminishing renal function. This rejection is not reversible. Acute and chronic rejection may be diagnosed by renal biopsy.

Complications of Renal Allotransplantation Complications may be renal-related or extrarenal. The most common renal-related include rejection (the dominant cause of graft loss), recurrent nephritis, acute tubular necrosis, or technical failure from genitourinary or vascular problems.

Extrarenal complications, usually caused by immunosuppressive or corticosteroid therapy, include infection (the leading cause of death on a long-term basis), pneumonitis, hepatitis, gastrointestinal bleeding, and psychological problems from perpetual fear of rejection. Immunosuppressive therapy must be used with caution.

Results of kidney transplantation are increasingly gratifying; life can be significantly prolonged. Causes for concern are vascular disease, a major cause of death in dialysis patients, which may occur in the long-term transplant patient, and the increasing incidence of malignant neoplasm in patients surviving renal transplantation more than a year. This incidence exceeds that expected in the general population.

Heart Allotransplantation

Heart transplantation may be performed in selected patients with terminal cardiac disease such as irreversible extensive myocardial failure and widespread atherosclerotic deterioration. These are patients with very limited life expectancy for whom no alternative therapy remains to sustain life. A brain-death donor with the heart preserved *in vivo* may be used. Optimum preservation of the donor heart is necessary as it must resume full activity after transplantation. As with renal transplantation, two teams operate in adjoining rooms, one of which harvests the donor organ at precisely the time it is needed. Thus ischemia time is kept to a minimum. After removal the donor heart is rapidly cooled and immediately implanted in the recipient. The operative procedure and postoperative care are similar to open-heart surgery, with anticoagulation therapy and cardiopulmonary bypass utilized during operation. Two operative modalities are available: total orthotopic heart replacement, or insertion of a transplanted heart as an assist device without removal of the recipient's heart.

Most fatalities occur in the first 2 postoperative months, the crucial period of immunologic rejection. Electrocardiogram changes such as drop in voltage, reduced cardiac output, arteritis, myocardial ischemia, and myocardial necrosis occur during rejection. Diagnosis and monitoring of acute rejection may be facilitated by serial transvenous endomyocardial biopsies, which also may confirm effectiveness of therapy. Under fluoroscopy, a forceps is passed through the catheter into the apex of the right ventricle via the right internal jugular vein and a small sample of myocardium removed for histologic study. A major obstacle to long-term survival is the development of obliterative coronary artery disease in the transplanted heart. The rejection process accelerates atherosclerosis. Improvement in survival rates is attributed to more accurate early diagnosis of rejection and vigorous measures to prevent atherosclerosis, thought to be due to immunologic injury to the intima of the coronary vessels. An increase in malignant neoplasms in heart-transplant patients has been observed. These patients need psychological support to maintain a will to live and to adjust to problems that may arise at any time.

Research continues in an effort to develop a suitable mechanical heart for cardiac substitution. The device must be fatigue-resistant and compatible with the body, with a nonthrombogenic inner surface. A temporary, left ventricular assist pump to aid postoperative heart patients with a weak ventricle is being clinically evaluated.

Liver Allotransplantation

Hepatic transplantation is a formidable procedure accompanied by a high mortality rate. It may be performed in selected patients with end-stage liver disease, both malignant and nonmalignant. Ideal recipients are patients with primary liver disease. Preexisting infection in any part of the body is a distinct contraindication, since the patients' preoperative status is poor and they lack the protective proteins normally produced by the liver. There is marked danger of postoperative infection.

Organ preservation presents a problem as hepatic tissue is very susceptible to damage from ischemia. While the liver can be preserved up to 6 hours outside the body, a brain-death cadaver donor with intact circulation is preferred. Donor and recipient hepatectomies should be synchronized so the recipient site is ready before circulation to the donor liver is arrested.

Complexity and friability of the liver contribute to technical hazards. In addition, extensive dissection is required. The majority of transplants are orthotopic.

Rejection may be noted by changes in laboratory findings, such as alterations in serum enzyme levels and elevated serum bilirubin. Cellular infiltration of the graft causes impairment of clotting factors, liver-cell necrosis, and impaired function. Complications from reconstruction of the biliary tract may lead to graft failure.

Pancreas Allotransplantation

A variety of techniques have been used in clinical endocrine transplantation in the treatment of patients with severe diabetes with associated systemic complications. These techniques utilize the ureter or the duodenum for exocrine drainage. The goal is to provide physiological islet function. Many technical problems remain.

Lung Allotransplantation

Lung transplant may be performed in patients with terminal respiratory failure such as insufficiency from emphysema. Patient selection is difficult since other organ systems, especially the heart, often are damaged by pulmonary failure.

Optimum preservation of the donor organ is vitally important because most recipients have inadequate pulmonary reserve. Moreover, the transplanted lung must assume oxygenation immediately, with respirator aid. Adequate preservation of donor lungs, more difficult than preservation of other organs, remains a problem. Brain-death cadaver donors afford minimum ischemia time.

Many special problems affect the success of clinical transplantation.

1 Recipients usually have some degree of pulmonary infection at the time of operation. The recipient's remaining lung, if diseased, may be a source of infection.

2 Ventilation-perfusion imbalance between the transplanted lung and the remaining lung may result in reduced function in the transplant.

3 Imminent rejection is not recognized easily.

4 Vascular and fibrotic changes produced by rejection create ischemia and anoxia.

5 Problems arise postoperatively at the site of bronchial anastomosis.

6 The procedure is technically difficult.

Bone Marrow Allotransplantation

This procedure is a tissue rather than an organ transplantation, but it follows the protocol of organ transplant since it is fraught with hazards. It is performed only after conventional methods of treatment have failed. Indications are severe combined immune deficiency disease (SCID), acute leukemia or chronic myelocytic leukemia in blastic phase, and aplastic anemia. The aim is to reconstitute the host's immune system. Contraindications are renal or cardiac disease, or previous maximum radiation dosage. The usual blood-typing and antigen-compatibility testing are essential. The donor usually is a sibling, with an identical twin definitely preferred.

Problems impeding progress in bone marrow transplantations are the high risk of infection during the prolonged period of immunologic insufficiency and the scarcity of compatible living donors. Successful transplants can prolong life in previously terminal patients.

Stem cells are collected from leukemic patients in remission and stored to be given back to these patients during subsequent relapse, as part of therapy.

Prior to transplantation, which consists of marrow infusion, the recipient is given a high-dose regimen of antineoplastic drugs to eradicate leukemic and bone marrow cells, thus inducing marrow depression. Three to five days later the recipient receives total body irradiation (TBI) to penetrate areas resistant to the drugs. He or she is then wrapped in sterile linens and placed in reverse isolation to receive the marrow infusion. Meanwhile the donor, hospitalized prior to the operation, is taken to the operating room where under general or spinal anesthesia 500 to 700 ml of bone marrow are aspirated at multiple sites from pelvic bones. The marrow is filtered, heparinized, and placed in sterile plastic bags for infusion. The donor is watched for bleeding and may be transfused with his or her own blood withdrawn prior to operation.

The marrow is infused into the recipient intravenously within 4 hours after donation and within 24 hours after TBI. The patient is constantly attended and closely monitored for adverse reaction during this time. By an unknown process, the marrow migrates into the marrow cavities of the bones. For 25 days after transplant the recipient receives daily transfusions of lymphocytes, platelets, and granulocytes preferably taken from the donor twin to counteract the predictable side effects (mainly hemorrhage and infection) of the immunosuppressive therapy. If it is not from an identical twin, the blood is irradiated before transfusion to destroy lymphocytes. Mature blood cells and platelets are unaffected. Daily marrow aspirations and complete blood counts are done on the host. Success or failure of transplantation usually is decided 10 to 20 days afterward when the new marrow begins to function.

Complications include leukemic relapse or graft versus host disease (GVHD), the rejection of the host by transplanted tissue. This does not occur in an identical twin, but may occur when antigenetically different cells are introduced into a host unable to reject foreign material. Meanwhile attempts to develop reliable functional artificial organs continue.

Transplantation Societies and Registries

The American Society of Transplant Surgeons (ASTS) and the International Society of Transplantation (IST) meet regularly to exchange ideas and information among persons of different scientific backgrounds. The aim is the best possible patient survival rather than merely transplant survival.

The Organ Transplant Registry of the American College of Surgeons/National Institutes of Health collects data on transplant operations and approves and funds various registries. The Human Kidney Transplant Registry collects information on worldwide renal transplantation.

Future Hope in Transplantation

Important areas of clinical transplantation investigation include:

1 Identification of host responses on an immune level and ability to identify posttransplant immune status on a daily basis.
2 Improvement in donor-recipient matching.
3 Increase in supply of good cadaver organs that would provide better tissue matching. Improvements in procedures for arranging during lifetime for organ gifts by potential donors.
4 Long-term storage of organs in a viable state.

Immunologic rejection and permanent shortage of all donors remain the principal deterrents in transplantation.

REPLANTATION OF SEVERED EXTREMITIES

Replantation may be attempted to salvage a traumatically amputated digit, hand, or entire upper extremity. Severing of a foot or lower extremity presents more formidable problems because of the necessity of weight bearing. Using microsurgical techniques, the replanted digit(s) or extremity can survive with varying degrees of effectiveness. Functional recovery, up to 80 percent of normal in some patients, may take up to a year or longer, since it takes time for nerves to regenerate. A team of specialists in hand surgery, plastic, and orthopaedic surgeons with microvascular skill, is vital to success in these arduous procedures. Experienced teams are on call in replantation centers.

Correct care and preservation of the severed part for transport with the patient also are vital to success. The amputated part should be placed dry into a plastic bag, which is then sealed and immersed in ice inside an insulated container (e.g. styrofoam) to retard melting of ice during travel. *The part should NOT be warmed, frozen, or packed in dry ice.* Rapid transport and cooling with ice buys time.

Initial treatment involves assessment of the total patient while the severed part is cleansed with isotonic solution under sterile technique. The injured extremity should be elevated. The patient and family should be supported emotionally but not given definitive promises in regard to outcome.

In judging whether or not to perform replantation, the surgeon considers numerous factors: need for the part, associated disease and injuries, economic and psychological factors, and age. Two criteria are of special significance.

1 The replanted part must have potential for being useful.

2 There should be no undue risk to the general safety of the patient if the procedure is performed.

Replantation is more successful in young patients. Also, incomplete amputations are more successful because they have intact subcutaneous venous circulation in the skin bridges. Restoration is much more difficult in crush injuries than in sharp, clean amputations.

Contraindications to replantation include prolonged warm ischemia, severe bruising or crushing injury, multiple fractures or injury at different levels in the same digit, or associated injuries that preclude the effort.

Supportive therapy following injury includes tetanus toxoid, intravenous antibiotics and fluids or blood products, and judicious administration of anticoagulants.

Preoperative patient preparation is in anticipation of a long procedure. Operation may take from 4 to 16 hours. The patient is placed on an air or water mattress. The head, scapulae, sacrum, and heels are padded. A footboard may be used and antiembolic stockings applied. An indwelling catheter is inserted or the patient draped in a way to make insertion possible. Most replants of the hand are done under preoperative sedation and axillary or supraclavicular block with an agent such as Marcaine. General anesthesia may be used for a long procedure.

These operations usually involve a two-team approach; one team prepares the recipient site and the other prepares the severed or distal part. In the OR, debridement of crushed tissue is carried out. Vessels are isolated for repair, and vessel patency ensured. The basic steps of replantation include:

1 Identifying proximal and distal tendons, nerves, and vessels.

2 Shortening bone within acceptable limit necessary for tension-free repair of blood vessels, nerves, and soft tissues.

3 Stabilizing skeletal structure such as with internal wire-fixation techniques to maintain joint continuity and fusion in functional position.

4 Suturing tendons and ligaments, both extensors and flexors, appropriately to lessen the junctional scar process that can inhibit motion.

5 Reanastomosing veins. A general rule is that more veins are reanastomosed than arteries to provide sufficient venous return and thereby minimize edema. Swelling creates pressure that impedes circulation, leading to necrosis.

6 Reanastomosing arteries. The vessels may be flushed with heparin solution, and systemic anticoagulants instituted. Antispasmotic agents may be needed.

7 Repairing nerves and soft tissues.

8 Skin grafting if necessary.

NOTE. 1. Microsurgical techniques are necessary for nerve, artery, and vein repairs of structures that have an external diameter of 1 mm or less.

2. Backup replantation teams must be available for lengthy procedures. This is especially important when the patient has multiple amputations or requires repeat of replantation soon after initial operation.

To avoid constriction, a circular bandage is not applied. Instead, foam bandage is used and the extremity suspended from a bedside IV pole with stockinet wrapped around the arm. The dressing is padded to prevent pressure sores and nerve damage. The original dressing is not changed for 10 days unless indicated.

Postoperative care is extremely important. Dressings must be checked carefully, since even slight manipulation can cause great damage. Checking just the tip of the digit for circulation is not adequate. Circulation is verified by *cautiously* going into the dressing to check capillary refill, color, temperature, and drainage. A Doppler flow meter and a temperature probe may be used to evaluate circulation. Patients are not permitted to smoke, as tobacco is a vasoconstrictor. Constriction of vessels may reduce circulation.

The many hours expended by the OR teams initially to achieve a successful repair of all structures can relieve the patient of subsequent operations. The objective is to obtain maximal return of function by minimizing permanent disability. Physical and occupational therapy are important in rehabilitation.

Chapter 29

Potential Complications in Surgical Patients

INTRODUCTION

No operative procedure, even the most simple, is without risk. The patient faces potential complications from the moment he or she is premedicated. For example, the patient may experience an anaphylactic reaction to a preoperative medication. A bowel obstruction secondary to adhesions may occur months to years after bowel surgery. However, pulmonary embolism is the major cause of death during operation and in the immediate postoperative period. Wound infections occur all too frequently. By being aware of possible complications, the operating room nurse must observe for and help prevent them.

PULMONARY COMPLICATIONS

One of the primary areas of postoperative complications is the respiratory tract. The patient's potential for developing pulmonary problems depends on several factors. Any preexisting lung disease such as emphysema, infection, or asthma predisposes the patient. Heavy smokers have the highest risk of succumbing to postoperative pulmonary problems, due to chronic irritation of the respiratory tract with consequent production of excess mucus. Chest wall deformities, obesity, and extremes of age are other pertinent preoperative influences.

Intraoperative factors include:

1 Type of preoperative medications
2 Type and duration of anesthesia
3 Type and duration of assisted ventilation
4 Position of the patient during operation
5 Extent of operation

Postoperatively, one of the most critical factors is the patient's ability to mobilize secretions by deep breathing, coughing, and ambulation. Patients undergoing chest and abdominal surgery are most likely to breathe shallowly, due to pain, and not adequately raise accumulated secretions. The development of one pulmonary complication frequently predisposes the patient to the development of another.

Airway Obstruction

Airway obstruction is the most frequent cause of respiratory embarrassment in the immediate postoperative period. This serious complication may lead to cardiac arrest if not relieved in seconds. The tongue may block the oral airway in a patient who is semiconscious, weak from muscle relaxants, or experiencing a convulsion. If the airway is totally obstructed, breath sounds will be absent; if partially obstructed, a snoring sound will be elicited. The patient may exhibit paradoxical respiration—downward movement of the diaphragm occurring with contraction rather than expansion of the chest. Use of accessory muscles for breathing also may be evident. The pulse is rapid and thready. As the condition worsens, the patient becomes restless, confused, delirious, diaphoretic, cyanotic, and finally unconscious.

To relieve obstruction, gently hyperextend the patient's neck and elevate the chin. If obstruction is still present, ventilate the patient with an Ambu bag and suction any obstructing blood, mucus, or emesis. Finally, nasal airway or endotracheal intubation may be necessary.

Hypoventilation

Inadequate or reduced alveolar ventilation can lead to hypoxemia. Pain, a faulty position, a short thick neck, or a full bladder are also contributing factors. Hypoventilated patients often are restless, or have an anxious facial grimace, and increased pulse rate. The acid-base balance can be affected. Treatment consists of alleviating the cause, if possible, encouraging coughing and deep breathing, and administering oxygen therapy as indicated. An endotracheal tube may be left in place postoperatively to support assisted ventilation.

NOTE. 1. Oxygen is a medication requiring proper dosage. Patients with chronic obstructive pulmonary disease (COPD) cannot tolerate large oxygen concentrations; therefore, to prevent cardiac arrest, a 2- to 3-liter flow is recommended for them.
2. Patients who have received Narcan need close watching. They may awaken too rapidly, cough, and inadvertently extubate.

Atelectasis or Pulmonary Collapse

Partial collapse of the lung is one of the most common postoperative problems. If mucus obstructs a bronchus, air in the alveoli distal to the obstruction is resorbed. That segment of lung then collapses and consolidates. The retained mucus, although initially sterile, becomes contaminated by inhaled bacteria; the patient may develop bronchopneumonia. Factors that promote increased production of mucus, e.g., certain irritating anesthetics, and decreased mobilization of mucus, e.g., a tight abdominal dressing, predispose the patient to pulmonary collapse. Furthermore, normal respiration includes a very deep sigh several times an hour to help keep the lungs expanded. This natural sigh is inhibited by anesthetics, narcotics, and sedatives.

Atelectasis is evidenced by rapid pulse, increased temperature, and increased respiratory rate. The patient may appear cyanotic and uncomfortable, with shallow respirations and pain upon coughing. Breath sounds are diminished, with fine rales. Chest x-ray reveals the collapsed areas of the lung as patch opacities, generally involving the lung bases.

Measures to help prevent or treat atelectasis are abstention from smoking, a regimen of coughing and deep breathing, and early ambulation. The upright position allows for better lung expansion. Medicating the patient for pain, when appropriate, before breathing exercises or ambulation improves ability to deep-breathe and cough effectively. Splinting chest or abdominal incisions with a pillow also aids in decreasing the pain of coughing. Coughing is contraindicated in selected patients, e.g., those who have had cataract extraction, craniotomy, or herniorrhaphy.

Pulmonary Embolism

The most important factor leading to pulmonary emboli is stasis of blood, particularly in the deep veins of the legs and pelvis where the majority of thrombi arise. These become detached and are carried to the lungs. Two other important factors are changes in the vessel wall and coagulative changes in the blood. Bedrest may decrease the blood flow to the lower extremities by more than 50 percent, with decreased pumping action of the muscles. Blood flow is impaired further if the knee is raised or a pillow is placed under the knees, putting pressure on the vessels. Venous stasis also is correlated with obesity, congestive heart failure, and certain cardiac arrythmias. Local trauma to the vein or venous disease enhances the chance of thrombus formation. Hypercoagulability may exist with certain conditions such as pregnancy, fever, myocardial infarction, and certain malignancies, and after abrupt cessation of anticoagulant therapy.

Prevention consists of a regimen of prophylactic anticoagulants or antiplatelets for high-risk patients and routine measures to prevent venous stasis such as elevation of the foot of the bed, antiembolic stockings, and avoidance of the Valsalva maneuver, which can dislodge a thrombus on the wall of a vein. For example, this maneuver accompanies straining at stool. Because of the origin of thrombi in the deep veins, it is important to observe for thrombophlebitis, evidenced by heat, edema, redness, pain in the calf, or a positive Homan's sign, which is pain in the calf upon forceful dorsiflexion of the foot.

The symptoms exhibited are nonspecific, and depend on whether the embolism is mild or massive. The patient may have dyspnea, pleural pain, hemoptysis, tachypnea, rales, tachycardia, mild fever, or persistent cough. Patients with massive emboli have air hunger, hypotension, shock, and cyanosis. Treatment of pulmonary emboli consists of bedrest, oxygen, anticoagulant therapy, thrombolytic agents, and sometimes operation, when indicated, to remove emboli or prevent their recurrence.

Fat Embolism; Other Emboli

Fat embolism occurs primarily following fractures of the long bones, pelvis, and ribs. However, it sometimes occurs after blood transfusion, cardiopulmonary bypass, or renal transplant. Fat globules enter the bloodstream, and the patient becomes symptomatic when the globules block the pulmonary capillaries, causing interstitial edema and hemorrhage. Frequently, adult respiratory-distress syndrome ensues, with hypoxia and decreased surfactant production, resulting in collapse of the alveolar membrane and microatelectasis. The syndrome develops most frequently in patients after the age of 10, especially those who have traveled long distances with an immobilized fracture.

Symptoms include disorientation, increased pulse and temperature, tachypnea, dyspnea, rales, and pleuritic chest pain. Other significant signs are fat in the sputum and urine and a petechial rash on the anterior chest. Treatment is supportive. The mortality rate is high.

Air embolism may follow the injection of air into a body cavity, or a bolus of air in an intravenous or intra-arterial infusion. Another portal of entry is transection of large veins with the patient in a sitting position. The pull of gravity on the blood column exerts a significant negative pressure that sucks air down the veins and into the heart.

Intrauterine fetal death or placenta previa may precipitate an *embolism of amniotic fluid.* Also, tumors may cause emboli from primary or metastatic sites.

Pulmonary Edema

Pulmonary edema may result from congestive heart failure or fluid overload. Blood becomes backed up in the pulmonary circulation, with fluid exuding from the pulmonary capillaries into the alveoli. When mixed with air, frothy pink sputum is produced. Reduction of capillary membrane perfusion leads to hypoxia.

Bounding rapid pulse, rales, dyspnea, apprehension, and engorged peripheral veins should alert the nurse to the possibility of pulmonary edema. Treatment includes digitalization, diuretics, upright position, oxygen, and rotating tourniquets to the extremities to decrease circulatory overload.

Other Pulmonary Complications

Adult respiratory-distress syndrome, also known as *progressive pulmonary insufficiency* or *shock lung,* may develop in the first 24 to 48 hours following a traumatic injury. Beginning with dyspnea, grunting respirations, and tachycardia, the signs progress to cyanosis, hypoxemia, and alveolar infiltration. The mortality rate is high.

Other potential pulmonary complications are pneumothorax, hemothorax, and pleural effusion. Aspiration of emesis may cause aspiration pneumonia and lung abscess with necrosis of the pulmonary parenchyma.

CARDIOVASCULAR COMPLICATIONS

The array of emotional and physical stresses to which the patient is subjected may lead to cardiovascular complications. These include cardiac arrest, congestive heart failure, myocardial infarction, thromboembolism and/or thrombophlebitis, hypotension, and various arrhythmias. Patients with a history of cardiac problems or those undergoing cardiovascular surgery are prone to develop these complications, as discussed in previous chapters. Cerebral thrombosis or embolism may result in prolonged coma. Patients who receive blood transfusions should be watched closely for transfusion reactions. Other problems may occur, including the following.

Venous Stasis

The venous stasis that develops in the lower extremities during operation can be effectively counteracted in most patients. This is especially important in patients with thromboembolic disease to prevent thrombophlebitis and pulmonary embolism postoperatively. Methods of augmenting venous flow from the legs during operation include:

1 *Elevation of the legs.* An elevation of 15° above horizontal is effective in preventing venous stasis. Surgeons frequently order this position for potentially susceptible patients postoperatively.

2 *Galvanic stimulation of the calf muscles.* Galvanic stimulation can be carried out only on anesthetized patients because it is too painful to be tolerated by patients who are awake. Through an electric charge administered externally, the velocity of venous return from the lower extremities is increased.

3 *Intermittent pneumatic compression.* Inflatable, double-walled vinyl boots use alternating compression and relaxation to reduce the risk of deep vein clotting in the legs of high-risk patients undergoing general anesthesia. Pressure between 40 and 50 mm of mercury applied quickly for 12 seconds, then released for 48 seconds, empties the blood from the deep leg veins.

Postoperatively, flexion and extension of the legs and feet, frequent turning, and early ambulation, unless contraindicated, aid circulation.

Hypertension

An abnormal elevation of blood pressure may occur, especially in the hypertensive or arteriosclerotic patient. Hypertension, if not controlled, may precipitate a cardiovascular accident (CVA). Etiologic factors include pain, hypoxia, hypercapnia, effects of vasopressor drugs, hypervolemia or overreplacement of fluid losses, and shivering. Treatment consists of administration of oxygen, diuretics, and antihypertensive drugs as indicated.

Vascular Accidents

Various types of vascular accidents may occur at any time in patients with cerebrovascular disease. Severe hypotension can predispose to cerebral thrombosis due to the slow flow of blood through arteriosclerotic vessels. Hypertension may be followed by cerebral hemorrhage. Acute arterial occlusion may result from embolization or *in situ* thrombosis.

Following Cardiopulmonary Bypass

Improvements in extracorporeal circulation have reduced the incidence of complications following cardiopulmonary bypass, but the patient may still encounter a number of serious problems. Alterations in clotting may occur due to heparinization of the blood, mechanical damage to platelets and clotting factors, and direct exposure of the blood to oxygen. When red blood cells are hemolyzed due to trauma or transfusion reaction, viscosity in the renal tubules may cause tubular necrosis and renal failure.

Inadequate or extended perfusion and oxygenation may promote tissue anoxia and metabolic acidosis. Fluid and electrotyle balance merit close watching, particularly for hypervolemia. When nonblood fluids are used to prime the pump, they may diffuse into the interstitial spaces. As this fluid returns to the circulation postoperatively, hypervolemia may result. Furthermore, the increased levels of aldosterone and antidiuretic hormone induced by the stress of surgery cause retention of sodium and water. Fluids are restricted for 24 hours postoperatively. Cerebral edema and brain damage at times ensue, for unknown reasons. However, these developments are generally temporary.

Another problem is "post-pump psychosis," which consists of visual and auditory hallucinations and paranoid delusions. This often terminates when the patient is transferred from the intensive care unit.

The most severe pulmonary complication of extracorporeal circulation is postperfusion lung syndrome. The etiology is unknown. It is often fatal, due to the development of atelectasis, pulmonary edema, and hemorrhage. Metabolic acidosis during the bypass may lead to the "low cardiac output" syndrome postoperatively. This occurs most frequently in patients with long histories of cardiac disease. Finally, cardiac tamponade is another potential complication, reflected by a drop of more than 10 mm of mercury in the systolic blood pressure upon inspiration.

SHOCK

Shock is a state of inadequate blood perfusion to the different parts of the body. If untreated, it will become irreversible and result in death. All forms of shock carry high mortality rates. The best treatment is prevention. There are five main classifications of shock as follows:

Hypovolemic or Hemorrhagic Shock

Decrease in circulating blood volume may be due to loss of blood, plasma, or extracellular fluid. Fluid loss is excessive when it is greater than the compensatory absorption of interstitial fluid into the circulation. Shock resulting from hemorrhage or inadequate blood volume replacement is often seen in the OR and recovery room. It usually is reversed by prompt restoration of circulating blood volume.

Cardiogenic Shock

In cardiogenic shock, the pumping action of the left ventricle is insufficient to pump enough blood to the vital organs. It may be precipitated by congestive heart failure, myocardial infarction, serious arrhythmias, or mechanical venous obstruction. Drugs used to treat this and the other types of shock are similar to those used for hypovolemic shock (refer to Chap. 9). In addition, various mechanical devices may be used, such as the auxiliary ventricle or counterpulsation with the intraaortic balloon to temporarily increase left ventricular function.

Neurogenic Shock

Loss of neurogenic tone in peripheral blood vessels leads to sudden vasodilatation and pooling of blood. Peripheral resistance is too great for compensation by increased cardiac output. Causes may be brain damage, deep anesthesia, emotional trauma, or vagal reflex from pain or operative manipulation.

Traumatic Shock

Damage to the capillaries due to bodily trauma causes increased capillary permeability, with loss of volume into the tissues. This state is aggravated by pain, which inhibits the vasomotor center, leading to vasodilatation.

Vasogenic Shock

In vasogenic shock, vasodilatation is caused by drugs such as histamine or alcohol. The two most common forms of vasogenic shock are anaphylaxis and septic shock.

Anaphylaxis This is a *severe allergic reaction* in which cells release histamine or a histaminelike substance, causing vasodilatation, hypotension, and bronchiolar constriction. Within seconds after the introduction of the antigenic substance, the patient will exhibit edema and itching around the site of injection or contact, and sneezing, followed by edema of the hands and face, wheezing, cyanosis, and dyspnea. Treatment includes epinephrine, antihistamines, and oxygen by positive pressure to control bronchospasm. Isoproterenol, vasopressors, corticosteroids, and aminophylline also may be administered.

Septic Shock Septic shock is a state of widely disseminated infection, generally of gram-negative bacterial origin, and often borne in the bloodstream. Early septic shock may begin with fever, restlessness, sudden unexplained hypotension, a cloudy sensorium, hypoxia, tachycardia, rapid breathing, and/or oliguria. One or more of these possible symptoms may be present. Toxic or metabolic by-products increase capillary permeability permitting loss of circulating fluid into the interstitial fluid. Endotoxins released by the bacteria promote vasodilatation and hypotension.

Septic shock differs from most of the other types of shock in its abrupt onset and high cardiac output. As shock progresses, the patient develops cold clammy skin, sharply diminished urinary output, respiratory insufficiency, cardiac decompensation, disseminated intravascular coagulation, and metabolic acidosis. The high-risk category comprises patients with severe infection (e.g., peritonitis), trauma, burns, impaired immunological state, diabetes mellitus, age-extreme patients, or patients who have undergone any invasive procedures.

Treatment consists of control of the infectious process, early administration of antibiotics, fluid-volume replacement, and oxygen. The use of diuretics, sodium bicarbonate, vasoconstrictors, vasodilators, inotropic agents, or heparin also may be indicated. Corticosteroids may be used, but their use is controversial.

HEMORRHAGE

Severe bleeding into or from a wound is a major contributing factor to operative and postoperative morbidity and mortality. If uncontrolled, the patient can exsanguinate. Massive hemorrhage may cause hypovolemic shock, ventricular fibrillation, or death due to the marked decrease in cardiac output.

Common symptoms are arterial hypotension, pale or cyanotic moist skin, oliguria, bradycardia from hypoxia, or tachycardia after moderate to marked blood loss, restlessness, and thirst in the conscious patient. In the operating room, hemorrhage is readily visible.

Meticulous hemostasis during every step of the operation and good nutritional status of the patient preoperatively are crucial to prevention. Preoperative evaluation of clotting time and history of bleeding (personal and familial), type and cross match of blood, and insertion of an intravenous line prior to incision are necessary precautions.

In treating hemorrhage, the surgeon locates the source of bleeding and applies digital compression to the severed or traumatized vessels until non-crushing vascular clamps can be placed to occlude the vessel proximally and distally to the site of bleeding. The vessel is then ligated, electrocoagulated, or sutured. Meanwhile, circulating blood volume must be restored promptly. If much blood is transfused, it must be fresh, and warmed to limit electrolytic changes. Sodium bicarbonate may be given intravenously to reduce acidosis. Multiple intravenous infusion routes can be utilized, by cutdown if necessary, to infuse blood under pressure. Lactated Ringer's solution or plasma expanders are used when blood is contraindicated, e.g., for religious reasons. Oxygen is administered to combat hypoxia. Accurate measurement of blood and fluid losses intraoperatively, followed by adequate replacement, will help prevent hypovolemic shock.

Hemorrhage can be detected postoperatively by observation of blood-soaked dressings. The patient must be checked frequently for both observable and nonobservable symptoms of hemorrhage. Internal bleeding can be caused by slipping or sloughing of a ligature or by the blowout of clots from vessels ligated or coagulated at the time of operation.

DISSEMINATED INTRAVASCULAR COAGULATION (DIC)

Disseminated intravascular coagulation is a life-threatening syndrome. It can follow many conditions, for example, hemorrhagic or septic shock, extracorporeal circulation, certain complications of pregnancy such as abruptio placentae, severe infection, and massive tissue damage of extensive burns. Coagulation is initiated throughout the bloodstream, especially in the microcirculation. Vital organs become ischemic, and the body's supply of platelets and major clotting factors is exhausted. As the blood becomes depleted of these factors, massive hemorrhaging ensues throughout the body. Cutaneous petechiae then appear, and bleeding may be noted from various sites, such as through a nasogastric tube. The patient also may have hypotension, nausea and vomiting, severe muscular pain, convulsions, oliguria, and coma. Diagnosis is based on blood laboratory studies.

Treatment should begin with control of the primary condition. If given early, heparin may help prevent coagulation and thus prevent depletion of clotting factors. In addition, blood, plasma, dextran, and clotting factors can be administered intravenously.

POSTOPERATIVE WOUND INFECTIONS

The patients most prone to develop wound infections are those listed under septic shock. Compromised patients are highly likely to develop endogenous infection. Operations on potentially contaminated areas, such as the gastrointestinal tract, are more apt to result in postoperative infections (refer to Chap. 4 for detailed discussion of predisposing factors and infection control).

The following measures, in addition to those previously discussed under infection control, may help prevent wound infections.

1 Some surgeons prefer to irrigate potentially contaminated wounds with topical antibiotics intraoperatively.

2 Cultures obtained during operation, rather than those obtained postoperatively, should be used for antibiotic sensitivity testing.

3 Indwelling catheters should be discontinued as soon as possible to prevent urinary tract infection, which increases in incidence the longer the catheter is in the patient.

4 Special precautions must be taken when prostheses such as porcine heart valves, total hip prostheses, or intraocular lenses are implanted. Infection can have disastrous effects, for example, the loss of an eye.

Gram-negative bacteria are the primary contaminants in wound infection. They are the predominant flora of the gastrointestinal tract and the primary pathogens in urinary tract, abdominal, and intravenous catheter infections, as well as in pneumonia. These infections carry a high risk of bacteremia and therefore require prompt intervention.

Nonbacterial opportunists such as fungi and viruses are a particular hazard to trauma or burn patients. Likelihood of infection is related to severity of injury. Initial gram-positive infection frequently is followed by a virulent gram-negative or fungal infection. Candida is a common fungal colonizer and invader.

Staphylococci species of gram-positive cocci are common pathogens that may occur as normal flora of the skin, hair, and upper respiratory tract.

Staphylococci wound infections acquired in the operating room are characterized by pus deep beneath a cleanly healed wound. A red wound accompanied by pus and fever within 7 days after operation may indicate such an infection. Infections appearing more than 7 days postoperatively usually are acquired on the unit.

Streptococci species of gram-positive cocci are found primarily in the upper respiratory tract. Beta-hemolytic streptococci are the pathogenic strain of this group.

Pseudomonas aeruginosa is an aerobic gram-negative bacillus found in water, soil, and intestinal tracts. It is becoming an increasing problem, particularly because of its ability to survive in plain water. It is readily recognized by a bluish-green fluorescent color and characteristic odor.

Difficult to eradicate, these infections often progress to septicemia and multiple-abscess formation in the viscera or body areas, resulting in fatality.

Isolation precautions may be required for staphylococcal, streptococcal, or gram-negative wound infections.

Enteric organisms normally are found in the intestinal tract. Gram-negative bacilli often are resistant to long-established antibiotics. Peritoneal contamination can result from visceral manipulation without mechanically entering the gastrointestinal tract in patients with cancerous lesions. A bowel wall can erode permitting intestinal organisms to escape into the peritoneal cavity.

Anaerobic organisms thrive in unoxygenated tissues. They outnumber aerobic organisms in the intestinal tract, and are less susceptible to antibiotics than aerobes. Often present in the lower genital tract of females, they cause severe pelvic infection. Anaerobic infections are caused by:

1 Peptostreptococcus and peptococcus.
2 *Bacteroides* species and fusobacteria are the most frequently isolated microorganisms from blood cultures. These are common bacteria in the colon.
3 *Clostridium perfringens, C. welchii,* is found in the colon. This is a species of highly resistant gas-producing spore formers, contributing to a high mortality rate.

Investigation of Postoperative Wound Infections

A special form is used to record specific data. Investigation, usually by the infection control coordinator, includes:

1 Analysis of each infection to seek the cause
2 Consultation with all persons who cared for the patient
3 Review of any problem encountered intraoperatively, such as a break in sterile technique
4 Review of possible contributory factors
5 Evaluation of procedures relating to the patient
6 Review of the chart, symptoms, bacterial cultures
7 Review of postoperative dressing changes

WOUND DISRUPTION

Failure of the wound to heal or closure material to secure the wound during the healing process leads to wound disruption, a separation of the wound edges. Disruption may occur after any operation and usually occurs on the fifth to tenth postoperative day. This is the lag period in healing, the time when the wound is not yet strong. Wound disruption is caused not by a single factor but by a combination of predisposing factors that influence healing.

Although it may occur in any body area, acute wound disruption most frequently follows abdominal operations. It is thought that wound disruption starts by a small opening in the peritoneum, allowing a wedge of omentum to slip into it. This omentum becomes edematous and extends the opening along the line of incision and upward through the other layers of the abdominal wall. Disruption is usually precipitated by distention or a sudden strain such as vomiting, coughing, or sneezing. Terms used to describe abdominal wound disruption include:

1 *Dehiscence*—the partial or total splitting open or separation of the layers of the wound. "Cutting out" of the sutures is the most important cause of dehiscence. The strength of the tissues and extent of the separation determine whether or not the wound must be reclosed.
2 *Evisceration*—a protrusion of the viscera through the abdominal incision. *While a wound disruption of any degree calls for emergency care,* an evisceration is a catastrophe requiring immediate replacement of the viscera and reclosure of the incision.

Symptoms

Frequently patients who disrupt do not present a smooth immediate postoperative course. They may have undue pain, discomfort, nausea, drainage, slight fever, vomiting, or hiccups. Acute symptoms include:

1 Tachycardia.
2 Vomiting.
3 Abnormal serosanguineous discharge.
4 Change in contour of the wound.
5 Sudden pulling pain during straining. The patient feels something give. Suspect any seepage of serosanguineous fluid after a sudden, sharp pain that lasts only momentarily after an effort. It is well to send some of this fluid for culture and smear.

Any of these symptoms should be investigated at once. Examination of the wound may show it gaping somewhat, or the viscera may appear at the skin surface.

Treatment at the Bedside

1 Put in an emergency call for the surgeon. Have a nasogastric tube ready for insertion to relieve distention.
2 Reassure the patient.
3 Apply sterile, moist saline dressings over the wound, and a loose binder.
4 Give drugs according to surgeon's order.
5 Do not give patient anything by mouth.
6 Prepare the patient for return to the operating room. Treatment in the OR consists of secondary wound closure.

Prevention of Wound Disruption

Factors that may contribute to wound disruption are eliminated as nearly as possible. Treatment and care are given to promote healing. Preoperatively:

1 Malnutrition and avitaminosis are corrected.
2 Obesity is reduced.
3 Anemia is corrected.
4 Operation is postponed, if possible, in the presence of transient illness, such as cold or influenza.
5 Antibiotics may be given prophylactically. While antibiotics cannot supplant sterile technique, some can render the operative field more free of microorganisms than it normally would be, as in operation on the gastrointestinal tract.

Precautions during Operation

1 The surgeon gives meticulous attention to sterile technique, hemostasis, tissue handling and approximation, and selection of wound closure materials.
2 The entire OR team carefully carries out strict aseptic and sterile techniques to prevent infection.

COMPLICATIONS OF ABDOMINAL SURGERY

Patients who have undergone abdominal surgery are particularly prone to *pulmonary complications.* They also are subject to a variety of *fluid and electrolyte imbalances* for several reasons. For example, they are generally on nothing by mouth postoperatively. They may be losing sodium, potassium, chloride, and water through nasogastric suction. If great quantities of alkalotic pancreatic secretions are lost through decompression of the small bowel, metabolic acidosis may result. Loss of acidic stomach secretions may lead to metabolic alkalosis.

Peritonitis and wound infection are more common after abdominal surgery because of spillage of contaminants from the lumen of the gastrointestinal tract. Another complication that may occur months to years postoperatively is *adhesions.* These may cause no problem, or may cause a mechanical bowel obstruction. The formation of this scar tissue is enhanced by peritonitis or postoperative radiation therapy. Increased intra-abdominal pressure even years postoperatively may induce an *incisional hernia* through an old, weakened scar.

RENAL COMPLICATIONS

Oliguria is frequently seen postoperatively. Water and sodium are conserved by antidiuretic hormone, aldosterone, epinephrine, and norepinephrine secreted during stress. This decreases urinary output. Dehydration, shock, cardiac failure, renal failure, or third-space loss such as edema or ascites may contribute to oliguria. Because prolonged oliguria may result in renal failure, urinary output of less than 30 ml an hour should be reported to the surgeon. Treatment depends on the cause.

The patient should be watched for infection following all urinary tract procedures because of the introduction of instruments into the sterile system. Cloudy urine, dysuria, frequency, urgency, and pain or burning upon urination are symptoms of urinary tract infections. Damage to the bladder sphincters from instrumentation or urethral infection may lead to incontinence. Sharp abdominal pain following cystoscopy or manipulation of the ureter in removal of calculi may suggest peritonitis from bladder or ureteral perforation. Particular susceptibility to infection accompanies urinary diversion.

WITHDRAWAL SYMPTOMS

Symptoms of withdrawal from either alcohol or drugs may appear postoperatively in habitual users. Unexplained agitation, disorientation, and/or hallucinations may be symptomatic of the body's reaction to deprivation of accustomed intake of chemical substances.

ELECTROLYTE IMBALANCES

Fluid and electrolyte imbalances may be caused by many different factors. Maintenance of correct balance is a very relevant aspect of postoperative care, which greatly influences outcome of operative intervention.

Chapter 30

Liability and Accountability

Most mistakes or accidents are preventable. Some are so slight that patients are never aware of them. Others, however, can cause injury resulting in pain, disfigurement, prolonged hospitalization and/or rehabilitation, and can even prove fatal. If negligence or malpractice is established, a nurse or technician can be held liable for his or her own acts of omission or commission.

Along with the development of *consumerism,* a movement that focuses on consumer rights, a well-informed American public has developed an increasingly litigious attitude, demanding compensation for bodily injuries or damages to personal property. The quality of health care in this country is assessed through the outcome of services rendered. However, there is an increasing tendency for patients to take grievances to court. The severity of an injury usually determines whether a claim will arise, but other contributing factors include a breakdown of rapport between the patient and the health care team members and unrealistic expectations about the outcome of care.

The welfare and safety of the patient constitute the principles around which nursing care is built. Safe care of the patient results in safety to the nurse, the technician, the surgeon, and the hospital. It also upholds the reputation of the professions by maintaining the confidence of the consumer public. Safeguards against the hazards peculiar to the care of patients in the operating room have been stressed throughout this text. Most incidents that could endanger the patient and lead to legal action can be prevented by following the accepted procedures as presented.

HISTORICAL EVOLUTION

Over 4000 years ago, King Hammurabi of Babylonia codified the laws of human behavior. These codes included penalties for physician/surgeons who did not cure. "If a physician has treated a man with a metal knife for a severe wound and has caused the man to die, or has opened a man's tumor with a metal knife and destroyed the man's eye, his hands shall be cut off."* Although this ancient punishment seems severe by contemporary judgment, it should remind the OR team that their primary consideration is still to do patients no harm, *primum non nocere.*

The first recorded medical malpractice suit was tried in England in the thirteenth century. The first one in the United States occurred in 1790. Throughout the nineteenth century and the early

*Code of Hammurabi, from the translation by Charles Edwards.

part of the twentieth, litigation against physicians was quite uncommon and rarely affected nurses. Malpractice suits began to increase markedly after World War II. They flourished in the 1960s and 1970s as the rising standard of living enabled an increasing number of people to seek medical and nursing care. This automatically increased exposure to incidents that could lead to lawsuits. A fundamental cause for litigation lies in the thinking of patients and their families that physicians have not provided appropriate diagnosis, treatment, or results. Although the physician is professionally responsible for patient care, other professionals and paraprofessionals act as part of the health care team. Ancillary personnel and suppliers of equipment and drugs also are indirectly involved in treatment, and may be held liable.

Medical care and professional liability have become institutional problems. The primary cause of professional liability claims is *iatrogenic medical injury,* an injury or other adverse result sustained by a patient during the course of hospital and medical treatment. Many of the serious incidents that are brought to suit occur in the operating room.

In the past, the surgeon was considered the "captain of the ship" in the operating room. If the surgeon had supervisory control and the right to give orders during the operation, then the operating room was like a ship and the surgeon like its captain. The captain or master was liable for the negligent acts of his servants. Courts held that this doctrine, based on the master-servant relationship, was applicable by the mere presence of the surgeon. Once having entered the OR, the surgeon was considered to have complete control over other team members. Courts now recognize that the surgeon does not have complete control over the acts of the nurses and technicians on the OR team. The surgeon usually is not held responsible when a nurse or technician fails to carry out a routine procedure as expected, since the courts have decided that these procedures do not need to be supervised by the surgeon. The hospital as the employer may be held responsible for its employees under the master-servant relationship. However, the most recent trend is to hold an individual responsible for his or her own acts under the principle of an independent contractor.

LIABILITY

To be *liable* is to be legally bound, as to make good any loss or damage that occurs in a transaction; to be answerable; to be responsible. A *tort* is a legal wrong committed by one person involving injury to another person, loss of or damage to personal property. When a tort has been committed, a patient or family member may institute a civil action against the person or persons who caused the injury, loss, or damage.

Statutory laws (laws by legislation) and *common laws* (laws based on court decisions) differ from state to state. Courts differ at times in their interpretation of the laws. A nurse or technician who is caring for a patient and is in some manner responsible for injury to that patient may be sued. The supervisor or instructor responsible for assigning duties to this individual may be included in the suit. Nurses and technicians may be considered employees of the hospital and, if the court so rules, the hospital is considered liable. However, the court may rule a learner or an experienced practitioner liable for his or her own acts. A learner may be held responsible in proportion to the amount and type of instruction received and judged by the standard of other learners in training. An individual can be held responsible for carrying out a wrong procedure if he or she has received sufficient instruction so that the correct procedure should be known.

An unqualified, unconditional general rule of law is that every person is liable for the torts he or she commits. *There is no exception to this rule.* However, liability may be imposed under one of several legal doctrines or common law precedents.

Doctrine of the Reasonable Man

A patient has the right to expect all professional and technical nursing personnel to utilize knowledge, skill, and judgment in performing duties that meet the standards exercised by other *reasonably prudent persons* involved in a similar circumstances. Every professional nurse and technician must always carry out duties in accordance with the national standards of care established by federal statutes, state practice acts, the professional organizations and regulatory agencies, and maintained in common practice throughout the country. Deviation from these standards of practice that cause injury to the patient can result in liabilities for negligence or malpractice.

Negligence is the lack of care or skills that any nurse or technician in the same situation would be expected to use. It has been legally defined as "the omission to do something which a reasonable person, guided by those ordinary considerations which ordinarily regulate human affairs, would do, or as doing something which a reasonable and prudent person would not do."* These acts of omission or commission may give rise to tort action, which is a civil liability, as a result of injury to a patient that can be traced directly to the breach of duty.

Malpractice is "any professional misconduct, unreasonable lack of skill or fidelity in professional or judiciary duties, evil practice, or illegal or immoral conduct."* Malpractice claims usually are settled in a civil court but, depending on the severity of the injury and the extent of the misconduct, they may be taken to criminal court. Legally from the point of view of damages or fault, professional negligence usually is synonymous with malpractice in a tort action. Factors contributing to actionable negligence have been called the *four D's of malpractice:*

1 Duty to demonstrate and deliver a high standard of care directly proportional to the degree of specialty training received
2 Dereliction of that duty by omission or commission
3 Damage to a patient or personal property
4 Direct cause of a personal injury or damage because of dereliction of duty

Doctrine of *Res Ipsa Loquitor*

Translated literally from the Latin, *res ipsa loquitor* means "the thing speaks for itself." Before this doctrine can be applied, three conditions must exist:

1 The type of injury does not ordinarily occur without a negligent act.
2 The injury was caused by the conduct or instrumentality within the exclusive control of the person or persons being sued.
3 The injured person could not have contributed to the negligence nor voluntarily assumed the risk.

This doctrine frequently applies to injuries sustained by patients while in the operating room suite.

Doctrine of *Respondeat Superior*

An employer may be liable for an employee's negligent conduct under the *respondeat superior* master-servant employment relationship. This implies that the master will answer for the acts of a servant. A hospital protects the patient, its personnel, and itself by maintaining good working conditions for a well-oriented staff. The professional and technical nursing staff members are chosen after careful screening of educational preparation and licensure or certification credentials. The staff should be adequate in size, and properly trained and assigned. A continuous program of staff orientation and education should be provided. Hospital procedures and routines are established in a manner consistent with the standards of competent nursing performance and patient safety.

*H Creighton, *Law Every Nurse Should Know,* 3d ed, Philadelphia: Saunders, 1975, p. 119.

Assault and Battery

In legal terms, *assault* is an unlawful threat to harm another physically. *Battery* is the carrying out of threatened physical harm. The lack of consent is an important aspect of an assault and battery charge. Consent may be given by words or implied by conduct, but it must be given voluntarily with full understanding of the implications. Witnessed written consent for operation is obtained before the patient is premedicated and transported to the OR suite. The purpose of a consent is to protect the surgeon, OR team members, and the hospital against claims of unauthorized operations and to protect the patient against unsanctioned procedures. If a surgeon goes beyond the limits to which the patient consented, liability for assault and battery may be charged.

The surgeon must explain the procedure to the patient or a member of the family or both, in understandable lay language, without details that might unnecessarily frighten the patient. When a patient signs an agreement, consent is given for the specific procedure that the patient understands will be done. The patient must sign the consent unless he or she is a minor, unconscious, mentally incompetent, or in the situation of a life-threatening emergency. The nearest of kin or other authorized person must sign for these patients. A witness is necessary to testify, if needed, that the patient signed without coercion after the surgeon explained the details of the procedure. The patient has the right to waive an explanation of the nature and consequences of the procedure, and also the right to refuse treatment (refer to Chap. 3, pp. 43–45, for discussion of the patient-physician relationship and written operative consents).

Human experimentation with new drugs and devices requires patient consent. Department of Health, Education and Welfare (HEW) regulations require a very specific informed consent for research carried out under HEW auspices, with strong emphasis on the need for a clear explanation of the experiment, its possible dangers, and the patient's complete freedom to refuse or withdraw from the regime at any time.

The surgeon may be approved by the Federal Food and Drug Administration (FDA) and the hospital as a clinical investigator in the controlled experimental use of new drugs and chemical agents or medical devices. Prior written, voluntary consent based on an informed decision to participate in the research must be obtained from the patient. The surgeon completes an investigator's report that is returned to the supplier of the drug or device and eventually filed with the FDA.

Invasion of Privacy

The patient's right to privacy exists either by statutory law or by common law. Patient charts and medical records, x-rays, and photographs are considered confidential information for use by physicians and other hospital personnel directly concerned with that patient's care. Lawsuits can be, and have been, brought to the courts by patients for violation of this right. Unauthorized persons are not permitted to observe or photograph operations or procedures of interest only to professional persons without the patient's written consent.

The patient has the right to expect that all communications and records pertaining to individualized care will be treated as confidential and will not be misused. This includes the right to privacy during interview, examination, and treatment. Every health care worker has a moral obligation to hold in confidence any personal or family affairs learned from patients.

> NOTE. If a patient has been criminally assaulted or is being held in criminal custody, team members are required by law to divulge voluntarily any information concerning the patient to legal authorities. Withholding known information is punishable by law.

ACCOUNTABILITY

Accountability is the expectation that an individual may be called to account for actions taken which were consistent with the responsibilities for which he or she contracted by virtue of employment or learner experience. Stated more succinctly, to be accountable means to answer to someone else for something one has done. OR nurses and technicians, both practitioners and learners, are accountable to:

1 Patients receiving services.
2 Hospital employing practitioners and educational institutions providing learning experiences.
3 Profession or vocation to uphold established standards of practice.
4 Public to whom nurses are licensed and technicians are certified to serve.
5 Self and other team members. The adages "to thine own self be true" and "do unto others" apply in all interpersonal relationships. Trust, honesty, and confidence are the essence of valid team member relationships.

Accountability is concerned with both *efficiency and effectiveness.* Patients and the public demand quality-care assurance. Documentation of nursing care given can attest to efficiency or protect against liability when an unusual incident occurs. Audit and peer review are methods for evaluating effectiveness by comparing actual care with established standards for the nursing care process. OR nursing process should include a systematic series of actions directed toward preoperative assessment of patient needs; development and implementation of a written, individualized, intraoperative nursing care plan; and postoperative evaluation of the effectiveness of the nursing care plan for continuity of each surgical patient's care.

Documentation in Patient Records

Verbal communications between patients and health care providers do not provide legal evidence in a court of law. However, the patient's medical records can be subpoenaed as legal evidence of care received or omitted. Documentation of the care that has been given, including the teaching provided, and the patient's response to care must be complete and accurate. Some hospitals allow patients access to their records so they can review them for reliability of subjective data and clarity of plans for treatment and teaching.

During a preoperative visit, the OR nurse should be alert to signs that a patient does not clearly understand what is going to happen as a result of surgical intervention. This must be brought to the attention of the surgeon. Significant observations or information must be recorded on the chart and reported to the unit nurse in charge. For example, if a patient verbally withdraws consent for operation or expresses a fear of death in the OR, the OR nurse is responsible for communicating this information.

The professional nursing role includes preoperative patient assessment and teaching, and postoperative evaluation of intraoperative care and reinforcement of preoperative teaching. All visits with patients are documented on the patient's chart, either in the nurses' notes or progress notes. The format for recording in the patient's chart varies from hospital to hospital. Some hospitals use problem-oriented records; others use integrated patients' progress records, and/or written nursing care plans.

Problem-oriented Medical Record With the problem-oriented, goal-directed approach to care, the patient's chart is organized on the basis of problems rather than on the source of the data about them such as radiology, laboratory reports, etc. Each problem is numbered in a problem list with the initial plan for meeting each. Progress notes are charted corresponding to the problem number to facilitate assessment of the patient's response to planned intervention. Briefly, the record utilizes:

1 A defined data base of information from history, examination, laboratory reports, etc., to formulate a complete problem list

2 Plans for diagnostic, therapeutic, teaching, and follow-up care for each problem

3 Progress notes and flow sheets for multiple parameters that contain both subjective (symptoms) and objective (signs) information

The advantages of problem-oriented medical records are that they:

1 Check efficiency, reliability, thoroughness, and analytic sense of the professional. The nurse acquires selected assessment and communicative skills, and bases nursing judgments on scientific knowledge rather than on intuitive observations.

2 Provide better communication among health care professionals.

3 Provide systematic management of patient care by assessing, recording, and evaluating. This establishes the concept of team patient care as opposed to nursing versus medical care.

4 Enhance continuity of care and recorded data; document practice and quality of care.

5 Permit qualified participants in patient care to cooperate in compiling patient records.

6 Bring to immediate attention all essential information. Specific problems are identified, thereby furnishing immediate relevancy to data. This avoids inadvertent omission and obviates unnecessary repetition of data.

7 Facilitate audit for efficiency, performance, and effectiveness.

Problem-oriented records document information needed to accurately diagnose illness and treat patients. Some hospitals use a combined, some a separate, problem list for nurses and physicians. Critics of the system cite its emphasis on symptoms rather than prevention or improvement, and its neglect of individual strengths.

Integrated Patient's Progress Record Documentation is a vitally important aspect of continuity in patient care. A record of the patient's progress from admission to discharge guides all health care providers in planning and coordinating care. Entry of a progress note may be made by a physician or nurse on the same record. This promotes the team concept of total patient care by sharing knowledge and observations made by each team member who cares for the patient. A note is made after a treatment or procedure is initiated to document the condition and tolerance of the patient. Any change in condition, any unusual incident, complication, or deviation from the usual pattern or course of the patient must be recorded as a progress note. The nurse must document any nursing intervention and management, as well as the time the physician was notified, if this is indicated.

Written Nursing Care Plan Statements of identified patient needs and planned approaches for nursing care to meet these needs are formalized into a nursing care plan. This may become a permanent part of the patient's chart or may be used as an accessory guideline for implementation of nursing care. If this tool is used to document care given, it should be incorporated into the patient's medical record.

Procedure for All Entries Regardless of the format of the patient's record, all entries must be:

1 Written legibly in ink without erasures.

2 Stated factually as to what happened. Documentation of services rendered or unusual incidents should be very specific.

3 Stated in complete words. Abbreviations should be used only for very commonly accepted medical terms, e.g., T&A, D&C, TUR, O.D., etc.

4 Dated, including the time note is written.

5 Signed with full legal signature and status of the writer.

Intraoperative Nurses' Notes

Specific care given in the OR should be documented on the patient's chart, not only for legal reasons, but also for the benefit of recovery room and unit nurses who provide postoperative care. Information documented by the circulating nurse in the nurses' notes or progress record should include:

1 Times patient arrived in and departed from the OR
2 Level of consciousness or anxiety manifested by observable physical responses
3 Site, time started, type of needle or cannula and solutions administered intravenously, including blood products
4 Position and types of restraints and supports used for maintaining position of patient on operating table
5 Skin condition and antiseptics used for skin preparation
6 Location of electrosurgical grounding devices and monitoring electrodes
7 Operation performed
8 Specimens and cultures sent to the laboratory
9 Medications given, including local anesthetic agents, and irrigating solutions used.
10 Site and types of drains and catheters
11 Type of dressing applied
12 Any unusual incident or complication

Incident Report

An injury may occur to a patient due to lack of proper care. When an accident or unusual incident occurs, whether or not it involves an injury, the person who knows the factual details should notify the supervisor at once and write an incident report. Details must be complete and accurate. The patient is given whatever care is needed as a result of accidental injury. This is recorded on the incident report and the patient's record. Incident reports are filed by administration as they can become legal evidence if the case goes to court.

Keep the Supervisor Informed

Policies pertaining to patients and personnel apply to nursing personnel in the operating room suite as well as to those on other units. It is very disconcerting to the OR supervisor to learn from someone outside the OR suite about events within the department that should have been communicated by the OR staff. For the safety and welfare of patients and the efficient management of the OR suite, the supervisor should learn what goes on in the department through the proper channels. Keep the supervisor informed of:

1 Any unexpected complication or change in the condition of the patient.
2 Any injury to a patient.
3 Any unusual incident, including infraction of policies or procedures by a surgeon, anesthesiologist, nurse, or technician. Every member of the OR team has both a moral and legal obligation to report a flagrant violation of accepted standards of patient care through appropriate administrative channels.
4 Complaints about any instruments, equipment, or other supplies.
5 Broken instruments and equipment.
6 Requests for equipment not available for change of procedure.
7 Criticism that can lead to friction between team members or departments. The supervisor will discuss problems concerning another nursing unit or hospital department with the respective supervisor.
8 Any other problems that might impair efficiency within the department or leave the supervisor open to criticism if not informed about them. Seek advice and discuss minor problems before they develop into major incidents.

PATIENT SAFETY PROGRAMS

Patient safety refers to a systematic, hospital-wide program designed to minimize preventable iatrogenic physical injuries, accidents, and undue psychological stress during hospitalization. Focus is on human behavior; what people are supposed to do and what they actually do. For example, whether or not a nurse or techncian is responsible for an injury to a patient due to defective equipment might depend upon whether or not the defect was noticeable and remained unrepaired when the equipment was used. Could the injury have been prevented by foresight, alertness, and good judgment? Potential hazards can be identified and eliminated, thereby reducing risks to patients.

Standards of Care

Standards provide a basic model to measure the quality of patient care. They are broad in scope, relevant, attainable, and definitive. Standards enunciate for both the practitioner and the consumer/public what the quality of health care should be. They are the criteria used in evaluating the quality of patient care rendered. Those established by national associations and agencies are recognized norms in most courts of law. For operating room nursing practice, these include:

1 *Standards of Nursing Practice: Operating Room*,* which are based on the nursing process, utilizing principles and theories of biophysical and behavioral sciences

*Association of Operating Room Nurses, Inc., and American Nurses' Association Division on Medical-Surgical Nursing Practice, *Standards of Nursing Practice: Operating Room,* Kansas City: American Nurses' Association, 1975.

2 *Standards of Technical and Aseptic Practice for the Operating Room,** which are based on principles of microbiology and validated research, and are directed toward providing a safe environment for the patient in the OR suite

3 Joint Commission on Accreditation of Hospitals (JCAH) standards,† which are the fundamental criteria used as the basis for hospital accreditation

4 Standards, guidelines, and regulations of other agencies, such as the National Fire Protection Association (NFPA), which are utilized for environmental and patient safety

5 Standards and controls established by the Food and Drug Administration (FDA) through the federal medical device legislation, which regulate the manufacture, sale, and use of many implantable medical devices

NOTE. The label, manufacturer's lot number, and product description of implanted devices should be attached to or included in the patient's chart, whenever feasible. If technique of implantation is inadequate, according to the manufacturer's instructions for use as approved by FDA, the surgeon is liable. If the device fails, the manufacturer is liable.

Policies and Procedures

Hospital policies and procedures are established as a protection for employees and learners as well as for patients. You can protect yourself by conscientious effort and meticulous attention to learning, knowing, and following hospital policies and procedures. These vary from one hospital to another, but all are established for patient safety in that specific physical facility. Particular attention is given to policies and procedures pertaining to potentially litigious duties. Some of these are repeated here for emphasis because of the potential legal implications.

Identification of the Patient When a patient enters the hospital, an identification wristband is put on in the admitting office before the patient goes to the unit. The unit nurse and OR nursing assistant check the label on the identification wristband before the patient leaves the unit. The circulating nurse and anesthesiologist always check the label with the patient and surgeon, the patient's chart, and the operating schedule. The surgeon sees the patient before anesthetic agents are administered.

*Established by AORN, Inc., and published in issues of *AORN Journal* during 1975 and 1976.

†*Accreditation Manual for Hospitals,* Chicago: JCAH, 1976.

Protection of Personal Property Generally, it is the responsibility of unit personnel to remove valuables and prostheses before the patient leaves the unit for the OR suite. It is the circulating nurse's responsibility to double-check the patient for contact lenses or eyeglasses, dentures, artificial extremity or glass eye, wig, wristwatch, rings, or religious medals. Besides the danger of losing these items, some of them constitute a hazard for the anesthetized patient.

The most frequently overlooked item on the unit seems to be dentures. These or any other item should be placed in a rigid container and labeled with the patient's name, hospital number, and room number. They should never be wrapped in a paper or linen towel, which could inadvertently be discarded in the trash or laundry hamper. The circulating nurse should immediately ask a nursing assistant to return the container to the unit. This person should obtain a receipt for the patient's personal property from the person receiving it. The receipt is given to the circulating nurse to put in the patient's chart along with a notation of the transaction in the nurses' notes.

Patients place a value on any of their property. Personnel and hospitals are liable for the care of it. A nurse can be held liable for loss of or damage to a patient's personal property.

Observation of the Patient Unattended patients may fall from a stretcher or the operating table. Falls are one of the most frequent causes of avoidable injuries. Siderails and restraint straps must be used to protect patients, especially children, disoriented or sedated adults. Observe special care when moving all patients to and from the operating table.

A child or disoriented patient left alone or unguarded may sustain injury by an electric shock from a nearby outlet, or by other hazard within reach. *Abandonment* may be a cause for a lawsuit.

Since many patients in the OR receive a general anesthetic and therefore are unconscious, constant vigilance is essential to safeguard patients unable to protect themselves. If a patient receives an injury while unconscious, such as a brachial nerve palsy from hyperextension of an arm on the armboard, negligence on the part of one or all team members may have to be disproved in court. Liability on someone's part would be difficult to dispute.

Dedication to Meticulous Technique Infection is a serious postoperative complication that may become life-threatening for the patient. OR team members must know and apply the principles of aseptic and sterile techniques at all times. An emergency situation in which asepsis becomes a secondary concern is a rare occurrence.

Postoperative wound infection can originate in the OR from a break in technique by a team member, from airborne contaminants of improperly cleaned floors, furniture, and ventilating systems, or from inadequately sterilized instruments and supplies. Reuse of disposable items is indefensible, as is use of a disinfected endoscope introduced into a body cavity or organ through an incision in tissues. Always carry out strict asepsis yourself and be alert to technique of other team members. Remember the principle: when in doubt about sterility, consider unsterile.

Execution of Accurate Counts Sponges left in wounds after closure are the most frequent cause for lawsuits following operations. A piece of a broken needle or a whole needle is more frequently left in the patient than an instrument; however, instruments have been left in also. The responsibility for accounting for all sponges, needles, and instruments, *before operation and at the time of closure,* rests with the circulating and scrub nurses. The surgeon and assistant take the field count before closure. If they have done their part in the count procedure, and a sponge is left in the wound because of a miscount by the circulating nurse, this nurse may be held solely responsible. In such a case the surgeon, hospital, and scrub nurse may be exonerated. Likewise the scrub nurse may be deemed responsible for an incorrect needle or instrument count. Because exemplary hospitals recognize sponge, needle, and instrument counts to be essential to safe practice, an OR team that omits counts, and a hospital that has not established counting procedures would be in a difficult legal position. The circulating nurse should document in writing the outcome of the final counts and any unusual incidents concerning them.

Instruction for Use of Equipment All equipment and appliances must be set up and used according to the recommendations and instructions of the manufacturer. Electrical equipment also must pass inspection of the hospital engineers. Exercise due caution in carrying out procedures for the use of equipment in areas of explosive or combustible agents. Electrical equipment must be properly grounded to prevent electric shock and burns.

Prevention of Burns Burns are one of the most frequent causes of lawsuits. A burn may occur from the use of a hot instrument such as a mouth gag or a large retractor. The scrub nurse should immerse a hot instrument in a basin of cool sterile water before handing it to the surgeon.

A patient may be burned during use of the electrosurgical unit. Inadequate skin contact or improper placement of the grounding pad or plate can cause an electrical burn. Alcohol and other flammable solutions can be ignited if pooled under the patient or allowed to saturate drapes. A thermal burn also can occur from other types of electrical equipment if improperly used or maintained.

Administration of Drugs Any drug that the surgeon uses in the operative site, such as an antibiotic or local anesthetic, is recorded by the circulating nurse and by the surgeon in the operative note. The drug is checked by two nurses, or the circulating nurse with the anesthesiologist or surgeon if a technician is scrubbed, before it is transferred to the sterile field. The scrub nurse (or technician) repeats the name of the drug to the surgeon when passing it. The surgeon is not held responsible if he or she is handed the wrong drug. The scrub nurse frequently has more than one drug on the instrument table. Each must be correctly identified and administered.

Preparation of Specimens All tissue removed from a patient is sent to pathology, with very few exceptions. The loss of a tissue biopsy could mean the possibility of a second operative procedure to obtain another. Specimens labeled incorrectly could mean a mistaken diagnosis, with possible critical implications for two patients. Also, the loss of a specimen could prevent determination of a diagnosis and subsequent initiation of definitive therapy. The pathological report becomes part of the patient's chart as an added record of the tissue removed and of the diagnosis.

Care for foreign bodies according to hospital policy. They may have legal significance and frequently are claimed by police, especially if the foreign body is a bullet. A receipt from the person taking them protects personnel and the hospital.

Patient Teaching

The patient and family members expect to be informed about the illness or condition and how to deal with it to restore or maintain optimum health. The patient has the right to make decisions about his or her own care. The OR nurse can assist, however, through preoperative teaching of deep-breathing exercises, for example, which will help the patient's postoperative recovery. Information should be provided so the patient knows how to respond appropriately. Patient teaching should be documented in the chart.

Audits

Quality assurance has been defined as the establishment of the degree of excellence in practice that constitutes quality, and the assurance that the consumer receives this level of care. The 1972 amendment to the federal Social Security Act creating the Professional Standard Review Organization (PSRO) for medical audits and utilization review in hospitals receiving federal reimbursement, followed by the JCAH requirements for auditing patient care, mandated the initiation of quality assurance programs in all hospitals. An *audit* is a program designed to measure the care received by patients as judged by professional standards. The purpose is to identify both strengths and weaknesses of policies and procedures, and ultimately to correct deficiencies or deviations from accepted standards. The focus is on the patient care *process* and the *outcome* of care.

A *process audit* focuses on a systematic series of actions that brings about an outcome. The major components of the nursing process are assessing, planning, implementing, and evaluating patient care. Through observation, a process audit determines whether or not the actions taken are consistent with the established standards for care in a given setting such as the operating room. This usually includes evaluation of the environment as well as of the care rendered. Operating room nursing care is usually evaluated through process audit.

An *outcome audit* focuses on the end result of nursing care or a measurable change in the actual state of the patient's health as a result of care received. This audit usually is done retrospectively through review of patient records. Unless every detail of nursing care is documented, an outcome audit may not reflect the actual care given in the OR, except when complications attributable to intraoperative care occur, for example, postoperative infection, nerve palsy from poor positioning, infiltration of an IV, and other complications. These may be difficult to identify unless unusual occurrences are recorded in the patient's record. Accurate and complete documentation is essential for meaningful outcome audits.

Any method that systematically examines the quality of nursing care can be termed a nursing audit. The audit must enable nurses to evaluate in an objective way the patient care they provide and to take corrective action for improvement of practice patterns on the basis of documented findings. The audit focuses on specific diagnoses and nursing tasks associated with their specific nursing problems rather than on broad, general nursing measures that apply to any patient. Preprinted audit forms used in the OR evaluate:

1 The written nursing care plan and note recorded on the patient's chart after the preoperative visit
2 Actions taken to protect the welfare and safety of the patient and to meet the identified physiological and psychological needs
3 The environment of the room used in the OR suite, including equipment and supplies
4 Records pertaining to the procedure
5 Personnel involved in care rendered

Audits encourage nurses and surgeons to coordinate their plans for patient care, improve their communications with other departments, identify needs for revision of policies and procedures, and reassess equipment, personnel, and other aspects of patient care.

EMPLOYEE SAFETY PROGRAMS

Orders, Judgment, and Appropriate Action

It is imperative that physicians' orders are understood and evaluated in relation to the patient's condition at the time of execution. If you do not understand an order, find out what is required of you before carrying it out. Always observe the patient closely and, if a change in condition is seen, report it at once to the surgeon, anesthesiologist, or supervisor. Do not carry out an order without checking or questioning it if in your judgment it is not in the best interests of the patient. If a patient shows an adverse reaction to a medication, report this at once. You can be held liable for not reporting a patient's symptoms, since they may indicate the need for special medication or treatment.

Do not assume responsibility for tasks or duties you have not been instructed or prepared to perform. For example, the circulating nurse can refuse an anesthesiologist's request to pump the reservoir bag in the ventilating system of the anesthesia machine, or to recover a patient postoperatively. Report requests outside of your written job description to your supervisor. Your professional and legal responsibilities as well as the patient's rights dictate this course of action. The patient entrusts his or her life to others when undergoing surgical intervention. Nursing personnel must act as patient advocates when patients' rights are compromised.

Peer Review

The development of review mechanisms used for peer assessment of performance are designed to evaluate the quality and quantity of care patients receive. Peer review differs from patient care audit in that it looks at the strengths and weaknesses of an individual practitioner's performance rather than appraising the quality of care rendered by a group of professionals to a group of patients.

Peer review for OR nurses has been defined as the ongoing process whereby registered nurses with the same role expectations and job descriptions examine the nursing care provided by other individual nurse practitioners in the OR setting. The review should offer constructive criticism of the performance observed. Broad categories of tasks examined in the review should include those concerned with:

1 Patient's physiological and psychosocial needs. Are nursing actions directed toward meeting these needs?

2 Accountability and responsibility for own actions in relation to self, patient, hospital, team members, and profession.

3 Skills utilizing knowledge in application of technical, interpersonal, teaching, leadership, and communication principles.

4 Personal attributes the nurse possesses that affect professional relationships with patients.

Safe Working Conditions

The Occupational Safety and Health Act (OSHA) became public law in 1970. The major purpose of OSHA is to assure safe and healthful working conditions for working men and women. Although explicitly designed to protect employees rather than patients, patients do receive secondary benefits from the regulations. Reducing the frequency of work-related injuries and illnesses and making hospitals as safe as possible benefit both patients and personnel. Some of the OSHA regulations require:

1 Minimizing exposure to ionizing radiation

2 Safeguarding exposure from instruments that emit sound or radio waves, visible light, infrared, ultraviolet, and nonionizing electromagnetic radiation

3 Meeting standards of approved electrical codes

4 Installing ventilating systems that maintain no more than maximum allowable concentrations of atmospheric contamination from toxic and flammable chemical vapors

5 Initiating procedures for safe use, handling, storage, and dispensing of flammable and combustible liquids

6 Monitoring procedures for infection control

The OR suite is one of the most critical areas of the hospital, if not the most critical, as it relates to safety control. Obvious hazards to the physical well-being of any employee should be brought to the attention of the supervisor. If the employer fails to correct a condition an employee believes to be a violation of a safety or health standard, a threat of physical harm, or an imminent danger, the employee may request an inspection by an OSHA compliance officer.

Inservice Education

Orientation of all new employees and regularly scheduled, ongoing, inservice educational programs are necessary to keep the nursing staff informed of policies, procedures, new techniques, and nursing care practices. If the process audits indicate deficiencies in nursing care because of lack of knowledge about a specific group of patients, corrective action must be taken to improve performance. Audits and peer review provide specific direction for educational programs. Deficiencies in hospital policies and procedures also should be reviewed by the staff and recommendations made to revise them as necessary.

Formally organized programs of environmental safety should be included in general orientation and inservice education. Personnel must be aware of specific job hazards, and familiar with occupational safety and health programs.

Continuing Education

Professional nurses and OR technicians have a personal responsibility for continued learning through reading and attending workshops, seminars, conferences, and other educational offerings. Education never ends with basic training. Continued learning helps the practitioner keep abreast of current trends and practices. Evidence of continuing education is mandatory in some states for renewal of RN licensure. Technicians must have evidence of continuing education for certification maintenance. Although continuing education is not a measurement for proven competence in practice, it is the most widely accepted method of self-development. Moreover, it helps maintain and update theoretical knowledge as a basis for sound practice and judgment.

Insurance

Liability of hospitals and individuals varies according to state laws and statues. It is advisable to find out your own liability and that of your employer, and to protect yourself as necessary in your place of employment.

Since any patient can sue any nurse or technician, the cost of defense may be more than you can afford even if you are not found guilty. As protection against possible financial loss from malpractice claims, nurses and technicians should have their own insurance policies. An employee may be sued individually or, if the employer has to pay damages, the hospital's insurance company may seek restitution. When insured by the employer, an employee should have a certificate of insurance from the hospital. The hospital policy protects the employee on the job only. Nurses and technicians also should have a policy that protects them off the job.

Nurses involved in new procedures and techniques, as in teaching hospitals, are especially vulnerable to lawsuits. The hospital's insurance carrier may provide basic coverage, but hold individual employees named in a lawsuit liable for amounts that exceed this coverage.

Bibliography

The references included in the bibliography represent the most recent and relevant content when the manuscript was written. Medical technology and research change rapidly. References in the bibliography are cited in the form adopted by the National Library of Medicine for its indexes including the official abbreviations for periodicals.

MULTIPLE SOURCES—BOOKS

American Cancer Society: *1977 Cancer Facts and Figures,* New York: 1976 (Annual publication).

American College of Surgeons, Committee on Control of Surgical Infections: *Manual on Control of Infection in Surgical Patients,* Philadelphia: Lippincott, 1976.

Association of Operating Room Nurses and American Nurses' Association Division on Medical-Surgical Nursing Practice: *Standards of Nursing Practice: Operating Room,* Kansas City, Mo.: American Nurses' Association, 1975.

Ballinger WF et al: Alexander's Care of the Patient in Surgery, 5th ed, St. Louis: Mosby, 1972.

Brunner LS, Suddarth DS: *Textbook of Medical-Surgical Nursing,* 3d ed, Philadelphia: Lippincott, 1975.

Clemente CD: *Anatomy: A Regional Atlas of the Human Body,* Philadelphia: Lea & Febiger, 1975.

Ethicon, Inc.: *Nursing Care of the Patient in the O.R.,* Somerville, N.J.: 1975.

Ethicon, Inc.: *Suture Use Manual: Use and Handling of Sutures and Needles,* Somerville, N.J.: 1977.

Gardner E et al: *Anatomy: A Regional Study of Human Structure,* 4th ed, Philadelphia: Saunders, 1975.

Gruendemann BJ et al: *The Surgical Patient: Behavioral Concepts for the Operating Room Nurse,* 2d ed, St. Louis: Mosby, 1977.

Hardy JD (ed): *Rhoads Textbook of Surgery: Principles and Practice,* 5th ed, Philadelphia: Lippincott, 1977.

Hoeller ML: *Surgical Technology: Basis for Clinical Practice,* 3d ed, St. Louis: Mosby, 1974.

Joint Commission on Accreditation of Hospitals: *Accreditation Manual for Hospitals,* Chicago: 1976.

LeMaitre GD, Finnegan JA: *The Patient in Surgery: A Guide for Nurses,* 3d ed, Philadelphia: Saunders, 1975.

McWilliams RM et al, comps.: *Every OR Supervisor Should Know,* Denver: The Association of Operating Room Nurses, Inc., 1974.

National Fire Protection Association: *Nonflammable Medical Gas Systems,* (NFPA No. 56F), Boston: 1974.

National Fire Protection Association: *Safe Use of High-Frequency Electricity in Health Care Facilities,* (NFPA No. 76C), Boston: 1975.

National Fire Protection Association: *Standard for the Use of Inhalation Anesthetics,* (NFPA No. 56A), Boston: 1973.

Schoenrock DF, Kneedler JA: *Operating Room Orientation Program for the New Graduate Nurse,* Denver: The Association of Operating Room Nurses, Inc., 1974.

Shafer K et al: *Medical-Surgical Nursing,* 6th ed, St. Louis: Mosby, 1975.

MULTIPLE SOURCES—JOURNALS

AORN Standards for OR sanitation, AORN J 21(7): 1228–1231, June 1975.

AORN Standards: OR wearing apparel, draping and gowning materials, AORN J 21(4):594–596, 598, Mar 1975.

Barratt-Boyes BG et al: Repair of ventricular septal defect in the first two years of life using profound hypothermia-circulatory arrest techniques, Ann Surg 184(3):376–390, Sep 1976.

Beck WC: Editorial: Barrier standards are statements of principle, AORN J 21(6):983–984, May 1975.

Caruthers B: Lumbar discectomy, OR Tech 8(2):24, 26–28, 39, Mar–Apr 1976.

Castle M: Isolation: Precise procedure for better protection, Nursing (Jenkintown) 5(5):50–57, May 1975.

Day JL, Lightfoot DA: OR radiation hazards, AORN J 20(2):249–256, Aug 1974.

Driscoll J: Establishing, implementing, and enforcing OR policies, AORN J 21(6):1031–1037, May 1975.

Fee NF et al: Gas gangrene complicating open forearm fractures, J Bone Joint Surg [Am] 59(1):135–138, Jan 1977.

Lawson BN: A nurse's guide to electro-surgery, AORN J 25(2):314–329, Feb 1977.

Mallison GF: Housekeeping in operating suites, AORN J 21(2):213–220, Feb 1975.

Marcinek MB: Stress in the surgical patient, Am J Nurs 77(11):1809–1811, Nov 1977.

Meakins JL: Body's response to infection, AORN J 22(1):37–44, July 1975.

Mehaffy NL: Rationale for asepsis standards, AORN J 21(7):1213–1216, June 1975.

Nora PF: OR environment: a surgeon's view, AORN J 24(2):266–267, 270–271, Aug 1976.

Oliver JD: Staff needs considered in OR design, AORN J 22(2):212–217, Feb 1976.

Pratt ML: Blood bank's link to OR, AORN J 25(6): 1058–1068, May 1977.

Scott HW Jr et al: Surgical experience with Cushing's disease, Ann Surg 185(5):524–534, May 1977.

Symposium on Perspectives in Operating Room Nursing (M.G. Nolan, Guest Editor): Nurs Clin North Am 10(4):613–686, Dec 1975.

Yablon IG, Paul GR: The augmentive use of methyl methacrylate in the management of pathologic fractures, Surg Gynecol Obstet 143(2):177–183, Aug 1976.

CHAPTER 1
INTRODUCTION FOR THE LEARNER

American Medical Association Council on Medical Education: *Essentials of an Approved Educational Program for the Operating Room Technician,* Chicago: American Medical Association, 1972.

American Nurses' Association: *Educational Preparation for Nurse Practitioners and Assistants to Nurses,* A position paper, New York: 1965.

AORN Statement Committee: Definition and objective for clinical practice of professional operating room nursing, AORN J 10(5):43–48, Nov 1969.

Ernst CB: Surgery, the abused word, Surg Gynecol Obstet 140(4):608, Apr 1975.

Essentials of an approved educational program for the surgeon's assistant, Bull Am Coll Surg 58(8):58–61, Aug 1973.

Fagin C et al: Can we bring order out of the chaos of nursing education? Am J Nurs 76(1):98–107, Jan 1976.

Horoshak I: Outpatient surgery: R.N. grows with the field, RN 38(7): 47, 50, 52–56, July 1975.

Lindbergh AM: *Hour of Gold, Hour of Lead: Diaries and Letters of Anne Morrow Lindbergh 1929–1932,* New York: Harcourt Brace Jovanovich, 1973.

Nolan MG: O.R. clinical experience: Catalyst for student learning, Nurs Outlook 24(6):378–383, June 1976.

Nolan MG: Potentials in OR nursing, AORN J 23(4): 583–590, Mar 1976.

NSNA Resolution: Active student participation in the operating suite, AORN J 20(1):12, July 1974.

CHAPTER 2
THE HEALTH CARE TEAM

American College of Surgeons: Statement on qualifications for surgical privileges in approved hospitals, Bull Am Coll Surg 62(4):12–13, Apr 1977.

American College of Surgeons: Statements on principles, Nov 1, 1974, Bull Am Coll Surg 60(1):7–12, Jan 1975.

ANA clarifies practitioner definitions, AORN J 20(5): 878, Nov 1974.

Bicknell J: Introducing surgical assistants, Point View 13(2):16–17, Apr 1, 1976.

Creighton H: OR nurse as first assistant, Supv Nurs 8(7):82–83, July 1977.

Davis JE: Why a mandate for the circulator? AORN J 23(7):1185–1193, June 1976.

George AM: Editorial: Communication to PRR nurses means better care, AORN J 21(2):201–202, Feb 1975.

Kroner JA: OR/PAR cooperation for better patient care, AORN J 23(2):181–182, Feb 1976.

MacPhail, JL: A plea for the professional nurse in the OR, AORN J 19(4):872–873, 876, Apr 1974.

McWilliams RM et al: The experts research: Q&A: What constitutes a major or minor surgical case? AORN J 21(7):1241–1242, June 1975.

Morgan ME: Surgical nurse clinical specialist, AORN J 23(4):638, 640, 642, 644, Mar 1976.

Morris CR, Deen JR: Hospital provides rules for assistants' privileges, Hospitals 49(19):56–57, Oct 1, 1975.

Schrader ES: The clinical nurse specialist in the OR, AORN J 23(4):571-582, Mar 1976.

Surgical Team Forum: Are OR technicians qualified to circulate? Surg Team 5(1):14-19, Jan-Feb 1976.

Thur MP: OR/Pharmacy drug quality assurance, AORN J 23(4):624-628, Mar 1976.

CHAPTER 3 THE PATIENT: THE REASON FOR YOUR EXISTENCE

Alexander C et al: Preoperative visits: The OR nurse unmasks, AORN J 19(2):401-412, Feb 1974.

American College of Surgeons: College issues statement on unnecessary surgery, Bull Am Coll Surg 61(5):3, May 1976.

American Nurses' Association: *Standards of Medical-Surgical Nursing Practice,* Kansas City, Mo.: 1974.

AORN Statement Committee: The first steps are crucial, AORN J 12(1):43-50, July 1970.

Barnett LA: Preparing your patient for the operating room, AORN J 18(3):534-539, Sep 1973.

Beard JM: What is your attitude saying? AORN J 24(4): 782, 784, 786, 788, Oct 1976.

Beletz EE, Covo GA: The case of the hidden infections in the elderly, Nursing (Jenkintown) 6(8):14-16, Aug 1976.

Bill of rights for patients, Nurs Outlook 21(2):82, Feb 1973.

Bray GA et al: Evaluation of the obese patient, JAMA 235(14):1487-1491, Apr 5, 1976.

Cahall JB, Smith D: Considerate care of the elderly, Nursing (Jenkintown) 5(9):38-39, Sep 1975.

Conway A, Williams T: Care of the critically ill newborn: parenteral alimentation, Am J Nurs 76(4): 574-577, Apr 1976.

Cook ET: *The Life of Florence Nightingale,* vol 2, London: Macmillan, 1913.

Damsteegt D: Pastoral roles in presurgical visits, Am J Nurs 75(8):1336-1337, Aug 1975.

Dobbie RP, Hoffmeister JA: Continuous pump-tube enteric hyperalimentation, Surg Gynecol Obstet 143(2):273-276, Aug 1976.

Englert DM, Dudrick SJ: Principles of intravenous hyperalimentation, AORN J 25(7):1253-1267, June 1977.

Galton L: Drugs and the elderly, Nursing (Jenkintown) 6(8):38-43, Aug 1976.

Gordon M: Nursing diagnoses and the diagnostic process, Am J Nurs 76(8):1298-1300, Aug 1976.

Grant MM, Kubo WM: Assessing a patient's hydration status, Am J Nurs 75(8):1306-1311, Aug 1975.

Irion F: The mourning of the caring professional, Point View 13(2):8-9, Apr 1, 1976.

Kaminski MV Jr: Hyperalimentation: Who what and why, Surg Team 5(3):22-25, 29, 32-33, June 1976.

Kaminski MV Jr, Burke WA: Parenteral hyperalimentation: Prevention and treatment of complications part II, Surg Team 6(1):30-36, Feb 1977.

Kuenzi SH, Fenton MV: Crisis intervention in acute care areas, Am J Nurs 75(5):830-834, May 1975.

The law of informed consent, Bull Am Coll Surg 59(5): 21-27, May 1974.

Little DE, Carnevali DL: *Nursing Care Planning,* 2d ed, Philadelphia: Lippincott, 1976.

McBeath AA: Counseling in elective operations, Surg Gynecol Obstet 143(2):270, Aug 1976.

McCloskey JC: How to make the most of body image theory in nursing practice, Nursing (Jenkintown) 6(5):68-72, May 1976.

McWilliams RM: The balance of caring, AORN J 24(2): 314, 316-317, 320 passim, Aug 1976.

Meisel A: Informed consent—the rebuttal, JAMA 234(6):615, Nov 10, 1975.

Moser RH: Ruminations: People aren't diseases, JAMA 233(1):62, July 7, 1975.

Munn HE Jr: Are you a skilled listener? AORN J 25(5): 994, 996, 998, 1000, Apr 1977.

Murray R, Zentner J: Guidelines for more effective health teaching, Nursing (Jenkintown) 6(2):44-53, Feb 1976.

Nick WV: Informed consent—the new decisions, Bull Am Coll Surg 59(5):12-14, May 1974.

Nightingale F: *Notes on Nursing: What It Is, and What It Is Not,* London: Harrison, 1860.

Nolan MG: The consumer's view of the O.R. nurse, Point View 12(2):15-17, Mar 1, 1975.

Richards F: Do you care for or care about? AORN J 22(5):792, 794, 796, 798, Nov 1975.

Ridgeway M: Preop interviews assure quality care, AORN J 24(6):1083-1085, Dec 1976.

Riella MC, Scribner BH: Five years' experience with a right atrial catheter for prolonged parenteral nutrition at home, Surg Gynecol Obstet 143(2):205-208, Aug 1976.

Saylor DE: Understanding presurgical anxiety, AORN J 22(4):624, 626, 628, 630, 632, 634, 636, Oct 1975.

Schoenberg DH: Informed consent—the rejoinder, JAMA 234(6):616, Nov 10, 1975.

Snyder JC, Wilson MF: Elements of a psychological assessment, Am J Nurs 77(2):235-239, Feb 1977.

Starr BB, Goldstein H: *Human Development and Behavior Psychology in Nursing,* New York: Springer, 1975.

Surgical progress reported at ACS Congress: Nutrition in the surgical patient, AORN J 21(1):37-38, 43, Jan 1975.

Wells RW: Body image and surgical alterations, AORN J 21(5):812-815, Apr 1975.

CHAPTER 4 ASEPSIS AND PRINCIPLES OF STERILE TECHNIQUE

American College of Surgeons Panel, Laufman H, Moderator: *How Can We Improve the O.R. Environment?* Chicago: American College of Surgeons, 1972 (Clinitape).

Anderson CB et al: Anaerobic infections in surgery: Clinical review, Surgery 79(3):313-324, Mar 1976.

Bernard HR, Beck WC: Operating room barriers—idealism, practicality, and the future, Bull Am Coll Surg 60(9):16, Sep 1975.

Burke J: Pinpointing the critical hours in wound sepsis: Timing is the key to preoperative antibiotics use, Surg Team 5(1):30, Feb 1976.

Burrows W: *Textbook of Microbiology,* 20th ed, Philadelphia: Saunders, 1973.

Carson DR: The role of the hospital administrator in implementing and monitoring an infection control program, Hosp Top 53(4):24, 41, 46, July-Aug 1975.

Castle M: Help stamp out infections: Be an infection-control coordinator, Nursing (Jenkintown) 6(9):90, 92, 95, Sep 1976.

Clark RE et al: Infection control in cardiac surgery, Surgery 79(1):89-96, Jan 1976.

Clemons B: Lister's day in America, AORN J 24(1): 43-51, July 1976.

Crawford ML: Surgical instruments in America, AORN J 24(1):150, 152-154, 156, July 1976.

Curti JF: Antibiotics and gram-negative bacteremia, JAMA 231(13):1361-1363, Mar 31, 1975.

Dineen P: Personnel, discipline, and infection, Arch Surg 107(4):603-604, Oct 1973.

DiPalma JR: The ubiquitous anaerobe: Cause for concern in OBG, RN 38(12):61-62, 65, Dec 1975.

Drake CT et al: Environmental air and airborne infections, Ann Surg 185(2):219-223, Feb 1977.

Eickhoff TC: Nosocomial infections, Am J Epidemiol 101(2):93-97, Feb 1975.

Fitzwater J: Nursing protocols for reducing sepsis rates in cancer patients, Surg Team 5(3):34-43, June 1976.

Gardner P, Provine, HT: *Manual of Acute Bacterial Infections,* Boston: Little, Brown, 1975.

Garner JS: Nurse epidemiologist instrumental in infection control, AORN J 20(2):261-262, 264, 266, 268, 270, 274-275, Aug 1974.

Hughes GB et al: Staphylococci in community acquired infections: Increased resistance to penicillin, Ann Surg 183(4):355-357, Apr 1976.

Hunt TK et al: Antibiotics in surgery, Arch Surg 110(2): 148-155, Feb 1975.

Huth ME: Principles of asepsis, AORN J 24(4):790, 792-793, 796, Oct 1976.

Kaslow RA et al: Nosocomial pseudo-bacteremia: Positive blood cultures due to contaminated benzalkonium antiseptic, JAMA 236(21):2407-2409, Nov 22, 1976.

Laufman H: Letter: Operating room infection control, Surgery 79(6):726-727, June 1976.

Laufman H: Surgical infection control: Basic definitions and current status, J Surg Practice 7(2):60-64, Apr 1978.

Leveen HH et al: Effects of prophylactic antibiotics on colonic healing, Am J Surg 131(1):47-53, Jan 1976.

MacClelland DC: The evolution of sterilization, AORN J 24(1):37-41, July 1976.

MacClelland DC: Laminar air unit: Achiever or appeaser? AORN J 23(5):766-771, Apr 1976.

Marino AWM Jr et al: Wound infection: Methods of prevention in colon and rectal surgery, Point View 12(3):3-5, May 1, 1975.

Nelson JP: Effectiveness, costs of clean rooms, helmet aspirators, AORN J 27(4):718, 720, 722, 724, 726, 728, 730, 732, 734, Mar 1978.

O'Brien TF et al: Computer surveillance of shifts in the gross patient flora during hospitalization, J Infec Dis 131(2):88-96, Feb 1975.

Phanauf MC: Model for quality: A matrix, AORN J 23(5):759-765, Apr 1976.

Schrader ES: ACS Clinical Congress reports: From design to evaluation of OR suite, AORN J 23(1):110-117, Jan 1976.

Schrader ES: The Center for Disease Control, AORN J 24(2):333-334, 336, 338 passim, Aug 1976.

Schrader ES: Editorial: What price asepsis? AORN J 25(1):136-142, Jan 1977.

Schultz J et al: The experts research: Q&A: Does routine sampling have a purpose in the operating room? AORN J 26(1):143, July 1977.

Standards of administrative nursing practice: Operating room, AORN J 23(7):1202-1208, June 1976.

Stone HH et al: Antibiotic prophylaxis in gastric, biliary and colonic surgery, Ann Surg 184(4):443-452, Oct 1976.

Vidt DG: Use and abuse of intravenous solutions, JAMA 232(5):533-536, May 5, 1975.

Walter CW: Role of bacteriologic survey cultures in control of nosocomial infection, JAMA 229(5):578-579, July 29, 1974.

Walter CW, Kundsin R: The airborne component of wound contamination and infection, Arch Surg 107(4):588-595, Oct 1973.

CHAPTER 5
STERILIZATION AND DISINFECTION

Association for the Advancement of Medical Instrumentation, Subcommittee on Ethylene Oxide Sterilization: *Recommendation for Proper Use of Ethylene Oxide Sterilization in Hospitals and other Medical Facilities,* Arlington, Va.: 1976.

Beck WC: Editorial: Abridged sterility—a level of disinfection, AORN J 26(2):242, 244, Aug 1977.

Boger W: A better understanding of ethylene oxide sterilization, Hosp Top 54(5):12, 14-16, Sep-Oct 1976.

Brown RS: A disinfectant label: What it means, OR Tech 6(2):8-9, Mar-Apr 1974.

Halleck FE: Hazards of EO sterilization in hospitals, Hosp Top 53(6):45-52, Nov-Dec 1975.

Halleck FE: Packaging materials for EO gas sterilization, AORN J 21(1):104, 106-108, 110-114, 116-118, Jan 1975.

Litsky BY: Microbiology of sterilization, AORN J 26(2):334, 337, 339-340, 342, 344, 346, 348, 350, Aug 1977.

Litsky BY, Litsky W: Thermocouple-pyrometer data for evaluating inhospital packaging material, AORN J 23(7):1175–1176, June 1976.

Mabbett AN, Flynn MM: Infection control: A self evaluation, Hosp Top 53(6):29–34, Nov–Dec 1975.

Mallison GF, Standard PG: Safe storage times for sterile packs, Hospitals 48(20):77–80, Oct 16, 1974.

Owins R: Ultraviolet radiation in the O.R., Point View 8(7):14–15, 1971.

Perkins JJ: *Principles and Methods of Sterilization in Health Sciences,* 2d ed, Springfield, Ill.: Thomas, 1969.

Revised guidelines for EO (ethylene oxide) sterilization, AORN J 24(6):1086–1088, Dec 1976.

Roberts RB: y-Rays + PVC + EO = OK, Respir Care 21(3):223–224, Mar 1976.

Ryan P: Basics of packaging, AORN J 21(7):1091–1092, 1094, 1096, 1098, 1100, 1102, 1104–1108, 1110, 1112, May 1975.

Ryan P: Inhospital packaging rationale, AORN J 23(6): 980–988, May 1976.

Schultz, J et al: The experts research: Back to basics steam sterilization, AORN J 25(1):67–68, Jan 1977.

Schultz J et al: The experts research: Q&A: Single-, double-wrapped packs vary in shelf life, AORN J 24(4):729–730, Oct 1976.

Spaulding EH: Uses and abuses of disinfectants, Hosp Top 52(5):7–8, 12–14, May 1974.

Standards for inhospital packaging material, AORN J 23(6):978–979, May 1976.

Walstrom P: Instrumentation, OR Tech, 6(6):23–25, Nov–Dec 1974.

Wisler MG: Guidelines for use of ethylene oxide, AORN J 19(6):1286–1287, 1290–1291, 1294–1295, June 1974.

CHAPTER 6
PHYSICAL FACILITIES

Anderson G: How others do it: Meridian Park Hospital uses new concepts for flexibility, Hosp Top 53(3): 41–43, May–June 1975.

Chvala C: OR supervisor's role in planning the surgical suite, AORN J 23(7):1238–1239, 1242–1243, 1246–1247, 1252, 1254, June 1976.

Fitzwater J: Preventing sepsis: Environmental factors, Surg Team 5(1):36–40, Feb 1976.

Friesen GA: Environmental control: Planning and design, AORN J 14(1):52–63, July 1971.

Laufman H, Rosenberg N: Television in the operating room, Surgery 78(3):273–275, Sep 1975.

Martin JT: An anesthesiologist looks at OR design, AORN J 21(2):259, 261, 264–265, 268–269, 272–273, 276, 278, Feb 1975.

Richmond LI: A closed case cart system, AORN J 19(1): 101–104, Jan 1974.

Rosenkoetter MM, Price DL: OR of the future: Implications for design, AORN J 24(2):241–245, Aug 1976.

CHAPTER 7
SURGICAL SCRUB, GOWNING AND GLOVING

Alford DJ et al: Your OR gown: Barrier or gateway for bacteria? RN 38(1):OR-12, Jan 1975.

Beck WC, Nora PF: ASTM standard for surgical gloves, AORN J 25(5):869–872, Apr 1977.

Dineen P, Drusin L: Epidemics of postoperative infections associated with hair carriers, Lancet 2(7839): 1157–1159, Nov 24, 1973.

Fried DA et al: The cotton gown as a barrier against contamination in the operating room, Am Surg 43(1): 52–54, Jan 1977.

Huth ME: Rationale for OR attire standards, AORN J 21(7):1217–1221, Jan 1975.

Jager, RM: Glove-starch granulomatous disease, JAMA 235(24):2583–2584, June 14, 1976.

Lee RM: Early operating room nursing, AORN J 24(1): 124, 126–128, 131–132, 134, 136, 138, July 1976.

McWilliams RM et al: The experts research: Q&A: Are lab coats acceptable to cover scrub attire? AORN J 23(2):177–178, Feb 1976.

McWilliams RM et al: The experts research: Q&A: Misuse of masks reduces effectiveness, AORN J 21(4): 691–692, Mar 1975.

Moylan JA et al: Intraoperative bacterial transmission, Surg Gynecol Obstet 141(5):731–733, Nov 1975.

National Nosocomial Infections Study Quarterly Report: *Methods for Prevention and Control of Nosocomial Infections,* Atlanta: Center for Disease Control, 1975.

Peterson AF et al: Comparative evaluation of surgical scrub preparations, Surg Gynecol Obstet 146(1):63–65, Jan 1978.

Schrader ES: From apron to gown: A history of OR attire, AORN J 24(1):52–67, July 1976.

Schultz J et al: The experts research: Q&A: Should masks be changed between cases? AORN J 25(4):763–764, Mar 1977.

Schultz J et al: The experts research: Q&A: Wet method preferred for preop shaves, AORN J 25(2):293, Feb 1977.

Standards for surgical hand scrubs, AORN J 23(6): 976–977, May 1976.

Tucci VJ et al: Studies of the surgical scrub, Surg Gynecol Obstet 145(3):415–416, Sep 1977.

White JJ, Duncan A: The comparative effectiveness of iodophor and hexachlorophene surgical scrub solutions, Surg Gynecol Obstet 135(6):890–892, Dec 1972.

CHAPTER 8
DIVISION OF DUTIES: SETUP, PROCEDURE, CLEANUP

Atkinson LJ et al: Blood loss replacement, Point View 14(1):18–19, Jan 1, 1977.

Autotransfusion: Dusting off an old technic, Surg Team 5(2):18–21, Apr 1976.

Beck WC: AORN technical standards guides to good practice, AORN J 24(4):650-651, Oct 1976.
Bonfils-Roberts EA et al: Autologous blood in the treatment of intraoperative hemorrhage, Ann Surg 185(3):321-325, Mar 1977.
Crooks LC: Aseptic technic—when, why and how, Point View 11(4):3-5, May 15, 1974.
Glover JL et al: Intraoperative autotransfusion: An underutilized technique, Surgery 80(4):474-479, Oct 1976.
Horoshak I: Autotransfusion: Promising alternative to donor blood, RN 38(5):33-40, May 1975.
Kent P: Intraoperative autotransfusion: Methodology and problems, Surg Team 5(2):29, 32-33, 38-41, Apr 1976.
Kneedler JA: Solution to the solutions used for OR decontamination, AORN J 24(2):329-330, Aug 1976.
Litsky BY: Microbiology and postoperative infections, AORN J 19(1):37-52, Jan 1974.
McWilliams RM et al: The experts research: Q&A: In OR, mop buckets, wringers dirty hazard, AORN J 23(7):1299-1300, June 1976.
McWilliams RM et al: The experts research: Q&A: Instrument count: Physician says no, nurses say yes, AORN J 23(4):565-566, Mar 1976.
Mehaffy NL: Implementing counts in the OR, AORN J 25(7):1275-1280, June 1977.
Peers JG: Cleanup techniques in the operating room, Arch Surg 107(4):596-599, Oct 1973.
Snider MA: Helpful hints on I.V.'s, Am J Nurs 74(11): 1978-1981, Nov 1974.
Standards for sponge, needle and instrument procedures, AORN J 23(6):971-973, May 1976.
Temes SP et al: A direct vasoconstriction effect of mannitol on the renal artery, Surg Gynecol Obstet 141(2):223-226, Aug 1975.
Ungvarski PJ: Parenteral therapy, Am J Nurs 76(12): 1974-1977, Dec 1976.
Wall W et al: Intraoperative autotransfusion in major elective vascular operations: A clinical assessment, Surgery 79(1):82-88, Jan 1976.
Weber DO et al: Influence of operating room surface contamination on surgical wounds, Arch Surg 111(4): 484-488, Apr 1976.
Wells P: "Confine and Contain" approach to OR cleanup, AORN J 25(1):60-65, Jan 1977.
Zett S: Safe handling and accountability, a routine procedure with sharps, OR Tech 6(6):12-13, Nov-Dec 1974.

CHAPTER 9
ANESTHESIA

Adams NR: Reducing the perils of intracardiac monitoring, Nursing (Jenkintown) 6(4):66-74, Apr 1976.
American Heart Association: *Advanced Cardiac Life Support,* Dallas: 1975.
American Society of Anesthesiologists: *Annual Refresher Course Lectures, 1975-1976,* Park Ridge, Ill.: 1975-1976.
Balasaraswathi K, El-Etr AA: Preop evaluation of drug history, AORN J 23(4):616, 618, 620, Mar 1976.
Barclay WR: Editorial: Adverse drug reactions and associated deaths, JAMA 236(6):592, Aug 9, 1976.
Beeson PB, McDermott W (eds): *Cecil-Loeb Textbook of Medicine,* 14th ed, Philadelphia: Saunders, 1975.
Betson C: The nurse's role in blood gas monitoring, Cardiovasc Nurs 7(6):83-86, Nov-Dec 1971.
Bruce DL, Bach MJ: Psychological studies of human performance as affected by traces of enflurane and nitrous oxide, Anesthesiology 42(2):194-205, Feb 1975.
Burrell LO, Burrell ZL: *Intensive Nursing Care,* 2d ed, St Louis: Mosby, 1973.
Collins VJ: *Principles of Anesthesiology,* 2d ed, Philadelphia: Lea & Febiger, 1976.
Corbett TH et al: Birth defects among children of nurse-anesthetists, Anesthesiology 41(4):341-344, Oct 1974.
Dahle JS: Caring for the patient with local anesthesia, AORN J 27(5):985, 986, 988, 990, Apr 1978.
Dougherty RD: Arterial blood gas interpretations, AORN J 20(4):669-670, 672, 674, 676, Oct 1974.
Dripps RD et al: *Introduction to Anesthesia: The Principles of Safe Practice,* 5th ed, Philadelphia: Saunders, 1977.
Dryden GE: Uncleaned anesthesia equipment, JAMA 233(12):1297-1299, Sep 22, 1975.
Electrical stimulation provides pain relief, AORN J 23(2):257, Jan 1976.
Etling T et al: Invasive monitoring of heart, circulation, AORN J 23(2):199-204, Feb 1976.
Extubation critical in endotracheal anesthesia: Abstracts, AORN J 25(6):1204, May 1977.
Floyd CC: Drugs for childbirth: Your guide to their benefits—and risks, RN 40(5):41-47, May 1977.
Geraci CL Jr: Operating room pollution: Governmental perspectives and guidelines, Anesth Analg (Cleve) 56: 775-777, Nov-Dec 1977.
Harrison DC: Practical guidelines for the use of lidocaine: Prevention and treatment of cardiac arrhythmias, JAMA 233(11):1202-1204, Sep 15, 1976.
Hrizo R: "My family's fight with malignant hyperthermia," RN 40(2):20-22, Feb 1977.
Hussar DA: Drug interactions: Good and bad, Nursing (Jenkintown) 6(9):61-65, Sep 1976.
Irey NS: Adverse drug reactions and death: A review of 827 cases, JAMA 236(6):575-578, Aug 9, 1976.
Katz JD et al: Pulmonary artery flow—guided catheters in the perioperative period: Indications and complications, JAMA 237(26):2832-2834, June 27, 1977.
Lee PK et al: Treatment of chronic pain with acupuncture, JAMA 232(11):1133-1135, June 16, 1975.
Manzi CC: Cardiac emergency! How to use drugs and C.P.R. to save lives, Nursing (Jenkintown) 8(3):30-39, Mar 1978.
'Older society' will mean new medical challenges, JAMA 235(18):1941-1942, May 3, 1976.

Salem MR et al: Cardiac arrest related to anesthesia: Contributing factors in infants and children, JAMA 233(3):238–241, July 21, 1975.

Seufert HJ: A review of occupational health hazards associated with anesthetic waste gases, AORN J 24(4): 744, 746, 748–749, 752, Oct 1976.

Stallings JO, Lines JA: Malignant hyperpyrexia anesthesia complication, AORN J 21(4):642, 644–645, 647, Mar 1975.

Standards for cardiopulmonary resuscitation (CPR) and emergency cardiac care (ECC), JAMA 227(7[suppl]): 833–868, Feb 18, 1974.

Standards for cleaning and processing anesthesia equipment, AORN J 25(7):1268–1274, June 1977.

Taylor G, Larson CP Jr: Unexpected cardiac arrest during anesthesia and surgery: An environmental study, JAMA 236(24):2758–2760, Dec 13, 1976.

Thomas E: Bacterial hazards and control in anesthesia, AORN J 19(1):88, 90, 94–95, Jan 1974.

West JB: New advances in pulmonary gas exchange, Anesth Analg (Cleve) 54(4):409–418, July–Aug 1975.

Whitcher C, Piziali RL: Monitoring occupational exposure to inhalation anesthetics, Anesth Analg (Cleve) 56:778–785, Nov–Dec 1977.

Woods, SL: Monitoring pulmonary artery pressures, Am J Nurs 76(11):1765–1771, Nov 1976.

CHAPTER 10
POSITIONS

MacClelland DC: A modified stirrup for lithotomy position, Point View 14(2):13, Apr 1, 1977.

Minckley BB: Physiologic hazards of position changes in the anesthetized patient, Am J Nurs 69(12):2606–2611, Dec 1969.

CHAPTER 11
PREPARATION OF THE OPERATIVE SITE AND DRAPING

Belkin NL: The rationale for re-usables: The other side of the drape, Hosp Top 53(1):45–48, 50–51, Jan–Feb 1975.

Castle M, Osterhout S: Urinary tract catheterization and associated infection, Nurs Res 23(2):170–174, Mar–Apr 1974.

Driscoll J: Disposables in O.R., Southern Hosp 43(2): 10–13, Feb 1975.

French MLV et al: The plastic surgical adhesive drape: An evaluation of its efficacy as a microbial barrier, Ann Surg 184(1):46–50, July 1976.

Garibaldi RA et al: Factors predisposing to bacteruria during indwelling urethral catheterization, N Eng J Med 291(5):215–219, Aug 1, 1974.

How do you handle hair if found in a sterile pack or instrument tray when setting up for a procedure? Point View 12(5):9–10, Oct 15, 1975.

Johnson RM et al: Flammability of disposable surgical drapes, Arch Opthalmo 94(8):1327–1329, Aug 1976.

Kildea J: The great prep solution paradox, Point View 11(4):6–8, May 15, 1974.

Lach J: *O.R. Nursing: Preoperative Care and Draping Technique,* Chicago: Kendall Co., 1974.

Laufman H et al: Strike through of moist contamination by woven and nonwoven surgical materials, Ann Surg 181(1):857–862, June 1975.

Laufman H et al: Use of disposable products in surgical practice, Arch Surg 111(1):20–26, Jan 1976.

MacClelland DC: Are current skin preparations valid? AORN J 21(1):55–60, Jan 1975.

Minnesota Mining and Manufacturing Company, Medical Products Division, Dept. of Clinical Research: *Steri-Drape Surgical Drape: Clinical Efficiency,* St. Paul, Minn.: 1975.

Rosenberg A et al: Safety and efficacy of the antiseptic chlorhexidine gluconate, Surg Gynecol Obstet 143(5): 789–792, Nov 1976.

Schneckloth NW: Indwelling catheter nursing care, AORN J 21(4):695–699, Mar 1975.

Standards for preoperative skin preparation of patients, AORN J 23(6):974–975, May 1976.

CHAPTER 12
WOUND HEALING AND METHODS OF HEMOSTASIS

Abbott WM, Austen WG: The effectiveness and mechanism of collagen-induced topical hemostasis, Surgery 78(6):723–729, Dec 1975.

Abramson DJ: Charles Bingham Penrose and the Penrose drain, Surg Gynecol Obstet 143(2):285–286, Aug 1976.

Avicon, Inc.: Avitene, a new topical hemostatic agent, Surg Team 5(5):46, Oct 1976.

Baum M, Fletcher JC: Porcine dressing for ileostomy retraction, Am J Nurs 76(5):760–761, May 1976.

Brooks SM: *Fundamentals of Operating Room Nursing,* St Louis: Mosby, 1975.

Church R, Hamlin WT: Electrosurgery demands OR vigilance, AORN J 22(6):903–908, Dec 1975.

Dineen P: Antibacterial activity of oxidized regenerated cellulose, Surg Gynecol Obstet 142(4):481–486, Apr 1976.

Gaul AL, Hart GB: Baromedical nursing combines critical, acute, chronic care, AORN J 21(6):1038–1047, May 1975.

Glover JL, Link WJ: The plasma scalpel: A tool for bloodless surgery, Surg Team 4(3):17–21, May–June 1975.

Haljamae H, Enger E: Human skeletal muscle energy metabolism during and after complete tourniquet ischemia, Ann Surg 182(1):9–14, July 1975.

Hartley MB: Hypothermia, AORN J 24(4):764, 766–767, 769, Oct 1976.

Hunt TK: Diagnosis and treatment of wound failure, Adv Surg 8:287–309, 1974.

Kildea J: The evolution of surgical wound drainage, Point View 10(7):2–4, 1973.

Krieger JN et al: Surgery in patients with congenital disorders of blood coagulation, Ann Surg 185(3): 290–294, Mar 1977.

Ledgerwood AM, Lucas CE: Biological dressings for exposed vascular grafts: A reasonable alternative, J Trauma 15(7):567–574, July 1975.

McIlrath DC et al: Closure of abdominal incisions with subcutaneous catheters, Surgery 80(4):411–416, Oct 1976.

Potteiger WR: Use and significance of hypothermia, Point View 13(4):6–7, Oct 1, 1976.

Schittek A et al: Microcrystalline collagen hemostat (MCCH) and wound healing, Ann Surg 184(6): 697–704, Dec 1976.

Shapiro RM: Anticoagulant therapy, Am J Nurs 74(3): 439–443, Mar 1974.

State D, Peter MF: Clinical use of porcine xenografts in conditions other than burns, Surg Gynecol Obstet 138(1):13–16, Jan 1974.

Stellar S et al: Carbon dioxide laser debridement of decubitus ulcers: Followed by immediate rotation flap or skin graft closure, Ann Surg 179(2):230–237, Feb 1974.

Strauch GO: Should we attempt to salvage the injured spleen? RN 39(2):OR-1, 4, 6, Feb 1976.

Thompson V: Hemostasis in surgery: A matter of life or death, Point View 10(7):6–8, 1973.

Waitman AM et al: Fiberoptic-coupled argon laser in the control of experimentally produced gastric bleeding, Gastrointest Endosc 22(2):78–81, Nov 1975.

CHAPTER 13
WOUND CLOSURE MATERIALS

Craig PH et al: A biologic comparison of polyglactin 910 and polyglycolic acid synthetic absorbable sutures, Surg Gynecol Obstet 141(1):1–10, July 1975.

Dehnel W: Staple suturing vs. conventional suturing, AORN J 18(2):296–300, Aug 1973.

Karakousis CP et al: Abdominal wall replacement with plastic mesh in ablative cancer surgery, Surgery 78(4): 453–459, Oct 1975.

Kronenthal RL: Ethibond polyester sutures with polybutilate, Point View 14(1):11, Jan 1, 1977.

Kronenthal RL et al (eds): *Polymers in Medicine and Surgery:* Proceedings of the Johnson & Johnson Symposium held in Morristown, N.J., July 11–12 1974, New York: Plenum, 1975 (Polymer Science and Technology, vol 8).

Markgraf WH: Mesh repair of abdominal wound dehiscence, AORN J 22(2):272–278, Aug 1975.

Minnesota Mining and Manufacturing Company, Surgical Products Division: *Primary Wound Closure,* Med Assist Bull 103, St. Paul, Minn.: 1975.

Radzius JR: FDA regulation of drugs, devices, AORN J 24(2):254–255, 258–259, 262–263, Aug 1976.

Reckling FW, Dillon WL: The bone-cement interface temperature during total joint replacement, J Bone Joint Surg [Am] 59(1):80–82, Jan 1977.

Sullivan RB: Impact of device legislation, AORN J 25(4):658–661, Mar 1977.

Van Winkle W, Salthouse TN: *Biological Response to Sutures and Principles of Suture Selection,* Somerville, N.J.: Ethicon, Inc., 1976.

Wheater RH: Hazard of methyl methacrylate to operating room personnel, JAMA 235(24):2652, June 14, 1976.

CHAPTER 14
ECONOMY, WORK SIMPLIFICATION, AND SAFETY

Codman & Shurtleff, Inc.: *The Care and Handling of Surgical Instruments,* Randolph, Mass.: 1975.

Corson SL: Should there be safety control of electrosurgical devices? JAMA 235(24):2652, June 14, 1976.

Gilbert BH: Tricks and triumphs of an orthopedic technician, OR Tech 7(2):14–18, Mar–Apr 1975.

Hefferin EA, Hill BJ: Analyzing nursing's work-related injuries, Am J Nurs 76(6):924–927, June 1976.

McElmurry M, Byrd D: Surgical instruments: Manufacture and proper care, AORN J 19(5):1074, 1076, 1078, 1080, 1082–1083, 1085–1086, May 1974.

Mylrea KC, O'Neal LB: Electricity and electrical safety in the hospital, Nursing (Jenkintown) 6(1):52–59, Jan 1976.

Nicholson MJ: Case history number 82: "Nonflammable" fires in the operating room, Anesth Analg (Cleve) 54(1):152–153, Jan–Feb 1975.

Nolan MG: Problem solving is research in action, AORN J 20(2):225–231, Aug 1974.

Pencer G: What you should know about surgical instruments, Surg Team 3(3):39–45, May–June 1974.

Sabo, B: Hazards of macroshock, microshock in the OR, AORN J 24(5):892–898, Nov 1976.

Schrader ES: Editorial: What price quality assurance? AORN J 22(3):147–148, Aug 1975.

Yeakel AE: Ssh... your anesthetized patients may be eavesdropping, RN 38(12):OR-1-2, Dec 1975.

CHAPTER 15
DIAGNOSTIC PROCEDURES

Andrassy RJ et al: Localization of peripheral catheter emboli with xeroradiography, Surgery 79(3):340–341, Mar 1976.

Andrews GH, Edwards CL: Tumor scanning with gallium 67, JAMA 233(10):1100–1103, Sep 8, 1975.

Axelbaum SP et al: Intracerebral hematoma: Diagnosis with automatic computerized transverse axial (ACTA) scanning, JAMA 235(6):641–643, Feb 9, 1976.

Baker HL et al: Computerized tomography of the head, JAMA 233(12):1304–1308, Sep 22, 1975.

Baker RR: Outpatient breast biopsies, Ann Surg 185(5): 543-547, May 1977.

Barnes RW et al: Differentiation of primary from secondary varicose veins by Doppler ultrasound and strain gauge plethysmography, Surg Gynecol Obstet 14(2):207-211, Aug 1975.

Barnes RW et al: An index of healing in below-knee amputation: Leg blood pressure by Doppler ultrasound, Surgery 79(1):13-20, Jan 1976.

Bassett LW: Detecting early breast cancer, AORN J 27(5):850-853, Apr 1978.

Beck WC, Littleton JT: Diagnostic x-ray in the operating room and the new federal regulations, Bull Am Coll Surg 59(11):14-15, Nov 1974.

Belinsky I: Fiberoptic advances: Visualizing the pancreatic and biliary ducts, Am J Nurs 76(6):936-937, June 1976.

Bergqvist D et al: Thermography: A noninvasive method for diagnosis of deep venous thrombosis, Arch Surg 112(5):600-604, May 1977.

Blackwell CA: PEG and angiography: A patient's sensations, Am J Nurs 75(2):264-266, Feb 1975.

Bone GE, Barnes RW: Limitations of the Doppler cerebrovascular examination in hemispheric cerebral ischemia, Surgery 79(5):577-580, May 1976.

Borge J: Operative cholangiography, Arch Surg 112(3): 340-342, Mar 1977.

Boyce WH et al: Ultrasonography as an aid in the diagnosis and management of surgical diseases of the pelvis: Special emphasis on the genitourinary system, Ann Surg 184(4):477-489, Oct 1976.

Coats K: Non-invasive cardiac diagnostic procedures, Am J Nurs 75(11):1980-1985, Nov 1975.

Cogen R: Preventing complications during cardiac catheterization, Am J Nurs 76(3):401-405, Mar 1976.

Curtis C: Colonoscopy: The nurse's role, Am J Nurs 75(3):430-432, Mar 1975.

Davis RW: The fibroscopes, Point View 12(3):6-7, May 1, 1975.

Dietler PC et al: Localization of nonpalpable breast lesions detected by xeromammography, Am Surg 42(11):810-811, Nov 1976.

DiPalma JR: Radiopharmaceuticals: Nuclear-age drugs for diagnosis and treatment, RN 38(3):59-63, 64-65, Mar 1975.

Driscoll J: Criteria for selecting arthroscopes, AORN J 27(5):831-834, Apr 1978.

Duncan RE, Evans AT: Diagnosis of primary retroperitoneal tumors, J Urol 117(1):19-23, Jan 1977.

El-Domeiri AA, Srinivasarao S: Role of preoperative bone scan in carcinoma of the breast, Surg Gynecol Obstet 142(5):722-724, May 1976.

Fennell SE: Percutaneous renal biopsy, Am J Nurs 75(8):1292-1294, Aug 1975.

Grana WA, Pons S: Arthroscopy to diagnose knee disorders, AORN J 27(5):823-830, Apr 1978.

Guttman PH Jr: Good vibrations: Advances in diagnostic ultrasound, Biomed Commun 5(1):10, Jan 1977.

Hancke S, Pedersen JF: Percutaneous puncture of pancreatic cysts guided by ultrasound, Surg Gynecol Obstet 142(4):551-552, Apr 1976.

Kajanoja P, Procopé BJ: Nongenital pelvic tumors found at gynecologic operations, Surg Gynecol Obstet 140(4):605-606, Apr 1975.

Kessler RE et al: Indications, clinical value and complications of endoscopic retrograde cholangiopancreatography, Surg Gynecol Obstet 142(6):865-870, June 1976.

Lee TG, Reed TA: Ultrasonic diagnosis of the bladder as a symptomatic pelvic mass, J Urol 117(3):283-284, Mar 1977.

Levine RU: Hysteroscopy—no passing fad, RN 38(11): OR-1-2, Nov 1975.

Lewis JD et al: Which breast to biopsy: An expanding dilemma, Ann Surg 184(3):253-257, Sep 1976.

Lye CR et al: The accuracy of the supraorbital Doppler examination in the diagnosis of hemodynamically significant carotid occlusive disease, Surgery 79(1): 42-45, Jan 1976.

McWilliams RM et al: The experts research: Q&A: Debate continues on necessity of sterilizing laparoscopes, AORN J 23(5):835-836, Apr 1976.

Menzer L et al: Computerized axial tomography, JAMA 234(7):754-757, Nov 17, 1975.

Milligan C et al: Screening for cervical cancer, Am J Nurs 75(8):1343-1344, Aug 1975.

Moss CM et al: Isotope angiography: Technique, validation and value in the assessment of arterial reconstruction, Ann Surg 184(1):116-121, July 1976.

Moylan JA et al: Fiberoptic bronchoscopy following thermal injury, Surg Gynecol Obstet 140(4):541-543, Apr 1975.

O'Dell CW Jr et al: Ascending lumbar venography in lumbar-disc disease, J Bone Joint Surg [Am] 59(2): 159-163, Mar 1977.

Pohutsky LC, Pohutsky KR: Computerized axial tomography of the brain: A new diagnostic tool, Am J Nurs 75(8):1341-1342, Aug 1975.

Raines JK et al: Vascular laboratory criteria for the management of peripheral vascular disease of the lower extremities, Surgery 79(1):21-29, Jan 1976.

Reeves KR: This CAT is a revolutionary scanner, RN 39(8):40-43, Aug 1976.

Robinson HB, Smith GW: Applications for laparoscopy in general surgery, Surg Gynecol Obstet 143(5):829-834, Nov 1976.

Rosenfield AT, Taylor KJW: Gray scale nephrosonography: Current status, J Urol 117(1):2-6, Jan 1977.

Shanik G et al: Foot vascular resistance index: A noninvasive method to assess foot vasomotor tone, Surgery 78(4):446-452, Oct 1975.

Slaughter JC: Preoperative neurosurgical diagnostic studies, Point View 12(5):6-8, Oct 15, 1975.

Sommer PK: Operative cholangiography: Its pros and cons, RN 39(10):38-39, Oct 1976.

Sommer PK: Operative cholangiography: The subtle techniques that count, RN 39(10):OR-1-2, 6, Oct 1976.

Switz DM et al: Electrical malfunction at endoscopy: Possible cause of arrhythmia and death, JAMA 235(3):273-275, Jan 19, 1976.

Thompson JE, Talkington CM: Carotid endarterectomy, Ann Surg 184(1):1-15, July 1976.

Villar HV: Emergency diagnosis of upper gastrointestinal bleeding by fiberoptic endoscopy, Ann Surg 185(3):367-374, Mar 1977.

Vollmar J, Storz LW: Intraoperative control in vascular reconstruction, Contemp Surg 7(4):147-149, Oct 1975.

Wherry DC, Zehner J Jr: Fiberoptic endoscopy—and of the colon, RN 38(9):OR-4, 7, Sep 1975.

Wood RAB et al: Comparative value of four methods of investigating the pancreas, Surgery 80(4):518-522, Oct 1976.

CHAPTER 16 MICROSURGERY

Bush E et al: Care and use of microscope in OR, AORN J 20(3):392-397, Sep 1974.

Connolly ES et al: OR inservice in microneurosurgery, AORN J 20(3):452, 454, 456, Sep 1974.

Runnells JB: Adapting OR techniques to microneurosurgery, RN 38(8):OR-1-2, 4, Aug 1975.

Troutman RC: *Microsurgery of the Anterior Segment of the Eye,* vol 1, St Louis: Mosby, 1974.

CHAPTER 17 GENERAL SURGERY

American College of Surgeons: *Biliary Tract Surgery,* Postgraduate Course, fifth annual spring meeting, Mar 28-31, 1977 Los Angeles (ACS/Clinitapes: Audiotape cassette and program available for purchase from American College of Surgeons, Chicago, Ill.).

American College of Surgeons: *Recurrent and Incurable Cancers,* Postgraduate course, fifth annual spring meeting, Mar 28-31, 1977, Los Angeles (ACS/ Clinitapes: Audiotape cassette and program available for purchase from American College of Surgeons, Chicago, Ill.).

American College of Surgeons Clinical Congress: Mammography cutback draws surgeon's criticism, AORN J 25(4):767, 770-772, Mar 1977.

Arndt RD et al: Colon carcinoma and the cancer family syndrome, JAMA 237(26):2847-2848, June 27, 1977.

Bailey GL (ed): *Hemodialysis: Principles and Practice,* New York: Academic Press, 1972.

Baker RR: Outpatient breast biopsies, Ann Surg 185(5):543-547, May 1977.

Brunner LS: What to do (and what to teach your patient) about peptic ulcer, Nursing (Jenkintown) 6(11):27-34, Nov 1976.

Carey LC (ed): *The Pancreas,* St. Louis: Mosby, 1973.

Edwards EA et al: *Operative Anatomy of Abdomen and Pelvis,* Philadelphia: Lea & Febiger, 1975.

Esselstyn CB Jr: Selective surgery for breast cancer, AORN J 22(5):730-732, Nov 1975.

Ethicon, Inc.: *Anatomical Insights: The Abdomen,* Somerville, N.J.: 1968.

Forde KA: Colonoscopy for the general surgeon, Contemp Surg 10(6):21-25, June 1977.

Hallal JC: Thyroid disorders, Am J Nurs 77(3):418-432, Mar 1977.

Harrison RC: What's new in surgery: Gastrointestinal-biliary conditions, Bull Am Coll Surg 62(1):16-19, Jan 1977.

Isler C: If ileostomy is continent, the benefits are obvious, RN 40(4):39-45, Apr 1977.

Kerstein MD: The air prosthesis for amputees, RN 39(7):42-43, July 1976.

Leis HP Jr: The diagnosis of breast cancer, CA 27(4): 209-231, July-Aug 1977.

Madden JPL: *Atlas of Technics in Surgery,* 2d ed, New York: Meredith, 1964.

Marshak RH et al: Adenomatous polyps of the colon, JAMA 235(26):2856-2858, June 28, 1976.

Patterson CA: Nursing management: Jejunoileal bypass surgery, AORN J 27(7):1343, 1346-1347, 1350-1351, 1355-1357, June 1978.

Schultz J: Experts research: Q&A: Do instruments used on malignant tissues need special attention? AORN J 25(6):1135, May 1977.

Schwartz SI et al (eds): *Principles of Surgery,* 2d ed, New York: McGraw-Hill, 1974.

Smith DW, Germain CPH: *Care of the Adult Patient: Medical-Surgical Nursing,* 4th ed, Philadelphia: Lippincott, 1975.

Stahlgren LH, Morris NW: Intestinal obstruction, Am J Nurs 77(6):999-1002, June 1977.

Staudt AR: Femur replacement, Am J Nurs 75(8):1347-1348, Aug 1975.

CHAPTER 18 GYNECOLOGY

Ball B (ed): Easing the shock of a radical vulvectomy, Nursing (Jenkintown) 5(8):26-31, Aug 1975.

Banner EA: What's new in surgery: Gynecology and obstetrics, Bull Am Coll Surg 62(1):20-23, Jan 1977.

Burchell RC: Opinion: Hysterectomy, CA 27(4): 241-242, July-Aug 1977.

Cibils LA: *Gynecologic Laparoscopy: Diagnostic and Operatory,* Philadelphia: Lea & Febiger, 1975.

DeAlvarez PR (ed): *Textbook of Gynecology,* Philadelphia: Lea & Febiger 1977.

Green TH Jr: *Gynecology: Essentials of Clinical Practice,* 3d ed, Boston: Little, Brown, 1977.

Hamilton MS, Schlapper NB: Pelvic exenteration, Am J Nurs 76(2):266-272, Feb 1976.

Kopit S, Barnes AB: Patients' response to tubal division, JAMA 236(24):2761-2763, Dec 13, 1976.

Lee CM: Acute hypotension during laparoscopy: A case report, Anesth Analg (Cleve) 54(1):142-143, Jan-Feb 1975.

McWilliams RM et al: Experts research: Q&A: Debate continues on necessity of sterilizing laparoscopes, AORN J 23(5):835, Apr 1976.

Milligan C et al: Screening for cervical cancer, Am J Nurs 75(8):1343-1344, Aug 1975.

Novak ER et al: *Novak's Textbook of Gynecology,* 9th ed, Baltimore: Williams & Wilkins, 1975.

Romney SL et al: *Gynecology & Obstetrics: The Health Care of Women,* New York: McGraw-Hill, 1975.

Rowland WD: Surgery for sex reassignment, AORN J 22(5):735-736, 738-740, Nov 1975.

Willson JR et al: *Obstetrics and Gynecology,* 5th ed, St. Louis: Mosby, 1975.

CHAPTER 19 UROLOGY

Baker CRF Jr: Complications and management of methods of dialysis access for renal failure, Am Surg 42(11):859-862, Nov 1976.

Belzer FO et al: *Ex vivo* renal artery reconstruction, Ann Surg 182(4):456-463, Oct 1975.

Bredin HC, Prout GR: One-stage radical cystectomy for bladder carcinoma: Operative mortality, cost/benefit analysis, J Urol 117(4):447-451, Apr 1977.

Brosman SA, Paul JG: Trauma of the bladder, Surg Gynecol Obstet 143(4):605-608, Oct 1976.

Casey JD, Koerner S: OR care of hemodialysis patients, AORN J 20(5):817-821, Nov 1974.

Cerilli J et al: Renal transplantation in patients with urinary tract abnormalities, Surgery 79(3):248-252, Mar 1976.

Cook JH, Lytton B: Intraoperative localization of renal calculi during nephrolithotomy by ultrasound scanning, J Urol 117(5):543-546, May 1977.

Dowd JB: Methods of urinary diversion, AORN J 23(1): 37-44, Jan 1976.

Gault P: The prostate: Coping with dangerous and distressing complications, Nursing (Jenkintown) 7(4): 34-38, Apr 1977.

Gillenwater JY et al: Evaluation of research needs in nephrology and urology, obstructive and neuromuscular disorders affecting the urinary system, J Urol 117(2):227-230, Feb 1977.

Gonzalez R, Taullard JC: Surgical treatment of varicocele, Surg Gynecol Obstet 143(5):802-803, Nov 1976.

Gottesman JE et al: The Small-Carrion prosthesis for male impotency, J Urol 117(3):289-290, Mar 1977.

Heaney D et al: Bilateral renal artery stenosis causing acute oliguric renal failure, report of a case corrected by renovascular surgery, Arch Surg 112(5):641-643, May 1977.

Hutchin P et al: Bovine graft arteriovenous fistulas for maintenance hemodialysis, Surg Gynecol Obstet 141(2):255-258, Aug 1975.

Iglesias JJ et al: Hydraulic hemostasis in transurethral resection of the prostate using the Iglesias continuous suction resectoscope, J Urol 117(3):306-308, Mar 1977.

Lipshultz LI, Corriere JN Jr: Progressive testicular atrophy in the varicocele patient, J Urol 117(2):175-176, Feb 1977.

McCombs PR et al: Operative management of renovascular hypertension, Ann Surg 182(6):762-766, Dec 1975.

Mahoney EM et al: An improved non-intubated cutaneous ureterostomy technique for the normal and dilated ureter, J Urol 117(3):279-282, Mar 1977.

Mitchell ME, Kerr WS Jr: Experience with the electrohydraulic disintegrator, J Urol 117(2):159-160, Feb 1977.

Morel A, Wise GJ: *Urologic Endoscopic Procedures,* St. Louis: Mosby, 1974.

Nicholson TC, Richie JP: Pelvic lymphadenectomy for stage B_1 adenocarcinoma of the prostate: Justified or not? J Urol 117(2):199-201, Feb 1977.

Peirce SB et al: Slush technique in renal surgery, AORN J 25(2):223-226, Feb 1977.

Pressman PI: Technique of adrenalectomy for metastatic cancer of the breast, Surg Gynecol Obstet 142(5): 743-747, May 1976.

Redman JF: The short ileal conduit: Rationale and description of a technique, J Urol 117(2):156-158, Feb 1977.

Rolley RT et al: Arteriovenous fistulas for dialysis using modified bovine arteries, Surg Gynecol Obstet 142(5): 700-704, May 1976.

Sampson D: RR nursing for kidney recipients, AORN J 23(2):191-198, Feb 1976.

Sandoz IL et al: Complications with transureteroureterostomy, J Urol 117(1):39-42, Jan 1977.

Silber SJ et al: Microscopic vasovasostomy and spermatogenesis, J Urol 117(3):299-302, Mar 1977.

Simone CM: The transsexual patient: How you can help toward a successful surgical outcome, RN 40(3):37-44, Mar 1977.

Squires JW et al: The morbidity of vasectomy, Surg Gynecol Obstet 143(2):237-240, Aug 1976.

Toledo-Pereyra LH et al: Proximal radial artery-cephalic vein fistula hemodialysis, Arch Surg 112(2): 226-227, Feb 1977.

Tomlinson RL et al: Radical prostatectomy: Palliation for stage C carcinoma of the prostate, J Urol 117(1): 85-87, Jan 1977.

Van Poole M: Penile prosthesis in impotence, AORN J 22(2):207-209, Aug 1975.

Veenema RJ et al: Radical retropubic prostatectomy for cancer: A 20-year experience, J Urol 117(3): 330-331, Mar 1977.

Wilson CS et al: Pelvic lymphadenectomy for the staging of apparently localized prostatic cancer, J Urol 117(2):197–198, Feb 1977.
Wood JB: Prostatectomy—which type? Point View 14(2):4–7, Apr 1, 1977.
Yost AJ: Inflatable penile prosthesis, AORN J 26(1): 75–76, 80–81, 84, July 1977.

CHAPTER 20 ORTHOPAEDICS

Bicknell J: Orthopedic instruments, OR Tech 7(4): 6–7, July–Aug 1975.
Bisla RS et al: Joint replacement surgery in patients under thirty, J Bone Joint Surg [Am] 58(8):1098–1104, Dec 1976.
Enneking WF, Shirley PD: Resection-arthrodesis for malignant and potentially malignant lesions about the knee using an intramedullary rod and local bone grafts, J Bone Joint Surg [Am] 59(2):223–236, Mar 1977.
Flesch JR et al: Harrington instrumentation and spine fusion for unstable fractures and fracture-dislocations of the thoracic and lumbar spine, J Bone Joint Surg [Am] 29(2):143–153, Mar 1977.
Harrington KD et al: Methylmethacrylate as an adjunct in internal fixation of pathological fractures, J Bone Joint Surg [Am] 58(8):1047–1054, Dec 1976.
Hogan KM, Sawyer JR: Fracture dislocation of the elbow, Am J Nurs 76(8):1266–1268, Aug 1976.
Hoppenstein R: Acrylic/steel splint for spinal stabilization, Hosp Top 53(4):12, July–Aug 1975.
Howmedica, Inc.: *Introduction to Orthopaedics in the Operating Room,* Rutherford, N.J., 1975.
Kettlekamp DB: Editorial: Infected total joint replacement, Arch Surg 112(5):552–553, May 1977.
Mickelson MR, Bonfiglio M: Pathological fractures in the proximal part of the femur treated by Zickel-nail fixation, J Bone Joint Surg [Am] 58(8):1067–1070, Dec 1976.
Robb S: Bunion surgery, Am J Nurs 74(12):2181–2184, Dec 1974.
Ryan J: Compression in bone healing, Am J Nurs 74(11): 1998–1999, Nov 1974.
Shands AR Jr: Charles Fayette Taylor and his times—1827 to 1899, Surg Gynecol Obstet 143(5):811–818, Nov 1976.
Sher MH: Principles in the management of arterial injuries associated with fracture/dislocations, Ann Surg 182(5):630–634, Nov 1975.
Thompson VR: Injuries and the athlete, Point View 13(1):4–7, Jan 1, 1976.
Wilson PD Jr: What's new in surgery: Orthopaedic surgery, Bull Am Coll Surg 62(1):28–32, Jan 1977.
Zimmer Manufacturing Company: *Orthopaedic Instruments and Procedures: A Basic Handbook Designed as a Guide for the Personal Use of Operating Room Personnel New to Orthopaedic Surgery,* Columbus, Ohio: Schad, 1970.

CHAPTER 21 THORACIC AND CARDIOVASCULAR SURGERY

American College of Surgeons: Standards of care in thoracic surgery, Bull Am Coll Surg 61(2):16–17, Feb 1976.
American College of Surgeons Clinical Congress: Membrane oxygenator successful for prolonged perfusion, AORN J 25(4):772–776, Mar 1977.
Austen GW: Experience with the intra-aortic balloon, Surg Team 5(4):21–23, Aug 1976.
Barker WF: *Peripheral Arterial Disease,* 2d ed, Philadelphia: Saunders, 1975.
Barry WH, Goldman RH: The patient with a permanently implanted pacemaker, JAMA 236(10):1152–1153, Sep 6, 1976.
Blades B (ed): *Surgical Diseases of the Chest,* 3d ed, St. Louis: Mosby, 1974.
Coats K: Non-invasive cardiac diagnostic procedures, Am J Nurs 75(11):1980–1985, Nov 1975.
Chow RK: *Cardiosurgical Nursing Care,* New York: Springer, 1976.
D'Amico DB: What's new in surgery: Hypothermia essential to preserve heart during CP bypass, AORN J 27(1):101–102, Jan 1978.
DePalma RG: Optimal exposure of the internal carotid artery for endarterectomy, Surg Gynecol Obstet 144(2):249–250, Feb 1977.
DePalma RG: A technique for preparation of saphenous vein grafts, Surg Gynecol Obstet 143(5):800–801, Nov 1976.
Ethicon, Inc.: *Cardiovascular Surgery,* Somerville, N.J.: 1977.
Foraker G: Forming an open heart program, Point View 14(1):8–9, Jan 1, 1977.
Galmiche ML: Abdominal left ventricular assist device, AORN J 25(4):678–682, Mar 1977.
Glenn WWL et al: *Thoracic and Cardiovascular Surgery with Related Pathology,* 3d ed, New York: Appleton-Century-Crofts, 1975.
Hershey FB, Calman CH: *Atlas of Vascular Surgery,* 3d ed, St. Louis: Mosby, 1973.
Hutson DG et al: The effect of the distal splenorenal shunt on hypersplenism, Ann Surg 185(5):605–612, May 1977.
Israel L, Chahinian AP (eds): *Lung Cancer,* New York: Academic Press, 1976.
Long ML et al: Cardiopulmonary bypass, Am J Nurs 74(5):860–867, May 1974.
McCarty DT: Esophagus replacement, AORN J 23(6): 1115–1130, May 1976.
Manwaring M: What patients need to know about pacemakers, Am J Nurs 77(5):825–830, May 1977.
Medical News: Closed chest lung biopsy proves useful in diagnosis, JAMA 237(1):10, Jan 3, 1977.

Metal coils in heart monitor function status, AORN J 23(2):226, Feb 1976.

Mulder DG: New developments in cardiothoracic surgery, JAMA 237(21):2315–2317, May 23, 1977.

Mulder DG: What's new in surgery: Cardio-thoracic surgery, Bull Am Coll Surg 62(1):12–15, Jan 1977.

Ottinger LW: Ruptured arteriosclerotic aneurysms of the abdominal aorta, JAMA 233(2):147–150, July 14, 1975.

Redman HC: Thoracic, abdominal, and peripheral trauma, JAMA 237(22):2415–2418, May 30, 1977.

Reed EA: Intra-aortic balloon pump, AORN J 23(6): 995–1001, May 1976.

Sabiston DC Jr, Spencer FC (eds): *Gibbon's Surgery of the Chest,* Philadelphia: Saunders, 1976.

Stertzer SH: Insertion of transvenous permanent pacemaker, Point View 11(5):6–7, July 1, 1974.

Stiles QR: *Myocardial Revascularization: A Surgical Atlas,* Boston: Little, Brown, 1976.

Strauss RA et al: Facilitation of exchange transfusions with Scribner shunts in Reye's syndrome, Am J Surg 131(6):772–774, June 1976.

Winslow EH, Marino LB: Temporary cardiac pacemakers, Am J Nurs 75(4):586–591, Apr 1975.

CHAPTER 22 OPHTHALMOLOGY

Alpar JL: Some considerations concerning care of ophthalmic patients in modern general community hospital practice, Ophthalmic Surg 6(4):66–70, Winter 1975.

Boyd-Monk H: Cataract surgery, Nursing (Jenkintown) 7(6):56–61, June 1977.

Driscoll J: Vitrectomy: A new approach to an old problem, Point View 13(3):4–5, July 1, 1976.

Emery JM: Cataract treatment and rehabilitation, AORN J 20(6):992–995, Dec 1974.

Fernsebner W: Early diagnosis of acute angle-closure glaucoma, Am J Nurs 75(7):1154–1155, July 1975.

Jaffe NS: *Cataract Surgery and its Complications,* 2d ed, St. Louis: Mosby, 1976.

Jennings B: Intraocular lens for cataracts, AORN J 23(4):664, 666–667, 670, 672, Mar 1976.

Levenson L, Levenson J: Corneal transplantation, Am J Nurs 77(7):1160–1163, July 1977.

Mayer W: Cryopreserved corneal grafting, AORN J 20(6):973–976, Dec 1974.

Mazzocco TR: Microsurgery of cataracts, AORN J 24(6):1091–1092, 1094, 1096, 1098, 1100, 1103, 1106, 1108, Dec 1976.

Newell FW: Current trends in ophthalmic anesthesia, Ophthalmic Surg 6(2):15–22, Summer 1975.

Shiery S: Insight into the delicate art of eye care, Nursing (Jenkintown) 5(6):50–56, June 1975.

Slight JR: Causes, management of glaucoma, AORN J 27(4):760, 762, 764, 766, Mar 1978.

Soll DB et al: A guide to emergency care of eye injuries, Bull Am Coll Surg 61(10):15–17, Oct 1976.

CHAPTER 23 OTORHINOLARYNGOLOGY

Attia R et al: Transtracheal ventilation, JAMA 234(11): 1152–1153, Dec 15, 1975.

Brewster EM: OR care for epistaxis patients, AORN J 22(3):373–378, Sep 1975.

Cantrell RW: Current concepts, head and neck cancer surgery, AORN J 22(2):253–254, 256, 258, 260, 262, Aug 1975.

Conner GH et al: Tracheostomy, Am J Nurs 72(1): 68–74, Jan 1972.

Ewing DM: Electronic larynx for aphonic patients, Am J Nurs 75(12):2153–2156, Dec 1975.

Greene DA: Tracheostomy or not? JAMA 234(11): 1150–1151, Dec 15, 1975.

Havener WH et al: *Nursing Care in Eye, Ear, Nose and Throat Disorders,* 3d ed, St. Louis: Mosby, 1974.

Lawless CA: Helping patients with endotracheal and tracheostomy tubes communicate, Am J Nurs 75(12): 2151–2153, Dec 1975.

McConnell EA: How to truly help the patient with a radical neck dissection, Nursing (Jenkintown) 6(11): 58–65, Nov 1976.

Nauton RF: What's new in surgery: Otolaryngology, Bull Am Coll Surg 62(1):33–35, Jan 1977.

Nicholson EM: Personal notes of a laryngectomee, Am J Nurs 75(12):2157–2158, Dec 1975.

Nursing Grand Rounds: Caring for the cancer patient, Nursing (Jenkintown) 7(8):30–33, Aug 1977.

Palmer ED: Backyard barbecue syndrome: Steak impaction in the esophagus, JAMA 235(24):2637–2638, June 14, 1976.

Saunders WH, Pararella MM: *Atlas of Ear Surgery,* 2d ed, St. Louis: Mosby, 1971.

Surgery vs packing for posterior nosebleed, AORN J 22(7):268, Jan 1976.

Tierney EA: Accepting disfigurement when death is the alternative, Am J Nurs 75(12):2149–2150, Dec 1975.

Up-to-date survey of tracheal tubes, Nursing (Jenkintown) 6(11):66–72, Nov 1976.

White HA: Tracheostomy: Care with a cuffed tube, Am J Nurs 72(1):75–77, Jan 1972.

White N: OR nursing in otomicrosurgery, AORN J 22(6): 889–897, Dec 1975.

Winawer SJ et al: Endoscopic brush cytology in esophageal cancer, JAMA 232(13):1358, June 30, 1975.

CHAPTER 24 NEUROSURGERY

Alexander MM, Brown MS: Physical examination: Part 17: Neurological examination, Nursing (Jenkintown) 6(6):38–43, June 1976.

Apuzzo MLJ et al: Neurosurgical endoscopy using the side-viewing telescope, J Neurosurg 46(3):398-400, Mar 1977.

Ballenger OM et al: Prognosis of surgically treated intracranial arterial aneurysm patients, JAMA 237(17):1845-1847, Apr 25, 1977.

Carini E, Owens G: *Neurological and Neurosurgical Nursing,* 6th ed, St. Louis: Mosby, 1974.

Caruthers B: Head injuries, OR Tech 7(5):23-25, Sep-Oct 1975.

DiTullio MV Jr, Rand RW: Efficacy of cryohypophysectomy in the treatment of acromegaly, J Neurosurg 46(1):1-11, Jan 1977.

Dooley DM: Spinal cord stimulation, AORN J 23(7): 1209-1212, June 1976.

Harris LO, Park E: Transsphenoidal approach to pituitary adenomas, AORN J 23(6):989-994, May 1976.

Johnson M, Quinn J: The subarachnoid screw, Am J Nurs 77(3):448-450, Mar 1977.

Kandel EI, Peresedov VV: Stereotaxic clipping of arterial aneurysms and arteriovenous malformations, J Neurosurg 46(1):12-23, Jan 1977.

Kildea J Jr: Conquering an obstacle; pituitary, Point View 12(5):3-5, Oct 15, 1975.

Linchitz R: Nursing care of the patient with brain stimulation for pain control, AORN J 25(4):651-657, Mar 1977.

Loetterle BC et al: Cerebellar stimulation: Pacing the brain, Am J Nurs 75(6):958-960, June 1975.

Mazzola R, Jacobs GB: Brain tumors: Diagnosis and treatment, RN 38(3):42-45, Mar 1975.

Ostrow LS: New hope for patients with trigeminal neuralgia, Am J Nurs 76(8):1301-1303, Aug 1976.

Penn RD, Etzel ML: Chronic cerebellar stimulation and developmental reflexes, J Neurosurg 46(4):506-511, Apr 1977.

Petrie TD: Intracranial tumor: Patient assessment, Point View 12(5):18-19, Oct 15, 1975.

Samson DS et al: Surgical management of unruptured asymptomatic aneurysms, J Neurosurg 46(6):731-734, June 1977.

Stauffer ES, Kelly EG: Fracture-dislocations of the cervical spine, J Bone Joint Surg [Am] 59(1):45-48, Jan 1977.

Stibitz MA: Intraoperative care during spinal cord stimulation, AORN J 23(7):1213-1216, June 1976.

Tindall GT: What's new in surgery: Neurologic surgery, Bull Am Coll Surg 62(1):24-27, Jan 1977.

Vandercook LJ: Diagnosis: L-5 disk rupture operation: Lumbar laminectomy, OR Tech 9(2):22-24, Mar-Apr 1977.

VanPoole M: Percutaneous electrocoagulation for tic douloureux, AORN J 24(5):887-891, Nov 1976.

Wheeler P: Care of a patient with a cerebellar tumor, Am J Nurs 77(2):263-266, Feb 1977.

CHAPTER 25
PLASTIC AND RECONSTRUCTIVE SURGERY

Ames, AEL: Craniofacial surgery, OR Tech 8(6):7-10, Nov-Dec 1976.

Baxter C: The challenge of the massively burned patient, Surg Team 5(1):40-41, 45-46, Jan-Feb 1976.

Beckman JS et al: For lip cancer—better results with surgery, RN 39(1):OR-6-7, Jan 1976.

Buncke H et al: Free osteocutaneous flap from a rib to the tibia, Plast Reconstr Surg 5(6):799-805, June 1977.

Burke JF et al: Immunosuppression and temporary skin transplantation in the treatment of massive third degree burns, Ann Surg 182(3):183-197, Sep 1975.

Castaneres S: Classification of baggy eyelids deformity, Plast Reconstr Surg 59(5):629-633, May 1977.

Castillo P: Blepharoplasty for baggy eyelids, AORN J 21(1):78-84, Jan 1975.

Collentine, G: How to reduce mortality from burns by proper therapy, Hosp Top 53(5):55-58, Sep-Oct 1975.

Dinner MI, Chait LA: Preventing the high-riding nipple after McKissock breast reductions, Plast Reconstr Surg 59(3):330-333, Mar 1977.

Drever JM: The epigastric island flap, Plast Reconstr Surg 59(3):343-346, Mar 1977.

Dunn EJ et al: Parotid neoplasms: A report of 250 cases and review of the literature, Ann Surg 184(4):500-506, Oct 1976.

Edgerton MT et al: New surgical concepts resulting from cranio-orbito-facial surgery, Ann Surg 182(3): 228-239, Sep 1975.

Fitzwater J: Nursing implications in the care of the burn patient, Surg Team 5(1):47-48, 50-51, Jan-Feb 1976.

Flagg SV et al: Ring avulsion injury, Plast Reconstr Surg 59(2):241-248, Feb 1977.

Fox CL et al: Zinc sulfadiazine for topical therapy of pseudomonas infection in burns, Surg Gynecol Obstet 142(4):553-559, Apr 1976.

Frank HA: Modern day burn therapy, OR Tech 8(5): 11-12, 14-15, 18, 30, Sep-Oct 1976.

Halversen RC: Total care concept for burns, AORN J 26(2):328, 330, 332, Aug 1977.

Hamit HF et al: The use of nylon net in the management of skin grafts applied to burn wounds, Surg Gynecol Obstet 143(5):809-810, Nov 1976.

Hart GB et al: Treatment of burns with hyperbaric oxygen, Surg Gynecol Obstet 139(5):693-696, Nov 1974.

Jabaley ME et al: Myocutaneous flaps in lip reconstruction, applications of the Karapandzic principle, Plast Reconstr Surg 59(5):680-688, May 1977.

Jurkiewicz MJ, Arnold PG: The omentum: An account of its use in the reconstruction of the chest wall, Ann Surg 185(5):548-554, May 1977.

Lewis JR: Facial scars resulting from vehicular accidents, Clin Plast Surg 2(1):143-166, Jan 1975.

McDowell F: The classic reprint: Commentary by the editor, Plast Reconstr Surg 59(5):730-732, May 1977.

Magil B: Exciting changes in grafting techniques, Contemp Surg 10(3):11-17, Mar 1977.

Markley JM: The preservation of close two-point discrimination in the interdigital transfer of neurovascular island flaps, Plast Reconstr Surg 5(6):812-816, June 1977.

Mendelson BC et al: Experience with the deltopectoral flap, Plast Reconstr Surg 59(3):360-365, Mar 1977.

Miller P: Initial burn care, Surg Team 5(4):26-30, July-Aug 1976.

Miller SH et al: Breast reconstruction following mastectomy, AORN J 25(5):945, 948-949, 952-953, 956-957, 960, Apr 1977.

Monafo WW et al: Cerium nitrate: A new topical antiseptic for extensive burns, Surgery 80(4):465-473, Oct 1976.

Mulliken JB: Biographical sketch of Charles Conrad Miller, "featural surgeon," Plast Reconstr Surg 59(2):175-184, Feb 1977.

Murray JE et al: Evaluation of craniofacial surgery in the treatment of facial deformities, Ann Surg 182(3): 240-265, Sep 1975.

Ninman C, Shoemaker P: Human amniotic membranes for burns, Am J Nurs 75(9):1468-1469, Sep 1975.

Rempel JH: Surgical treatment of the burn patient, AORN J 24(4):775-776, 778, 780, Oct 1976.

Stark RB: A rhytidectomy series, Plast Reconstr Surg 59(3):373-378, Mar 1977.

Woods JE et al: Use of muscular, musculocutaneous, and omental flaps to reconstruct difficult defects, Plast Reconstr Surg 59(2):191-199, Feb 1977.

Zarem HA: What's new in surgery: Plastic, reconstructive and maxillofacial surgery, Bull Am Coll Surg 62(1):36-38, Jan 1977.

CHAPTER 26
PEDIATRIC SURGERY

Agarwala B, Baffes T: Congestive heart failure in the infant, Heart Lung 5(1):63-70, Jan-Feb 1976.

Baker BA: The fetal circulatory system, OR Tech 8(1):20-24, Jan-Feb 1976.

Bell RH et al: Intestinal anastomoses in neonatal surgery, Ann Surg 183(3):276-281, Mar 1976.

Bender HW et al: Selective operative treatment for tetralogy of Fallot: Rationale and results, Ann Surg 183(6):685-690, June 1976.

Cox NC: Psychological effects of surgery on children, AORN J 24(3):425-432, Sep 1976.

Cross PS: Ureteral reimplantation: Nursing care of the child, Am J Nurs 76(11):1800-1803, Nov 1976.

Diamond LS: Pediatric orthopedic surgery rehabilitates handicapped children, AORN J 19(5):1039-1045, May 1974.

Drencsko S: Anterior spine fusion to correct scoliotic deformities, AORN J 19(5):1066-1072, May 1974.

Edgerton MT: The treatment of hemangiomas: With special reference to the role of steroid therapy, Ann Surg 183(5):517-532, May 1976.

Edmunds LH Jr, et al: Transatrial repair of tetralogy of Fallot, Surgery 80(6):681-688, Dec 1976.

Eoff MJF et al: Temperature measurement in infants, Nurs Res 23(6):457-460, Nov-Dec 1974.

Gatch G: Intraoperative nursing care of pediatric patients, AORN J 25(5):873-877, Apr 1977.

Graivier L: Abdominal masses in infants, children, AORN J 24(6):1076-1082, Dec 1976.

Guttman FM et al: The pathogenesis of intestinal atresia, Surg Gynecol Obstet 141(2):203-206, Aug 1975.

Janosko EO et al: Congenital anomalies of the umbilicus, Am Surg 43(3):177-185, Mar 1977.

Kalamchi A et al: Halo-pelvic distraction apparatus: An analysis of one hundred and fifty consecutive patients, J Bone Joint Surg [Am] 58(8):1119-1125, Dec 1976.

Kilman JW et al: Respiratory distress: Surgery in the newborn, RN 38(6):OR-1-2, June 1975.

Lopez-Perez GA: A modified method for the repair of esophageal atresia with tracheoesophageal fistula, Surgery 79(5):499-503, May 1976.

Lorig J: Localizer cast, fusion for scoliosis, AORN J 22(3):360-371, Sep 1975.

Myers MS: Mature or immature? Assessing gestational age, RN 38(1): 22-25, Jan 1975.

O'Brien ET, Fahey JJ: Remodeling of the femoral neck after *in situ* pinning for slipped capital femoral epiphysis, J Bone Joint Surg [Am] 59(1):62-68, Jan 1977.

Othersen HB Jr: Prevention and treatment of tracheal injuries in children, Am Surg 43(2):108-113, Feb 1977.

Parker RK et al: Repair of truncus arteriosus in patients with prior banding of the pulmonary artery, Surgery 78(6):761-767, Dec 1975.

Ragheb MI et al: Management of corrosive esophagitis, Surgery 79(5):494-498, May 1976.

Raimondi AJ, Gutierrez FA: A new surgical approach to the treatment of coronal synostosis, J Neurosurg 46(2):210-214, Feb 1977.

Salanitre E, Rackow H: Considerations in neonatal anesthesia, AORN J 25(5):879-887, Apr 1977.

Stewart DR et al: Malrotation of the bowel in infants and children: A 15-year review, Surgery 79(6):716-720, June 1976.

Wolfer JA, Visintainer MA: Pediatric surgical patients and parents' stress responses and adjustment, Nurs Res 24(4):244-255, July-Aug 1975.

CHAPTER 27
ONCOLOGY

Bochow AJ: Cancer immunotherapy: What promise does it hold? Nursing (Jenkintown) 6(10):50-56, Oct 1976.

Breeding MA, Wollin M: Working safely around implanted radiation sources, Nursing (Jenkintown) 6(5): 58-63, May 1976.

Carter J: Role of the oncology nurse in regional infusion chemotherapy, AORN J 25(4):662-668, Mar 1977.

Degenshein GA: Editorial: A new look at surgical ablation for advanced cancer of the breast, Surg Gynecol Obstet 142(4):578-579, Apr 1976.

DiPalma JR: Cancer chemotherapy, RN 39(4):85-88, Apr 1976.

Einhorn LH et al: Improved chemotherapy for small-cell undifferentiated lung cancer, JAMA 235(12): 1225–1229, Mar 22, 1976.

El-Domeiri AA et al: Effectiveness of systemic BCG therapy in advanced melanoma, Arch Surg 112(3): 257–259, Mar 1977.

Englert DM, Dudrick SJ: Principles of intravenous hyperalimentation, AORN J 25(7):1253–1267, June 1977.

Fisher B et al: Ten year follow-up results with carcinoma of the breast in a cooperative clinical trial evaluating surgical adjuvant chemotherapy, Surg Gynecol Obstet 140(4):528–534, Apr 1975.

Fortner JG, Pahnke LD: A new method for long term intrahepatic chemotherapy, Surg Gynecol Obstet 143(6):979–980, Dec 1976.

Greco RS: Application of transfer factor to clinical immunotherapy, Surg Gynecol Obstet 142(5):765–778, May 1976.

Gullo S: Chemotherapy: What to do about side effects, RN 40(4):30–32, Apr 1977.

Holt JA et al: Hormone receptors and breast cancer, AORN J 27(5):841–849, Apr 1978.

Isler C: Newest treatment for cancer: Immunotherapy, RN 39(4):35–38, Apr 1976; 39(5):29–51, May 1976.

Jackson BS, Armenaki DW: A tumor classification system, Am J Nurs 76(8):1320–1322, Aug 1976.

Kane RD et al: Multiple drug chemotherapy regimen for patients with hormonally unresponsive carcinoma of the prostate: A preliminary report, J Urol 117(4): 467–471, Apr 1977.

Ketcham AS: What's new in surgery: Tumors, Bull Am Coll Surg 62(1):48–53, Jan 1977.

Kim DK et al: Tumor vascularity as a prognostic factor for hepatic tumors, Ann Surg 185(1):31–34, Jan 1977.

Krementz ET et al: Chemotherapy of sarcomas of the limbs by regional perfusion, Ann Surg 185(5):555–564, May 1977.

McCarthy S: Cancer complicated in growth, treatment, AORN J 21(4):706–707, 710–711, Mar 1975.

Marino EB, LeBlanc DH: Cancer chemotherapy, Nursing (Jenkintown) 5(1):22–33, Nov 1975.

Mayer A: Extent of disease: A philosophic approach to its determination and significance, Bull Am Coll Surg 61(6):14–17, June 1976.

Minton JP: Precise selection of breast cancer patients with bone metastasis for endocrine ablation, Surgery 80(4):513–517, Oct 1976.

Montie JE et al: Immunotherapy of disseminated renal cell carcinoma with transfer factor, J Urol 117(5): 553–556, May 1977.

Morton DL et al: Limb salvage from a multidisciplinary treatment approach for skeletal and soft tissue sarcomas of the extremity, Ann Surg 184(3):268–278, Sep 1976.

Rapp MA et al: Hyperalimentation: Special nutrition therapy for the cancer patient, RN 29(8):55–61, Aug 1976.

Sasaki GH et al: Therapeutic value of nafoxidine hydrochloride in the treatment of advanced carcinoma of the human breast, Surg Gynecol Obstet 142(4):560–564, Apr 1976.

Scott W: Surgical radiation therapy with Vicryl-125_I absorbable sutures, Surg Gynecol Obstet 142(5): 667–670, May 1976.

Seigler HF, Fetter BF: Current management of melanoma, Ann Surg 186(1):1–12, July 1977.

CHAPTER 28 TRANSPLANTATION AND REPLANTATION

Belzer FO: What's new in surgery: Transplantation, Bull Am Coll Surg 62(1):46–47, Jan 1977.

Bergan JJ: A review of human solid organ transplantation, Bull Am Coll Surg 60(3):24–26, Mar 1975.

Bernstein DM: The organ donor, JAMA 237(24):2643–2644, June 13, 1977.

Bone marrow transplantation from donors with aplastic anemia: A report from the ACS/NIH Bone Marrow Transplant Registry, JAMA 236(10):1131–1135, Sep 6, 1976.

Cahan MP, Lyddane NR: Bone marrow transplantation at UCLA, Ca Nursing 1(1):47–51, Feb 1978.

Castro JE (ed): *Immunlogy for Surgeons,* Baltimore: University Park Press, 1976.

D'Amico DB: What's new in surgery: Antigen skin tests indicate transplantation response, AORN J 27(1): 112–114, Jan 1978.

Developments in transplantation, AORN J 23(2):218, 220–222, 224, 226, Feb 1976.

Donley DL: The immune system: Nursing the patient who is immunosuppressed, Am J Nurs 76(10): 1619–1625, Oct 1976.

Extending preservation of transplant organs, AORN J 23(1):92, Jan 1976.

Ferrone S et al: Humoral immunity in kidney transplant recipients, Transplantation 23(2):113–118, Feb 1977.

Foot replantation attempt encouraged, AORN J 25(5): 980, Apr 1977.

Kobrzycki P: Renal transplant complications, Am J Nurs 77(4):641–643, Apr 1977.

Lee RM (ed): Developments in transplantation, AORN J 23(2):218, Feb 1976.

Losman JG, Rautenback MA: Status of heart transplantation, Point View 14(1):4–6, Jan 1, 1977.

Mahony JF et al: Renal transplantation: Effect on the ischemic heart disease of essential malignant hypertension, JAMA 235(21):2318–2319, May 24, 1976.

May JW Jr et al: Amputation: Injury to replantation, AORN J 27(1):35–43, Jan 1978.

Medical News: Rare operation reimplants toddler's foot severed by lawnmower, JAMA 237(14):1413–1414, 1417–1418, Apr 4, 1977.

New drug therapy improves kidney transplant outlook, AORN J 24(4):702, Oct 1976.

Nysather JO et al: The immune system: Its development and functions, Am J Nurs 76(10):1614-1619, Oct 1976.

Organ transplant registry report, AORN J 25(4):800, Mar 1977.

Poznanski EO et al: Quality of life for long-term survivors of end-stage renal disease, JAMA 239(22): 2343-2347, June 2, 1978.

Putnam CW et al: Liver transplantation for Budd-Chiari syndrome, JAMA 236(10):1142-1143, Sep 6, 1976.

Rapaport FT et al: Recent advances in clinical and experimental transplantation, JAMA 237(26):2835-2840, June 27, 1977.

Schröter GTJ et al: Acute bacteremia in asplenic renal transplant patients, JAMA 237(20):2207-2208, May 16, 1977.

Shumway NE: Third annual Paul D. White lecture—Human cardiac transplantation—1975 in *Cardiovascular Problems: Perspectives and Progress,* ed A Russek, Baltimore: University Park Press, 1976, pp. 427-431.

Starzl TE et al: Orthotopic liver transplantation in 93 patients, Surg Gynecol Obstet 142(4):487-505, Apr 1976.

Walker P: Bone marrow transplantation: A second chance for life, Nursing (Jenkintown) 7(1):24-25, Jan 1977.

Woodhall PB et al: Apparent recurrence of progressive systemic sclerosis in a renal allograft, JAMA 236(9): 1032-1034, Aug 30, 1976.

Zimmerman S et al: Bone marrow transplantation, Am J Nurs 77(8):1311-1317, Aug 1977.

CHAPTER 29
POSTOPERATIVE COMPLICATIONS

Blaisdell FW: What's new in surgery: Shock and metabolism, Bull Am Coll Surg 62(1):40-45, Jan 1977.

Brown C et al: Progression and resolution of changes in pulmonary function and structure due to pulmonary microembolism and blood transfusion, Ann Surg 185(1):92-99, Jan 1977.

Codd J, Grohar ME: Postoperative pulmonary complications, Nurs Clin North Am 10(1):5-15, Mar 1975.

Durham N: Looking out for complications of abdominal surgery, Nursing (Jenkintown) 5(2):24-31, Feb 1975.

Durkin DM: Pulmonary fat embolism: A complication of fracture, Heart Lung 5(3):477-481, May-June 1976.

Elbaum N: Mg: Detecting and correcting magnesium imbalance, Nursing (Jenkintown) 7(8):34-35, Aug 1977.

Ellis H: Postoperative pulmonary collapse, Nurs Times 71(3):100-101, Jan 16, 1975.

Fitzmaurice JB, Sasahara AA: Current concepts of pulmonary embolism: Implications for nursing practice, Heart Lung 3(2):209-218, Mar-Apr 1974.

Garrett JJ: Oliguria in postoperative patients, Nurs Clin North Am 10(1):59-67, Mar 1975.

Guyton AC: *Textbook of Medical Physiology,* 5th ed, Philadelphia: Saunders, 1976.

Hirsh, J: Venous thromboembolism: Diagnosis, treatment, prevention, Hosp Prac 10(8):53-62, Aug 1975.

Hollan EL: Alcohol withdrawal: The unexpected post-op syndrome, RN 39(2):40-42, Feb 1976.

Holliday RL: Intra-abdominal sepsis, Heart Lung 5(5): 781-783, Sep-Oct 1976.

Johnson CF, Convery FR: Preventing emboli after total hip replacment, Am J Nurs 75(5):804-806, May 1975.

Libman RH, Keithley J: Relieving airway obstruction in the recovery room, Am J Nurs 75(4):603-605, Apr 1975.

McConnell EA: After surgery, Nursing (Jenkintown) 7(3):32-39, Mar 1977.

McConnell EA: Meeting the special needs of diabetics facing surgery, Nursing (Jenkintown) 6(6):30-37, June 1976.

McFarland MB: Fat embolism syndrome, Am J Nurs 76(12):1942-1944, Dec 1976.

Marr JJ et al: Isolation of mycobacteria species from porcine heart valve prostheses, Morbid Mortal Week Rep 26(6):42-43, Feb 11, 1977.

Metheny NA, Snively WD Jr: Perioperative fluids and electrolytes, Am J Nurs 78(5):840-845, May 1978.

Picklesimer L: D.I.C., the nurse-challenging syndrome, RN 37(6):46-47, June 1974.

Redding JS, Cooke JE: Management of pulmonary edema, AORN J 21(4):659-660, 662, 664, Mar 1975.

Rodman MJ: Thromboembolic disorders, Part 2: Arterial thrombosis & embolism, RN 39(7):61-66, July 1976.

Ryan R: Thrombophlebitis: Assessment and prevention, Am J Nurs 76(10):1634-1636, Oct 1976.

Sheridan JL: Obstructions of the intestinal tract, Nurs Clin North Am 10(1):147-155, Mar 1975.

Silva J Jr: Anaerobic infections, Heart Lung 5(3):406-410, May-June 1976.

Smith BJ: After anesthesia, Nursing (Jenkintown) 4(12): 28-32, Dec 1974.

Sweet K: Hiatal hernia: What to guard against most in postop patients, Nursing (Jenkintown) 7(8):36-43, Aug 1977.

Taylor CM: When to anticipate septic shock, Nursing (Jenkintown) 5(4):34-38, Apr 1975.

Tharp GD: Shock: The overall mechanisms, Am J Nurs 74(12):2208-2211, Dec 1974.

Twombly M: The shift into third space, Nursing (Jenkintown) 8(6):38-41, June 1978.

Walker BJ: Nursing care to assess and prevent common cardiovascular problems. Nurs Clin North Am 10(1): 43-48, Mar 1975.

Webb GE: Hyper and hypotension in the recovery room, AORN J 26(3):546, 548, 550, 554, 557, 559, 561, 564, 566, 570, 572, 574, Sep 1977.

Wiley L (ed): Confronting alcoholism: How one medical/surgical unit faced the problem, Nursing Grand Rounds, Nursing (Jenkintown) 7(5):56-61, May 1977.

Wiley L: Shock: Different kinds . . . different problems, Nursing (Jenkintown) 4(5):43-52, May 1974.

Wilson RF: The diagnosis and management of severe sepsis & septic shock, Heart Lung 5(3):422-429, May-June 1976.

Wyper M: Pulmonary embolism: Fighting the silent killer, Nursing (Jenkintown) 5(10):30-38, Oct 1975.

CHAPTER 30
LIABILITY AND ACCOUNTABILITY

Althouse HL: How OSHA affects hospitals and nursing homes, Am J Nurs 75(3):450-453, Mar 1975.

Baumann BA: The integrated progress record, Supv Nurse 8(8):29-35, Aug 1977.

Byrd JM: Peer review for quality charting, Supv Nurse 8(7):25-27, July 1977.

Creighton H: Captain of the ship doctrine, Supv Nurse 8(8):63, 66-67, Aug 1977.

Creighton H: *Law Every Nurse Should Know,* 3d ed, Philadelphia: Saunders, 1975.

Crooks LC: Are nurses abdicating their obligations? AORN J 22(4):523-529, Oct 1975.

Ellis GL: PSROs' background and perspective, AORN J 22(2):169-178, Aug 1975.

Gouge RL: OR nurses face potential liabilities, AORN J 20(4):660-661, 664-665, Oct 1974.

Gruendemann BJ et al: *Nursing Audit: Challenge to the Operating Room Nurse,* Denver: The Association of Operating Room Nurses, Inc., 1974.

Hanlon CR et al: Patient safety approach to professional liability, Bull Am Coll Surg 62(7):7-14, July 1977.

Kelly LY: The patient's right to know, Nurs Outlook 24(1):26-32, Jan 1976.

Kneedler JA: Corrective action completes audit cycle, AORN J 26(3):485-494, Sep 1977.

Lang NA: Quality assurance in nursing, AORN J 22(2): 180-186, Aug 1975.

McConnell EA: Nursing audit for recovery room, AORN J 26(3):525-528, 530, Sep 1977.

Mohr BJ: JCAH patient care audit, AORN J 22(2): 187-190, Aug 1975.

Ochsner HA: Legal implications of the C.S. operation, Hosp Top 53(4):14, 18, July-Aug 1975.

OR nursing notes form, guidelines, AORN J 26(3): 513, 516, 518, 520, Sep 1977.

Plourde C: The evolution of OR peer review, AORN J 24(4):754, 756, 758, 760, 762, Oct 1976.

Reed EA: OR nursing audit becomes a reality, AORN J 26(3):479-484, Sep 1977.

Regan WA: OR nursing law, AORN J 25(4):784, 786, 788, Mar 1977; 25(5):974, 976, 978, 980, Apr 1977; 25(6):1184, 1186, 1188, May 1977; 25(7):1242, 1244, 1246, June 1977; 26(2):352, 354, Aug 1977.

Schmidt A, Deets C: Writing measurable nursing audit criteria, AORN J 26(3):495-499, Sep 1977.

Scott HW Jr: Professional liability—the crisis and approaches to the solution, Bull Am Coll Surg 60(11): 7-15, Nov 1975.

Index